The Leukemic Cell

METHODS IN HEMATOLOGY

Volume 2

EDITORIAL BOARD

I. Chanarin MD, FRCPath, *Chairman*
  Northwick Park Hospital and Clinical Research Centre, Harrow, UK
Ernest Beutler MD
  Scripps Clinic and Research Foundation, La Jolla, California, USA
Elmer B. Brown MD
  Washington University School of Medicine, St Louis, Missouri, USA
Allan Jacobs MD, FRCPath
  University of Wales College of Medicine, Cardiff, UK

Also in the series

Volume 1: Iron, James D. Cook, *Guest Editor*
Volume 2: The Leukemic Cell, D. Catovsky, *Guest Editor*
Volume 3: Leucocyte Function, Martin J. Cline, *Guest Editor*
Volume 4: Quality Control, I. Cavill, *Guest Editor*
Volume 5: The Hemophilias, Arthur L. Bloom, *Guest Editor*
Volume 6: The Thalassemias, D. J. Weatherall, *Guest Editor*
Volume 7: Disorders of Thrombin Formation, Robert Colman, *Guest Editor*
Volume 8: Measurements of Platelet Function, Laurence A. Harker and Theodore S. Zimmerman, *Guest Editors*
Volume 9: The Immune Cytopenias, Robert McMillan, *Guest Editor*
Volume 10: The Cobalamins, Charles A. Hall, *Guest Editor*
Volume 11: Hematopoietic Stem Cells, David W. Golde, *Guest Editor*
Volume 12: Acquired Immune Hemolytic Anemias, Hugh Chaplin, *Guest Editor*
Volume 13: Monoclonal Antibodies, P. C. L. Beverley, *Guest Editor*
Volume 14: Radionuclides in Haematology, S. M. Lewis and R. J. Bayly, *Guest Editors*
Volume 15: Hemoglobinopathies, T. H. J. Huisman, *Guest Editor*
Volume 16: Red Cell Metabolism, Ernest Beutler, *Guest Editor*
Volume 17: Blood Transfusion, T. J. Greenwalt, *Guest Editor*
Volume 18: Venous Thrombosis and Pulmonary Embolism: Diagnostic Methods, Jack Hirsh, *Guest Editor*
Volume 19: Red Cell Membranes, Stephen B. Shohet and N. Mohandas, *Guest Editors*
Volume 20: Molecular Genetics, Edward J. Benz, Jr, *Guest Editor*
Volume 21: Perinatal Hematology, Blanche P. Alter, *Guest Editor*
Volume 22: Quality Control, I. Cavill, *Guest Editor*

The Leukemic Cell

EDITED BY

D. Catovsky DSc (Med) FRCP FRCPath

Professor of Academic Haematology and Cytogenetics,
The Royal Marsden Hospital and Institute of Cancer Research, London.

SECOND EDITION

CHURCHILL LIVINGSTONE
EDINBURGH LONDON MELBOURNE NEW YORK TOKYO AND MADRID 1991

CHURCHILL LIVINGSTONE
Medical Division of Longman Group UK Limited

Distributed in the United States of America by Churchill Livingstone Inc., 1560 Broadway, New York, N.Y. 10036, and by associated companies, branches and representatives throughout the world.

© Longman Group UK Limited 1991

All rights reserved. No part of this publication may be reproduced, stored in a retrieval system, or transmitted in any form or by any means, electronic, mechanical, photocopying, recording or otherwise, without either the prior written permission of the publishers (Churchill Livingstone, Robert Stevenson House, 1-3 Baxter's Place, Leith Walk, Edinburgh EH1 3AF), or a licence permitting restricted copying in the United Kingdom issued by the Copyright Licensing Agency Ltd, 90 Tottenham Court Road, London, W1P 9HE.

First edition 1981
Second edition 1991

ISBN 0-443-03867-8
ISSN 0264-4711

British Library Cataloguing in Publication Data
The leukemic cell.
 1. Man. Blood. Leukaemia. Diagnosis. Laboratory techniques
 I. Catovsky, D. (Daniel) II. Series
 616.99419075

Library of Congress Cataloging in Publication Data
The Leukemic cell / edited by
D. Catovsky. — 2nd ed.
 p.   cm. — (Methods in hematology, ISSN 0264-4711; v. 2)
 Includes bibliographical references.
 Includes index.
 1. Leukemia—Cytodiagnosis.
2. Immunocytochemistry. 3. Nucleic acid hybridization. I. Catovsky, D. (Daniel)
II. Series.
 [DNLM: 1. Cytological Technics.
2. Leukemia—ultrastructure. W1 ME9615L
v. 2 / QZ 350 L652]
RC643.L47 1991
616.99'41907—dc20
DNLM/DLC
for Library of Congress

Produced by Longman Singapore Publishers Pte Ltd
Printed in Singapore

For Churchill Livingstone:
Publisher: Michael Parkinson
Editing: Editorial Resources Unit
Production Controller: Mark Sanderson
Design: Design Resources Unit
Sales Promotion Executive: Marion Pollock

Preface

The quest for a better understanding of the leukemic process has continued unabated since this book first came to light almost a decade ago. There have been major advances in technology and with it a more comprehensive view of the great heterogeneity of human leukemias and a wider application of more precise diagnostic methods. The greatest progress has been in the fields of immunology, with the development of an ever-growing range of monoclonal antibodies specific for leucocyte differentiation and functional antigens, and of molecular genetics, with new and highly sophisticated techniques. The advances in both areas have been nothing short of spectacular. For this reason we have included in this edition two chapters on cell markers and two on DNA analysis. As before, the methods are described as used in the laboratories of the authors, who are themselves actively involved in research and teaching in their respective fields. The classic disciplines of morphology, cytochemistry and bone marrow histology, which still form the basis of day-to-day diagnosis and practice, have been given a modern perspective to match the numerous clinicopathological entities included now under the broad term leukemia. The role of ultrastructural morphology and immunocytochemistry is examined in greater detail than before and we have now included a chapter on lymphoid malignancies. Chromosome analysis, which made significant strides in recognising leukemias of different prognosis and has led the way to molecular advances by discovering non-random translocations and consistent breakpoint regions, has also been expanded to two chapters. The book has been completely re-written and, as such, it bears little resemblance to the first edition apart from the same focus on methodology applied to the study of the leukemic cell. We hope that it will aid hematologists, oncologists, clinicians, pathologists and other scientists in their diagnostic and research work. The field moves very fast and new techniques replace old ones but the process is gradual. This book summarises the practice of leukemia diagnosis in today's leading laboratories and should serve as the basis for further developments.

D. Catovsky
London, 1991

Contributors

Reiner Bartl MD
Professor of Internal Medicine, Department of Knochenmarkdiagnostik, University of Munich, West Germany.

Vasantha Brito-Babapulle BSc MSc PhD
Research Scientist, Department of Academic Haematology and Cytogenetics, The Royal Marsden Hospital, London, UK.

Janine Breton-Gorius PhD
Director of Research INSERM (Institut National Sante et Recherche Medicale), Hospital Henri Mondor, Creteil, France.

Rolf Burkhardt MD
Former Head of Department of Knochenmarkdiagnostik, University of Munich and Department of Heamatomorphology, Gesellschaft fur Strahlen und Umweltforschung mbH, Munich, West Germany.

Dario Campana MD
Assistant Member Department of Hematology/Oncology, St Jude Children's Research Hospital Memphis, USA

Daniel Catovsky DSc(Med) FRCP FRCPath
Professor of Academic Haematology and Cytogenetics, The Royal Marsden Hospital, London, UK.

Mary Sue Coleman PhD
Professor of Biochemistry/Associate Provost and Dean of Research, University of North Carolina, NC, USA.

Alistair D. Crockard BSc PhD
Principal Scientist, Regional Immunology Laboratory, Royal Victoria Hospital, Queen's University of Belfast, N. Ireland, UK.

Marie-Therese Daniel MD
Chef de Travaux, Laboratoire Central d'Hematologie and Unite INSERM Hospital Saint-Louis, Paris, France.

Wendy N. Erber MB BS DPhil FRCPA
Haematologist, Department of Haematology, Royal Perth Hospital, Perth, Australia.

Georges Flandrin MD
Professor Laboratoire Central d'Hematologie and Unite INSERM Hospital Saint-Louis, Paris, France.

L. Foroni
Postdoctoral Fellow, MRC Laboratory of Molecular Biology, Cambridge, UK.

Bertha Frisch
Professor of Haematology Institute of Haematology, Jchilov Hospital, Sackler School of Medicine, Tel-Aviv University, Israel.

T. S. Ganesan MD PhD MNAMs MRCP
Consultant in Medical Oncology, Churchill Hospital, Oxford and ICRF Consultant Clinical Scientist, Institute of Molecular Medicine, John Radcliffe Hospital, Oxford, UK.

Lynne R. Hiorns PhD
Research Fellow, Academic Unit of Radiotherapy and Oncology, The Institute of Cancer Research, Surrey, UK.

George Janossy MD PhD MRCPath DSc
Professor of Immunology, Royal Free Hospital School of Medicine, London, UK.

Lucio Luzzatto MD
Honorary Director, MRC/LRF Leukaemia Unit, Department of Haematology, Royal Postgraduate Medical School, Hammersmith Hospital, London, UK.

David Y. Mason DM FRCPath
Lecturer in Haematology, John Radcliffe Hospital, Oxford, UK.

P. Mason PhD
Lecturer, Laboratory of Molecular Genetics, Department of Haematology, Royal Postgraduate Medical School, Hammersmith Hospital, London, UK.

Estela Matutes MD PhD
Lecturer in Haematology, The Royal Marsden Hospital, London, UK.

Donald Metcalf MD FRACP FRCPA FAA FRS
Research Professor of Cancer Biology, Walter and Eliza Hall Institute of Medical Research, Royal Melbourne Hospital, Australia.

Frank Miedema PhD
Head of Department of Clinical Viro Immunology, Central Laboratory of the Netherlands Blood Transfusion Service and the Laboratory for Expansion and Clinical Immunology, University of Amsterdam, The Netherlands.

Jennifer Kennedy Morrow PhD
Assistant Research Professor Department of Pathology, University of Kentucky, Lexington, KY, USA.

Lela K. Riley PhD
Assistant Professor, Department of Veterinary Pathology, University of Missouri, Columbia, MO, USA

Daniele S. F. Robinson BSc MPhil PhD
Research Fellow, Royal Postgraduate Medical School, Hammersmith Hospital, London, UK.

Dorothy L. Williams MD
Member, Department of Pathology and Laboratory Medicine, St Jude Children's Research Hospital; and Professor, Department of Pathology, The University of Tennessee College of Medicine, Memphis, Tennessee, USA.

Bryan D. Young BSc PhD MRCPath
Head of Laboratory, ICRF Medical Oncology Unit, St Bartholomew's Hospital, London, UK.

Contents

1. Overview — 1
   Daniel Catovsky
2. Cytochemistry in the classification of leukemias — 23
   Georges Flandrin   Marie-Therese Daniel   Alistair Crockard
3. Bone marrow histology — 47
   Reiner Bartl   Bertha Frisch   Rolf Burkhardt
4. Ultrastructure of the leukemic cell — 91
   Janine Breton-Gorius
5. The ultrastructure of lymphoid cells — 127
   Estela Matutes   Daniele Robinson
6. Monoclonal antibodies in the diagnosis of acute leukemia — 168
   George Janossy   D. Campana
7. Immunocytochemical labeling of leukemia samples with monoclonal antibodies by the APAAP procedure — 196
   David Y. Mason   Wendy N. Erber
8. Terminal deoxynucleotidyl transferase, adenosine deaminase and purine nucleoside phosphorylase: diagnostic tools and chemotherapeutic targets — 215
   Mary Sue Coleman   Lela K. Riley   Jennifer K. Morrow
9. Lymphocyte functional assays — 234
   Frank Miedema
10. The clonal culture in vitro of human myeloid cells — 253
    Donald Metcalf
11. Cytogenetics of acute leukemia — 288
    Dorothy L. Williams
12. Cytogenetic abnormalities of mature T-cell malignancies — 327
    Vasantha Brito-Babapulle
13. Immunoglobin and T-cell receptor gene analysis for the investigation of lymphoproliferative disorders — 339
    L. Foroni   P. Mason   L. Luzzatto
14. The analysis of molecular changes in leukemia — 392
    Bryan D. Young   Trivadi S. Ganesan   Lynne Hiorns

Index — 411

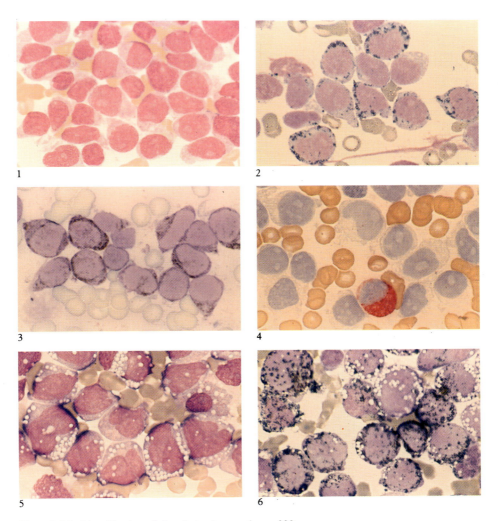

Plates 1–24 Magnification of the photomicrographs × 990.
Plates 1–4 Bone marrow films of a case of myeloblastic leukemia without maturation (M1).

Plate 1 May–Grünwald–Giemsa stain showing undifferentiated blast cells without azurophil granulations.
Plate 2 *Myeloperoxidase* in the same case with the majority of blast cells positive (myeloblasts).
Plate 3 *Sudan black B* in the same case, showing an equivalent positive result.
Plate 4 *NASD chloroacetate esterase* in the same case showing complete negativity of the blast cells with the exception of a promyelocyte (in this field as positive control for the reaction).
Plate 5 May–Grünwald–Giemsa stain showing large blast cells devoid of granulation and with cytoplasm filled with vacuoles, in a case of poorly differentiated myeloblastic leukemia (M1) – bone marrow.
Plate 6 Positive *myeloperoxidase* reaction in the same case demonstrating the myeloblastic nature of the vacuolated blast cells.

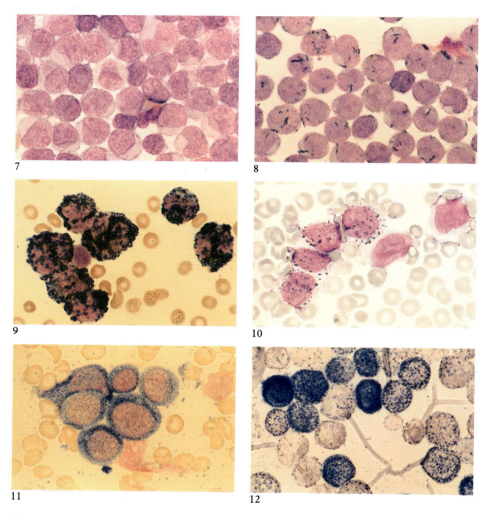

Plate 7 May–Grünwald–Giemsa stain from a buffy-coat preparation of peripheral blood in a case of acute myeloblastic leukemia. Very few Auer rods are visible with this staining.
Plate 8 *Myeloperoxidase* in the same case, showing numerous short sized Auer rods.
Plate 9 Peripheral blood of a case of variant of promyelocytic leukemia (M3-variant). In this case, as well as in cases of typical hypergranular promyelocytic leukemia (M3), the *myeloperoxidase* positivity is always very strong, covering up the whole cytoplasm.
Plate 10 Peripheral blood of a case of acute monocytic leukemia (M5B). *Myeloperoxidase* positive reaction with a typical monocytic pattern with small scattered granules.
Plate 11 Bone marrow film of a case of acute monocytic leukemia (M5A), *NASDA esterase* reaction showing a strong positivity in all blast cells. In this case, exposure to *sodium fluoride* would result in a marked inhibition of the NASDA reaction.
Plate 12 *NASDA esterase* reaction in a case of acute myelomonocytic leukemia (M4), showing strong positivity in some cells (presumably monocytic) and faint positivity in others.

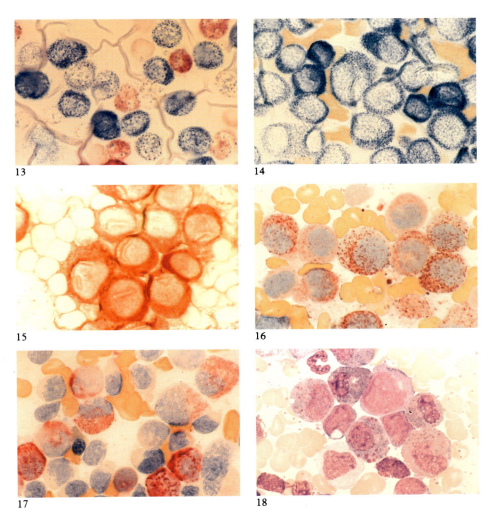

Plate 13 Double esterase staining using *NASDA esterase* technic with fast blue BB as coupler (blue staining), followed by *NASDCA* with pararosanilin as coupler (red staining). Blue staining occurs in monocytic cells and red staining in granulocytic cells.

Plate 14 Bone marrow film of a case of acute monocytic leukemia (M5A). Strong positivity in all blast cells for *NASDA esterase* reaction.

Plate 15 α-*Naphthyl butyrate esterase* from the same patient. Instead of the blue staining obtained by the preceding technic, the reaction product is a dense brown colour. It also shows a very strong positivity in all the blast cells.

Plate 16 *Chloroacetate esterase* reaction in bone marrow from the same case, showing a paradoxic strong positivity in ALL blast cells. Such cases of double esterase positivity give rise to problems in interpretation.

Plate 17 Bone marrow film of a case of acute myelomonocytic leukemia with an abnormal eosinophilic component (M4-EO). The *NASDCA esterase* reaction shows an unusual positive reaction in eosinophil precursors. (This reaction is negative in normal eosinophil precursors.)

Plate 18 Bone marrow film of another case of M4-EO. May–Grünwald–Giemsa stain showing a prominent abnormal eosinophil component.

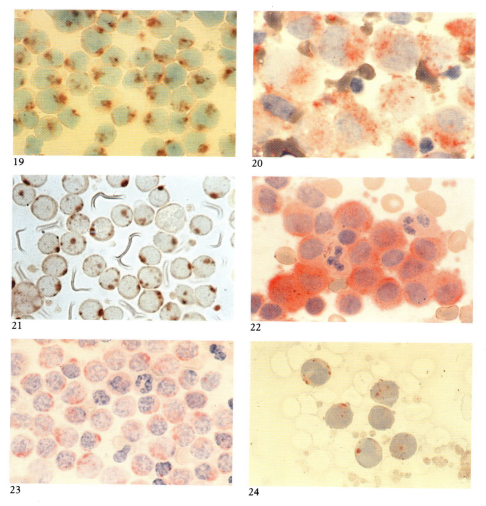

Plate 19 Peripheral blood buffy-coat preparation from a patient with T-ALL. *Acid phosphatase* reaction shows typical positivity in the Golgi zone.
Plate 20 Lymph node imprint from a case of peripheral T-large cell malignant lymphoma. *Acid phosphatase* reaction shows a strong multigranular positivity.
Plate 21 Peripheral blood buffy-coat preparation from a patient with T-PLL. *Acid α-naphthyl acetate esterase* reaction showing a characteristic dot-like activity.
Plate 22 Buffy-coat preparation from the peripheral blood of a case of hairy cell leukemia. *Acid phosphatase* reaction showing a strong positivity appearing as numerous small granules on a background of diffuse positivity. (Inhibition of this positivity is obtained in TRAP processed smears.)
Plate 23 Peripheral blood buffy-coat preparation of a patient with a large granular lymphocytic leukemia. *β-Glucuronidase* reaction showing a multigranular scattered positivity.
Plate 24 Peripheral blood film from a case of T-PLL. *β-Glucuronidase* showing a dot-like positivity.

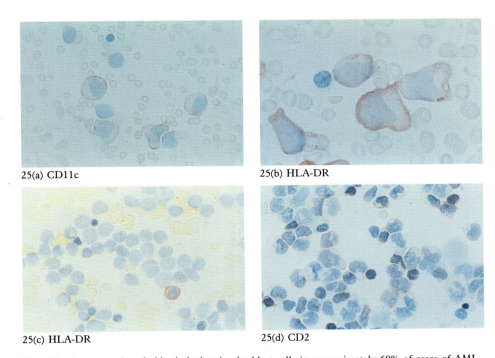

25(a) CD11c   25(b) HLA-DR

25(c) HLA-DR   25(d) CD2

Plate 25 Acute non-lymphoblastic leukemia: the blast cells in approximately 60% of cases of AML express CD11c (p150, 95) and, in 90% of cases, HLA-DR. About 10% of cases of AML express CD2 (anti-SRBC-receptor).

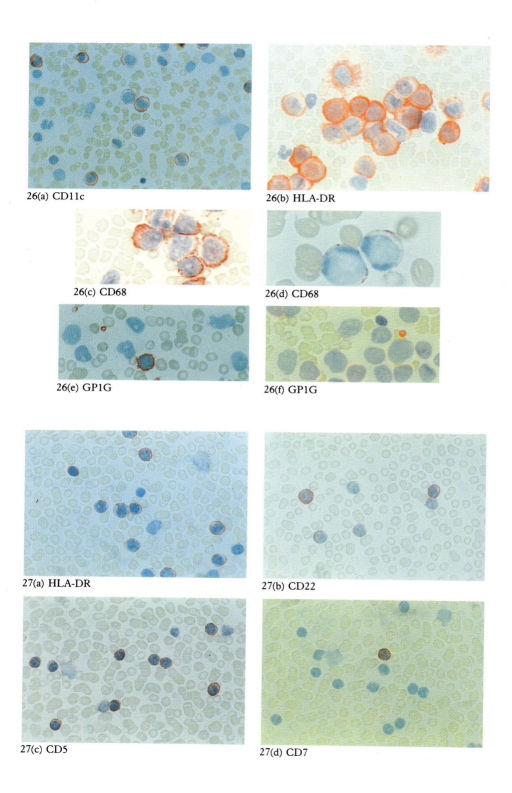

Plate 26 Acute non-lymphoblastic leukemia: In AMML almost all cases express CD11c (p150, 95) and HLA-DR. In addition the blast cells show intracytoplasmic labelling for the CD68 monocyte/macrophage associated antigen, the percentage of positive cells and the number of positive granules per cell varying between cases. In about 20% of cases micromegakaryblasts can be detected using antibodies to platelet glycoprotein Ib or IIIa, (although it should be noted that the former antigen is occasionally also expressed on myelomonoblasts).

Plate 27 B cell chronic lymphocytic leukemia: Cases of B-CLL characteristically express HLA-DR, B cell antigens such as CD19 or 22 (often weakly) and CD5 (T1). The CD7 pan-T cell antigen in this case is absent from the neoplastic B-CLL cells but present on normal T lymphocytes.

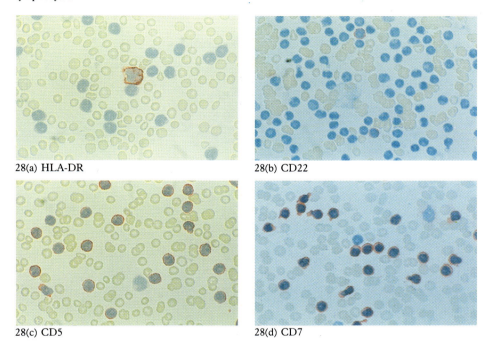

28(a) HLA-DR   28(b) CD22

28(c) CD5   28(d) CD7

Plate 28 T cell chronic lymphocytic leukemia: In contrast to B-CLL, cases of T-CLL lack HLA-DR and B cell antigens (note the two normal B cells, arrowed). The neoplastic lymphocytes in this case of T-CLL are strongly positive for CD5 (T1) and CD7.

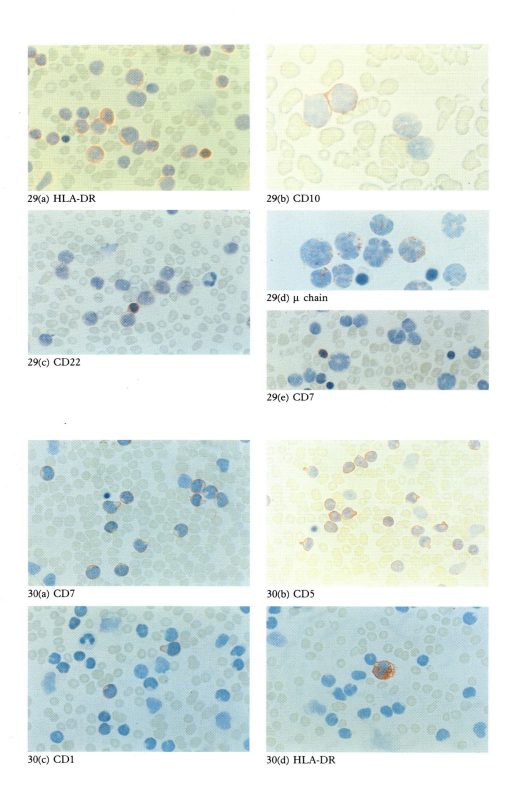

29(a) HLA-DR
29(b) CD10
29(c) CD22
29(d) μ chain
29(e) CD7

30(a) CD7
30(b) CD5
30(c) CD1
30(d) HLA-DR

Plate 29 Acute lymphoblastic leukemia: In common-ALL the majority of blast cells express HLA-DR (CALLA) and B-cell antigens, but lack T-cell antigens. In 20% of cases cytoplasmic μ chains are also found. Note the strongly labelled normal B lymphocytes in the HLA-DR and B-cell preparations, and the normal T cell labelled with anti-CD7.

Plate 30 Acute lymphoblastic leukemia: The expression of T-cell antigens in cases of T-ALL can be related to the maturation stage of the malignant thymocyte. The case of T-ALL illustrated shows the phenotype of an intermediate thymocyte expressing CD1, CD5 and CD7. HLA-DR is absent from leukemic cells in almost all cases of T-ALL (note the positive monocyte).

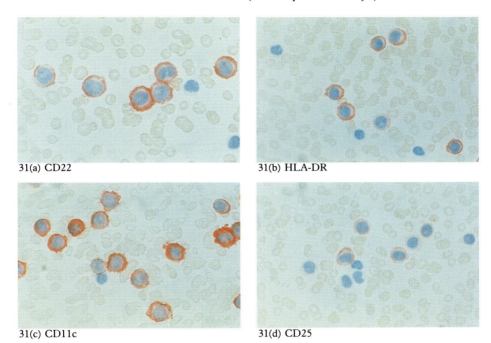

31(a) CD22

31(b) HLA-DR

31(c) CD11c

31(d) CD25

Plate 31 Hairy cell leukemia: The neoplastic cells in this disorder are of B-cell origin and show strong expression of CD19, CD22, HLA-DR and CD11c (p150, 95). The majority of cases also express CD25 (Tac, interleukin-2 receptor) with variable intensity.

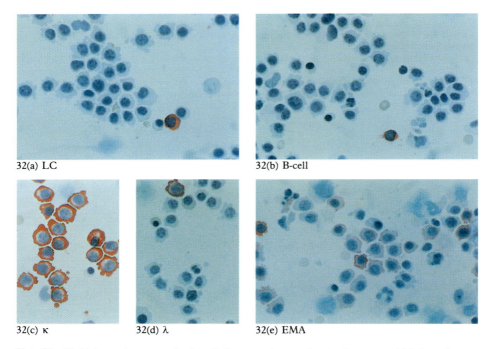

32(a) LC
32(b) B-cell
32(c) κ
32(d) λ
32(e) EMA

Plate 32 Multiple myeloma: neoplastic cells have a unique antigenic phenotype which is easily distinguished from that of the other chronic hematological neoplasms. These end-stage B-cells lack the leukocyte common antigen CD45 expressed in all other hematological malignancies and B-cell antigens. Myeloma cells express monoclonal κ or λ, light chains and, in the majority of cases, epithelial membrane antigen.

1
Overview

Daniel Catovsky

INTRODUCTION

Since the publication of the first edition of this book, we have witnessed significant advances in the methodology used to study leukemic cells. The main progress has been in the field of monoclonal antibodies, growth factors and DNA analysis. This decade has also seen a consolidation of the value of traditional methods which in some fields, such as morphology, have experienced a revival because they can now be correlated with immunological and cytogenetic findings and thus acquire a more precise meaning.

The methods which can be applied to study leukemic cells are summarized in Table 1.1. Some of these technics are often essential for diagnosis whilst others are necessary for research purposes and to advance our understanding of disease pathogenesis and molecular

Table 1.1 Methods for the study of leukemic cells

Morphology	Light microscopy (peripheral blood and bone marrow films) Transmission electron microscopy
Cytochemistry	Light microscopy methods Ultrastructural cytochemistry
Histology	Bone marrow, lymph nodes, spleen, etc. Plastic and paraffin embedding Immunohistochemistry

Cell markers	Monoclonal antibodies
	Membrane immunofluorescence (cell suspensions)
	    Fluorescence microscopy
	    Flow cytometry
	Immunocytochemistry (fixed cells/tissues)
	    Immunoperoxidase (IP)
	    Alkaline phosphatase anti-alkaline phosphatase (APAAP)

Enzyme assays	Terminal transferase (also by immunocytochemistry) Adenosine deaminase; others
Clonal assays	Hemopoietic growth factors Cultures in agar and in suspension Permanent cell lines
Cytogenetics	Banding techniques Cell cultures (with and without mitogens)
DNA analysis	Gene rearrangements and probes for oncogenes and chromosome breakpoints Southern blots Polymerase chain reaction
Cell kinetics	Autoradiography Flow microfluorimetry
New technics	Detection of multidrug resistance (P-glycoprotein), adhesion molecules and homing receptors

events, and for a classification based on objective criteria for identifying cell types and their true lineage.

The progress has been closely associated with technological advances, the production of monoclonal antibodies and their analysis by means of powerful and yet simple to use flow cytometers, remarkable new molecular biology technics including the revolutionary polymerase chain reaction, and sophisticated equipment like the Cytoscan, which is changing the outlook for chromosome analysis by providing a rapid search for metaphases and aid for karyotyping. The culture technics are now becoming more precise by using purified growth factors, in contrast with studies in the past where the nature of the factors was a matter of conjecture.

MORPHOLOGY

The examination of peripheral blood and bone marrow is still the mainstay for the diagnosis and classification of leukemia. Although the appearance of the cells does not change, cytological methods have benefited indirectly from the advances in electron microscopy and immunology. For example, the recognition of megakaryoblasts afforded by monoclonal antibodies (McAbs) and ultrastructural cytochemistry (see Ch. 4) has allowed us to define better the cytological and cytochemical profile of such cells.[1] A better immunological characterization of B- and T-lymphoid cells has facilitated the morphological classification of chronic lymphoproliferative disorders.[2]

ACUTE LEUKEMIAS

The proposals of the FAB group[3,4] are still widely used (see also Ch. 2). The different morphological types of acute lymphoblastic leukemia (ALL) are still considered useful to identify prognostic groups within childhood ALL.[5] Two new problems are worth mentioning: one is the recognition within cases of acute myeloid leukemia (AML) of myelodysplastic changes in neutrophils (hypogranular, Pelger-like), erythroblasts (dyserythropoiesis) and megakaryocytes (mononuclear, hypersegmented, etc.). Such patients, reported as AML with trilineage myelodysplasia,[6] represent 15% of all new AML and are associated with a lower remission rate than AML without myelodysplasia and, in some patients, with a unique type of relapse, as myelodysplastic syndrome (MDS), without the corresponding increase in blast cells as in all types of acute leukemia.[7] Others[8] have identified a similar group of cases by analysing only the morphology of megakaryocytes. It is interesting that the same proportion of AML cases is known to present with chromosome abnormalities characteristically found in MDS, e.g. -5, -7, $5q-$, $7q-$, and also has a lower remission rate.[9] Unfortunately, there is no published study correlating both features, MDS morphology and karyotypic changes in AML.

The other instance where morphology may contribute to our understanding of the nature of an acute leukemia is seen in cases of 'biphenotypic leukemia' (see below), where markers of more than one lineage are demonstrated on the same leukemic cells. It has been our experience, and that of others, that such cases may represent a very early (stem cell) leukemia with morphological differentiation in a lymphoid or myeloid direction or, not infrequently, with appearances of a double population, small blasts resembling lymphoblasts and typical myeloblasts or monoblasts. A closely related phenomenon in such leukemias is the so-called 'phenotypic switch' which again is often, but not always, manifested by a cytological change. Clearly, morphological analysis could contribute, as do the cell marker studies, to definition or suspicion of a leukemia showing dual differentiation features.

CHRONIC MYELOID LEUKEMIAS

In this group of disorders the most common disease is chronic granulocytic leukemia (CGL) in which the cells have the Philadelphia chromosome, as a result of the t(9;22) translocation and, at the molecular level, by the fusion of a truncated *bcr* gene (chromosome 22) with the *c-abl* gene (chromosome 9) which give rise to a chimeric protein with enhanced protein-tyrosine kinase activity, as demonstrated by many studies (reviewed in Chapter 13). A minority of CGL patients have a typical differential count with no cytogenetic evidence of t(9;22) — designated Ph-negative CGL — but who nevertheless show rearrangement of the *bcr* gene. Work pioneered by David Galton has shown that, overall, there is a good correlation between the cytogenetic and/or molecular evidence of t(9;22) and the typical CGL morphology, with a predominance in peripheral blood films of myelocytes, basophils, etc., in contrast to cases with Ph - /*bcr* - disease in which the differential counts show either features of chronic myelomonocytic leukemia with a predominance of neutrophils and monocytes, or cases of 'atypical' chronic myeloid leukemia with features of myelodysplasia, a higher proportion of immature granulocytes, few myelocytes, rare basophils, etc.[10] From the above, it is apparent that a greater focus on the analysis of peripheral blood films may contribute to a disease classification which will often be confirmed by cytogenetic and molecular analysis.

CHRONIC B-CELL LEUKEMIAS AND THE LEUKEMIC PHASE OF B-CELL NON-HODGKIN'S LYMPHOMAS

The great heterogeneity of these disorders is reflected in the immunological phenotype and the diverse morphology of the circulating cells.[2] It is unquestionable that the morphology of the peripheral blood lymphocytes is an important element in the diagnosis and classification of these lymphoproliferative disorders which often have, in addition, different clinical features, response to therapy and overall prognosis. In chronic lymphocytic leukemia (CLL), the demonstration of more than 10% circulating prolymphocytes and, in particular, an absolute number greater than $15 \times 10^9/l$, seems to be associated with a more aggressive clinical course and a short survival.[11] Interestingly the excess of prolymphocytes correlates with a larger spleen than in typical CLL cases, confirming the suggestion that the spleen is the main source of these cells, as is also the case in prolymphocytic leukemia (PLL).

Detailed morphological analysis of the peripheral blood cells has also allowed the recognition of two unique B-cell diseases in which the lymphoid cells display long villi, resembling, and being confused with, hairy cell leukemia (HCL). One of these disorders has been considered to be a variant form of HCL because its tissue expression in the spleen affects predominantly the red pulp. Morphologically, the HCL-variant cells appear to be a hybrid between hairy cells (wide cytoplasm) and prolymphocytes (prominent nucleolus). The author's group has recently studied a series of 17 patients with the variant form of HCL and has described the main clinical and laboratory features of this disease, namely: moderately high WBC, lack of monocytopenia and tartrate-resistant acid phosphatase (in contrast to HCL), poor response to therapy (in particular, resistance to α-interferon) and, despite this, a relatively good prognosis.[12] HCL-variant cells also differ from typical hairy cells in the class of immunoglobulin heavy chain class and the reactivity with several McAbs (see below).[12]

The other condition, splenic lymphoma with circulating villous lymphocytes (SLVL),[13] is relatively frequent and, from experience, is more common than PLL and HCL. This disease has been recognized in the past as distinct from HCL by the histology of the spleen in which the white pulp is predominantly involved, in contrast with typical HCL.[14] The importance of distinguishing SLVL from other B-cell disorders arises when patients require treatment, because splenectomy and, if this is contraindicated, splenic irradiation are, in the author's experience, the treatments of choice.

4 THE LEUKEMIC CELL

At least three types of non-Hodgkin's lymphoma (NHL) can evolve with a leukemic phase and, when this occurs, they present major problems of differential diagnosis with CLL or, in the case of large cell NHL, with monoblastic leukemia. The morphology of the circulating cells in follicular lymphoma[15] and in intermediate (mantle zone or centrocytic) NHL has been described in detail.[16] The importance of recognizing such cases is that, when they present with a high WBC (greater than $30 \times 10^9/l$), they appear to be associated with an aggressive clinical course and do not benefit from single agent chemotherapy.

MATURE T-CELL LEUKEMIAS

This is a less common group of disorders which comprises proliferations of post-thymic T-lymphocytes with different biological features. By morphology and membrane phenotype, it is possible to identify at least four disease entities, each with diverse clinical and laboratory manifestations.

The most common of these is T-cell prolymphocytic leukemia (T-PLL) in which the cells resemble 'classic' B-prolymphocytes or are smaller and have a nucleolus only visible under electron microscopy examination.[17,18] T-PLL runs an aggressive course with a median survival of 7 months; two-thirds of cases are associated with chromosome abnormalities involving chromosomes 14 and 8[19] (see Ch. 14). A number of cases of T-PLL show cells with a deep basophilic cytoplasm suggesting 'lymphoplasmocytic' differentiation, thus emphasizing that morphology alone, without immunological information, could be misleading in the diagnosis of the lymphoid leukemias.

Adult T-cell leukemia lymphoma (ATLL) is another T-cell disorder often recognized on morphological grounds by the presence of a polylobed nucleus, which led to the description of flower-like cells in the Japanese literature.[20] The importance of ATLL lies in its association with the retrovirus HTLV-I, its etiological agent, and its epidemiology which now includes south-western Japan, the Caribbean region, extending further to Brazil and to the south east of the USA.

Another form of T-cell malignancy — large granular lymphocyte (LGL) leukemia — is also recognized by the evidence of LGL in the peripheral blood and/or other affected tissues (e.g. the spleen). The variable clinical manifestations (benign or aggressive) depend on the immunophenotype, with the stable or chronic forms being characterized by CD4 − , CD8 + cells[18,21,22] whilst the more rare and severe forms have atypical phenotypes, e.g. CD4 + , CD8 − and/or express markers of natural killer cells, e.g. CD11b, CD16.[18,23] The association of rheumatoid arthritis in 20% of cases suggests an interesting pathogenesis that deserves further study.

The cutaneous T-cell lymphomas, which include Sézary syndrome and mycosis fungoides, are also identified morphologically when the malignant T-cells appear in peripheral blood films, a feature which is characteristic of Sézary syndrome.[2] In the small Sézary cell variant, the circulating cells may escape recognition by the light microscope. This is one of the few clear indications for the use of electron microscopy to establish a definitive diagnosis. A group of patients with circulating Sézary-like cells, but without pathological involvement of the skin, has recently been identified by the author's group.[24] This is a rare and clinically aggressive disorder which may be important with respect to pathogenesis, because one of the patients in that series was identified as HTLV-1 positive. A large review,[25] evaluating the significance of circulating Sézary cells in the peripheral blood of cutaneous T-cell lymphoma, concluded that patients with more than 20% large cells have a shorter survival than those in whom small cells predominated, and also correlated with more extensive visceral involvement and a worse histological picture.

TRANSMISSION ELECTRON MICROSCOPY

The contribution of ultrastructural studies to acute and chronic leukemias is described in Chapters 4 and 5. The role of electron microscopy is to define more precisely morphological characteristics of leukemic cells which are not apparent by conventional cytology or histology. This morphological refinement is relevant when there is a need to describe new disease entities and for evidence that the cells indeed have special features. Further progress can be made by quantitative analysis of some cell structures or organelles, which may be different in the various leukemias. For example, the morphometric analysis performed in circulating cells with villous projections found in HCL, HCL-variant and SLVL, was useful to characterize these different types of B-cell disorder.[26] In the leukemic phase of folicular lymphoma, the small lymphocytes can be seen by electron microscopy to be much more irregular and 'cleaved' than suspected on Romanovsky-stained films.[2,15] As described above, electron microscopy is also important to define morphological differences between the various types of post-thymic T-cell leukemias. The possibility of combining immunogold labeling with morphology has been applied to identify normal counterparts of the cells involved in some B- and T-cell malignancies (see Ch. 5).

CYTOCHEMISTRY

The cytochemical methods used by light microscopy are still widely employed to classify acute leukemias, in particular the two major types: ALL and AML (see Ch. 2). Results of immunophenotyping have allowed the characterization of megakaryoblastic leukemias (AML, M7) and, in turn, a description of the characteristic cytochemical profile of these cells which, as the erythroid precursors, share a localized pattern with reactions for two acid hydrolases — α-naphthyl acetate esterase and acid phosphatase.[1]

An interesting report by Scott et al[27] has recently clarified the nature of the atypical α-naphthyl acetate esterase reaction observed in promyelocytic leukemia cells (AML, M3). Despite this reactivity, these cells were shown to lack antigens characteristic of monocytes and showed, by isoelectric focusing, an esterase isoenzyme pattern identical to that of normal granulocytes and different from that of monocytes.[27]

ULTRASTRUCTURAL CYTOCHEMISTRY

Greater advances have also been made by cytochemical methods at electron microscopy level in the recognition of different types of blast cells (see Ch. 4). The role of ultrastructural cytochemistry is to detect, by sensitive technics, specific patterns of differentiation, e.g. early evidence of myeloperoxidase (MPO) activity in myeloblasts or platelet peroxidase in megakaryoblasts, and use this information to evaluate the results with more simple and widely used methods, such as immunophenotyping with McAbs.[28,29] A good example of such an application is in the diagnosis of early or immature myeloblastic leukemia or AML, M0. Such cases are undifferentiated by conventional light microscopy, morphology and cytochemistry, and the blast cells do not react with McAb against B- or T-lineage lymphoblasts, but instead express one or more antigens of myeloid cells. The author's experience in such cases is that, by sensitive ultrastructural methods, it is possible to detect MPO, thereby confirming the myeloid nature of the blast cells.[28] Small MPO+ granules were also reported in rare cases with an apparent lymphoid phenotype and reactive with a polyclonal antibody anti-MPO.[29] These more sensitive methods for detecting myeloid differentiation also include short-term cultures with phorbol esters as inducing agents[30] and the detection of MPO mRNA by Northern blot analysis.[31] In the experience of the author's group, murine stem cell lines which express MPO mRNA also show MPO activity by ultrastructural cytochemistry and, sometimes, also show reactivity with an McAb anti-MPO (V. Shetty & E. Matutes, unpublished; see below).

HISTOLOGY

The study of leukemias and lymphomas now also requires a precise description of the tissue expression of those tumors. Lymph node histology is an essential component of evaluation and diagnosis of the lymphomas. In the leukemias and related myelo- and lymphoproliferative disorders, bone marrow histology is important for diagnostic and classification purposes and for evaluating response to therapy. In CLL, the bone marrow histological pattern correlates with clinical staging, but is also an independent prognostic variable, and it is essential for the differential diagnosis with low grade NHL and to interpret the pathogenesis of anemia or thrombocytopenia. As described in Chapter 3, details of the bone marrow microenvironment and its cellular components are also highly informative. The morphological detail obtained in thin sections from plastic-embedded biopsies is also a major element which contributes to a more precise diagnosis.

Immunocytochemistry methods are increasingly used for the assessment of bone marrow biopsies. Most antigens are only susceptible to be tested in frozen sections, where the morphological detail may not be satisfactory. Fortunately, a wide range of reagents (monoclonal and some polyclonal), can now be used in paraffin-embedded sections, with the added advantage of good morphology and the possibility of performing retrospective studies in samples prepared by routine histological technics.[32-34] Occasionally, monoclonal antibodies appear to be reliable reagents also in plastic-embedded sections.[35] These new technologies will undoubtedly make more accurate the assessment of lineage of differentiation and, hopefully, will be applied more widely by practising hematopathologists.

CELL MARKERS

The methodology used for the detection of membrane and/or cytoplasmic antigens in normal and leukemic cells has expanded dramatically in the last 15 years, particularly since the development of the hybridoma technology. The number of McAbs grouped in well-defined clusters of differentiation (CD) has reached 78 after the Fourth International Workshop on Leukocyte Differentiation Antigens.[36,37] The importance of these workshops lies, not only in the standardization of nomenclature, but also in the parallel advances in the functional characterization of the membrane molecules defined by the CD markers. A good example is the integrin family of adhesion molecules, which are transmembrane glycoprotein heterodimers that interact with a wide variety of ligands and consist of a common β-chain non-covalently associated with distinct α-chains. Three McAbs recognize the leukocyte-associated molecules (LFA) or Leu-CAMS[38] that share a β_2-chain (CD18):

1. CD11a or LFA-1, which binds to ICAM-1 (CD54) and predominates on lymphocytes.
2. CD11b which acts as a receptor of the third component of complement (CR3) and predominates in granulocytes.
3. CD11c (McAb LeuM5) which predominates on macrophages (and is also expressed on hairy cells).

Many of the membrane antigens defined by the CD numbers have recently been found to have enzymatic activities,[39] a notable example being the CD10 or common-ALL antigen which was shown to correspond to neutral endopeptidase.[40] The clarification of the nature of this molecule will open the way to understanding its function in health and disease (for a review see LeBien and McCormack[41]).

The applications of McAbs to the diagnosis of acute leukemia are reported in detail in Chapters 6 and 7. The possibilities of testing these reagents are now extensive and include the study of cells in suspension and on fixed preparations (see Table 1.1). Methods such as immunoperoxidase or APAAP (see Ch. 7) have the advantage of being tested directly on blood or bone marrow slides and of correlating with morphology.[42] Immunofluorescence by flow cytometry allows rapid quantitation of large numbers of cells and performance of double or treble simultaneous labeling (see Ch. 6). Often both approaches need to be combined because the analysis of cells in suspension is not adequate to detect the early antigens which appear first in the cytoplasm of hemopoietic precursors, e.g. CD13 in AML,[43] CD3 in T-ALL[44-46] and CD22 in B-lineage ALL.[46]

MARKERS IN ACUTE LEUKEMIA

The contribution of McAbs to the identification of the type of blast cells has been very significant, and continues to improve all the time with the larger number of antigens being defined in the three main hemopoietic lineages: myeloid, B-lymphoid and T-lymphoid. The most recent progress has been the recognition of McAbs specific for the myeloid lineage (CD13, CD33), including reagents for the megakaryocytic and erythroid lineages. The possibility of combining one or more McAbs by flow cytometry, taking advantage of the presence of aberrant or asynchronous phenotypes, can be exploited to detect minimal residual disease, as detailed in Chapter 6, when combinations of markers not seen in the normal bone marrow, e.g. CD7 (normally a T-cell marker) or terminal transferase, are demonstrated in cells which also express CD13 or CD33.

Terminal deoxynucleotidyl transferase (TdT)

The significance of TdT estimations, fully described in Chapter 8, is one of the earliest differences reported between immature lymphoid (TdT+) and myeloid (TdT−) cells. Further studies over the years have shown that, whilst TdT is consistently positive in B- or T-lineage ALL, a proportion of AML (20–25%) also shows TdT activity in the nucleus of the blast cells. It is interesting to note that the relatively high proportion of TdT+ AML, by comparison with the original reports, includes at least 22% of AML cases which may also express other lymphoid antigens[47] and are now described as 'biphenotypic'. Thus, the value of TdT as a lymphoid marker remains high. In the author's experience, the more immature myeloblastic types of AML (M0 and M1) are more often TdT+ than the other FAB types.[47] This finding supports the view that TdT is expressed early on lymphoid and some myeloid progenitor cells. The data correlating TdT activity with gene rearrangements of T-cell receptor and immunoglobulin heavy chain genes are not clear cut, although the role of TdT during this functional rearrangement has been recognized.

TdT as a single marker has been found extremely valuable for the diagnosis of meningeal relapse in ALL as normal reactive lymphocytes are, as a rule, TdT−.[48] When the significance of TdT positivity (tested by indirect immunofluorescence) was compared with the morphological analysis of cerebrospinal fluid samples, the follow-up confirmed a meningeal relapse in the majority. When two consecutive samples were TdT+, all such cases had overt CNS relapse.[49] Assessment of TdT was also predictive in samples taken at diagnosis in that study. It seems that TdT should be assessed routinely in cerebrospinal samples as part of the investigation of patients with ALL, TdT+ AML and TdT+ lymphoblastic lymphoma.

Monoclonal antibody anti-MPO

A recent development with respect to myeloid markers is the availability of a McAb against the α-chain of MPO (55 kilodaltons) and its precursor polypeptide (89 kDa). Because of the reactivity against the proenzyme form, this McAb appears to be more sensitive for the diagnosis of AML than the corresponding cytochemical reactions of MPO and Sudan black B.[50] The author's group has tested 54 cases of AML with the anti-MPO reagent and found 50 (93%) positive including five cases which were Sudan black B and MPO negative by light microscopy (E. Matutes, unpublished data). Interestingly enough, when the reactivity of anti-MPO was combined with that of CD33 (64% positive) and cytoplasmic CD13 (92% positive), all the AML cases studied were positive with one or more of these reagents. Thus, the addition of this new anti-myeloid reagent has increased significantly the chances of a diagnosis of AML, including in cases like AML, M0 which are negative by conventional cytochemistry. The sensitivity of the anti-MPO McAb was compared with ultrastructural cytochemical methods for MPO and an excellent concordance was found, thus emphasizing further the importance of this reagent (V. Shetty, E. Matutes and V. Buccheri, unpublished observations). A similar comparison made by Vainchenker et al[29] suggests that the electron microscopy method is more sensitive. However, that study used a polyclonal antibody anti-MPO which is presumably less sensitive than the McAb.

BIPHENOTYPIC ACUTE LEUKEMIA

Independent of biological interpretation, genetic misprogramming or limited promiscuity of gene expression in hemopoietic progenitor cells,[51] there is now unequivocal evidence of the co-expression of lymphoid and myeloid antigens in cases presenting, or being classified, as AML or ALL. Furthermore, such cases may represent a special type of acute leukemia for two important reasons:

1. They are often associated with chromosome abnormalities, such as t(9;22),[52] t(4;11) and other aberrations affecting chromosome 11q,[53] known to correlate with poor prognosis.
2. Particularly in adults with ALL, the expression of myeloid antigens seems to identify a high-risk group of patients with low remission rates and short survival.[53,54]

Although frequently these cases of biphenotypic acute leukemia present as ALL and are more often adults, the expression of lymphoid antigens in cases presenting as otherwise typical AML is equally common.

It is not clear whether the 'aberrant' expression of one antigen is sufficient to define such cases, or whether the more full expression of two or more specific antigens (or enzymes) of the opposite lineage recognizes the true biphenotypic cases. Apart from this difference, the often confusing terminology employed — bilinear or mixed when the cells involved are apparently of two separate lineages and biphenotypic when the same blast cell expresses antigens from different lineages (which can now be demonstrated by double labeling with a FACS flow cytometer — see Ch. 6) — has not contributed to a better understanding of such cases. This problem is compounded by the lack of specificity of the markers used in some studies and the lack of strictness in the criteria employed by some authors. For example, 16% of cases included in the series of Sobol et al[54] correspond to what we would now call AML (M0), i.e. blasts expressing only myeloid antigens in cases which may resemble ALL morphologically; this point has also been criticized by others.[55] It is also unclear whether the rare cases (1.5%) of ALL, which co-express B- and T-cell antigens,[56] have the same biological and clinical significance as when myeloid and lymphoid are co-expressed. The study by Uckun et al[56] showed, by two-color immunofluorescence, the existence of biphenotypic lymphocyte precursors from which, presumably, the biphenotypic CD2 + (T), CD19 + (B) ALL arose.

The correct interpretation of biphenotypic acute leukemia may be relevant to therapy. For example, some cases of childhood AML expressing CD2 failed anti-AML therapy and responded to anti-ALL treatment.[57] This has been relevant to the related phenomenon of phenotypic switch,[58] i.e. cases which present as ALL or AML and relapse as AML or ALL, respectively. In such cases it is believed that the lineage-directed therapy modifies the differentiation drive of a leukemia involving early hemopoietic precursors with a multiple differentiation potential.

MARKERS IN MATURE B-CELL LEUKEMIAS AND NHL

As discussed above, immunological markers are essential nowadays for the diagnosis and classification of B- and T-cell leukemias and lymphomas.[2] Table 1.2 illustrates the diagnostic power of McAbs when applied to the heterogeneous group of chronic B-cell leukemias and NHL. Although all these represent disorders of mature B-lymphocytes, the expression of several B-cell-associated antigens varies with the stages of differentiation, and therefore can be exploited for this purpose. The two diseases at both extremes of the B-cell maturation pathway are CLL and hairy cell leukemia (HCL). CLL cells are characterized by weak staining for membrane immunoglobulin, reactivity with McAbs of the CD5 and CD23 groups and, in contrast with most other B-cell disorders, weak membrane expression of CD22 and FMC7.[11] HCL cells have a unique reactivity with four McAbs, two clustered (CD11c and CD25) and two antibodies not yet clustered (anti-HC2 and B-ly7). The latter is a recently described McAb with high specificity for HCL[59] within the B-cell disorders. These findings have been confirmed in a large number of cases[60] and it was also shown that a minority of HCL-variant cases[12] are B-ly7+. An unexpected finding was the expression of the B-ly7 antigen in some T-cell leukemias. With double-labeling studies it has, in fact, been shown that B-ly7 reacts with an activation antigen in normal CD8+ T-lymphocytes, although the three cases of T-cell leukemia positive with B-ly7 were CD4+.[60]

Currently, the author's group is exploiting this unique reactivity of HCL cells to investigate the value of the specific McAb for the detection of minimal residual disease in

Table 1.2 Immunophenotype of chronic B-cell leukemias and lymphomas

Marker	CLL	PLL/SLVL	HCL-V	HCL	NHL[b]
CD19/class II	++	++	++	++	++
FMC7; CD22 (m)[a]	-/+	++	++	++	++
SmIg (intensity)	+/-	++	++	++	++
Ig class	MD	MD	G	GAM	MDG
M-rosettes	++	-	-	-/+	-/+
CD5/CD23	++	-/+	-	-	-/+ [c]
CD25 (Tac)	-	-/+	-	++	-
HC2	-	-	-	++	-
CD11c	-	-/+	+	++	-
B-ly7	-	-	-/+	++	-

-/+ = weak expression or more frequently negative.

[a] m = membrane expression only; CD22 will otherwise be equally positive in the cytoplasm in most B-cell disorders. Note too that FMC7 has not been clustered in the CD22 group but the pattern of reactivity parallels the membrane binding of CD22.
[b] Follicular lymphoma and intermediate NHL (or diffuse centrocytic) in leukemic phase.
[c] CD5 is, as a rule, expressed in intermediate NHL lymphocytes; CD10 (not in table) is often positive in follicular lymphoma cells and weakly or not expressed in the other B-cell disorders.

frozen bone marrow sections after treatment with α-interferon and 2′-deoxycoformycin. It has already been seen that the HCL-specific McAbs, particularly B-ly7, detected foci of residual hairy cells when conventional histology suggests a complete remission.[60]

HEMOPOIETIC GROWTH FACTORS

Studies with clonal assays (see Ch. 10) have been essential for the isolation of glycoprotein hormones that function as hemopoietic growth factors and modulate the proliferation, activation and development of blood-forming cells.[61,62] The continued presence of these factors is required for the survival, in vitro, of hemopoietic cells and their maturation into functional cells. Most growth factors have now been purified, their genes cloned and active molecules have been produced on a large scale through DNA technology.[61, 62] These, in turn, have improved the precision of experiments with in vitro colony assays, which can now be performed under controlled serum-free culture conditions with the addition of the various factors individually or in combination.[63] In addition to the colony assays, some of the hemopoietic growth factors have now moved to the clinic and are actively used in therapeutic trials.[62] Some of the growth factors — the interleukins or lymphokines, numbered 1 to 6 — have a key role in the immune response and are responsible for the expansion and differentiation of antigen-specific lymphocytes. One of the lymphokines (interleukin-3) is one of the colony stimulating factors (CSF), also known as multi-CSF, produced by mitogen- or antigen-activated T-lymphocytes (see Ch. 10).

Alkaline phosphatase is an enzyme of neutrophils (NAP), which is better known in the field of leukemia because of its low levels in the neutrophils of chronic granulocytic leukemia CGL, and high levels in polycythemia rubra vera, within the myeloproliferative disorders. One of the growth factors — granulocyte colony-stimulating factor (G-CSF) — induces the synthesis of NAP in normal as well as in leukemic neutrophils, as shown in cultures in vitro,[64] by activation of the NAP gene. It is not clear, however, what the relationship between G-CSF and the very low NAP values in CGL neutrophils is.

The clinical applications of the recombinant growth factors are rapidly expanding. G-CSF has been used to treat the neutropenia induced by cytotoxics and produces high neutrophil levels with minor side effects.[62,65] Recombinant human granulocyte–macrophage colony-stimulating factor (GM-CSF) and G-CSF can also accelerate the myeloid recovery, but not that of platelets, after high-dose chemotherapy and autologous bone marrow transplantation,[66,67] and consequently reduces considerably the period during which patients are at risk of infection and the use of parenteral antibiotic therapy.

An extension of these applications is the demonstration that GM-CSF induces a significant expansion in the number of circulating granulocyte–macrophage progenitor cells which can then be harvested by leukapheresis and used for reinfusion together with autologous bone marrow.[68] This approach has also resulted in a more rapid hemopoietic recovery with the potential for greater therapeutic index following chemoradiotherapy. Perhaps more controversial is the use of recombinant GM-CSF in myelodysplastic syndromes. There is no question that GM-CSF can improve the cytopenias suffered by these patients,[69] but the effect on the blast cell population, whether stimulation or differentiation, is less clear, one study reporting a decrease in the percentage of bone marrow blasts,[69] whilst another showed an increase of such cells in the blood and bone marrow.[70]

CHROMOSOME ABNORMALITIES

The advances in the field of cytogenetics and molecular genetics have been considerable in the last decade. Non-random chromosome abnormalities have been demonstrated in most types of leukemia and lymphoma and the analysis of breakpoints by molecular technics has resulted in remarkable discoveries and a greater understanding of the pathogenesis of these human malignancies. In addition to drawing attention to specific DNA lesions, the demonstration of specific chromosome abnormalities in the acute leukemias, chiefly ALL, has great prognostic significance (Table 1.3 and see Ch. 11). The correlation of some abnormalities with morphological subtypes of AML and immunological subtypes of ALL have, pari passu, contributed to the diagnostic precision of many of the acute leukemias. The concept of the MIC (morphology, immunology and cytogenetics) classifications for ALL[71] and AML[72] is a recognition of the combined power of these three methodologies.

In leukemias and lymphomas involving B- and T-cell precursors or mature lymphocytes, the breakpoints nearly always affect functional genes according to the lineage involved. Thus, in B-cell tumors, the immunoglobulin heavy chain (IgH) gene in chromosome 14q32 is the most consistent breakpoint, whilst in T-cell lymphoid malignancies the most common breakpoint is also in chromosome 14 but at 14q11, loci of the T-cell receptor α- and δ-chain genes, and in chromosome 7, at 7q34, loci of the T-cell receptor β-chain gene;[73] (see Ch. 14).

A phenomenon of great importance is the evidence for subtle differences in the breakpoints at the molecular level between seemingly similar chromosome aberrations. For example, in Ph chromosome leukemias, the breakpoint in chromosome 22, affecting the *bcr* gene, is different in CGL and in 50% of cases of Ph + ALL (see Ch. 13). Similar differences have been reported in Burkitt's lymphoma where the breakpoint may involve, directly or indirectly, the *c-myc* gene. In the endemic form, the breakpoints are at the joining region of the Ig heavy chain gene (in chromosome 14) and 90 kilobases upstream of the first exon of *c-myc* (in chromosome 8), whereas, in the sporadic form and the Burkitt lymphoma seen in AIDS patients, the breakpoints in chromosome 14 are at the switch region of the Ig heavy chain gene and, in chromosome 8, in a region around the first exon of *c-myc*.[74]

Further examples of the power of molecular technics, once the breakpoint regions have been cloned and defined, is that they may detect molecular rearrangements without microscopic evidence of chromosome abnormalities. This is the case in the Ph − chronic myeloid leukemias[75] which, as discussed above, may have clinical and morphological similarities to Ph + CGL and show rearrangement of the *bcr* gene. A similar situation has now emerged with the translocation t(14;18), which is found in 70% of cases of follicular lymphoma with involvement of the IgH gene at 14q32 and the *bcl-2* gene at 18q21.[74,76] In some patients with B-cell CLL, a submicroscopic (molecular) rearrangement has been documented which involves the Ig light chain gene and a breakpoint in the *bcl-2* gene at the 5′ end,[77,78] distant from the standard *bcl-2* breakpoints (major and minor) of follicular lymphoma at the 3′ end of the gene.[76,79] This means that molecular rearrangements may be more common than hitherto suspected by chromosome abnormalities.

Table 1.3 Chromosome abnormalities in ALL according to immunophenotype and their relation to prognosis[a]

ALL-type	Karyotype	Prognosis
Early-B ('null')	t(4;11)(q21;q23)	Poor
Common	Hyperdiploidy	Good
	Ph +, t(9;22)(q34;q11)	Poor
Pre-B (cytμ)	t(1;19)(q23;p13)	Modest
B-ALL (SmIg)	t(8;14)(q24;q32)	Poor
T-ALL (CD2 +)	t(11;14)(p13;q11)	Variable

[a] Full details in Chapter 11.

Deletions involving the short arms of chromosome 9 at 9p21–22, where the α-interferon and β_1 genes are localized, have also been found more readily (29% of cases) by molecular technics using specific DNA probes than by the microscopic demonstration of chromosome rearrangements.[80] Nevertheless, the original demonstration of chromosome translocations or deletions of the 9p arm have been reported in 7–13% of cases and have, indeed, stimulated these important studies, which suggest that the loss of tumor-suppressor genes located on chromosome 9p may be important in the pathogenesis of ALL.[80]

Further developments are on the horizon with the use of new technics such as the combination of immunology (McAbs with the APAAP method) and karyotype in order to identify precisely the cell lineage of an abnormal metaphase.[81] With this technic it is possible to identify clonal chromosome abnormalities involving several cell lineages in a high proportion of AML cases.[81] The identification of trisomies (+ 12 in CLL) or monosomies (− 7 in myelodysplasia) may also be possible with chromosome-specific probes by in situ hybridization or Southern blotting.[82] Such advances will help answer important questions on pathogenesis and, at the same time, may result in simpler tests being applied in everyday practice.

ACUTE LYMPHOBLASTIC LEUKEMIA

Immunological and cytogenetic analysis of ALL has disclosed the great heterogeneity of this group of leukemias.[71] Many studies, particularly from the leading group at St Jude's Children's Hospital (see Ch. 11) and from the International Workshop on Chromosomes in Leukemia[83] have demonstrated the important role of karyotype in predicting survival in children and adults with ALL.

Patients with hyperdiploidy (especially with a modal number greater than 50 chromosomes) have the best prognosis.[83] The incidence of hyperdiploidy within adult ALL is 5% and in childhood ALL 14% in the analysis of the International Workshop,[83] but other studies seem to indicate that this proportion is higher in children (about 25%)[84] and lower in adults. This, and the higher incidence of some structural abnormalities, e.g. t(9;22) in adults, may be responsible for the worse prognosis of adult ALL. It appears, too, that even within the relatively good group with hyperdiploidy, the simultaneous presence of structural abnormalities may identify patients who do not respond to primary therapy.[84] For example, a relatively uncommon abnormality, isochromosome 17q (seen in 1.7% of cases) is often associated with hyperdiploidy and with failure to respond to treatment.[85]

Analysis of DNA content by flow cytometry may recognize cases with more than 50 chromosomes, and this may obviate the need for a karyotype to identify this group with a good prognosis.[85,86] Unfortunately, this methodology will not recognize the subset with structural abnormalities or, within the diploid cases, those with the abnormalities associated with very poor prognosis, namely t(4;11), t(8;14), t(9;22), etc.[83]

Abnormalities involving 11q23

Chromosome abnormalities with a breakpoint at chromosome 11q23 represent a distinct group of acute leukemia in childhood. In St Jude's series they represent 5.7% of all ALL cases.[88] The best known abnormality with a breakpoint at 11q23 is t(4;11) (q21;q23); other translocations include t(1;11), t(10;11), t(11;19) and t(9;11), the latter often presenting as AML, M5a (monoblastic type). In half of the cases, 11q23 is the only change.[88] Children with this abnormality tend to be young and with higher WBC than other ALL cases. In at least 50% of cases they are under the age of 2 years; half of the infants (<1 year of age) presenting with ALL or AML have demonstrable abnormalities involving 11q23.[89–91]

The most usual phenotype is null-ALL (early B without expression of CD10) but, not infrequently, there is co-expression of myeloid and early lymphoid antigens. When DNA analysis is performed, most cases show rearrangement of the Ig heavy chain gene.[88-90] A high proportion of cases also show rearrangement of T-cell receptor genes.[90] Even in cases presenting as AML, rearrangement of Ig or T-cell receptor genes can also be demonstrated by DNA analysis. Overall, the available evidence suggests that leukemias with abnormalities of 11q23 represent stem cell leukemias which may present either as ALL (with an early B-phenotype) or as biphenotypic acute leukemia, or as AML.[91] In infants presenting with AML the translocation t(9;11) (p21;q23), characteristic of monoblastic leukemia, is often seen.[91]

The features associated with the translocation t(4;11) are:

1. Poor prognosis with less than 15% of patients surviving longer than 2 years.[83,92]
2. A slight predominance of females (62%).
3. Presentation with a WBC greater than $100 \times 10^9/1$ and splenomegaly.[92]
4. Phenotypic characteristics of null-ALL and expression of myeloid antigens,[92,93] as all other cases with breakpoint 11q23.

An intriguing report from St Jude's Hospital describes the occurrence of 'secondary' AML in 13 children out of 733 cases of ALL studied after a median period of 3 years from diagnosis.[94] In 8 of the 13 children, the blast cells showed abnormalities of chromosome 11 in the 11q23 region which were, apparently, not detected at diagnosis. A number of these patients had a previous diagnosis of T-lineage ALL and received therapy which included etoposide. Unfortunately, there was no indication of any DNA analysis, comparing the original samples with the relapse ones, to ascertain beyond any doubt that the hypothesis of a second leukemogenic event is tenable. The evidence discussed above for 11q23 abnormalities is that they occur at a stem cell level and therefore an alternative hypothesis, that of a phenotypic switch, also needs to be considered. It would be important, in future cases, to test these hypotheses because they may have implications for therapy, namely the omission of some drugs in ALL therapy or the addition of anti-AML drugs in cases with high risk for a phenotypic switch. From a single case report, there is evidence that a phenotypic switch from typical T-ALL to typical AML could occur in adults with genotypic conservation, thus demonstrating the common clonal origin of both leukemias in that particular case.[95]

ACUTE MYELOID LEUKEMIA

Chromosome abnormalities in AML correlate closely with FAB morphological subtypes and are useful in identification of distinct entities such as t(8;21) in AML, M2; t(15;17) in both types of promyelocytic leukemia, M3 and M3 variant; inv(16) in myelomonocytic leukemia with bone marrow eosinophilia or M4Eo, etc.[72] In addition, a distinct pattern of prognosis and response to treatment is emerging for some of these abnormalities. For instance, inv(16) and t(8;21) are associated with the highest complete remission rate,[9,96] whilst complex abnormalities and involvement of chromosomes 5 and 7 ($-5, 5q-, -7, 7q-$), a feature of myelodysplastic syndromes and secondary leukemia,[97] have a significantly lower remission rate and worse prognosis. It is interesting, too, that monosomy 7 has also been reported in megakaryoblastic leukemia (AML, M7)[98,99] associated with myelodysplastic features suggestive of a leukemia affecting a multipotent stem cell.

The pathogenic importance of chromosome changes in AML and myelodysplasia is exemplified by the deletion of the long arm of chromosome 5 (5q−), frequently seen in such cases. It is now known that an important family of genes encoding growth factors and its receptors have been mapped in the deleted region q23–q31. These include GM-CSF, CSF-1, IL3 or multi-CSF, IL4, IL5, platelet-derived growth factor receptor, etc.[100]

ABNORMALITIES IN LYMPHOPROLIFERATIVE DISORDERS

The most common leukemia in adults over the age of 50 years, B-CLL, is associated with trisomy 12 in 25% of cases. Other less frequent abnormalities include 14q+, t(11;14) (q13;q32) and deletion of the long arm of chromosomes 6 (6q−), 11 (11q−) and 13 (13q−); trisomy 12 and 14q+ are associated with worse prognosis.[101] In the author's experience, 14q+ is the most frequent abnormality in B-cell prolymphocytic leukemia, with a number of cases showing the translocation t(11;14) with breakpoints in 11q13,[102] a region which may contain the candidate gene *bcl-1*, although not all the breakpoints documented seem to cluster within the same region.[103] t(11;14) (q13;q32) is not infrequent in aggressive myelomatosis, plasma cell leukemia and lymphoplasmacytic lymphoma, thus suggesting a relationship of this translocation with malignancies of B-cells at late stages of their maturation pathway.

The coexistence of t(14;18), characteristic of follicular lymphoma, with t(8;14), a feature of Burkitt's lymphoma, on the same cells has now been demonstrated in a number of cases, usually presenting as an ALL, frequently but not always of L3 (Burkitt type) morphology,[104,105] and sometimes as a follicular lymphoma undergoing transformation.[106,107] The authors recently studied a patient who presented as a B-ALL (SmIg+) with L3 morphology (Fig. 1.1) with a WBC of $41 \times 10^9/l$ and a bone marrow crowded with L3 lymphoblasts. It was of interest that, whilst 24 of the 25 metaphases had t(14;18) (q32;q21) and t(8;14)(q24;q32), one cell had only t(14;18), suggesting that the latter abnormality was the first to develop (Dr V. Brito-Babapulle, personal communication). Furthermore, the bone marrow biopsy showed foci of small lymphocytes, some of them cleaved, in the paratrabecular region, also consistent with a preceding phase (subclinical) of low-grade (follicular) NHL. Molecular analysis showed rearrangement of Ig heavy and light chain genes, *c-myc* and *bcl-2*. This case confirms that the aggressive (acute leukemic) transformation of follicular lymphoma is associated with new cytogenetic changes, similar to those seen in Burkitt

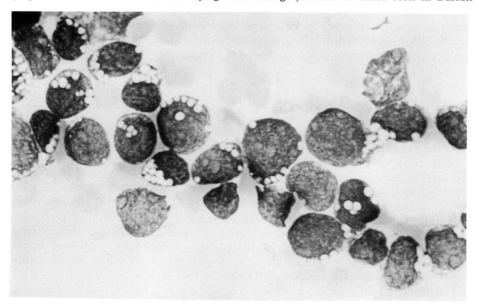

Fig. 1.1 Bone marrow cells from a case presenting as ALL, L3 with t(14;18) and t(8;14), presumably representing the transformation of a low grade follicular lymphoma to a high grade ALL (see text).

lymphoma, which result in deregulation of *c-myc* and lead to the rapid clonal expansion of L3 lymphoblasts.

DNA ANALYSIS

The remarkable progress in molecular biology technics cannot be given full justice in this overview. Chapters 12 and 13 outline in detail the applications of DNA technology to the study of leukemic cells. The applications of this work are expanding rapidly and have taken a significant leap forward with the development of the highly sensitive method of the polymerase chain reaction (PCR), which can be applied not only to DNA but also to RNA analysis[108] to investigate such problems as minimal residual disease,[109,110] early relapse after bone marrow transplantation, involvement of rare sites, etc. By analogy with McAbs that bind to particular antigens, DNA probes are increasingly used to search for complementary sequences of genes to which they will then hybridize.

In leukemia, the applications of molecular technics have been mainly in the study of rearrangements of functional genes of B- and T-lymphocytes, Ig heavy and light chain genes and T-cell receptor (TCR) β-, α- and δ-genes[111] and in the identification of specific breakpoints which often involve oncogenes such as *c-myc, c-abl, bcl-2*, etc. The frequent and interesting phenomenon of illegitimate recombinations of Ig and TCR with other genes, through target heptamer and nonamer sequences, as a result of mistakes during the physiological process of rearrangement, has provided new insights in understanding pathogenic mechanisms.[75] The applications of DNA analysis also extend to the study of etiological agents such as retroviruses, HTLV-I and -II, HIV, and DNA viruses such as Epstein–Barr virus (EBV), which may have a key role in the development of some lymphoid malignancies, and point mutations of some oncogenes, notably the members of the *ras* family,[112] which become activated through this aberration.

IG AND TCR GENE REARRANGEMENTS AS CLONAL MARKERS

One of the most useful applications of the study of gene rearrangement is the possibility of demonstrating clonality in seemingly 'benign' B or T lymphocytosis and reactive lymphadenopathies. The interest has focused particularly on the T-cell disorders where the need for a clonal marker is essential because it is not provided by immunological markers. This contrasts with the B-cell disorders which show light chain restriction as evidence of clonality by simple staining with anti-Ig reagents. In addition, the cells in a number of large cell NHLs, often T and sometimes B in nature, do not express, or do so only partially, lineage-specific markers, and their cellular origin has been shown only by the demonstration of Ig or TCR gene rearrangements.

Two examples in the chronic lymphoproliferative disorders are large granular lymphocyte leukemia and B-cell CLL. LGL proliferations were thought, for a long time, to be non-clonal due to their benign clinical course.[21] It has now been shown that, in the majority of cases of persistent lymphocytosis with a uniform marker profile, i.e. with a predominant subset such as CD4−, CD8+, CD57+, the study of TCR rearrangement will demonstrate clonality.[113-115] This, of course, does not necessarily indicate that the process is malignant in a clinical sense,[111] but should be considered as neoplastic in a wider context. Two caveats are important here:

1. Studies only with probes for the β-chain gene may give negative results in the rare cases of LGL leukemias derived from lymphocytes bearing TCRγδ and which need to be studied with δ-chain gene probes.[115]

2. Cases resulting from natural killer (NK) cell proliferations which do not express T-cell antigens, chiefly CD3, will show germ-line configuration with all the TCR probes.[23,113]

In CLL the transformation to a large cell immunoblastic NHL, known as Richter's syndrome, may result from a malignant event involving the same B-cell clone[116] or, in some cases, represents a new disease. It is necessary to study all such cases with the technics for Ig gene rearrangement to establish the true incidence and clinical significance of one or other event. By extrapolation from CLL, the transformation which occurs in all low grade NHL should be studied by comparing the original diagnostic material with that of the new tumor. Implicit in this statement is the value of freezing diagnostic samples of blood, bone marrow and lymph nodes for future studies.

DNA analysis is also an important tool for deciding whether or not an established cell line derives from the original malignancy. Although karyotypic analysis is also useful in this respect, looking for Ig light chain restriction may be misleading. In such instances information from the tumor cells' specific gene rearrangements will be crucial.[117]

Also discussed above is the need for gene rearrangement data when examining the problem of secondary leukemias or phenotypic switch to seek an explanation for apparent new leukemias supervening in previously treated ALL. Because most ALLs will show Ig or TCR rearrangements, and at least one-third of AMLs will show cross-lineage rearrangement of Ig heavy chain or TCR α-, δ- or β-chain genes, these may be used as clonal markers to study minimal residual disease,[118] particularly in relation to bone marrow transplantation. Similarly, these molecular tools should be applied to the analysis of the bone marrow to be reinfused in autotransplantation programs, and used to decide about the advantages of, or the need for, 'purging' procedures.

RAS MUTATIONS

The three *ras* genes (Harvey, Kirstein (*Ki*) and *N-ras*) acquire transforming activity through specific point mutations, usually affecting codons 12, 13 or 61.[112] Activation of *ras* genes has been documented in a variety of different human neoplasias and in chemically induced tumors in animals. *Ki-ras* mutations at codon 12 are a feature of carcinomas of the colon, pancreas and lung. Mutations of *N-ras* have been documented in 25% of AML, and MDS,[112] adult ALL, Ph − chronic myeloid leukemias (CMLs),[119] chronic myelomonocytic leukemia and, recently, in myelomatosis;[120] they are exceedingly rare in Ph + CML.[121] *Ras* mutations are investigated by polymerase chain reaction (PCR) for amplifying nucleic acid sequences and dot–blot hybridization with specific oligonucleotide probes. Although the strong association of *ras* mutations with certain types of human malignancy suggests a pathogenic role of the p21 *ras* proteins localized in the inner surface of the plasma membrane, there are still many questions to be answered about the precise role of these changes in leukemogenesis. The mutations at codon 12, 13 and 61 result in transformed proteins of reduced intrinsic guanosine triphosphatase activity, which is their main function.[112] The oncogene protein products do not perform as the normal *ras* proteins. *Ras* mutations may not be initiating malignant events and, if present at diagnosis, they may disappear following a relapse.[112,122] *Ras* mutations cannot, therefore, be used regularly as clonal markers of the leukemia. Although some reports suggest that *ras* mutations in MDS correlate with a higher rate of transformation to AML,[123] there is no information about any correlation of *ras* mutations in de novo AML and the morphological changes described as trilineage MDS in AML[6,7] and/or the abnormalities of chromosomes 5 and 7.[97]

NEW TECHNICS

The advances brought about by the hybridoma technology continue to provide tools to investigate the function of newly recognized surface molecules. Systematic studies with McAbs specific for a series of adhesion molecules may gradually clarify the patterns of tumor progression and preferential tissue distribution of certain leukemias and lymphomas. The degree of expression of LFA-1 (CD11a) molecules on cells from various lymphoid malignancies could explain their different anatomical distribution. Notably B-CLL cells lack LFA-1, whilst B-cell small lymphocytic lymphoma is nearly always LFA-1 positive; this subtle difference could provide a rationale for the recirculation pattern of CLL and the relatively fixed tissue expression of seemingly similar cells in lymphocytic NHL.[124]

Another recently discovered molecule, the lymphocyte homing receptor, may also be important to understand the spread of certain lymphoid tumors. In large cell NHL, this receptor is highly expressed in disseminated disease, whilst few of the patients with localized disease have tumors expressing this receptor.[125] It could probably be very useful to study this receptor in cases of large cell NHL presenting as leukemia, and to ascertain whether the cellular levels are even higher in such cases.

The study of cell kinetics in leukemia has lagged behind in the past due to the complexity of the early technics. It seems now that studies with the McAb Ki-67 and/or a reagent against the enzyme DNA-methyl transferase[126] may provide a simple tool to test systematically the proliferation kinetics of leukemic cells, and to identify proliferative grades: low, intermediate and high. This information may be used for correlation with other clinical and laboratory parameters.[127] In chronic disorders, these reagents may identify changes, e.g. during early transformation, which can then be applied to suggest alternative treatment approaches, e.g. with drugs which are more active for cells in particular stages of the cell cycle.

Finally, the demonstration of the multidrug resistant (*mdr*) phenotype in cells which have a high expression of the P-glycoprotein, p170, can now be determined also by specific McAbs.[128,129] This glycoprotein, which acts as a drug efflux pump, has internal and external domains and the methodology used for its detection by McAbs needs to be selected carefully. Reagents against external epitopes can be tested on cell suspensions by flow cytometry, whilst McAbs against internal epitopes can only be tested on fixed preparations by immunocytochemistry. The use of this and similar technics will provide a more rational approach to therapy and indicate ways to overcome resistance to cytotoxic drugs by manipulation of the efflux pump with agents such as verapamil and cyclosporin A. Recent studies have shown that there are two *mdr* genes (*mdr1* and *mdr3*) with 80% homology. Whilst most reports so far have associated *mdr1* with clinical drug resistance, a recent paper suggests that high levels of *mdr3*, but not of *mdr1*, determined by RNA dot-blot analysis, were found in all six patients with B-cell PLL tested.[130] This finding may indeed explain the refractory nature of B-PLL and provide a rationale for better treatments of this disease. Thus, more studies on basic differences between leukemic cells are likely to have important clinical implications for patient management in the near future.

REFERENCES

1 Pombo de Oliveira M S, Gregory C, Matutes E, Parreira A, Catovsky D 1987 Cytochemical profile of megakaryoblastic leukaemia: a study with cytochemical methods, monoclonal antibodies and ultrastructural cytochemistry. Journal of Clinical Pathology 40: 663–669
2 Bennett J M, Catovsky D, Daniel M-T et al 1989 The French–American–British (FAB) Cooperative Group. Proposals for the classification of chronic (mature) B and T lymphoid leukaemias. Journal of Clinical Pathology 42: 567–584
3 Bennett J M, Catovsky D, Daniel M-T et al 1985 Criteria for the diagnosis of acute leukemia of megakaryocyte lineage (M7). Annals of Internal Medicine 103: 460–462

4 Bennett J M, Catovsky D, Daniel M-T et al 1985 Proposed revised criteria for the classification of acute myeloid leukemia. Annals of Internal Medicine 103: 620–625
5 Lilleyman J S, Hann I M, Stevens R F, Eden O B, Richards S M 1986 French American British (FAB) morphological classification of childhood lymphoblastic leukaemia and its clinical importance. Journal of Clinical Pathology 39: 998–1002
6 Brito-Babapulle F, Catovsky D, Galton D A G 1987 Clinical and laboratory features of de novo acute myeloid leukaemia with trilineage myelodysplasia. British Journal of Haematology 66: 445–450
7 Brito-Babapulle F, Catovsky D, Galton D A G 1988 Myelodysplastic relapse of de novo acute myeloid leukaemia with trilineage myelodysplasia: a previously unrecognised correlation. British Journal of Haematology 68: 411–415
8 Jinnai I, Tomonaga M, Kuriyama K et al 1987 Dysmegakaryocytopoiesis in acute leukaemias: its predominance in myelomonocytic (M4) leukaemia and implication for poor response to chemotherapy. British Journal of Haematology 66: 467–472
9 Samuels B L, Larson R A, Le Beau M M et al 1988 Specific chromosomal abnormalities in acute nonlymphocytic leukemia correlate with drug susceptibility in vivo. Leukemia 2: 79–83
10 Shepherd P C A, Ganesan T S, Galton D A G 1987 Haematological classification of the chronic myeloid leukaemias. Bailliere's Clinical Haematology 1: 887–906
11 Melo J V, Catovsky D, Galton D A G 1987 Chronic lymphocytic leukaemia and prolymphocytic leukaemia: a clinicopathological reappraisal. Blood Cells 12: 339–353
12 Sainati L, Matutes E, Mulligan S P et al 1990 A variant form of hairy cell leukemia resistant to alpha-interferon: clinical and phenotypic characteristics of 17 patients. Blood 76:157–162
13 Melo J V, Robinson D S F, Catovsky D 1987 Splenic B-cell lymphoma with circulating 'villous' lymphocytes in the peripheral blood: a disorder distinct from HCL. Leukemia 1: 294–299
14 Neiman R S, Sullivan A L, Jaffe R 1979 Malignant lymphoma simulating leukemic reticuloendotheliosis. A clinicopathologic study of ten cases. Cancer 43: 329–342
15 Melo J V, Robinson D S F, de Oliveira M P et al 1988 Morphology and immunology of circulating cells in leukaemic phase of follicular lymphoma. Journal of Clinical Pathology 41: 951–959
16 Pombo de Oliveira M S, Jaffe E S, Catovsky D 1989 Leukaemic phase of mantle zone (intermediate) lymphoma: its characterisation in 11 cases. Journal of Clinical Pathology 42: 962–972
17 Matutes E, Garcia Talavera J, O'Brien M, Catovsky D 1986 The morphologic spectrum of T-prolymphocytic leukaemia. British Journal of Haematology 64: 111–124
18 Matutes E, Brito-Babapulle V, Worner I, Sainati L, Foroni L, Catovsky D 1988 T-cell chronic lymphocytic leukaemia: the spectrum of mature T-cell disorders. Nouvelle Revue Française d'Hematologie 30: 347–351
19 Brito-Babapulle V, Pomfret M, Matutes E, Catovsky D 1987 Cytogenetic studies on prolymphocytic leukemia. II. T-cell prolymphocytic leukemia. Blood 70: 926–931
20 Takatsuki K, Uchiyama J, Sagawa K, Yodoi J 1977 Adult T-cell leukaemia in Japan. In: Seno S, Takaku F, Imino S (eds) Topics in hematology. Excerpta Medica, Amsterdam, p. 73–77
21 Newland A C, Catovsky D, Linch D et al 1984 Chronic T-cell lymphocytosis: a review of 21 cases. British Journal of Haematology 58: 433–446
22 Lougran T P, Kadin M E, Starkebaum G et al 1985 Leukemia of large granular lymphocytes: association with clonal chromosomal abnormalities and autoimmune neutropenia, thrombocytopenia and hemolytic anemia. Annals of Internal Medicine 102: 169–175
23 Imamura N, Kusinoki Y, Kawa-Ha K et al 1990 Aggressive natural killer cell leukaemia/lymphoma: report of four cases and review of the literature. British Journal of Haematology 75: 49–59
24 Matutes E, Kelling D M, Newland A C et al 1990 Sézary cell-like leukaemia: a distinct type of mature T-cell malignancy. Leukemia 4: 262–266
25 Schechter G P, Sausville E A, Fishmann A B et al 1987 Evaluation of circulating malignant cells provides prognostic information in cutaneous T-cell lymphoma. Blood 69: 841–849
26 Robinson D, Lackie P, Aber V, Catovsky D 1989 Morphometric analysis of chronic B-cell leukemias — an aid to the classification of lymphoid cell types. Leukemia Research 13: 357–365
27 Scott C S, Patel D, Drexler H G, Master P S, Limbert H J, Roberts B E 1989 Immunophenotypic and enzymatic studies do not support the concept of mixed monocytic–granulocytic differentiation in acute promyelocytic leukemia (M3): a study of 44 cases. British Journal of Haematology 71: 505–509
28 Matutes E, Pombo de Oliveira M, Foroni L, Morilla R, Catovsky D 1988 The role of ultrastructural cytochemistry and monoclonal antibodies in clarifying the nature of undifferentiated cells in acute leukaemia. British Journal of Haematology 69: 205–211
29 Vainchenker W, Villeval J L, Tabilio A et al 1988 Immunophenotype of leukemic blasts with small peroxidase-positive granules detected by electron microscopy. Leukemia 2: 274–281

30 Heil G, Ganser A, Raghavachar A et al 1988 Induction of myeloperoxidase in five cases of acute unclassified leukaemia. British Journal of Haematology 68: 23–32
31 Ferrari S, Mariano M T, Tagliafico E et al 1988 Myeloperoxidase gene expression in blast cells with a lymphoid phenotype in cases of acute lymphoblastic leukemia. Blood 72: 873–876
32 Hall P A, Lindeman R, Bulter M G, Amess J A L, d'Ardenne A J 1987 Demonstration of lymphoid antigens in decalcified bone marrow trephines. Journal of Clinical Pathology 40: 870–873
33 Mason D Y, Cordell J, Brown M et al 1989 Detection of T-cells in paraffin wax embedded tissue using antibodies against a peptide sequence from the CD3 antigen. Journal of Clinical Pathology 42: 1194–1200
34 Ralfkaier, Pulford K A F, Lauritzen A F, Avnstrom S, Guldhammer B, Mason D Y 1989 Diagnosis of acute myeloid leukaemia with the use of monoclonal anti-neutrophil elastase (NP57) reactive with routinely processed biopsy samples. Histopathology 14: 637–643
35 Chan J, Beckstead J H 1987 Leu-M1 antigen as a marker of acute nonlymphoid leukemia. Hematologic Pathology 1: 209–215
36 Knapp W, Dorken B, Rieber P, Schmidt R E, Stein H, von dem Borne A E G Kr 1989 CD antigens 1989. International Journal of Cancer 44: 190–191
37 Knapp W, Dorken B, Gilks W R et al eds 1989 Leucocyte typing IV. White cell differentiation antigens. Oxford University Press, Oxford, p. 1–1182
38 Patarroyo M, Makgoba M W 1989 Leucocyte adhesion to cells in immune and inflammatory responses. Lancet ii: 1139–1141
39 Kenny A J, O'Hare M J, Gusterson B A 1989 Cell surface peptidases as modulators of growth and differentiation. Lancet ii: 785–787
40 Letarte M, Vera S, Tran R et al 1988 Common acute lymphocytic leukemia antigen is identical to neutral endopeptidase. Journal of Experimental Medicine 168: 1247–1253
41 LeBien T W, McCormack R T 1989 The common acute lymphoblastic leukemia antigen (CD10) — Emancipation from a functional enigma. Blood 73: 625–635
42 Hanson C A, Gajl-Peczalska K J, Parkin J L, Brunning R D 1987 Immunophenotyping of acute myeloid leukemia using monoclonal antibodies and the alkaline phosphatase–antialkaline phosphatase technique. Blood 70: 83–89
43 Pombo de Oliveira M S, Matutes E, Rani S, Morilla R, Catovsky D 1988 Early expression of MCS2 (CD13) in the cytoplasm of blast cells from acute myeloid leukaemia. Acta Haematologica 80: 61–64
44 Rani S, de Oliveira M S P, Catovsky D 1988 Different expression of CD3 and CD22 in leukemic cells according to whether tested in suspension or fixed on slides. Hematologic Pathology 2: 73–78
45 Van Dongen J J M, Krissansen G W, Wolvers-Tettero I L M et al 1988 Cytoplasmic expression of the CD3 antigen as a diagnostic marker for immature T-cell malignancies. Blood 71: 603–612
46 Janossy G, Coustan-Smith E, Campana D 1989 The reliability of cytoplasmic CD3 and CD22 antigen expression in the immunodiagnosis of acute leukemia: a study of 500 cases. Leukemia 3: 170–181
47 Parreira A, Pombo de Oliveira M S, Matutes E, Foroni L, Morilla R, Catovsky D 1988 Terminal deoxynucleotidyl transferase positive acute myeloid leukaemia: an association with immature myeloblastic leukaemia. British Journal of Haematology 69: 219–224
48 Bradstock K F, Papageorgiou E S, Janossy G 1981 Diagnosis of meningeal involvement in patients with acute lymphoblastic leukaemia. Cancer 47: 2478–2481
49 Hooijkaas H, Hahlen K, Adriaansen H J, Dekker I, van Zanen G E, van Dongen J M 1989 Terminal deoxynucleotidyl transferase (TdT)-positive cells in cerebrospinal fluid and development of overt CNS leukemia: a 5-year follow-up study in 113 children with a TdT-positive leukemia or non-Hodgkin's lymphoma. Blood 74: 416–422
50 Van der Schoot C E, von dem Borne A E G K, Tetteroo P A T 1987 Characterization of myeloid leukemias by monoclonal antibodies, with an emphasis on antibodies against myeloperoxidase. Acta Haematologica 78 (suppl. 1): 32–40
51 Greaves M F, Chan L C, Furley A J W, Watt S M, Molgaard H V 1986 Lineage promiscuity in hemopoietic differentiation and leukemia. Blood 67: 1–11
52 Chen S J, Flandrin G, Daniel M-T et al 1988 Philadelphia positive acute leukemia: lineage promiscuity and inconsistently rearranged breakpoint cluster regioin. Leukemia 2: 261–273
53 Childs C C, Hirsch-Ginsberg C, Walters R S et al 1989 Myeloid surface antigen-positive acute lymphoblastic leukemia (My + ALL): immunophenotypic, ultrastructural, cytogenetic and molecular characteristics. Leukemia 3: 777–783
54 Sobol R E, Mick R, Royston I et al 1987 Clinical importance of myeloid antigen expression in adult acute lymphoblastic leukemia. New England Journal of Medicine 316: 1111–1117

55 Drexler H G 1987 Myeloid-antigen expression in adult acute lymphoblastic leukemia. New England Journal of Medicine 317: 1156
56 Uckun F M, Muraguchi A, Ledbetter J A et al 1989 Biphenotypic leukemic lymphocyte precursors in CD2+ CD19+ acute lymphoblastic leukemia and their putative normal counterparts in human fetal hemopoietic tissues. Blood 73: 1000-1015
57 Mirro J, Zipf T F, Pui C-H et al 1985 Acute mixed lineage leukemia: clinicopathologic correlations and prognostic significance. Blood 66: 1115-1123
58 Nosaka T, Ohno H, Doi S et al 1988 Phenotypic conversion of T lymphoblastic lymphoma to acute biphenotypic leukemia composed of lymphoblasts and myeloblasts. Journal of Clinical Investigation 81: 1824-1828
59 Visser L, Shaw A, Slupsky J, Vos H, Poppema S 1989 Monoclonal antibodies reactive with hairy cell leukemia. Blood 74: 320-325
60 Mulligan S P, Travade P, Matutes E et al 1990 B-ly7, a monoclonal antibody reactive with hairy cell leukemia, also defines an activation antigen on normal CD8+ T-cells. Blood 76:959-964
61 Metcalf D 1989 Haemopoietic growth factors 1. Lancet i: 825-827
62 Metcalf D 1989 Haemopoietic growth factors 2: clinical applications. Lancet i: 885-887
63 Salem M, Delwel R, Mahmoud L A, Clark S, Elbasousy E M, Lowenberg B 1989 Maturation of human acute myeloid leukaemia in vitro: the response to five recombinant haematopoietic factors in a serum-free system. British Journal of Haematology 71: 363-370
64 Chikkappa G, Wang G J, Santella D, Pasquale D 1988 Granulocyte colony-stimulating factor (G-CSF) induces synthesis of alkaline phosphatase in neutrophilic granulocytes of chronic myelogenous leukemia patients. Leukemia Research 12: 491-498
65 Morstyn G, Campbell L, Souza L M et al 1988 Effect of granulocyte colony stimulating factor on neutropenia induced by cytotoxic chemotherapy. Lancet i: 667-672
66 Brandt S J, Peters W P, Atwater S K et al 1988 Effect of recombinant human granulocyte-macrophage colony-stimulating factor on haematopoietic reconstitution after high-dose chemotherapy and autologous bone marrow transplantation. New England Journal of Medicine 318: 869-876
67 Sheridan W P, Morstyn G, Wolf M et al 1989 Granulocyte colony-stimulating factor and neutrophil recovery after high-dose chemotherapy and autologous bone marrow transplantation. Lancet ii: 891-895
68 Gianni A M, Siena S, Bregni M et al 1989 Granulocyte–macrophage colony-stimulating factor to harvest circulating haemopoietic stem cells for autotransplantation. Lancet ii: 580-585
69 Vadhan-Raj S, Keating M, LeMaistre A et al 1987 Effects of recombinant human granulocyte–macrophage colony-stimulating factor in patients with myelodysplastic syndromes. New England Journal of Medicine 317: 1545-1552
70 Herrmann F, Lindemann A, Klein H, Lubbert M, Schulz G, Mertelsmann R 1989 Effect of recombinant human granulocytemacrophage colony-stimulating factor in patients with myelodysplastic syndrome with excess blasts. Leukemia 3: 335-338
71 First MIC Cooperative Study Group 1986 Morphologic, immunologic and cytogenetic (MIC) working classification of acute lymphoblastic leukemias. Cancer Genetics and Cytogenetics 23: 189-197
72 Second MIC Cooperative Study Group 1988 Morphologic, immunologic and cytogenetic (MIC) working classification of the acute myeloid leukemias. Cancer Genetics and Cytogenetics 30: 1-15
73 Smith S D, Morgan R, Gemmell R et al 1988 Clinical and biologic characterization of T-cell neoplasias with rearrangements of chromosome 7 band q34. Blood 71: 395-402
74 Krolewski J J, Dalla-Favera R 1989 Molecular genetic approaches in the diagnosis and classification of lymphoid malignancies. Hematologic Pathology 3: 45-61
75 Greaves M F 1989 The contribution of molecular genetics to the study of leukemia. Cancer Genetics and Cytogenetics 40: 217-230
76 Lipford E, Wright J J, Urba W et al 1987 Refinement of lymphoma cytogenetics by the chromosome 18q21 major breakpoint region. Blood 70: 1816-1823
77 Adachi M, Cossman J, Longo D, Croce C M, Tsujimoto Y 1989 Variant translocation of the bcl-2 gene to immunoglobulin light chain gene in chronic lymphocytic leukemia. Proceedings of the National Academy of Sciences of the USA 86: 2771-2774
78 Adachi M, Tefferi A, Greipp P R, Kipps T J, Tsujimoto Y 1990 Preferential linkage of bcl-2 to immunoglobulin light chain gene in chronic lymphocytic leukemia. Journal of Experimental Medicine 171: 559-564
79 Ngan B-Y, Nourse J, Cleary M L 1989 Detection of chromosomal translocation t(14;18) within the minor cluster region of bcl-2 by polymerase chain reaction and direct genomic sequencing of the enzymatically amplified DNA in follicular lymphomas. Blood 73: 1759-1762
80 Diaz M O, Rubin C M, Harden A et al 1990 Deletions of interferon genes in acute lymphoblastic leukemia. New England Journal of Medicine 322: 77-82

81 Keinanen M, Griffin J D, Bloomfield C D, Machnicki J, de la Chapelle A 1988 Clonal chromosomal abnormalities showing multiple-cell-lineage involvement in acute myeloid leukemia. New England Journal of Medicine 318: 1153-1158
82 Kere J, Ruutu T, de la Chappelle A 1987 Monosomy 7 in granulocytes and monocytes in myelodysplastic syndrome. New England Journal of Medicine 316: 499-503
83 Bloomfield C, Secker-Walker L M, Goldman A I et al 1989 Six-year follow-up of the clinical significance of karyotype in acute lymphoblastic leukemia. Cancer Genetics and Cytogenetics 40: 171-185
84 Pui C-H, Raimondi S C, Dodge R K et al 1989 Prognostic importance of structural chromosomal abnormalities in children with hyperdiploid (>50 chromosomes) acute lymphoblastic leukemia. Blood 73: 1963-1967
85 Pui C-H, Raimondi S C, Williams D L 1988 Isochromosome 17q in childhood acute lymphoblastic leukemia: an adverse cytogenetic feature in association with hyperdiploidy. Leukemia 2: 222-225
86 Smets L A, Homan-Blok J, Hart A et al 1987 Prognostic implication of hyperdiploidy as based on DNA flow cytometric measurement in childhood acute lymphocytic leukemia – a multicenter study. Leukemia 1: 163-166
87 Look A T, Roberson P K, Murphy S B 1987 Prognostic value of cellular DNA content in acute lymphoblastic leukemia of childhood. New England Journal of Medicine 317: 1666
88 Raimondi S C, Peiper S C, Kitchingman G R et al 1989 Childhood acute lymphoblastic leukemia with chromosomal breakpoints at 11q23. Blood 73: 1627-1634
89 Katz F, Malcolm S, Gibbons B et al 1988 Cellular and molecular studies on infant null acute lymphoblastic leukemia. Blood 71: 1438-1447
90 Ludwig W-D, Bartram C R, Harbott J et al 1989 Phenotypic and genotypic heterogeneity in infant acute leukemia. I. Acute lymphoblastic leukemia. Leukemia 3: 431-439
91 Koller U, Haas O A, Ludwig W-D et al 1989 Phenotypic and genotypic heterogeneity in infant acute leukemia. II. Acute non-lymphoblastic leukemia. Leukemia 3: 708-714
92 Lampert F, Harbott J, Ludwig W-D et al 1987 Acute leukemia with chromosome translocation (4;11): 7 new patients and analysis of 71 cases. Blut 54: 325-335
93 Hagemeijer A, van Dongen J J M, Slater R M et al 1987 Characterization of the blast cells in acute leukemia with translocation (4;11): Report of eight additional cases and of one case with a variant translocation. Leukemia 1: 24-31
94 Pui C-H, Behm F G, Raimondi S C et al 1989 Secondary acute myeloid leukemia in children treated for acute lymphoid leukemia. New England Journal of Medicine 321: 136-142
95 Scott C S, Vulliamy T, Catovsky D, Matutes E, Norfolk D R 1989 DNA genotypic conservation during phenotypic switch from T-cell acute lymphoblastic leukaemia to acute myeloblastic leukaemia. Leukaemia and Lymphoma 1: 21-28
96 Fenaux P, Preudhomme C, Lay J L, Morel P, Beuscart R, Bauters F 1989 Cytogenetics and their prognostic value in de novo acute myeloid leukaemia: a report on 283 cases. British Journal of Haematology 73: 61-67
97 Le Beau M M, Albain K S, Larson R A et al 1986 Clinical and cytogenetic correlations in 63 patients with therapy-related myelodysplastic syndromes and acute nonlymphocytic leukemia: further evidence for characteristic abnormalities of chromosomes no. 5 and 7. Journal of Clinical Oncology 4: 325-345
98 Berger R, Flandrin G, Bernheim A et al 1987 Cytogenetic studies on 519 consecutive de novo acute nonlymphocytic leukemias. Cancer Genetics and Cytogenetics 29: 9-21
99 Cuneo A, Mecucci C, Kerim S et al 1989 Multipotent stem cell involvement in megakaryoblastic leukemia: cytologic and cytogenetic evidence in 15 patients. Blood 74: 1781-1790
100 Le Beau M M, Lemons R S, Espinosa R, Larson R A, Arai N, Rowley J D 1989 Interleukin-4 and Interleukin-5 map to human chromosome 5 in a region encoding growth factors and receptors and are deleted in myeloid leukemias with a del (5q). Blood 73: 647-650
101 Juliusson G, Gahrton G 1990 Chromosome aberrations in B-cell chronic lymphocytic leukemia: pathogenetic and clinical implications. Cancer Genetics and Cytogenetics 45: 143-160
102 Brito-Babapulle V, Pittman S, Melo J V, Pomfret M, Catovsky D 1987 Cytogenetic studies on prolymphocytic leukemia. 1. B-cell prolymphocytic leukemia. Hematologic Pathology 1: 27-33
103 Rabbitts P H, Douglas J, Fischer P et al 1988 Chromosome abnormalities at 11q13 in B-cell tumours. Oncogene 3: 99-103
104 Mufti G J, Hamblin T J, Oscier D G, Johnson S 1983 Common ALL with pre-B-cell features showing (8;14) and (14;18) chromosome translocations. Blood 62: 1142-1146
105 Pegoraro L, Palumbo A, Erikson J et al 1984 A 14;18 and an 8;14 chromosome translocation in a cell line derived from an acute B-cell leukemia. Proceedings of the National Academy of Sciences of the USA 81: 7166-7170

106 de Jong D, Voetdijk B M H, Beverstock G C, van Ommen G J B, Wilemze R, Kluin P M 1988 Activation of the c-myc oncogene in a precursor-B-cell blast crisis of follicular lymphoma, presenting as composite lymphoma. New England Journal of Medicine 318: 1373–1378
107 Gauwerky C E, Hoxie J, Nowell P C, Croce C M 1988 Pre-B-cell leukemia with a t(8;14) and a t(14;18) translocation is preceded by follicular lymphoma. Oncogene 2: 431–435
108 Peake I 1989 The polymerase chain reaction. Journal of Clinical Pathology 42: 673–676
109 Hansen-Hagge T E, Yokota S, Bartram C R 1989 Detection of minimal residual disease in acute lymphoblastic leukemia by in vitro amplification of rearranged T-cell receptor δ-chain sequences. Blood 74: 1762–1767
110 Gabert J, Thuret I, Lafage M, Carcassone Y, Maraninchi D, Mannoni P 1989 Detection of residual bcr/abl translocation by polymerase chain reaction in chronic myeloid leukaemia patients after bone-marrow transplantation. Lancet ii: 1125–1128
111 Griesser H, Tkachuk D, Reis M D, Mak T W 1989 Gene rearrangements and translocations in lymphoproliferative diseases. Blood 73: 1402–1415
112 Toksoz D, Farr C J, Marshall C J 1989 Annotation: ras genes and acute myeloid leukaemia. British Journal of Haematology 71: 1–6
113 Rambaldi A, Pelicci P-G, Allavena P et al 1985 T-cell receptor B-chain gene rearrangements in lymphoproliferative disorders of large granular lymphocytes/natural killer cells. Journal of Experimental Medicine 162: 2156–2162
114 Loughran T P, Starkebaum G, Aprile J A 1988 Rearrangement and expression of T-cell receptor genes in large granular lymphocyte leukemia. Blood 71: 822–824
115 Foroni L, Laffan M, Boehm T, Rabbitts T H, Catovsky D, Luzzatto L 1989 Rearrangement of the T-cell receptor genes in human T-cell leukemias. Blood 73: 559–565
116 Bertoli L F, Kubagawa H, Borzillo G V et al 1987 Analysis with antiidiotype antibody of a patient with chronic lymphocytic leukemia and a large cell lymphoma (Richter's syndrome). Blood 70: 45–50
117 Melo J V, Foroni L, Brito-Babapulle V, Luzzatto L, Catovsky D 1988 The establishment of cell lines from chronic B-cell leukaemias: evidence of leukaemic origin by karyotypic abnormalities and Ig gene rearrangement. Clinical Experimental Immunology 73: 23–28
118 Bregni M, Siena S, Neri A et al 1989 Minimal residual disease in acute lymphoblastic leukemia detected by immune selection and gene rearrangement analysis. Journal of Clinical Oncology 7: 338–343
119 Cogswell P C, Morgan R, Dunn M et al 1989 Mutations of the ras protooncogenes in chronic myelogenous leukemia: a high frequency of ras mutations in bcr/abl rearrangment-negative chronic myelogenous leukemia. Blood 74: 2629–2633
120 Neri A, Murphy J P, Cro L et al 1989 Ras oncogene mutation in multiple myeloma. Journal of Experimental Medicine 170: 1715–1725
121 Collins S J, Howard M, Andrews D F, Agura E, Radich J 1989 Rare occurrence of N-ras point mutations in Philadelphia chromosome positive chronic myeloid leukemia. Blood 73: 1028–1032
122 Senn H P, Jiricny J, Fopp M, Schmid L, Moroni Ch 1988 Relapse cell population differs from acute onset clone as shown by absence of the initially activated N-ras oncogene in a patient with acute myelomonocytic leukemia. Blood 72: 931–935
123 Harai H, Kobayashi Y, Mano H et al 1987 A point mutation at codon 13 of the N-ras oncogene in myelodysplastic syndrome. Nature 327: 430–432
124 Inghirami G, Wieczorek R, Zhu B-Y, Silber R, Dalla-Favera R, Knowles D M 1988 Differential expression of LFA-1 molecules in non-Hodgkin's lymphoma and lymphoid leukemia. Blood 72: 1431–1434
125 Pals S T, Horst E, Ossekoppele G J, Figdor C G, Scheper R J, Meijer C J L M 1989 Expression of lymphocyte homing receptor as a mechanism of dissemination in non-Hodgkin's lymphoma. Blood 73: 885–888
126 Neubauer A, Serke S, Siegert W, Kroll W, Musch R, Huhn D 1989 A flow cytometric assay for the determination of cell proliferation with a monoclonal antibody directed against DNA-methyltransferase. British Journal of Haematology 72: 492–496
127 Scott C S, Ramsden W, Limbert H J, Master P S, Roberts B E 1988 Membrane transferrin receptor (TfR) and nuclear proliferation-associated Ki-67 expression in hemopoietic malignancies. Leukemia 2: 438–442
128 Bell D R, Gerlach J H, Kartner N, Buick R N, Ling V 1985 Detection of P-glycoprotein in ovarian cancer: a molecular marker associated with multidrug resistance. Journal of Clinical Oncology 3: 311–315
129 Kaye S B 1988 The multidrug resistance phenotype. British Journal of Cancer 58: 691–694
130 Nooter K, Sonneveld P, Janssen A et al 1989 Expression of the mdr3 gene in prolymphocytic leukemia: association with cyclosporin-A-induced increase in drug accumulation. International Journal of Cancer 45: 626–631

2
Cytochemistry in the Classification of Leukemias

*Georges Flandrin   Marie-Therèse Daniel
Alistair Crockard*

INTRODUCTION

Despite the recent contribution of immunological technics and gene rearrangement studies in the precise description of leukemic populations, cytochemical studies remain useful for the classification of leukemias, particularly in the acute types.[1-4]

Results of cytochemical reactions cannot be used for classification of leukemias without taking into consideration cell morphology on May–Grünwald–Giemsa (MGG) stained films, as well as the presence of different antigens expressed by these cells and studied with specific monoclonal antibodies (McAbs).

Among the various cytochemical reactions which could help to distinguish different leukemia cell types, seven cytoenzymatic reactions have been selected, namely myeloperoxidase (MPO), alkaline phosphatase (APL), acid phosphatase (ACP), non-specific esterase (NSE), naphthol AS-D chloroacetate esterase (NASDCA), β-glucuronidase (β-G) and dipeptidylaminopeptidase IV (DAP IV). In addition the results from the Sudan black B (SB) and period acid-schiff (PAS) reactions[5] are mentioned.

Since it is often difficult to compare results obtained in different laboratories due to the variety of technics used, the International Committee for Standardization in Haematology (ICSH) recommended standardization of cytochemical procedures for five enzymes (MPO, APL, ACP, NSE, NASDCA).[6] In this chapter the technics used routinely in the authors' laboratories are mentioned with modifications recommended by the ICSH reference methods. Detailed technical recommendations are given in the Appendix.

PRINCIPLES OF THE CYTOCHEMICAL METHODS[7,8]

MYELOPEROXIDASE (MPO)

Peroxidases catalyse the oxidation of a variety of substances via a mechanism involving hydrogen peroxide (H_2O_2). The classic benzidine base (BB) technic is being used (see Appendix); however, the ICSH did not adopt this method as a reference, because of restrictions of manufacture and distribution of BB in some countries and because of its potential carcinogenicity. If the BB method is used, solutions must be prepared with appropriate safety precautions (air flow hood, mask and gloves). The ICSH compared the BB method with two others, namely 3-aminocarbazole (3AC) and diaminobenzidine (DAB). The DAB reaction has the advantages of excellent localization and no diffusion, and is better for identifying Auer rods. None of these three methods has major advantages and selection may depend on availability of substrate, concern over potential carcinogenicity and personal satisfaction with the visual appearance of the reaction product.[6] With some restrictions, the Sudan black B reaction may be proposed instead of MPO.[7]

ALKALINE PHOSPHATASE (APL)

Alkaline phosphatases include different isoenzymes able to liberate phosphate from various phosphomonoesters under alkaline conditions.[8] In making their recommendations the ICSH recognized that the main use of APL in hematology is to study mature granulocytes in myeloproliferative disorders. The authors have stopped using α-naphthyl phosphate because the reaction product is not very chromogenic. In its place the ICSH recommendation has been adopted in using a technic employing the substituted naphthol phosphates.[6] The cytochemical method from Kaplow has been used utilizing naphthol AS-BI phosphate.[9] A technic from Tomonaga et al using naphthol AS-MX phosphate[10] is also recommended by the ICSH. Tomonaga's method gives better enzymatic staining in the leukocytes but is more time consuming than Kaplow's method.

ACID PHOSPHATASE (ACP)

Acid phosphatases are enzymes that are able to hydrolyse phosphate esters under acidic conditions. The acid phosphatase reaction has two applications in hematology, namely the diagnosis of hairy cell leukemia[11] and discriminating between different lymphoid cell categories.[12] The ICSH assessed two sets of methods for these two specific purposes. Naphthol AS-BI phosphate was the recommended substrate because of its strong chromogenic properties, good localization and lack of diffusion.[6] For the diagnosis of hairy cell leukemia, after Yam et al,[11] the ICSH recommended the use of fast Garnet GBC as the coupler. Hexa-azotized pararosaniline is particularly suitable for demonstration of ACP in lymphocytes and is also recommended for use in tissue sections.

NON-SPECIFIC ESTERASE (NSE)

The esterases are a group of enzymes capable of hydrolysing a variety of aliphatic or aromatic esters under acidic or neutral conditions.[13] Acetate and butyrate esterases, acting with a preference for short-chain esters, are called non-specific esterases. These NSEs have been identified in a variety of hemopoietic cells including megakaryocytes and plasma cells, but are mainly employed for their positivity in mononuclear phagocytes.[14] NSE activity can be inhibited by sodium fluoride (NaF) in monocytic cells,[15] but not in cells of the granulocytic series. For the identification of monocytic and megakaryocytic cells, α-naphthyl butyrate and α-naphthyl acetate are the preferred substrates for their respective esterases, showing the strongest reactions in mononuclear phagocytes. The suitable pH for this reaction is 6.3, with hexa-azotized pararosaniline as the coupler. The reaction using naphthol AS-D acetate (NASDA) as substrate and fast blue BB as the coupler gives a granular reaction product which may be useful for a quantitative estimation of the reaction in monocytes and granulocytes. With this method NaF inhibition is necessary for the positive identification of monocytic cells; in contrast, α-naphthyl acetate and α-naphthyl butyrate positivity is not observed in mature granulocytes. Some exceptions to this have been noted in pathological situations, the additional use of NaF may enhance the specificity of these reactions for monocytic cells. For the identification of acid esterase activity in lymphoid cells (T-cells), use of α-naphthyl acetate esterase at pH 5.0 is recommended.[16]

NAPHTHOL AS-D CHLOROACETATE ESTERASE (NASDCA)

NASDCA is an esterase which shows a specific activity in granulocytes and mast cells.[6] Unlike the MPO reaction, which is positive in all stages of the granulocytic series as well as in monocytes, NASDCA esterase activity is more specific for mature granulocytes (including promyelocytes and more mature stages) and does not stain monocytes. Interestingly, in contrast to MPO and Sudan black B, NASDCA is still reactive after histological processing of fixed and decalcified bone marrow biopsies.

β-GLUCURONIDASE (β-G)

β-Glucuronidase catalyses the hydrolysis of a number of biosynthetically prepared glucuronides including β-naphthyl glucuronide.[17] The enzyme is localized in the lysosomes. The β-G reaction is used to discriminate between different types of lymphoid cells.[18,19]

DIPEPTIDYLAMINOPEPTIDASE IV (DAP IV)

Glycyl-proline-naphthylamidase (dipeptidyl (amino) peptidase IV) (DAP IV) is an aminopeptidase. DAP IV releases N-terminal glycyl-proline from various tri- and tetrapeptides and from naphthylamides. DAP IV is optimally active at neutral pH.[20]

SUDAN BLACK B

Sudan black B is well known as a specific stain for free or combined lipid but it will also stain granules of granulocytes. It appears that the staining of granulocytes results from a cytochemical combination of the dye with non-lipid constituents. The pattern of positivity is similar to that produced by the peroxidase reaction; however there is some difference in the pattern of staining.[7] Sudan black B positivity is present in neutrophilic and eosinophilic series as well as in mature monocytes and monocytic precursors.

PERIOD ACID–SCHIFF (PAS)

Period acid (HIO_4) acts specifically to oxidise the 1,2-glycol grouping (CHOH–CHOH) or its amino or alkylamino derivatives to produce a dialdehyde. The oxidation does not proceed further and with the addition of Schiff's reagent the resulting aldehydes give a magenta-colored substituted dye.[7] A positive reaction may be given by several classes of carbohydrates including monosaccharides, polysaccharides, glycoprotein and mucoprotein conjugates, phosphorylated sugars, inositol derivatives and cerebrosides.

PRACTICAL VALUE OF CYTOCHEMICAL REACTIONS FOR THE CLASSIFICATION OF LEUKEMIAS[5,7,21-24]

Different problems arise depending on the myeloid or the lymphoid nature of leukemic cells.

ACUTE AND CHRONIC MYELOID PROLIFERATIONS

Acute granulocytic leukaemia (M1, M2 and M3 of the FAB classification) and myelodysplastic syndromes (MDS)[1,2,25]

Myeloperoxidase reaction and/or Sudan black B staining (Plates 1–9)
Myeloperoxidase is an enzyme localized exclusively in the azurophil granules of both granulocytic and monocytic series. Despite uncertainties concerning the specificity of Sudan black B reactions, a positive Sudan reaction is closely related to peroxidase activity (see Plates 2 and 3); both are usually positive in the same samples.[7] At least 5% and usually more blast cells are positive in acute myeloblastic leukemia (AML), with a strongly localized or

heavy overall reaction.[1,2] This type of positivity should be distinguished from the more finely granular type found in monoblastic leukemia.[7,26] Although myeloperoxidase is located in the azurophil granules, positivity may be seen in the cytoplasm of undifferentiated cells totally devoid of granules.[5] This cytoplasmic staining in the absence of granules probably represents myeloperoxidase reaction in the perinuclear space, endoplasmic reticulum and Golgi apparatus as demonstrated by ultrastructural cytochemistry.[27] (See also Ch. 4.) Because azurophil granules are almost always present in AML this reaction is usually not essential for its diagnosis. There are, however, a few cases of poorly differentiated AML (among the M1 class of the FAB classification) where the blast cells have little or no granulation (Plate 1). In those cases the striking peroxidase positivity (Plate 2) establishes the diagnosis of AML and rules out acute lymphoblastic leukemia (ALL). The myeloperoxidase reaction is then more often useful in M1 than in the M2 class of the FAB classification. The other finding when using the myeloperoxidase reaction in AML is loss of the enzyme in some mature cells of the granulocytic series.[28] Immunological studies have demonstrated the myeloid nature of blast cells by using specific McAbs;[29] these have shown exceptions to the MPO positivity of AML that was previously believed to be constant.[30] Such cases, which are completely devoid of MPO positivity but demonstrated to be of myeloid nature by McAb myeloid markers, were previously classified as acute undifferentiated leukemia or erroneously classified as ALL before the systematic use of lymphoid markers (see Chs 6 and 7). The frequency of these AML cases, better defined as AML,MO, seems to be low. Interestingly, bilineage markers (lymphoid and myeloid markers) have been demonstrated in rare cases by the presence of lymphoid McAb markers in addition to MPO positivity.[31-33] Another feature of the MPO reaction is observed in 'hypergranular' promyelocytic leukemia (M3 in the FAB classification). In these cases myeloperoxidase is always strongly positive in all blast cells (Plate 9), with the reaction product covering up the whole cytoplasm and very often the nucleus too.[1]

Naphthol AS-D chloroacetate esterase
This esterase is positive in the granulocytic series, its reactivity increasing with cell maturity.[16,34] Thus this reaction is less sensitive than myeloperoxidase for the diagnosis of AML. Some of the more immature AMLs (among the M1 group) may be totally negative for NASDCA (Plate 4). In particular this reaction was of no help in patients where the May–Grünwald–Giemsa failed to show azurophil granules although the myeloperoxidase reaction was positive. In 'hypergranular' promyelocytic leukemia (M3), the NASDCA reaction is strongly positive, more intensely so than in all other types of AML.[5]

Naphthol AS-D acetate esterase
The positivity of this reaction in AML depends on the degree of maturation. Acute promyelocytic leukemia (M3) shows the most positive reaction.[5] In these cases the esterase reaction is unaffected by exposure to NaF as it is in cases of monocytic leukemia. α-Naphthyl acetate and α-naphthyl butyrate esterase activities are not usually observed in the granulocytic series. However, in some cases of AML (M1 or M2) some immature forms may demonstrate positivity with these substrates. Using a double esterase method[35] with successive reactions by NASDCA and α-naphthyl acetate esterase (ANAE), atypical ANAE reaction (so-called monocytic specific reaction) can be demonstrated in primary and therapy-related myelodysplastic syndrome (MDS).[36,37] This positivity is considered a distinctive feature of dysgranulopoieses. Similar results are obtained in some non-malignant conditions, mainly megaloblastic anemias.[36] Some authors do not consider the cells with double esterase positivity as atypical granulocytes. Rather they believe them to be ambiguous cells supporting characteristics of both granulocytic and monocytic cells, arising from their common origin – the colony forming unit cell – granulocyte macrophage (CFU-GM).[38] (See also Ch. 10.)

PAS reaction
Many blast cells in AML are PAS negative; some others may show a faint cytoplasmic tinge with or without fine superimposed granules.[5,7] The 'typical' single coarse-granular pattern of ALL[7,39] is very unusual in AML.

Acid phosphatase
Acid phosphatase activity in AML is ordinarily greater than in ALL,[5] but seems to be variable and is without sufficient specificity to help in diagnosis or subclassification. The acid phosphatase reaction in AML is usually diffusely positive in the cytoplasm with or without superimposed granules, whilst in ALL it is granular. The positive versus negative acid phosphatase subclassification is relevant only in the context of ALL.[1]

Acute monocytic leukemia (M5 of the FAB classification)

Myeloperoxidase and/or Sudan black B
Very variable results are seen in M5 with these methods.[5,7] In some cases the reaction is totally negative in all blast cells, in some the majority of cells are positive and in others only a few cells are positive, with variable degrees of reaction. The pattern of myeloperoxidase reaction in monocytic cells differs, however, from those observed in granulocytic precursors.[7] The positivity is more finely granular (Plate 10) and discretely scattered than in AML. The myeloperoxidase reaction of cells of monoblastic (M5A) and monocytic (M5B) leukemias differs from the reaction of cells of the normal monocytic series. Normal immature monocytes are more strongly positive than mature monocytes; the latter may even be negative. In contrast, M5A monoblasts are often, but not always, peroxidase negative, probably reflecting in the negative cases a myeloperoxidase deficiency. In the differentiated type (M5B) both features can be observed with peroxidase positive cells often predominating.

Naphthol AS-D acetate esterase (Plates 11-14)
Acute monocytic leukemia is characterized by a strong NASDCA activity inhibited by NaF.[16,26] In the absence of NaF this reaction is very strong and uniform in the majority of cells.

α-Naphthyl butyrate esterase (ANBE)
It is now preferable to use α-naphthyl butyrate as the substrate because its greater degree of specificity and stronger reaction in monocytic cells (Plate 15) can eliminate the need for systematic use of an additional reaction with NaF inhibition.[6] With both NSE reactions, ANBE and α-naphthyl acetate esterase (ANAE), M5 cells are strongly positive, although there are a few cases which have not shown the typical positivity. These rare M5 cases have demonstrated monocytic antigens in specific McAb studies but were cytochemically unreactive.[37]

Naphthol AS-D chloroacetate esterase (Plate 16)
This reaction is always negative in M5 but positive in the granulocytic series. However, this is of little practical value in distinguishing M5 from immature AML (M1) because, as mentioned earlier, NASDCA esterase is negative in the less differentiated granulocytic cells.[5]

PAS reaction
This reaction is rather variable in M5. Some blast cells are entirely negative whilst others give a reaction like normal monocytes, showing fine granulation with a background of diffuse cytoplasmic staining. In other cases some cells are strongly positive with coarse granules or blocks of PAS positivity.[7]

Acid phosphatase
This reaction is usually strongly positive with a diffuse and granular pattern but, since it can sometimes also be strongly positive in AML as well as in M5, it may not represent a distinctive feature of M5.[5]

Acute myelomonocytic leukemia (M4 of the FAB classification)
In M4 both granulocytic and monocytic differentiation are present in varying degrees in the bone marrow and peripheral blood. The authors consider that, when the proportion of monocytes and promonocytes exceeds 20% of the bone marrow cells, M4 can be separated from AML (M2). However, when the percentage of monocytic cells is high, M4 can be distinguished from M5 only when the monocytic precursors are lower than 80%.[1,2] The cytochemical reactions, NSE (Plates 12 and 13) and MPO, are often helpful in making this distinction.[16,26] However, in some patients, even with these cytochemical reactions a sharp distinction between cell lines may be difficult because of intermediate staining reactions occurring in both series or because of double esterase positivity in some cases.[35] Comparison of bone marrow and peripheral blood is often of great importance in diagnosing M4. Monocytic differentiation is often more obvious in the peripheral blood than in the bone marrow. In contrast, the bone marrow appearance stained with May–Grünwald–Giemsa, if taken alone, may often suggest a diagnosis of AML (M2) rather than M4.

Erythroleukemia (M6 of the FAB classification)
In the FAB classification the diagnosis of M6 requires a minimal percentage of 50% of erythroblasts in the bone marrow, and that of the remaining non-erythroblast bone marrow cells more than 30% blast cells of other types.[2] This definition is mainly based on somewhat arbitrary cytological criteria and does not heavily depend on the results of cytochemical studies. Erythroblasts may show heavy PAS positivity, generally granular in early erythroblasts and diffuse in late ones.[5,7] In the blast cells, the cytochemical results are those expected for each cell type. Most often they are myeloblasts with typical myeloperoxidase positivity, sometimes possibly monocytic precursors or rarely undifferentiated blasts, with no distinguishing cytochemical features. Among these so-called undifferentiated blast cells, it has been demonstrated (cytochemically at electron microscopic level and by using specific McAbs) some micromegakaryoblasts can be seen in addition to erythroblastic precursors.[40] Recently it has been shown that some cases of otherwise undifferentiated blast cells in rare cases of acute leukemia belong to the erythroblastic series. The nature of these 'early precursors' of erythroblasts ('cryptic erythroleukemias') is recognized by using specific McAbs and comparing their immunological phenotype with those of early steps of maturing cells obtained by in vitro culture of erythroid colony forming cells, i.e. cells at the CFU-E stage of differentiation.[40]

Megakaryoblastic leukemia (M7 of the FAB classification)
In the rare cases of acute leukemia with predominant megakaryoblastic differentiation[3] the precise identification of these blast cells is often difficult or sometimes impossible by light microscopy alone.[41,42] MPO is constantly negative. Megakaryoblasts in M7 show a positive reaction for ANAE and ACP with a predominant localization in the Golgi zone and a negative reaction for ANBE.[43,44] The ANAE reaction is NaF sensitive (similar findings are demonstrated in early erythroblastic precursors). The PAS positivity of normal mature megakaryocytes can also be found in the megakaryoblasts of some acute leukemias.[5] The PAS reaction may, however, be negative and cannot therefore be considered a reliable marker. Such otherwise undifferentiated megakaryoblasts are diagnosed by their unique immunological phenotype determined by specific McAbs and by the presence of a specific platelet peroxidase activity (PPO) detected by electron microscopy.[45-49] (See also Ch. 4)

Eosinophilic leukemia (Plates 17 and 18)

Rare cases of acute myelomonocytic leukemias with a high content of abnormal eosinophils in the bone marrow (M4EO) have been identified (Plate 18). These cases of M4EO are otherwise identical cytologically and cytochemically with other cases of M4, but are consistently positive with the NASDCA reaction in the eosinophilic precursors (promyelocytes and myelocytes) of the bone marrow[21,50,51] (Plate 17), a positive reaction which is not seen in normal eosinophilic precursors or in the eosinophils of other AML subtypes.[52] This special M4EO with NASDCA positive eosinophils has been shown to be associated with a chromosome abnormality (inv 16).[53,54]

Basophilic leukemia

Basophilic leukemia is most often seen as a blastic transformation of chronic myeloid leukemia with a high percentage of basophils. The basophilic cells can easily be identified by their metachromatic granules on May–Grünwald–Giemsa stained films or after toluidine blue staining. True acute basophilic leukemia seems to be exceptionally rare.[55] In such rare cases the majority of blast cells are negative for the MPO reaction.

Mast cell leukemia

The very exceptional cases of mast cell leukemia which have been reported in the literature[56] show in the blast cell, the absence of MPO activity, a strong NASDCA positivity and NSE activity.

Chronic myeloid leukemia (CML)

Leukocyte alkaline phosphatase (LAP)
LAP is usually found to be markedly depressed in CML.[57-59] Absent or low LAP levels are characteristic although not pathognomonic of CML. However, an elevated LAP may be seen in CML during remission, bacterial infection, blast crisis and pregnancy.[60] A high LAP is usually associated with non-malignant leukemoid reactions and with myeloproliferative syndromes other than CML, such as polycythemia rubra vera and myelofibrosis and myeloid metaplasia. However, in no instance is an LAP level alone of diagnostic value since other causes of a low LAP have been found: paroxysmal nocturnal hemoglobinuria; viral infections; infectious mononucleosis and idiopathic thrombocytopenic purpura.[60]

Blast crisis of CML

The blast crisis of CML is characterized by the presence of blast cells which show very variable morphological and cytochemical characteristics. Attempts have been made to classify these diverse patterns of acute phase CML. The most noticeable cytochemical change is the appearance of myeloid precursors containing PAS material.[61,62] Frequently mixed features are observed with myeloblasts, monoblasts with their own specific cytochemical reactions,[63] and megakaryocyte precursors.[64] Undifferentiated blast crises with strong basophilic cytoplasm may correspond to the 'cryptic erythroleukemia' recently defined as having a very early erythroblastic immunological phenotype.[40] Concomitant studies using both cytochemistry and McAbs may help to determine the precise composition of the blast cell mixtures of blast crises in CML and other chronic myeloproliferative disorders. In some blast crises the cells have a lymphoblastic cytological appearance with PAS positivity and peroxidase negativity. The lymphoid nature of the blasts in this form of blast crisis has been confirmed by appropriate immunological studies, mostly showing early B-lineage cell markers.[65]

ACUTE AND CHRONIC LYMPHOID PROLIFERATIONS

Acute lymphoblastic leukemia (ALL)

The primary use of cytochemistry in ALL diagnosis is in helping to distinguish ALL from other non-lymphoblastic leukemias. Secondly, and to a lesser extent, particular cytochemical reactions can help in distinguishing subtypes of ALL. It is now clear that in ALL the leukemic cells have composite phenotypes corresponding to B- or T-lymphocyte precursors. On this basis the following subtypes of the disease have been recognized:

1. *B progenitor malignancies:* null-ALL; common-ALL; B-ALL. (B-ALL is probably more characteristic of a disseminated B-cell lymphoma.)
2. *T progenitor malignancies:* T-ALL; T-lymphoblastic lymphoma (T-LbLy).

The cytochemistry of ALL will be discussed in relation to these disease subtypes and is summarized in Table 2.1.

Myeloperoxidase and Sudan black B

The myeloperoxidase reaction is negative in ALL lymphoblasts irrespective of the immunological phenotype and therefore provides an important means of distinguishing lymphoblasts from myeloblasts, particularly in cases of poorly differentiated AML. In general, Sudan black staining parallels that of myeloperoxidase; however, it has been reported that Sudan black positivity may occasionally be observed in lymphoblasts in cases of common-ALL.[66] Consequently, a negative myeloperoxidase reaction remains the most satisfactory cytochemical method for diagnosing ALL.

PAS reaction

Lymphoblasts show great variability with the PAS reaction. When present PAS positivity is usually seen as coarse granular or block-like staining. However, in a minority of cases of ALL the PAS reaction produces a fine scattered granular appearance similar to that which can be observed in cases of acute non-lymphoblastic leukemia. The lack of reaction specificity, and the occurrence of negative PAS reactions in ALL, make this stain of little value in the differential diagnosis of ALL.

Acid phosphatase (Plates 19 and 20)

The acid phosphatase reaction is of considerable importance in identifying the acute T-cell malignancies (T-ALL, pre-T-ALL and T-LbLy),[67] where a focal deposition of reaction product in a small paranuclear region of the blast cell is characteristic (Plate 19). This reaction pattern contrasts with that of B-cell-derived ALL (null, common and B) where a

Table 2.1 Cytochemical profile of acute lymphoblastic leukemias

	Myeloperoxidase Sudan black	Acid phosphatase	DAP IV	Esterases		β-Glucuronidase
				NASDA/CA	ANAE	
T-Lineage						
T-ALL }	–	+ +[a]	+/–	–	±/+	±/+
T-LbLy }						
B-Lineage						
Null } ALL	–[b]	±/+	–	–	–/+	±/–
Common }						
B-ALL	–	–/±	–	–	–/+	–

[a] Focal reaction.
[b] Sudan black positive in rare cases

more variable pattern of reactivities ranging from negative to weak scattered granular positivity is observed.[68] Thus the acid phosphatase reaction allows a broad distinction to be made between T- and non-T-ALL, but does not help in the further subclassification of these disease subtypes.

Dipeptidylaminopeptidase IV (DAP IV)
The serine peptidase DAP IV displays a more selective reactivity in ALL than other lysosomal hydrolases. DAP IV cannot be demonstrated cytochemically in null-, common- or B-ALL.[69,70] Variable reactions (negative to strong granular positivity) are observed in T-ALL and T-LbLy cells, the positivity corresponding to cells at a later stage of differentiation.[70,71]

Additional cytochemical reactions
Although β-glucuronidase is positive in the majority of T-ALL, the enzyme also displays positivity in cases of non-T-ALL, and thus its value as a means of distinguishing T-ALL from non-T-ALL is extremely limited.[68] The distribution of the reaction product in lymphoblasts (granular) differs from that observed in myeloblasts (diffuse).[72]

The esterases, naphthol AS-D acetate (NASDA) esterase and naphthol AS-D chloroacetate (NASDCA) esterase, display negative reactions in virtually all cases of ALL. Variable reactivity is observed with ANAE in T-ALL and non-T-ALL; consequently this reaction as thus is not useful in distinguishing T-derived ALL.

β-Glucosaminidase activity can be demonstrated in lymphoblasts of B- or T-cell origin.

It is clear that a spectrum of cytochemical reactivities can be observed in ALL. However certain reactions, in combination with morphological, immunological and cytogenetic investigations, are of diagnostic value. The prognostic implications of the various cytochemical patterns recorded in ALL are not clear, although some evidence has indicated that, in non-T-ALL, lack of cytochemically demonstrable acid hydrolase activities is a good prognostic feature.[73]

Chronic lymphoid leukemias

Immunological and molecular analyses of the chronic lymphoid leukemias have shown that these neoplasms usually represent clonal expansions of relatively mature B- or T-lymphocyte populations detectable in normal lymphoid tissue.[74] Chronic B-cell leukemias comprise a spectrum of diseases ranging from disorders of immunologically incompetent small lymphocytes in B-cell chronic lymphocytic leukemia (B-CLL) to immunoglobulin-secreting plasma cells in multiple myeloma (MM). The subset affiliation or level of differentiation of the proliferating cells in B-cell prolymphocytic leukemia (B-PLL) and hairy cell leukemia (HCL) is less clearly defined. The chronic T-cell leukemias similarly comprise several distinct entities. T-cell chronic lymphocytic leukemia (T-CLL) lymphocytes may be broadly subclassified on the basis of reactivity with the so-called helper–inducer (CD4 + ; Fcμ +) or suppressor–cytotoxic (CD8 + ; Fcγ +) markers. T-PLL cells and Sézary cells can be recognized by characteristic morphological and immunological features. Adult T-cell leukemia (ATL) cells (HTLV-I +) have been identified as arising from within the CD4 + suppressor–inducer subset. The cytochemical reactivities of these diseases is discussed below and summarized in Table 2.2.

α-Naphthyl acetate esterase (ANAE)
ANAE has proved to be a useful cytochemical reaction in the differential diagnosis of the chronic B- and T-cell disorders. Its value in this regard has developed from early work demonstrating that T-cells from blood and lymphoid tissue were rich in ANAE activity whereas B-cells showed a relative paucity of activity.[75] Furthermore, T-cell subsets as defined by membrane receptors for IgM (Tμ) and IgG(Tγ) were shown to display characteristic

Table 2.2 Cytochemical profile of chronic lymphoid leukemias

	ANAE	ACP	DAP IV	β-G
T-Lineage				
T-CLL (CD4+)	++	++	++	++
(CD8+)	±	++	−	++
T-PLL	++	+	++[b]	++
SS	+	++	−[c]	++
ATL	±/+	±/+	−	±/+
B-Lineage				
B-CLL	−/±	−/±	−	−/±
B-PLL	−/±	−/±	−	−/±
HCL	−/±	++[d]	−	++
MM	++	++	−	++

[a] Strength of reaction = ++ strong; + moderate; ± weak; − negative
[b] negative in CD8+ T-PLL.
[c] positive in some cases.
[d] Tartrate resistant.

dot-like or scattered diffuse activities, respectively.[76,77] More recently, studies on McAb-defined lymphocyte subsets, using a variety of technics including flow cytometric separations,[78-80] immunogold and immunorosette labeling,[81] have attempted to define the reactivity of the enzyme in T helper-inducer (CD4+) and T suppressor-cytotoxic (CD8+) cells. Although some trends are observed in the reaction patterns in the respective subpopulations (dot-like activity in the majority of CD4+ cells; diffuse reactions in CD8+ cells), and overlapping of the distinctive reactivities between the subsets prevents a clear distinction being made on the basis of ANAE activity.

ANAE reactions are weak or negative in B-CLL and B-PLL;[82,83] however both normal and malignant plasma cells display strong ANAE reactivity.[84] In hairy cell leukemia (HCL) weak or moderately positive ANAE or ANBE reactions have been reported in the hairy cells with the reaction product (fine or coarse granules) being distributed in a semicircular pattern around the nucleus.[85,86] In some cases the ANAE activity may be inhibited by NaF.[87] Electron microscopic evidence indicates that in hairy cells the enzyme is present in the plasma membrane and associated vesicles.[88]

In the chronic T-lymphoproliferative diseases, ANAE is generally strongly expressed in the malignant cells. The strongest reactions (block-like, multigranular) are observed in T-PLL cells (Plate 21) irrespective of morphological or immunological subtype.[82,89] Ultrastructurally, the enzyme is located in large granules and gall bodies.[90] In those conditions where there is an expansion of Fcγ+, CD8+ lymphocytes (termed 'T-CLL' in this article),[91] the cells characteristically display weak or scattered granular ANAE reactivity.[82] In T-cell leukemias of the helper-inducer phenotype (CD4+), a dot-like ANAE reaction is observed.[92] Thus, these patterns of reactivity broadly reflect those observed in normal T-cell subpopulations. Sézary cells are strongly positive for ANAE;[82,92] a less intense reaction is observed in ATL cells.[82,93]

Acid phosphatase (ACP)
Acid phosphatase reactions are generally weak or negative in B-CLL and B-PLL, in contrast to the granular positivity seen in T-CLL and in the majority of cases of T-PLL.[68,83] Ultrastructurally, the enzyme is located in granules in T-CLL and T-PLL cells and in parallel tubular array complexes in T-CLL lymphocytes.[90] Strong acid phosphatase reactions are also characteristic of Sézary, ATL and myeloma cells.[68] In HCL, a tartrate-resistant acid

phosphatase (TRAP) reaction in the hairy cells was almost considered pathognomonic of the disease (Plate 22). This resistance to tartaric acid, conferred by the presence of isoenzyme 5,[94] has been observed in other cell types. Consequently, TRAP cannot be considered specific for hairy cells although the reaction remains a useful diagnostic test in this disease.

Dipeptidylaminopeptidase IV (DAP IV)
The cytochemical demonstration of DAP IV in human lymphocytes was first described by Lojda[20] who reported that DAP IV reactivity was associated with E-rosette-forming T-lymphocytes. Subsequently it has been shown that the enzyme is more selectively expressed in Tμ lymphocytes, the majority of this subpopulation (90%) displaying granular positivity, with only a minority of Tγ cells (13%) being reactive.[95] The majority of McAb-defined T helper–inducer cells (CD4 +) have DAP IV positivity, whereas DAP IV reactions are negative or expressed in a minority of CD8 + cells.[96,97] B-cells are DAP IV negative.[20,95] Within the spectrum of B-cell disorders (CLL, B-PLL, HCL and MM), DAP IV staining is consistently negative in the malignant cells.[70] In T-PLL and T-CLL, the enzyme reaction appears to distinguish those leukemias which display Fcμ; CD4 positivity (DAP IV +) from those which are Fcγ; CD8 + (DAP IV −).[70,98,99] Sézary cells, in most cases, are DAP IV − although rare patients displaying DAP IV reactive cells have been reported.[70,96] As the Sézary cells in those cases tested displayed CD4 positivity in addition to the small numbers of CD4 + ATL cases reported to be DAP IV −,[97] it is evident that not all CD4 + leukemias are DAP IV +.

β-Glucuronidase (β-G) (Plates 23 and 24)
β-Glucuronidase reactivity broadly parallels that of acid phosphatase in the chronic lymphoid leukemias. Strong granular reactions are a feature of the mature T-cell leukemias (T-CLL, T-PLL, Sézary syndrome and ATL), whereas weak or negative reactions are observed in B-CLL, B-PLL and hairy cells.[68,100] Myeloma cells are rich in β-glucuronidase activity.

Additional cytochemical reactions
β-Glucuronidase reactions are strongly positive in chronic (mature) T-cell leukemias irrespective of cellular phenotype or stage of differentiation, in contrast to the negative or weak reactions observed in B-CLL, B-PLL and HCL.[68] Myeloma cells are β-glucosaminidase positive.

Strong granular DAP II positivity has been reported in both CD4 + and CD8 + T-CLL, with weak or negative reactions being observed in malignant cells from B-CLL, B-cell non-Hodgkin's lymphoma and HCL.[101] The DAP II reaction may be of potential prognostic significance in B-CLL, in that patients with progressive disease have higher numbers of circulating DAP II reactive cells than those with stable disease.[102]

APPENDIX: METHODS

MYELOPEROXIDASE

The technic used is a modification of the Graham–Knoll peroxidase method.[6,103,104]

Reagents and preparation of solutions

1. *Solution A* (stored in the dark):
   0.25 g of benzidine base in 100 ml 95° ethanol
2. *Solution B:*
   0.25 g sodium nitroprusside in 100 ml distilled water

3. *Solution C:*
   100 ml solution A + 2 ml solution B
4. *Diluted H_2O_2*
   3% H_2O_2 0.1 ml
   Distilled water to make   50 ml
5. Giemsa solution at 10% in Sörensen buffer pH 6.4.

Procedure

1. *Fixation:* cover films with solution C for 3 min. Shake off excess fixative.
2. Incubate for 5 min in the following solution:
   Solution C   50 ml
   H_2O_2 solution   50 ml prepared and filtered immediately before use
3. Wash with Sörensen buffer pH 6.4
4. Counterstain with filtered buffered Giemsa solution
5. Wash with tap water and dry.
6. Mount in Eukitt.

Result

The cytochemical reaction product is blue-green (Plates 2, 6, 8–10). Alternative technics avoiding the use of benzidine base are available. (See ICSH report–Diaminobenzidine method and 3-amino-9-ethyl carbazole method.)[6]

ALKALINE PHOSPHATASE (MODIFIED FROM KAPLOW[9] AND FROM ICSH[6])

Reagents and preparation of solutions

1. *Fixatives:*
   (a) Acetone in citrate buffer: Add 300 ml acetone, while stirring, to 0.03 mol/l citrate buffer with 168 ml 0.03 mol/l citric acid and 32 ml 0.03 mol/l sodium citrate. The final pH should be 4.2–4.5. Store at room temperature.
   (b) Formalin in methanol: Add 900 ml methanol to 100 ml formaldehyde. Mix well. Store in freezing compartment of refrigerator. Make up fresh every 2–4 weeks.
2. *Buffer solutions:*
   (a) Stock buffer (0.2 mol/l propanediol): Dissolve 21 g 2-amino-2-methyl-1,3-propanediol (Eastman Kodak) in distilled water and dilute to 100 ml with distilled water. Store in refrigerator.
   (b) Working buffer (0.05 mol/l propanediol pH 9.4–9.6): Add 70 ml 0.1 mol/l HCl to 250 ml stock buffer. Dilute to 1 litre with distilled water and store in a refrigerator. Warm to room temperature before use.
3. *Incubation solution:*
   Dissolve 5 mg sodium naphthol AS-BI phosphate and 40 mg fast violet B salt in 60 ml working propanediol buffer. Mix well. Filter into a Coplin jar. Use immediately after preparation.
4. *Counterstain:*
   Add 1 g Mayer's hematoxylin to 500 ml distilled water. Heat to boiling, then dilute to 900 ml with distilled water. Add 0.2 g sodium iodate and 50 g aluminium potassium sulphate. Dilute to 1 litre with distilled water. Filter and store in a brown bottle at room temperature.

Procedure

1. Prepare films from capillary blood or heparinized venous blood. Dry in air

2. Fix films in buffered acetone solution at room temperature for 10 s or in formol–methanol for 30 s at 0–5°C. Wash with gently running tap water and dry in air.
3. Incubate films at room temperature for 15 min in the freshly prepared substrate mixture.
4. Wash with tap water.
5. Counterstain with hematoxylin 2–8 min
6. Wash in tap water. Mount in a drop of water and examine with an oil immersion lens
7. Remove cover slip after examination. Wash, dry and store slide unmounted.

Results
Enzyme activity is seen as bright red granules in cytoplasm of both segmented and stab forms of human neutrophils. (See method using naphthol AS-MX phosphate in ICSH report.)[6]

ACID PHOSPHATASE REACTIONS
FAST GARNET GBC METHOD (FROM YAM ET AL[11] AND FROM ICSH[6])

Reagents and preparation of solutions

1. *Fixative* (methanol–acetone mixture): Add 10 ml methanol to 90 ml 60% acetone in 0.03 mol/l citrate buffer. Adjust the pH of this solution to 5.4 with 1 mol/l NaOH or HCl. Store at about 4°C. This fixative is stable for at least 1 month
2. *Substrate solution:* Dissolve 10 mg naphthol AS-BI phosphoric acid in 0.5 ml N,N'-dimethylformamide. Add 0.1 mol/l acetate buffer pH 5.0, to a final volume of 10 ml. This solution is stable at about 4°C for 2 months
3. *Incubation medium:* Dissolve 5 mg fast Garnet GBC in 10 ml substrate solution. Filter before use. Tartrate-containing medium is prepared by adding 75 mg/l (+) tartaric acid and 5 mg fast Garnet GBC to 10 ml substrate solution. Adjust pH of this solution to 5.0 with concentrated NaOH solution. Filter and use immediately.

Procedure

1. Fix smears with cold methanol–acetone mixture for 30 s. Wash briefly with distilled water. Air dry
2. Incubate smears in incubating medium with or without tartaric acid at 37°C for 45 min
3. Wash with tap water. Counterstain with Mayer's hemalum for 1–5 min
4. Wash with tap water, dry and mount in glycerin jelly.

Results
Positivity appears as numerous small red granules in a background of diffuse positivity in hairy cells (Plate 22).

Inhibition of positivity is obtained in TRAP-processed films. (See Fast Red ITR Method in ICSH Report.)[6]

PARAROSANILIN METHOD (MODIFIED FROM GOLDBERG AND BARKA[105])

Reagents and preparation of solutions

1. *Fixative:* 60% aqueous acetone
2. *Solution A:*
    1 ml pararosanilin 4% in HCl
    1 g pararosanilin acridine-free dissolved in 20 ml distilled water to which is added

5 ml concentrated HCl. This is stored in the dark at 4°C
   1.5 ml freshly prepared solution of 4% $NaNO_2$ in distilled water
3. *Solution B:* Michaelis buffer pH 5 90 ml
4. *Solution C:* 30 mg naphthol AS-BI phosphate in 3 ml N,N'-dimethylformamide
5. Harris' hematoxylin.

Procedure

1. Fix films for 30 s
2. Rinse in tap water; dry in air
3. The working solution is prepared and filtered just before use:
   Solution A 2.5 ml. 60 s after solution A has been prepared, add solution B 90 ml
   Solution C 3 ml. Readjust pH to 5 with 1 mol/l NaOH
4. Incubate films at 37°C for 90 min
5. Rinse in abundant tap water
6. Counterstain with Harris' hematoxylin for 10 min (or with methyl green)
7. Wash in tap water for 10 min
8. Mount in glycerin jelly.

Results

The reaction product is dark red; nuclei are stained blue (or green) (Plates 19 and 20).

NON-SPECIFIC ESTERASE REACTIONS

α-NAPHTHYL BUTYRATE ESTERASE (MODIFIED FROM ISCH[6])

Reagents and preparation of solutions

1. Buffered formolacetone pH 6.6 (keep at 4°C)
2. Buffer pH 6.3 Sorensen
3. α-Naphthyl butyrate (1 g) in 50 ml dimethylformamide (keep at −20°C)
4. Pararosanilin solution 1 g in 25 ml hot HCL (2N); keep at 4°C
5. Aquaeous sodium nitrate solution 4%.

Procedure

1. Fix air-dried films in formolacetone for 30 s
2. Wash briefly in tap water and dry
3. Mix pararosanilin and sodium nitrate solutions for 1 min
4. Prepare working solution and filter
   Sorensen buffer 89 ml
   Pararosanilin and sodium nitrate 0.5 ml
   Solution of α-Naphthylbutyrate 6 ml
5. Immerse slides for 45 min at 37°C in working solution.
6. Wash briefly in tap water
7. Counterstain 10 min in methyl green
8. Mount in Eukitt.

Results

The cytochemical reaction production is brown (Plate 15).

NAPHTHOL AS-D ACETATE ESTERASE (NASDA) (AFTER LÖFFLER[34] AND SCHMALZL AND BRAUNSTEINER[15])

Reagents and preparation of solutions

1. *Fixative:* 40% formalin
2. 0.1 mol/l phosphate buffer pH 6.9
3. Propylene–glycol (1:2)
4. Naphthol AS-D acetate solution
   Naphthol AS-D acetate   11 mg
   Acetone   2 ml
5. Fast blue BB salt

Procedure

1. Fix air-dried peripheral blood or bone marrow films with formalin vapor at room temperature for 5 min
2. Wash with tap water and dry
3. Immerse slides for 70 min at room temperature in the following solution, prepared and filtered just before use:
   Phosphate buffer   100 ml
   Propylene–glycol   2 ml
   Naphthol AS-D acetate solution   1.9 ml
   (add the substrate solution dropwise while slowly shaking the buffer propylene–glycol mixture)
   Fast blue BB salt   200 mg
4. Wash in running tap water briefly. Dry in air
5. Counterstain with Feulgen reaction
6. Mount in glycerin jelly.

Results

The cytochemical reaction product is blue: the nuclei are stained red (Plates 11, 12 and 14).
    For the inhibition of NASDA, add 1.5 mg/ml sodium fluoride (NaF) to the buffer.

ACID α-NAPHTHYL ACETATE ESTERASE (ANAE)

This method from Mueller et al[16] has a long incubation time in acid medium.

Reagents and preparation of solutions

1. *Fixative:* cold Baker's formol–calcium pH 6.7. (Kulenkampff et al[75] recommended fixing the film while wet in 2.5% glutaraldehyde/saline pH 7.2 for 10 min at 4°C)
2. *Solution A:* 1 g pararosanilin acridine-free dissolved in 20 ml distilled water to which 5 ml HCl is added. This is stored in the dark at 4°C
3. *Solution B:* freshly prepared 4% sodium nitrite solution ($NaNO_2$) in distilled water
4. 0.067 mol/l phosphate buffer pH 5
5. α-Naphthyl acetate
6. Acetone
7. 2 mol/l NaOH
8. Methyl green 1% as counterstain.

Procedure

1. Fix air-dried films at 4°C for 10 min and wash in distilled water for 20 min
2. Incubate for 3 h at room temperature in the following freshly prepared and filtered solution:
   2.4 ml hexazonium pararosanilin (mix 1.2 ml solution A and 1.2 ml solution B and shake for a few seconds)
   40 ml phosphate buffer
   10 mg α-naphthyl acetate in 0.4 ml acetone. The mixture is adjusted to pH 5.8 using 2 mol/l NaOH
3. Wash in distilled water for 10 min
4. Counterstain with methyl green
5. Mount in glycerin jelly.

Results

The cytochemical reaction product is brown (Plate 21).

CHLOROACETATE ESTERASE (NASDCA) (FROM MOLONEY ET AL[106])

Reagents and preparation of solutions

1. *Fixative:* methanol–formalin (9:1)
2. 0.1 mol/l Michaelis buffer pH 7.4:
   0.1 mol/l Veronal   60 ml
   0.1 mol/l HCl   40 ml
3. Propylene–glycol
4. Naphthol AS-D (NASD) chloroacetate solution:
   NASD chloroacetate   40 mg
   Acetone   3.2 ml

Procedure

1. Fix films for 3 min. Rinse in tap water. Dry in air
2. Immerse slides for 30 min in the following solution, which is prepared and filtered just before use:
   Buffer   40 ml
   Distilled water   40 ml
   Propylene–glycol   2 ml
   NASD chloroacetate solution 3.2 ml
      (add the substrate solution dropwise while slowly shaking the buffer/propylene–glycol mixture)
   Fast Garnet GBC   80 mg
3. Rinse and dry in air
4. Counterstain with Harris' hematoxylin for 10 min
5. Rinse in running tap water for 10 min
6. Mount in glycerin jelly.

Results

The cytochemical reaction product is red; nuclei are stained blue (Plate 16).

Double esterase staining (DE) may be processed by using first the NASDA technic with fast blue BB as coupler, followed by NASDCA with pararosanilin as coupler. The reaction product in monocytic cells is blue, and red in granulocytic cells (Plate 13). It can also be performed by using ANAE with pararosanilin as coupler, followed by NASDCA with fast blue BB as coupler.

β-GLUCURONIDASE (MODIFIED FROM HAYASHI ET AL[17] AND LORBACHER ET AL[18])

Reagents and preparation of solutions

1. *Fixative:* methanol–formalin (7:3) stored at 4°C
2. *Solution A:*
    1.5 ml pararosanilin 4% in HCl
    1 g pararosanilin acridine-free dissolved in 20 ml distilled water to which is added 5 ml concentrated HCl. This is stored in the dark at 4°C
    2 ml freshly prepared solution of $NaNO_2$ 4% in distilled water
3. *Solution B:* acetate buffer pH 5.2
4. *Solution C:* sodium bicarbonate ($NaHCO_3$) 420 mg in 100 ml H_2O (store at 4°C)
5. *Solution D:* 14 mg naphthol AS-BI-B-D glucuronic acid in 0.6 ml solution C + solution B to 50 ml.

Procedure

1. Fix films for 45–60 s at 4°C (for marrow films, rinse in acetone to dissolve fat)
2. Rinse in tap water
3. Dry for 30 min
4. Freeze slides for 1 h at −20°C
5. Keep at 4°C until incubation
6. Immerse slides for 1 h at 37°C in the working solution, prepared and filtered just before use as follows:
    3.5 ml solution A
    50 ml solution D
    Adjust pH to 5.2 with 1 mol/l NaOH; add distilled water to make 100 ml
7. Rinse in distilled water
8. Counterstain with Harris' hematoxylin
9. Rinse in tap water for 10 min
10. Mount in glycerin jelly.

Results

The cytochemical reaction product is red (Plates 23 and 24).

DIPEPTIDYLAMINOPEPTIDASE IV (DAP IV) (MODIFIED FROM LODJA[20])

Reagents and preparation of solutions

1. *Fixative:* acetone–formaldehyde (2:1) in 50 mol/l phosphate buffer pH 6.6 stored at 4°C
2. 0.1 mol/l phosphate buffer pH 7.0
3. N,N'-Dimethylformamide
4. Glycyl-L-proline-4-methoxy-β-naphthylamide
5. Fast blue BB salt
6. 1% methyl green (chloroform extracted).

Procedure

1. Fix air-dried films at 4°C for 30 s, wash in cold distilled water and dry
2. Dissolve 8 mg glycyl-L-proline-4-methoxy-β-naphthylamide in 1 ml dimethylformamide and add to 20 ml phosphate buffer containing 20 mg fast blue BB salt. Mix and filter solution
3. Incubate slides for 45 min at room temperature in the above solution
4. Wash briefly in distilled water
5. Counterstain with 1% methyl green solution for 5–10 min
6. Wash in distilled water. Dry and mount in glycerin jelly.

Results

The cytochemical reaction product is red.

SUDAN BLACK B (AFTER SHENAN AND STOREY, QUOTED IN HAYHOE AND QUAGLINO[7])

Reagents and preparation of solutions

1. Sudan black B 0.3 g in 100 ml absolute ethanol
2. *Buffer:* dissolve 16 g crystalline phenol in 30 ml absolute ethanol. Add to 100 ml distilled water in which 0.3 g hydrated disodium hydrogen phosphate ($Na_2HPO_2 \cdot 12H_2O$) has been dissolved
3. *Working stain:* add 40 ml buffer to 60 ml Sudan black B solution and filter by suction. Keep 2–3 months.

Procedure

1. Fix air-dried films in formalin vapor 5–10 min
2. Wash in running tap water 10 min
3. Immerse in working stain 1 h
4. Wash with 70% ethanol
5. Wash with tap water 2 min
6. Blot dry and counterstain with Leishman or May-Grünwald-Giemsa.

Results

The cytochemical reaction product is black; nuclei are stained blue.

PERIODIC ACID–SCHIFF (PAS) (MODIFIED FROM MACMANUS, QUOTED IN HAYHOE & QUAGLINO[7])

Reagents and preparation of solutions

1. *Fixative:* methanol–formol (9:1) stored at 4°C
2. Periodic acid solution prepared by dissolving 1 g in 100 ml distilled water. The solution can be stored for several months in a dark bottle
3. Schiff's reagent is purchased commercially but it can be prepared[7,8]
4. Sodium metabisulfite solution 10 g in 100 ml distilled water
5. 1 mol/l hydrochloric acid (HCl)
6. Mayer's solution

Procedure

1. Air-dried, thinly spread peripheral blood or bone marrow films are fixed in cold fixative for 10 min and rinsed in running tap water
2. Immerse in periodic acid solution for 10 min. Wash again and dry
3. Immerse in Schiff's basic fuchsin in the dark for 30 min
4. Rinse three times in the following solution:
Metabisulfite	6 ml
HCl	5 ml
Distilled water to make	100 ml
5. Wash with tap water. Dry in air
6. Counterstain with Mayer's hemalum for 10 min. Rinse in running water for 10 min
7. Mount in Eukitt (Vitromed-Basel).

Results

The cytochemical reaction product is red; nuclei are stained blue.

OIL RED O (ORO)[8]

Reagents and preparation of solutions

1. *Fixative:* 40% formalin
2. 2-Propanol (50% diluted in distilled water)
3. Oil red O.

Procedure

1. Fix in formalin vapor 15 min. Rinse gently in running tap water
2. Rinse in 2-propanol
3. Immerse films for 30 min in the following solution:
   30 ml oil red O solution at 0.2% in 2-propanol
   20 ml distilled water
   Cover up; do not filter
4. Rinse with 2-propanol to shake off excess staining
5. Rinse in distilled water
6. Counterstain with Harris' hematoxylin 10 min
7. Rinse in running tap water 10 min
8. Mount in glycerin jelly.

Results

The cytochemical reaction product is orange.

REFERENCES

1 Bennett J M, Catovsky D, Daniel M T et al 1976 Proposals for the classification of the acute leukaemias. British Journal of Haematology 33: 451–458
2 Bennett J M, Catovsky D, Daniel et al 1985 Proposed revised criteria for the classification of acute myeloid leukemia. A report of the French–American–British Cooperative Group. Annals of Internal Medicine 103: 620–625
3 Bennett J M, Catovsky D, Daniel M T et al 1985 Criteria for the diagnosis of acute leukemia of megakaryocyte lineage (M7). A report of the French–American–British Cooperative Group. Annals of Internal Medicine 103: 460–462

4. Brouet J C, Valensi F, Daniel M T, Flandrin G, Preud'Homme J L, Seligmann M 1976 Immunological classification of acute lymphoblastic leukaemia. British Journal of Haematology 33: 319-328
5. Flandrin G, Daniel M T 1973 Practical value of cytochemical studies for the classification of acute leukemias. Recent Results in Cancer Research 43: 43-56
6. Shibata A, Bennett J, Castoldi G L et al 1985 International Committee for Standardization in Haematology (ICSH). Clinical and Laboratory Haematology 7: 55-74
7. Hayhoe F G J, Quaglino D 1980 Haematological cytochemistry. Churchill Livingstone, London
8. Pearse A G E 1960 Histochemistry theoretical and applied, 2nd edn. Little Brown, Boston
9. Kaplow L S 1955 A histochemical procedure for localizing and evaluating leukocyte alkaline phosphatase activity in smears of blood and bone marrow. Blood 10: 1023-1029
10. Tomonaga M, Sasaki T, Okuzaki E 1963 Studies on leukocyte alkaline phosphatase. I. Use of naphthol AS-MX phosphate; fast blue RR staining method. Acta Haematologica Japonica 26: 179-192
11. Yam L T, Li C Y, Lam K W 1971 Tartrate-resistant acid phosphatase isoenzyme in the reticulum cells of leukemic reticulo-endotheliosis. New England Journal of Medicine 284: 357-360
12. Catovsky D, Galetto J, Okos A, Miliani E, Galton D A G 1974 Cytochemical profile of B and T leukaemic lymphocytes with special reference to acute lymphoblastic leukaemia. Journal of Clinical Pathology 27: 767-771
13. Li C Y, Lam K W, Yam L T 1973 Esterases in human leucocytes. Journal of Histochemistry and Cytochemistry 21: 1-12
14. Yam L T, Li C Y, Crosby W H 1971 Cytochemical identification of monocytes and granulocytes. American Journal of Clinical Pathology 55: 283-290
15. Schmalzl F, Braunsteiner H 1968 Zur Diagnose Monozytärer Leukämien mit Zytochemischen Methoden. Acta Haematologica 40: 121-133
16. Mueller J, Brun Del Re G, Buerki H, Keller H U, Hess M W, Cottier H 1975 Non specific acid esterase activity: a criterion for differentiation of T and B lymphocytes in mouse lymph nodes. European Journal of Immunology 5: 270-274
17. Hayashi M, Nakajima Y, Fishman W H 1964 The cytologic demonstration of beta-glucuronidase employing naphthol AS-BI glucuronide and hexazonium pararosanilin; a preliminary report. Journal of Histochemistry and Cytochemistry 12:293-297
18. Lorbacher P, Yam L T, Mitus W J 1967 Cytochemical demonstration of beta-glucuronidase activity in blood and bone marrow cells. Journal of Histochemistry and Cytochemistry 15: 680-687
19. Flandrin G, Daniel M T 1974 Beta-glucuronidase in Sézary cells. Scandinavian Journal of Haematology 12: 23-31
20. Lodja Z 1977 Studies on glycyl-proline naphthylamidase in lymphocytes. I. Histochemistry 54: 299-309
21. Löffler H 1973 Indications and limits of cytochemistry in acute leukaemias. Recent Results in Cancer Research 43: 57-62
22. Löffler H 1973 Biochemical properties of leukemic blast cells revealed by cytochemical methods: their relation to prognosis. Advances in the Biosciences 14: 163-173
23. Scott C S 1978 Cytochemical applications in haematology, with particular reference to acute leukaemias: a review. Medical Laboratory Sciences 35: 111-136
24. Löffler H 1969 Zytochemische Klassifizierung der Akuten Leukosen in Chemo und Immunotherapie der Leukosen und malignen lymphoma Ed. Stacher Wien. Bohmann
25. Bennett J M, Catovsky D, Daniel M T et al 1982 Proposals for the classification of the myelodysplastic syndromes. British Journal of Haematology 51: 189-199
26. Daniel M T, Flandrin G, Lejeune F, Liso P, Lortholary P 1971 Les estérases spécifiques monocytaires. Utilisation dans la classification des leucémies aiguës. Nouvelle Revue Française d'Hématologie 11: 233-240
27. Breton-Gorius J, Guichard T 1969 Etude au microscope électronique de la localisation des péroxydases dan les cellules de la moelle osseuse humaine. Nouvelle Revue Fançaise d'Hématologie 9: 678-687
28. Catovsky D, Galton D A G, Robinson J 1972 Myeloperoxidase deficient neutrophils in AML. Scandinavian Journal of Haematology 9: 142-148
29. Griffin J D, Mayer R J, Weinstein H J et al 1983 Surface marker analysis of acute myeloblastic leukaemia: identification of differentiation-associated phenotypes. Blood 62: 557-563
30. Ganser A, Heil G, Bohm T et al 1987 Human acute unclassifiable leukemia with a unique t(4;17) chromosomal translocation expresses T lymphoid and myeloid surface antigens after in vitro culture. Blood 69: 271-277

31 Takagi S, Morita R, Morita T et al 1980 Peroxidase positive acute leukemia with T-cell markers. Blut 41: 397–398
32 Mirro J, Zipf T F, Pui C H et al 1985 Acute mixed lineage leukemia: clinicopathologic correlations and prognostic significance. Blood 66: 1115–1123
33 Murphy S B, Stass S, Kalwinsky D, Rivera G 1983 Phenotypic conversion of acute leukemia from T-lymphoblastic to myeloblastic induced by therapy with 2′ deoxycoformycin. British Journal of Haematology 55: 285–286
34 Löffler H 1961 Zytochemischer Nachweis von unspezifischer Esteras in Austricher. Klinische Wochenschrift 39: 1220–1227
35 Tavassoli M 1984 Combined esterase in acute myelomonocytic leukaemia. British Journal of Haematology 57: 178
36 Scott C S, Cahill A, Bynoe A G, Ainley M J, Hough D, Roberts B E 1983 Esterase cytochemistry in primary myelodysplastic syndrome and megaloblastic anaemias: demonstration of abnormal staining patterns associated with dysmyelopoiesis. British Journal of Haematology 55: 411–418
37 Milligan D W, Roberts B E, Limbert H J, Jalihal S, Scott C S 1984 Cytochemical and immunological characteristics of acute monocytic leukaemia. British Journal of Haematology 58: 391–397
38 Mastrangelo D, Orrico A, Pasqui A L, Capecchi P L, Ceccatelli L, Laghi Pasini F 1987 Double esterase (DE) positivity in AML cells. British Journal of Haematology 65: 119
39 Astaldi G, Verga L 1957 Glycogen content of the cells of lymphatic leukaemia. Acta Haematologica 17: 129–135
40 Villeval J L, Cramer P, Lemoine F et al 1986 Phenotype of early erythroblastic leukemias. Blood 68: 1167–1174
41 Breton-Gorius J, Daniel M T, Flandrin G, Kinet-Denoel G 1973 Fine structure and peroxidase activity of circulating micromegakaryoblasts and platelets in a case of acute myelofibrosis. British Journal of Haematology 25: 331–339
42 Den Ottolander G J, Te Velde J, Brederoo P et al 1979 Megakaryoblastic leukemia (acute myelofibrosis): a report of three cases. British Journal of Haematology 42: 9–20
43 Grusovin G D, Castoldi G L 1976 Characterization of blast cells in acute non-lymphoid leukemias by consecutive cytochemical reactions. Acta Haematologica 55: 338–345
44 Polli N, O'Brien M, Tavares de Castro J, Matutes E, San Miguel J F, Catovsky D 1985 Characterization of blast cells in chronic granulocytic leukaemia in transformation, acute myelofibrosis and undifferentiated leukaemia. I. Ultrastructural morphology and cytochemistry. British Journal of Haematology 59: 277–296
45 Breton-Gorius J, Reyes F, Duhamel G, Najman A, Gorin N C 1978 Megakaryoblastic acute leukaemia: identification by the ultrastructural demonstration of platelet peroxidase. Blood 51: 45–60
46 Bain B J, Catovsky D, O'Brien M et al 1981 Megakaryoblastic leukemia presenting as acute myelofibrosis. A study of four cases with the platelet-peroxidase reaction. Blood 58: 206–213
47 Vainchenker W, Deschamps J F, Bastin J M et al 1982 Two monoclonal antiplatelet antibodies as markers of human megakaryocyte maturation: immunofluorescent staining and platelet peroxidase detection in megakaryocyte colonies and in in vivo cells from normal and leukemic patients. Blood 59: 514–521
48 Koike T 1984 Megakaryoblastic leukemia: the characterization and identification of megakaryoblasts. Blood 64: 683–692
49 Tabilio A, Vainchenker W, Van Haecke D et al 1984 Immunological characterization of the leukemic megakaryocytic line at light and electron microscopic levels. Leukaemia Research 8: 769–781
50 Leder L D 1970 Acute myelo-monocytäre Leukämie mit atypischen Naphtol AS-D chloroacetate-Esterase positiven Eosinophilen. Acta Haematologica 44: 52–62
51 Schaefer H E, Hellriegel K P, Hennekeuser H H et al 1973 Eosinophilenleukämie, eine unreifzellige Myelose mit chloroacetatesterase positiven Eosinophilie. Blut 26: 7–19
52 Berger R, Berheim A, Daniel M T, Valensi F, Sigaux F, Flandrin G 1985 Cytogenetic studies on acute myelomonocytic leukaemia (M4) with eosinophilia. Leukaemia Research 9: 279–288
53 Arthur D C, Bloomfield C D 1983 Partial deletion of the long arm on chromosome 16 and bone marrow eosinophilia in acute nonlymphocytic leukaemia. A new association. Blood 61: 994–998
54 Le Beau M, Larson R A, Bitter M A, Vardiman J W, Golomb H M, Rowley J D 1983 Association of an invasion of chromosome 16 with abnormal marrow eosinophils in acute myelomonocytic leukemia. New England Journal of Medicine 309: 630–636
55 Quattrin N 1973 Leucémies aiguës à basophiles. Nouvelle Revue Française d'Hématologie 13: 745–754

56 Daniel M T, Flandrin G, Bernard J 1975 Leucémie aiguë à mastocytes. Etude cytochimique et ultrastructurale à propos d'une observation. Nouvelle Revue Française d'Hématologie 15: 319–332
57 Wachstein M 1946 Alkaline phosphatase activity in normal and abnormal human blood and bone marrow cells. Journal of Laboratory and Clinical Medicine 31: 1–17
58 Valentine W N, Beck W Q, Folette J H, Mills H, Lawrence J S 1952 Biochemical studies in chronic myelocytic leukemia, polycythemia vera and other idiopathic myeloproliferative disorders. Blood 7: 959–977
59 Tanaka K R, Valentine W N, Fredicks R E 1960 Diseases or clinical conditions associated with low alkaline phosphatase. New England Journal of Medicine 262: 912–918
60 Okun D B, Tanaka K R 1978 Leukocyte alkaline phosphatase. American Journal of Hematology 4: 293–299
61 Pederson B 1973 Period acid–Schiff positive myeloblasts in chronic myelogenous leukaemia. Relation to karyotype evolution. Scandinavian Journal of Haematology 11: 112–121
62 Hammouda F, Quaglino D, Hayhoe F G J 1964 Blastic crisis in chronic granulocytic leukaemia. Cytological, cytochemical and autoradiographic studies of four cases. British Medical Journal i: 1275–1281
63 Castoldi E L, Grusovin E D, Scapoli E L 1975 Consecutive cytochemical staining for the analysis of the blastic population of the acute phase of chronic myeloid leukemia. Biomedicine 23: 12–16
64 Breton-Gorius J, Reyes F, Vernant J P, Tulliez M, Dreyfus B 1978 The blast crisis of chronic granulocytic leukaemia: megakaryoblastic nature of cells as revealed by the presence of platelet-peroxidase-a cytochemical ultrastructural study. British Journal of Haematology 39: 295–304
65 Janossy G, Greaves M F, Revesz T 1976 Blast crisis of chronic myeloid leukaemia (CML). II. Cell surface marker analysis of 'lymphoid' and myeloid cases. British Journal of Haematology 34: 179–192
66 Stass S A, Pui C H, Melvin S, Rovigatti U, Williams D, Motroni T, Kalwinsky D, Dahl G V 1984 Sudan black B positive acute lymphoblastic leukaemia. British Journal of Haematology 57: 413–421
67 Catovsky D, Crockard A D, Matutes E, O'Brien M 1981 Cytochemistry of leukaemic cells. In: Stoward P J, Polack J M (eds) Histochemistry – the widening horizons of its application in the biomedical sciences. Wiley, Chichester p 67–87
68 Crockard A D 1984 Cytochemistry of lymphoid cells: a review of findings in the normal and leukaemic state. Histochemical Journal 16: 1027–1050
69 Feller A C, Parwaresch M R 1981 Specificity and polymorphism of dipeptidylaminopeptidase IV in normal and neoplastic Tμ lymphocytes. Journal of Cancer Research and Clinical Oncology 101: 59–63
70 Andrews C, Crockard A D, San Miguel J F, Catovsky D 1985 Dipeptidylaminopeptidase IV (DAP IV) in B and T cell leukaemias. Clinical and Laboratory Haematology 7: 359–368
71 Feller A C, Parwaresch M R, Lennert K 1984 Cytochemical distribution of dipeptidylaminopeptidase IV (DAP IV: EC 3.4.14.5) and T lymphoblastic lymphoma/leukaemia characterised with monoclonal antibodies. Leukaemia Research 8: 397–406
72 Mann J R, Simpson J S, Munkley R M, Stuart J 1971 Lysosomal enzyme cytochemistry in acute leukaemia. Journal of Clinical Pathology 24: 831–836
73 Basso G, Agostini C, Cocito M G et al 1984 Non-T, non-B childhood acute lymphoblastic leukaemia. Correlations between cytochemical markers and first complete remission. Cancer 54: 981–985
74 Greaves M F 1986 Differentiation-linked leukemogenesis in lymphocytes. Science 234: 697–700
75 Kulenkampff J, Janossy G, Greaves M F 1977 Acid esterase in human lymphoid cells and leukaemic blasts: a marker for T lymphocytes. British Journal of Haematology 36: 231–240
76 Grossi C E, Webb S R, Zicca A et al 1978 Morphological and histochemical analyses of two human T cell subpopulations bearing receptors for IgM or IgG. Journal of Experimental Medicine 147: 1405–1417
77 Ferrarini M, Cadoni A, Franzi A T et al 1980 Ultrastructure and cytochemistry of human peripheral blood lymphocytes. Similarities between the cells of the third population and T G lymphocytes. European Journal of Immunology 10: 562–570
78 Armitage R J, Linch D C, Worman C P, Cawley J C 1982 The morphology and cytochemistry of human T cell subpopulations defined by monoclonal antibodies and Fc receptors. British Journal of Haematology 51: 605–613

79 Crockard A D, Catovsky D 1983 Cytochemistry of normal human lymphocyte subsets defined by monoclonal antibodies and immunocolloidal gold. Scandinavian Journal of Haematology 30: 433–443
80 De Waele M, De Mey J, Moeremans M, Smet L, Broodaerts L, Van Camp B 1983 Cytochemical profile of immunoregulatory T lymphocyte subsets defined by monoclonal antibodies. Journal of Histochemistry and Cytochemistry 31: 471–478
81 Bernard J, Dufer J 1983 Cytochemical analysis of human peripheral blood lymphocyte subsets defined by monoclonal antibodies. Scandinavian Journal of Immunology 17: 89–93
82 Crockard A D, Chalmers D, Matutes E, Catovsky D 1982 Cytochemistry of acid hydrolases in chronic B and T cell leukemias. American Journal of Clinical Pathology 78: 437–444
83 Boesen A M, Hokland P, Jensen O M 1984 Acid phosphatase and acid esterase activity in neoplastic and non-neoplastic lymphoid cells. Scandinavian Journal of Haematology 32: 313–322
84 Halper J P, Tolidjian B, Knowles D M 1982 Acid alpha-naphthyl acetate esterase (ANAE) in human B cells: correlation of expression with stages of B cell differentiation. Cellular Immunology 72: 367–374
85 Higgy K E, Burns G F, Hayhoe F G J 1978 Identification of the hairy cells of leukaemic reticuloendotheliosis by an esterase method. British Journal of Haematology 38: 99–106
86 Tolksdorf G, Stein H 1979 Acid alpha-naphthyl acetate esterase in hairy cell leukaemia cells and other cells of the haematopoietic system. Blut 39: 165–175
87 Variakojis D, Vardiman J W, Golomb H M 1980 Cytochemistry of hairy cells. Cancer 45: 72–77
88 Boesen A M 1984 Ultrastructural localisation of acid alphanaphthyl acetate esterase in human normal and neoplastic lymphocytic and monocytic cells and in hairy cells. Scandinavian Journal of Haematology 32: 367–375
89 Matutes E, Garcia Talavera J, O'Brien M, Catovsky D 1986 The morphological spectrum of T-prolymphocytic leukaemia. British Journal of Haematology 64: 111–124
90 Matutes E, Crockard A D, O'Brien M, Catovsky D 1983 Ultrastructural cytochemistry of chronic T cell leukaemias. A study with four acid hydrolases. Histochemical Journal 15: 895–909
91 Pandolfi F 1986 T-CLL and allied diseases: new insights into classification and pathogenesis. Diagnostic Immunology 4: 61–74
92 Knowles D M, Halper J P 1982 Human T cell malignancies. American Journal of Pathology 106: 187–203
93 Tricot G J K, Van Orshoven A, Den Ottolander G J et al 1983 Adult T cell leukaemia: a report on two white cases. Leukaemia Research 7: 31–42
94 Li C Y, Yam L T, Lam K W 1970 Acid phosphatase isoenzymes in human leukocytes in normal and pathologic conditions. Journal of Histochemistry and Cytochemistry 18: 473–481
95 Feller A C, Heignen C J, Ballieux R E, Parwaresch M R 1982 Enzyme histochemical staining of Tμ lymphocytes for glycyl-proline-4-methoxy-beta-naphthylamide-peptidase (DAP IV). British Journal of Haematology 51: 227–234
96 Wirthmuller R, Dennig D, Oertel J, Gerhartz H 1983 Dipeptidylaminopeptidase IV (DAP IV) activity in normal and malignant T cell subsets as defined by monoclonal antibodies. Scandinavian Journal of Haematology 31: 197–205
97 Crockard A D, MacFarlane E, Andrews C, Bridges J M, Catovsky D 1984 Dipeptidylaminopeptidase IV activity in normal and leukaemic T cell subpopulations. American Journal of Clinical Pathology 82: 294–299
98 Feller A C, Parwaresch M R, Lennert K 1983 Subtyping of chronic lymphocytic leukaemia of T-type by dipeptidylaminopeptidase IV (DAP IV), monoclonal antibodies and Fc receptors. Cancer 52: 1609–1612
99 Chilosi M, Pizzolo G, Semenzato G, De Rossi G, Pandolfi F 1984 Heterogeneous expression of dipeptidylaminopeptidase IV (DAP IV) in T cell chronic lymphocytic leukaemia. Acta Haematologica 71: 277–281
100 Machin G A, Halper J P, Knowles D M 1980 Cytochemistry demonstrable beta-glucuronidase activity in normal and neoplastic human lymphoid cells. Blood 56: 1111–1119
101 Invernizzi R, Bertolino G, Girino M, Perseghin P, Michienzi M, Nano R 1985 Cytochemistry of dipeptidylaminopeptidase IV and II in normal and neoplastic lymphoid cells. Blut 50: 277–285
102 Klener P, Lodja Z, Haber J, Kvasnicka J, Cmunt E 1985 Problems with prognostic criteria in patients with chronic lymphocytic leukaemia with special reference to DPP II assessment. Neoplasma 32: 737–740
103 Kaplow L S 1965 Simplified myeloperoxidase stain using benzidine dihydrochloride. Blood 26: 215–219

104 Kaplow L S 1975 Substitute for benzidine in myeloperoxidase stains. American Journal of Clinical Pathology 63: 451
105 Goldberg A R F, Barka T 1962 Acid phosphatase activity in human blood cells. Nature 195: 297
106 Moloney W C, McPherson K, Fliegelman L 1960 Esterase activity in leukocytes demonstrated by the use of naphthol AS-D chloroacetate substrate. Journal of Histochemistry and Cytochemistry 8: 200–207

3
Bone Marrow Histology

Reiner Bartl   Bertha Frisch   Rolf Burkhardt

INTRODUCTION

Morphology has formed the basis of hematology from its inception as a medical speciality, bone marrow aspirated from the sternum together with peripheral blood films providing material for diagnosing leukemias. Cytochemistry and, in some cases, electron microscopy were then added as supplementary procedures to recognize and to characterize abnormal blood cells.

In recent years, the bone marrow has come to be regarded as an organ with its own complex structure and function as shown in a number of atlases and textbooks.[1-9] Its different components — stroma on the one hand and blood cell precursors on the other — have their own topography, interrelationships and spheres of influences; particular regions have specific effects on the differentiation and the egress of the blood cells: the 'hemopoietic inductive microenvironment'.[10-11] Once these facts were recognized, it became clear that the architecture of the bone marrow itself must be taken into account in the diagnosis and evolution of the leukemic process:[12-14] consequently the analysis of aspirates and of sections of bone marrow biopsies (BMB) are now regarded as complementary procedures.[15] Each method contributes specific information which helps to clarify abnormalities of the hemopoietic system.

The increasing use of BMB has been promoted by the introduction of improved instruments for taking biopsies and of better technics for their histological preparation.[1,8,16,17] Biopsies of more than 6000 patients with hematological malignancies were reviewed and the histological parameters relevant for diagnosis, prognosis and follow-up are summarized here.

BONE MARROW BIOPSIES

SITES

Leukemias are systemic disorders of the bone marrow and, therefore, bone marrow samples of adequate size obtained from any site of the skeleton containing red marrow may be used for investigation. In normal individuals about 18 years of age, hemopoietically active (red) marrow in normal individuals is located in the vertebrae, ribs, sternum, pelvic bones and proximal epiphyses of the long bones. Originally biopsies were taken from ribs or sternum, but the specimens obtained were too small.[18,19] The iliac crest constitutes an accessible site and few complications after biopsy have been reported.[8,20] Therefore, bone biopsies are now most frequently taken from the anterior and posterior iliac crests after local anesthesia (Fig. 3.1). Sequential biopsies are usually obtained from the opposite side to avoid the previously biopsied area. In choosing the site and mode of biopsy (i.e. left or right side; anterior or posterior iliac crest; horizontal or vertical approach), the variance of histological and histomorphometric parameters in the different regions must be considered.[21] When the

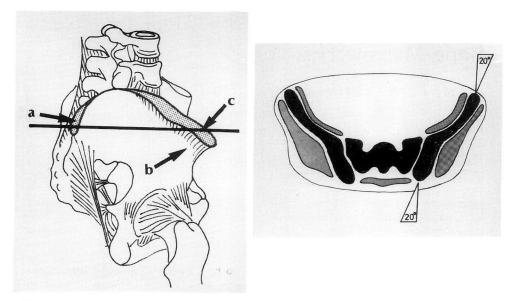

Fig. 3.1 Schematic representation of lateral aspect of the pelvic bones, left; positions for different iliac crest biopsies: (a) Jamshidi needle (posterior iliac spine): (b) Bordier needle (anterior iliac spine); (c) Burkhardt drill (anterior iliac crest). Thick horizontal line indicates orientation of the horizontal section of the pelvis, right.

area of investigation depends on a local manifestation of disease, a BMB can be taken using radiological, scintigraphic, computed tomographic or ultrasound guidance.[22]

Although there are differences in the volume percentages of marrow and of trabecular bone in different regions of the ilium, these have little practical significance.[17,21,23] There are no differences in the amount of trabecular bone and of marrow in sections of biopsies taken vertically and horizontally, whether from right or from left iliac crests. Studies comparing biopsy cores of the iliac crest with those of other skeletal sites have shown differences in absolute values of bone marrow but parallel deviations were found in each individual case.[6,21] To evaluate the representative nature of the iliac crest biopsy, bone marrow biopsies of 81 autopsy cases of accidental death were investigated. Biopsies were taken from the anterior and posterior iliac crest, sternum and second lumbar vertebra. The volume percentages of trabecular bone, hemopoiesis and fat cells were assessed by histomorphometry using the ZEISS integration disc I. The sternum and the iliac crest contained more fatty tissue than the vertebra. The results at different ages at the different sites are given in Table 3.1.

INSTRUMENTS

An optimal bone marrow biopsy method should have the following qualities: the biopsy site should be readily accessible; the procedure should be easy to perform (in hospitalized patients, as well as in outpatients); it should have a minimum of possible complications, the resulting core should be of adequate size and of good quality; and, most importantly, the procedure should be well tolerated with the least amount of pain and discomfort to the patient.[17] Finally, the choice of the biopsy instrument depends on the diagnostic requirements as well as on the clinician's skill and experience.

BONE MARROW HISTOLOGY

Table 3.1 Histomorphometry of normal bone and bone marrow in different skeletal regions

Skeletal site	Age group (years)	Hemopoiesis (vol.%)	Fatty tissue (vol.%)	Trabecular bone (vol.%)	Osteoid (vol.%)
Anterior iliac crest	2–19	62	10	22	6
	20–39	48	28	21	3
	40–59	43	35	21	1
	60–99	43	40	15	2
Posterior iliac crest	2–19	60	14	22	4
	20–39	47	30	21	2
	40–59	42	37	20	1
	60–99	38	43	18	1
2nd lumbar vertebra	2–19	64	14	17	5
	20–39	57	23	18	2
	40–59	55	28	16	1
	60–99	52	35	12	1
Sternum	2–19	65	13	17	5
	20–39	58	25	15	2
	40–59	49	36	14	1
	60–99	45	39	15	1

Values derived from 81 autopsy cases of accidental death.[24]

There are two main groups of instruments available: manual trephines and electric drills (Fig. 3.2). The trephines are of two general categories: iliac crest (vertical, unicortical) and transiliac (horizontal, bicortical). In most cases the manual Jamshidi needle (2 or 3 mm width), or various modifications thereof, are employed and the biopsies are taken vertically from the superior spinous process of the posterior iliac crest (Fig. 3.3a).[24–29] The length of these biopsies varies, but may reach 3–4 cm. In some pathological bone conditions (such as

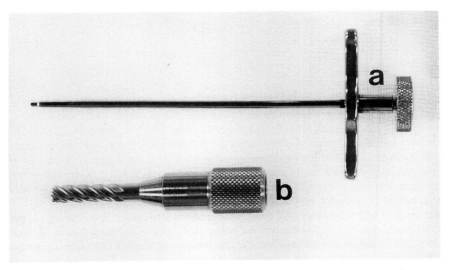

Fig. 3.2 Bone marrow biopsy instruments used by hematologists: (a) Jamshidi needle, 2 mm core diameter; (b) Burkhardt drill, 4 mm core diameter.

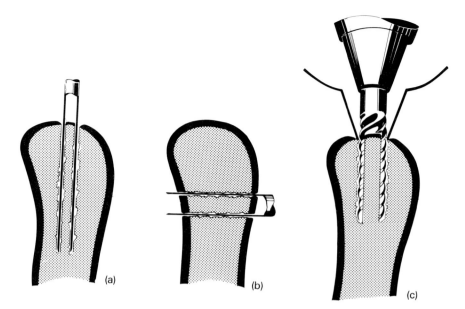

Fig. 3.3 Schematic representation of biopsy instruments: (a) Jamshidi needle (unicortical); (b) Bordier needle (bicortical); (c) Burkhardt drill (unicortical).

osteosclerosis and osteoporosis/lysis), a very sharp, wide bore needle is required. The manual trephine for horizontal transiliac biopsy (7–8 mm width, Bordier needle) is mainly used by nephrologists and osteologists for histomorphometric measurements of cortical and trabecular bone (Fig. 3.3b).[30,31] Excellent preservation of trabecular and hemopoietic tissue is obtained with an electrically driven trephine such as the Burkhardt drill (4 mm width) (Fig. 3.3c).[1] Practical details of how to take a biopsy using different procedures can be found in appropriate books and publications.[1,8,32]

PROCESSING

Biopsy cores with a diameter of 3 mm or more may be longitudinally halved with the aid of an especially designed plastic device (Fig. 3.4).[33,34] The cut surface is then used for imprints. One biopsy half (usually the longer one) is fixed in Schaffer's solution for embedding into plastic (methyl methacrylate) without decalcification (Fig. 3.5).[1,6,8] The other half is rapidly frozen after removal of small pieces if required for electron microscopy and/or chemical analysis. Both imprints and frozen sections may be used for rapid diagnosis (within 2 hours of taking the biopsy) after staining with Wright–Giemsa, as well as for supplementary enzyme and antigen–antibody reactions.[34] Biopsy cores 2 mm or less in diameter cannot be halved longitudinally. They should be cut into segments and treated as above.

After fixation and dehydration the cores are embedded into plastic, and sections are cut at 3 μm intervals (Fig. 3.6). Following removal of the plastic, the sections are stained by Giemsa for cytological detail, Gomori's stain for reticulin, periodic acid–schiff (PAS) for glycoprotein, Berlin blue for iron and Ladewig for mineralized bone and osteoid. Details of the technical processing have been published elsewhere.[1,8,35–44]

BONE MARROW HISTOLOGY 51

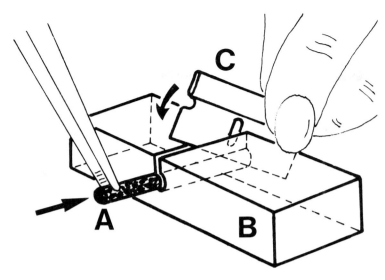

Fig. 3.4 Device for longitudinal halving of the biopsy core: the biopsy (A) is inserted into a plastic holder (B) and there cut by gentle sawing action of the razor blade (C) avoiding pressure and squeezing.

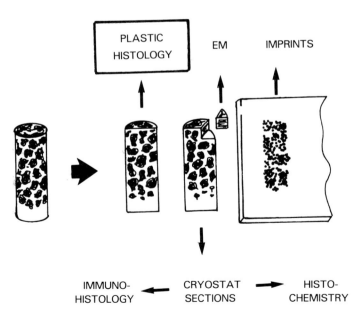

Fig. 3.5 Biopsy processing — steps and possibilities: after cutting, one half is used for plastic histology, while the other may be used for imprints (cytological details), cryostat sections (rapid diagnosis, immunohistology and histochemistry), electron microscopy (EM) and other technics (e.g. chemical analysis).

52 THE LEUKEMIC CELL

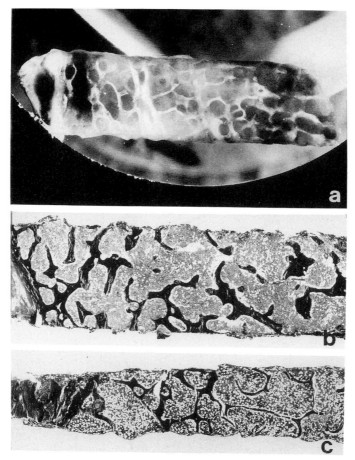

Fig. 3.6 (a) One biopsy half, embedded in plastic; (b) section of bone marrow biopsy, obtained by Burkhardt drill; and (c) by Jamshidi needle. (Gomori × 10)

INDICATIONS

In the past, the main indication for taking a marrow trephine biopsy was a 'dry tap' on aspiration. The availability of new biopsy instruments and histological technics as well as the clinician's need for detailed characterization and monitoring of hematological neoplasias have greatly increased the indications. The most frequent are listed below.

Indications for BMB in hematological neoplasias

- Dry tap on aspiration.
- Initial diagnosis.
- Minimal lesions.
- Hypocellular (smoldering) variants.
- Proliferation pattern.
- Evidence of systemic spread (staging).
- Degree of fibrosis.

- Stromal reactions.
- Degree of marrow atrophy.
- Residual hemopoiesis.
- Osseous reactions.
- Concomitant disorders.

- Evolution of disease.
- Transformation.
- Monitoring of therapy.
- Recognition of relapse.

EVALUATION OF BONE MARROW BIOPSIES

Initially, a morphological diagnosis is made on the basis of the histological findings. The clinical data and the results of other diagnostic investigations are then considered and a clinical interpretation given. When necessary, further information may be derived from marker studies, imprints or cryostat sections.

Sections of biopsies illustrating the normal range of hemopoiesis, bone and fatty tissue as well as their topographic arrangement are shown in Figs 3.6 and 3.7. It is mandatory first to scan the section at low magnification (× 4) to evaluate the technical quality and diagnostic representative nature of the biopsy (Fig. 3.8). The cortex shows a variable thickness and porosity. The subcortical zone is often occupied by fatty tissue, especially in older patients, and is therefore not representative, so the deeper parts (central zone) of the biopsy are the more informative. Consequently, 30 mm² (five or more marrow spaces) should be regularly available for diagnosis. However, even these regions may not present uniform cellularity and

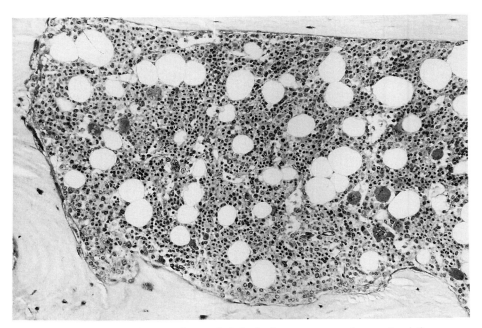

Fig. 3.7 Histotopography of normal hemopoiesis in the bone marrow: early granulopoietic precursors are situated in proximity to the trabeculae, while 'erythrons' and megakaryocytes are associated with the central sinusoids. (Giemsa × 100)

54 THE LEUKEMIC CELL

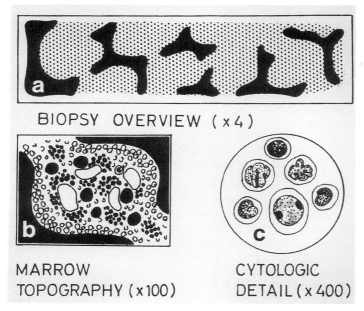

Fig. 3.8 Evaluation of bone marrow biopsy sections.

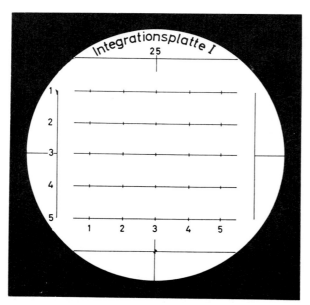

Fig. 3.9 ZEISS integration eyepiece I for quantitative assessment.

Table 3.2 Evaluation of bone marrow biopsy sections

1. Examination of the whole biopsy section (overview)
   Quality, artefacts
   Cortical bone and trabeculae
   Fatty tissue
   Cellularity
   Infiltration patterns?
2. Examination of trabecular bone
   Trabecular structure
   Osteoid
   Osteoblasts and osteocytes
   Osteoclasts
   Primitive bone?
3. Examination of hemopoiesis
   Eythropoiesis
   Megakaryopoiesis
   Granulopoiesis
   Topography of the cell lines
   Atypical blast forms?
4. Examination of bone marrow stroma
   Vasculature
   Macrophages
   Plasma cells
   Lymphocytes and lymphoid nodules
   Mast cells
   Fibers
   Iron content
   Granuloma?
5. Examination of malignant infiltrations
   Proliferative cell type
   Proliferative cell line(s)
   Growth pattern
   Tumor cell burden
   Stromal reactions
   Bone changes
6. Histopathological diagnosis
   Clinical interpretation
   Recommendations

alternating fatty and hyperplastic areas or concentrations of leukemic cells in single marrow spaces have been noted. It should be remembered that various artefacts are easily produced when taking a biopsy or when processing the specimen and misleading artefacts must be recognized and excluded. The sequence of evaluation of histological parameters used in the authors' departments is summarized in Table 3.2.

For morphometric assessment of the bone and marrow components, the ZEISS integration eyepiece I is used (Fig. 3.9).[45,46] Profile areas in the section (vol. %) are determined by the numbers of superimposed test points referred to as 'hits' and profile boundaries (surfaces) by numbers of intersections with the test lines. The grid must be calibrated for the magnification used (e.g. × 100), and usually 10–20 fields are assessed.[17] Comparative volumetric evaluation of trabecular bone, fatty tissue, hemopoiesis and other parameters such as tumor infiltration is useful, especially when sequential biopsies are compared.

The following sections describe the scope and value of BMB in the diagnosis and follow-up of hematological neoplasias. They are based on studies designed to derive diagnostic and prognostic information from bone marrow histology in large series of patients. Each section on one of the main diseases includes the relevant data for bone marrow histology, the histological subdivisions, evolution of disease and the diagnostic pitfalls.

MYELOPROLIFERATIVE DISORDERS (MPDs)

MYELODYSPLASTIC SYNDROMES (MDSs)

'Dysplasia comprises a loss in the regularity of the individual cells as well as a loss in their architectural orientation.'[47] When it occurs in the bone marrow, MDSs result. Hallmarks of the MDS include ineffective hemopoiesis, peripheral blood cytopenias and, frequently, a hypercellular bone marrow.[48–50] Primary MDS (preleukemia) represents a very early phase of hemopoietic stem cell disorder that may precede acute myeloid leukemia.[51,52] Secondary MDS constitutes hemopoietic reactions to exogenous agents.[53]

Bone marrow histology

The biopsies were divided into three groups according to the cellularity: (1) hypercellular (> 50 vol%) 60%; (2) normocellular (20–50 vol%) 25%; and (3) hypocellular (< 20 vol%) 15%.[54] The topographic distortion of the three hemopietic cell lines in MDSs proved to be the most important histological parameter (Fig. 3.10):[54] groups of myeloid precursors in the central areas of the marrow space (abnormal localization of immature precursors, ALIP), and erythrons and micromegakaryocytes (and others of variable size) at the trabecular surface (Fig. 3.11).[54,55] There were also a variety of cytological alterations in the hemopoietic precursors and alterations in the bone marrow stroma, e.g. inflammatory and fibrotic reactions.

The main diagnostic criteria of MDSs in BMB were:[54]

1. Marrow cellularity (H).
2. Topographic distortion (H).
3. Stromal reactions (H).
4. Ineffective hemopoiesis (H & C).
5. Predominant cell line(s) (H & C).
6. Cellular abnormalities (H & C).

(H = histology; C = cytology from smears and imprints.)

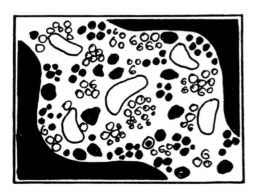

Fig. 3.10 Topographic distortion in MDS: distribution of precursors throughout the marrow space; granulopoiesis in the center (ALIP = abnormal localization of immature precursors); erythro- and megakaryopoiesis in the paratrabecular regions. Compare with normal histotopography in Figs. 3.7 and 3.8b.

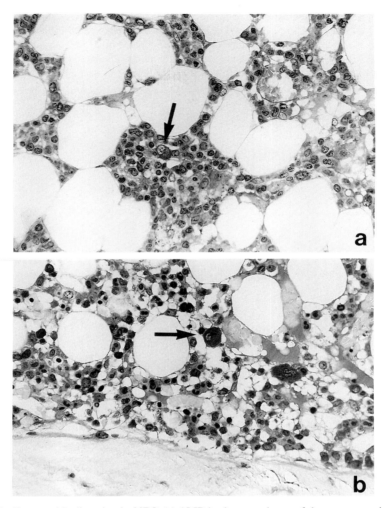

Fig. 3.11 Topographic distortion in MDS: (a) ALIP in the central area of the marrow cavity, micromegakaryocyte (arrow); (b) atypical, immature erythropoiesis and micromegakaryocyte (arrow) in the paratrabecular region. (Giemsa × 250)

Histological subdivisions

Recognition of different entities in the MDSs has been based on films of bone marrow aspirates and peripheral blood. The French–American–British (FAB) cooperative group addressed the confusion of nomenclature and suggested a division into five subtypes using the percentages of blast cells in the peripheral blood and in the bone marrow aspirates as one of the main criteria for separation of these subtypes.[56–58] However, this classification will probably need to be modified as more modern technics are used to characterize the MDS.[48,49] The same reservation applies to histology, so it is preferable to use only a tentative histological subdivision, although more specific information on dysplasia may be gained from sections of BMB than from aspirates. Topography and stromal reactions may also be evaluated.

58 THE LEUKEMIC CELL

The biopsies were each assigned to one of seven categories (the frequencies are given in brackets): MDS sideroblastic (19%); MDS megaloblastoid (13%); MDS inflammatory (10%); MDS fibrotic (6%); MDS hypocellular (15%); MDS proliferative (22%); and MDS blastic (15%) (Figs 3.12, 3.13a and 3.14a). Chronic myelomonocytic leukemia (CMML) — being by definition a leukemia — should be excluded from the MDSs (Fig. 3.13b).

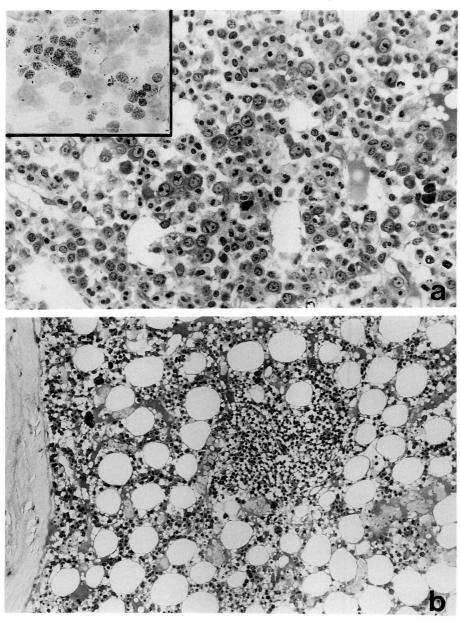

Fig. 3.12 (a) MDS sideroblastic with increased proerythroblasts; proof of 'ringed sideroblasts' in imprints. (Giemsa; Berlin blue × 250) (b) MDS inflammatory with topographic distortion, lymphoid nodule and edema (Giemsa × 100)

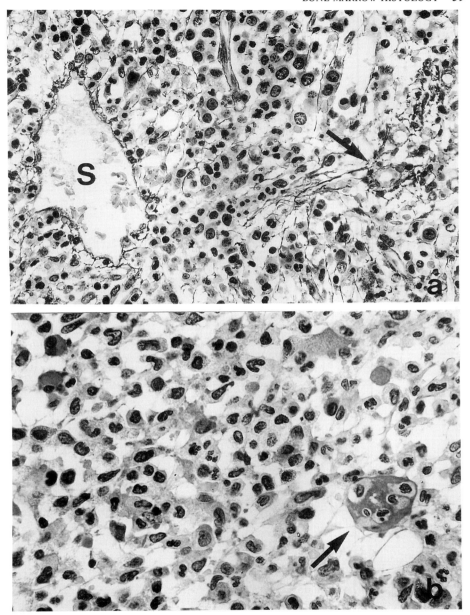

Fig. 3.13 (a) MDS fibrotic, 14 months later transition to acute leukemia; ectatic sinusoid (S) with sclerotic wall, pronounced perivascular fibrosis (arrow). (Gomori × 250) (b) CMML with emperipolesis (arrow). (Giemsa × 300)

Evolution of disease

The clinical outcome of the authors' MDS cases was as follows: unknown outcome (40%); detection of concurrent conditions such as infectious disorders, metastatic carcinoma or immune diseases (30%); preleukemic conditions with subsequent documentation of overt hematological neoplasia (20%); and pre-aplastic conditions with evolution to aplastic anemia (10%). The preleukemic MDSs showed transitions to acute and subacute leukemias, but also to myelofibrosis and chronic myeloproliferative disorders.[53,58,59]

Diagnostic pitfalls
Difficulties and even discrepancies in the histological diagnosis of MDSs are usually based on site discordance (e.g. discrepancies between sternal aspiration and iliac crest biopsy), temporal variability and overlapping of categories (e.g. ring sideroblasts in hypocellular type), and the presence of other conditions (e.g. solid tumors).[53]

ACUTE AND SUBACUTE LEUKEMIAS

Traditionally, the diagnosis of acute leukemia is based on values of peripheral blood counts and routinely stained blood and/or bone marrow films. A fundamental requirement for the diagnosis of acute leukemia is the presence of 30% or more blasts in smears of the bone marrow. Presence of Auer rods, cytochemistry, immunological markers and enzyme determinations are used for further categorization.[60-63] Although 'dry taps' and errors inherent in the technic of marrow aspiration have long been acknowledged, the supplementary value of BMB for initial diagnosis and for monitoring of therapy has only recently been fully recognized.[64-66]

Bone marrow histology
There were two main types of infiltration in the bone marrow biopsies investigated:

1. Hypercellular (85% of the cases), in which sheets of leukemic cells occupied the marrow cavities and presented a uniformly monomorphic picture; in some cases the infiltration was so dense ('packed marrow'), that a dry tap ensued.
2. Hypocellular (15% of the cases) (Fig. 3.14b), in which blasts were dispersed throughout the marrow, fat cells were increased and the residual hemopoiesis was dysplastic.

The degree of fibrosis varied widely in acute leukemia, from a slight increase in reticulin fibers to coarse fibrosis as in acute myelosclerosis. Cases with subacute leukemia revealed the typical topographic arrangement of the cell lines involved: promyelocytes in the paratrabecular and periarterial regions, erythroid and megakaryopoietic precursors in the central perisinusoidal zones. These were often less cellular than those of the acute hypocellular type (in 35% of the cases) but showed a tendency to differentiation, albeit with dysplastic features.

Histological subdivisions
The French–American–British working group proposed the morphological criteria for the classification of acute non-lymphocytic leukemias,[67,68] utilizing Wright–Giemsa staining of peripheral blood and bone marrow smears and special cytochemical stains. This system is now internationally used and a BMB is generally performed when aspiration is unsuccessful. However, as understanding of the role of the hemopoietic microenvironment and the stroma increases, BMB is likely to be included in future classifications of acute leukemia. Several studies have shown that the quantitative estimation of the leukemic infiltration and the degree of fibrosis have predictive value and thereby influence therapeutic considerations. In subacute leukemias, i.e. the promyelocytic, erythroblastic (diGuglielmo) and promegakaryocytic types, BMB is a prerequisite for cell line recognition because of the high incidence of subleukemic blood pictures and dry tap on aspiration, and the diagnostic value of the proliferation patterns in the bone marrow.[6,8]

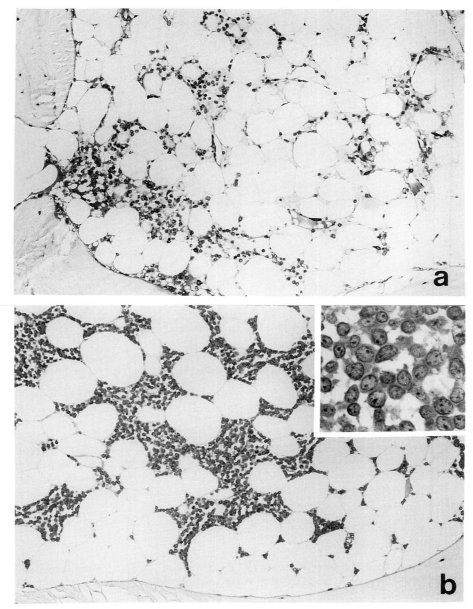

Fig. 3.14 Smoldering leukemia in a 72-year-old patient: (a) MDS hypocellular. (Giemsa × 100) (b) 12 months later — hypocellular type of acute myeloblastic leukemia, with subleukemic blood picture and smoldering course. (Giemsa × 100) **Inset:** higher magnification of myeloblasts. (Giemsa × 400)

Evolution of disease

Some patients with hypocellular acute leukemia had slow disease progression corresponding to 'smoldering' leukemia.[69,70] Development of coarse fibrosis indicated an unfavorable prognosis and a poor response to chemotherapy (Fig. 3.15).[71] Most cases of malignant myelosclerosis proved to be acute or subacute leukemias (often megakaryoblastic type) with

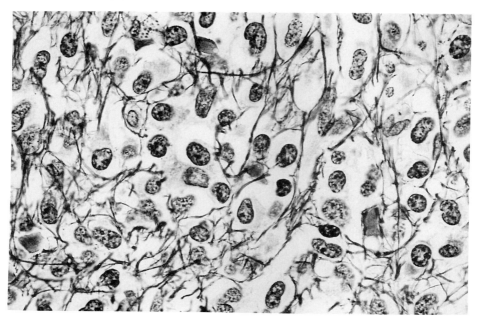

Fig. 3.15 Coarse fibrosis in AML (relapse), no response to therapy. (Gomori × 600)

a dominant fibrotic reactions.[172] BMBs are also more reliable for checking remission or documenting early relapse in acute leukemia, than examination of peripheral blood or aspirates alone.[8]

Diagnostic pitfalls
When the infiltration consists of undifferentiated blasts, bone marrow histology must be supplemented by cytochemistry and immunological methods in order to exclude malignant lymphomas and undifferentiated carcinomas. There is a diagnostic overlap between the hypocellular type of acute leukemia and MDS with a high percentage of blasts. Additional cytological and immunological studies, together with the clinical picture, will clarify the diagnosis.

POLYCYTHEMIA VERA (PV)

The chronic myeloproliferative disorders (MPDs) are clonal disorders of the hemopoietic stem cell and comprise a spectrum of more or less well-defined clinical entities.[73,74] In contrast to other neoplasias, there are no unequivocal cytological characteristics that distinguish the cells in MPDs from their normal counterparts in the bone marrow. There is still disagreement in the literature concerning the place of bone marrow biopsy in the diagnosis of the MPD. Their value in PV is still disputed by some,[75] and in some cases the recognition of secondary polycythemia may not be possible by clinical parameters alone. Nearly 20% of PV have a normal leukocyte and platelet count and the leukocytes are often raised in secondary erythrocytosis.

Bone marrow histology
The following histological findings are characteristic of PV:[76-83]

1. Increase in overall cellularity with a corresponding decrease in fat cells and hyperplasia of the affected cell lines in their normal topographic locations.
2. Polymorphism of the megakaryocytes ranging from 'giant' to 'micro' and pyknotic types.
3. Hyperplasia and hyperemia of sinusoids.
4. Depletion of iron stores.
5. Presence of variable amounts of reticulin fibers, lymphoid nodules and plasma cells and some degree of osteopenia.

However, not all these features are always present, so that the histology resembles that of secondary erythrocytosis.[6,8,82] The situation could be clarified in follow-up biopsies and by additional clinical data.

Histological subdivisions
The bone marrow histology in PV can be divided into four subtypes:[6,80,82]

1. The classic trilinear type (51% of cases) with numerous giant megakaryocytes (Fig. 3.16a).
2. The bilinear erythrocytic/megakaryocytic type (33%) with additional clusters of giant megakaryocytes.
3. The bilinear erythrocytic/granulocytic type (9%) with minimal megakaryocytic atypia.
4. The unilinear erythrocytic type with only erythroid hyperplasia, usually indistinguishable from hemolytic pictures (7%) (Fig. 3.16b).

In this group, clinical and laboratory data are necessary to establish the diagnosis.

Evolution of disease
As demonstrated in sequential biopsies, both the course and the metamorphosis of PV were largely influenced by the proliferative cell line(s) in the bone marrow.[6,8,80,82] Extensive myelofibrosis occurred almost exclusively in cases with marked proliferation of megakaryocytes (types 1 and 2); approximately 50% of our patients with PV developed myelofibrosis. On the other hand, administration of therapy, such as busulphan or radioactive phosphorus, did not carry a greater risk of inducing fibrosis. When 'spent' ('burned out') PV occurred, the peripheral blood levels fall and the bone marrow presents a fibrotic picture, with dysplastic hemopoiesis, stromal changes and an increase in fat cells. Metamorphoses to terminal blast crisis, to other MPDs and even to malignant lymphoma have been described.[6,8,80,82,83]

Diagnostic pitfalls
In secondary erythrocytosis there is hyperplasia of the erythroid line only, whilst megakaryocytes and fat cells are quantitatively normal. Usually iron stores are not depleted and reticulin fibers are not increased.

PRIMARY (ESSENTIAL) THROMBOCYTHEMIA
This is a myeloproliferative disorder in which very high platelet counts predominate and features of both PV and myelofibrosis are seen.[84,85]

Bone marrow histology
The bone marrow may be hyper-, normo- or hypocellular, with marked proliferation of polymorphic megakaryocytes ranging from micro to giant forms (Fig. 3.17).[6,8,80,82] When the cells are mature (megakaryocytic myelosis), with production of platelets and their release into the blood stream, very high platelet counts in the peripheral blood are observed. Coarse

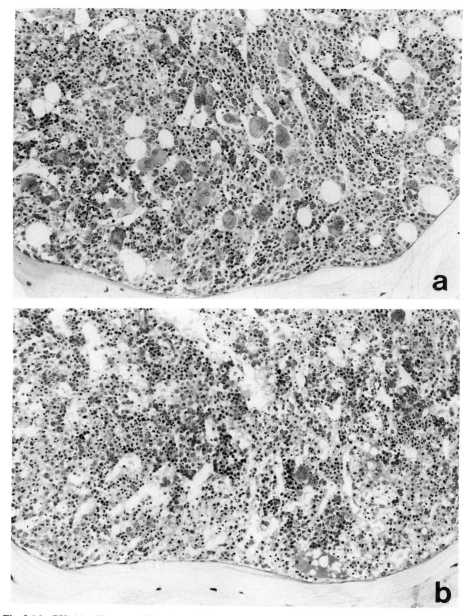

Fig. 3.16 PV: (a) trilinear proliferation with hyperplastic sinusoids. (Giemsa × 100) (b) Unilinear with proliferation of the erythroid cell line, hyperplastic sinusoids. (Giemsa × 100)

fibrosis was found in proximity to clusters of polymorphous megakaryocytes. Red and white cell precursors are often reduced, especially in a hypocellular marrow.

Histological subdivisions
Primary thrombocythemia can be grouped according to the distribution of the megakaryocytes into a diffuse subtype and a cluster subtype. However, the latter may represent a more advanced stage of megakaryocytic proliferation.

BONE MARROW HISTOLOGY 65

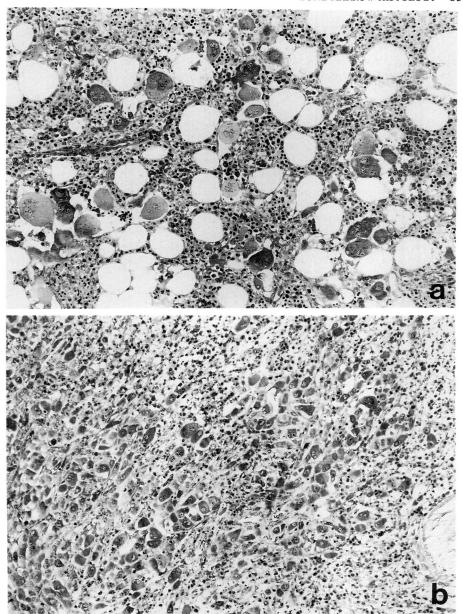

Fig. 3.17 Primary thrombocythemia: (a) unilinear proliferation of atypical, mature megakaryocytes, partly in clusters. (Giemsa × 100) (b) Transition to promegakaryocytic type 6 years later, with thrombocytopenia. (Giemsa × 100)

Evolution of disease
Patients with the clinical entity of thrombocythemia corresponded to the histological picture of megakaryocytic myelosis of the mature type. The disease usually follows a slow course, but eventually a falling platelet count signals the transition either to the immature (promegakaryocytic) subtype (Fig. 3.17b), or to myelofibrosis.[6,8,80,82]

Diagnostic pitfalls
The different bone marrow pictures found in patients with thrombocythemia demonstrate that essential thrombocythemia is a syndrome with a variable underlying bone marrow histopathology. It corresponds to a megakaryocytic myelosis in 60% of the cases. Patients with Philadelphia (Ph) chromosome positive thrombocythemia have also been reported and they illustrate the overlapping of clinical and histological entities in the MPDs.[86]

CHRONIC MYELOID LEUKEMIA (CML)
Bone marrow biopsies are not routinely performed in patients with CML, although they can provide useful information for diagnosis and treatment purposes.

Bone marrow histology
The marrow is densely cellular, dominated by granulocytic proliferation consisting of broad paratrabecular and perivascular seams of immature myeloid precursors and mature granulocytes in the central regions.[6,8,82] There are usually eosinophilia and macrophages are increased, many with crystalloid inclusions — the 'pseudo-Gaucher' cells. The number of megakaryocytes varies even within a single biopsy. They exhibit polymorphism and microfilms as well as heterotopia. A moderate increase of reticulin fibers is always present.

Histological subdivisions
CML also proved to be a heterogeneous group with respect to histology. It divides into two main subtypes according to the proliferative cell line(s) (Fig. 3.18):

1. The granulocytic type (45%) with a striking hyperplasia of granulopoiesis. The mean number of megakaryocytes was low and they were usually small. Neutrophilic CML was most common, but eosinophilic and basophilic types were also encountered. Reticulin fibers were slightly increased, a fact which may influence the cellular percentages in smears of marrow aspirates.
2. The megakaryocytic/granulocytic type (55%) with concomitant qualitative and quantitative alterations of megakaryopoiesis.[8,82,87]

The megakaryocytes, highly polymorphic and many immature, were found in all marrow regions. Many were close to hyperplastic sinusoids, as well as in their lumina (heterotopia). Fibers were prominent adjacent to megakaryocytic clusters and to blood vessels. Patients with mixed type CML may reveal a subleukemic blood picture at initial diagnosis sometimes making their clinical categorization under the heading of CML difficult.

Evolution of disease
The assessment of sequential biopsies clearly demonstrated that:

1. There were transitions between the two types.
2. Transformation to myelofibrosis occurred only in the mixed type.
3. Metamorphosis to a terminal blast crisis was seen predominantly in the unilinear type, which may be one reason for its less favorable prognosis.[82,88,89]

Expanding myeloblastic seams proved to be a reliable sign of the accelerated phase and imminent blast crisis, often recognizable before an increase of blasts in peripheral blood.[6] After aggressive chemotherapy, a hypocellular, even aplastic phase often ensues.[6]

Diagnostic pitfalls
The histological distinction of eosinophilic CML from reactive eosinophilia, or between CML and a leukemoid reaction, is not always possible from bone marrow biopsy. However, in a leukemoid reaction the abrupt transition from myeloblast seams to mature granulocytes,

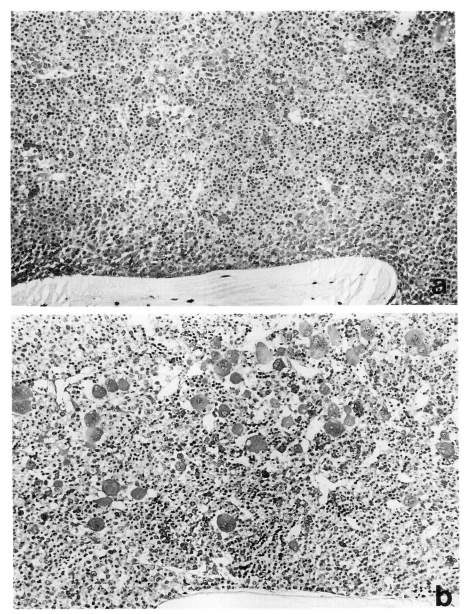

Fig. 3.18 CML: (a) granulocytic type. (Giemsa × 100); (b) granulocytic/megakaryocytic type. (Giemsa × 100).

polymorphism and heterotopia of megakaryopoiesis are absent. An overlapping of the mixed type CML with the histological pictures of essential thrombocythemia and PV is also observed.

MYELOFIBROSIS/OSTEOMYELOSCLEROSIS

Fibrosis of the bone marrow takes place in response to different toxic, osteolytic and malignant processes.[90,91] Reactive fibrosis on the basis of MPD is called myelofibrosis or (with presence of primitive bone) osteomyelosclerosis. Two pathogenic mechanisms have been proposed:

1. A chronic inflammatory reaction mediated by circulating immune complexes,[92,93] indicated by the presence of plasma cells, mast cells, lymphoid nodules and edema in the bone marrow undergoing fibrosis.
2. Production of fibroblast stimulating growth factor (PGDF) and of collagenase inhibiting factor (platelet factor 4) by megakaryocytes and platelets.[90-96]

Deposition of platelets into the interstitium instead of into the sinusoidal lumina in areas of incipient fibrosis has been observed, lending support to the second theory.

Bone marrow histology
The histologic picture of myelofibrosis is characterized by a diffuse network of coarse fibers (collagen type III).[6] Clusters of polymorphous megakaryocytes surrounded by fibrotic tissue are located close to the sclerotic walls of ectatic sinusoids (Fig. 3.19). Edema and platelets are found in the interstitial spaces (Fig. 3.20). Morphological signs of inflammation are always present and hemopoiesis is replaced by fibrosis and fatty tissue.

The diagnosis of osteomyelosclerosis (OMS) is made when woven bone is also present. The content of fat cells is usually higher in OMS than in myelofibrosis (MF).[96]

Histological subdivisions
MF/OMS generally developed in those cases associated with proliferation of megakaryocytes. Two grades were distinguished according to the degree of fibrosis.[91,96]

1. Both fine and coarse fibrosis around megakaryocytes and vessels.
2. Widespread coarse fibrosis.

When still recognizable, the underlying myeloproliferative process should be identified. At least the basic clinical diagnosis should be defined, e.g. 'MF secondary to PV'. The term 'idiopathic' MF should be used only when the patient presents with the full blown picture of MF/OMS and no cause can be determined.

Acute myelofibrosis (acute MF) originally referred to by Lewis and Szur as 'malignant MF',[97] is usually characterized by a rapidly progressive fibrosis on the basis of an immature or blastic myeloproliferation (Fig. 3.21c). Acute MF may terminate in acute leukemia.[97-100] In OMS, the extent of primitive bone production is variable. Three grades were distinguished:

1. Small foci of primitive bone.
2. Trabecular bone and increased woven bone in approximately equal proportions.
3. Almost complete replacement of the trabeculae by a network of primitive bone (Fig. 3.21a,b).

Evolution of disease
Transformation to MF/OMS was observed in approximately 50% of the patients with MPDs. The basic myeloproliferative process was known in 80% of the patients with MF/OMS. In the remaining 20% the underlying MPD could not be identified. Although there is a close relationship between MF and OMS, there are differences in the clinical courses and prognosis is more favourable in OMS than in MF.[6,8,80] On the basis of follow-up studies the authors were able to demonstrate that OMS is not necessarily a more advanced stage of MF; the two types should be regarded as different modes of stromal reactions to myeloproliferation.

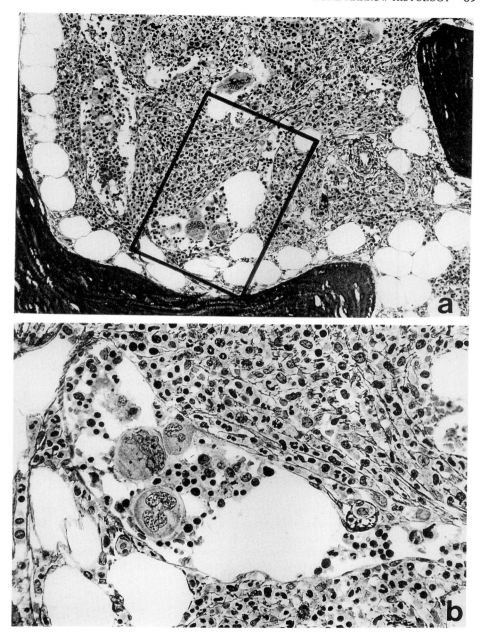

Fig. 3.19 MF on the basis of CML: (a) diffuse fibrosis with coarse fibers around a small artery (*rectangle*)–ectatic sinusoids with sclerotic walls and hemopoietic precursors in the lumina. (Gomori × 100) (b) Higher magnification of the rectangle in (a) showing megakaryocytes and erythroblasts in the lumen. (Gomori × 250)

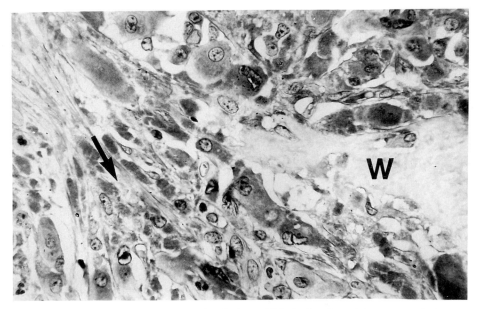

Fig. 3.20 MF on the basis of thrombocythemia: interstitial platelets (*arrow*) between atypical immature and heterotopic megakaryocytes; W, woven bone. (Giemsa × 400)

Diagnostic pitfalls

There are numerous conditions that may induce marrow fibrosis: metastatic carcinoma, osteopathies, Hodgkin's disease, sclerosing myelitis due to toxic agents and other unknown causes. In most cases causative agents are identifiable, but occasionally only fibrotic tissue is present. In these cases a second biopsy from another site may clarify the diagnosis.[91] It should be noted that marked differences in fibrosis and in myeloproliferation may be observed in the different marrow cavities.

LYMPHOPROLIFERATIVE DISORDERS

The value of bone marrow biopsies in the diagnostic and clinical assessment of lymphoproliferative disorders has now been fully established and they are routinely taken to estimate the stage of disease at initial diagnosis.[101-105] In this review of bone marrow histology the Kiel nomenclature, which is widely employed in Europe, was used to enable comparison of lymph node and bone marrow findings in malignant lymphomas.[106] The nomenclature of the lymphoid growth patterns is summarized schematically in Fig. 3.22.

CHRONIC LYMPHOCYTIC LEUKEMIA (CLL)

CLL, the most common leukemia, involves the pathological, systemic accumulation of long-lived lymphocytes. Histologically it is classified as malignant lymphoma lymphocytic, low grade malignancy, usually of B-cell type.

Bone marrow histology

The bone marrow is always involved and the infiltration showed three modes of spread called growth patterns: interstitial, nodular/interstitial and packed marrow (Fig. 3.23).[107-111] There was a thin network of fibers and only a few mast or plasma cells. There were variations in

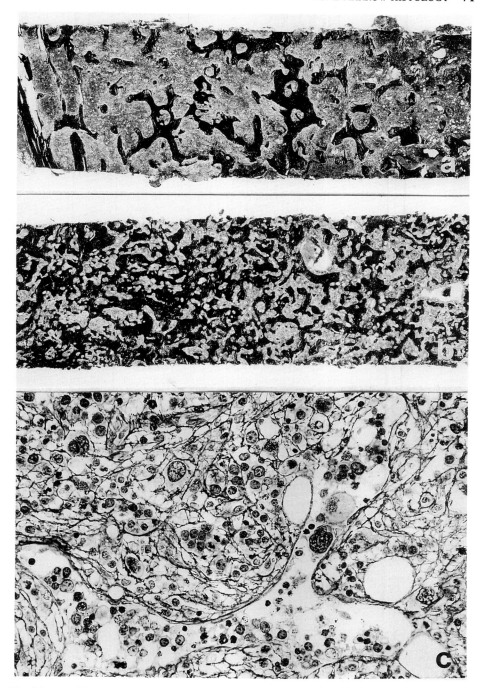

Fig. 3.21 (a) OMS, grade 2 (Gomori × 10) (b) OMS, grade 3. (Gomori × 10) (c) Malignant myelofibrosis, with precursors of erythro- and megakaryopoiesis between the fibers and within the lumen of the sinusoid. (Gomori × 250)

72 THE LEUKEMIC CELL

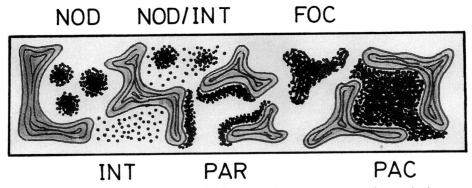

Fig. 3.22 Growth patterns of lymphoproliferative disease in the bone marrow (frequencies in brackets): NOD, nodular (9%); INT, interstitial (22%); NOD/INT, nodular/interstitial (29%); PAR, paratrabecular (2%); FOC, focal (10%); patchy, PAC, packed marrow (28%).

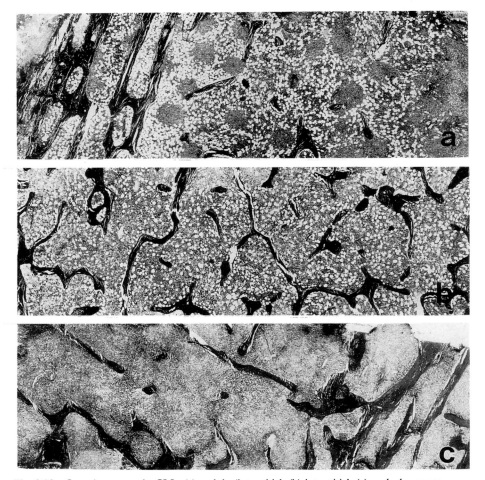

Fig. 3.23 Growth patterns in CLL: (a) nodular/interstitial; (b) interstitial; (c) packed marrow. (Gomori × 10)

lymphocyte size, number of nucleolated cells and nuclear configuration. B2 lymphocytes have predominantly notched nuclei, whereas in the rare T-CLL the lymphocytes in the bone marrow have convoluted nuclei and a striking perivascular localization.[105] In prolymphocytic leukemia the lymphoid cells have small nuclei, moderate amounts of cytoplasm and a positive acid phosphatase reaction (on smears, imprints or cryostat sections).[113,114]

Histological subdivisions
The proliferation pattern in the bone marrow proved to be the most significant prognostic factor and three easily recognizable and reproducible groups have been described: interstitial (45%), nodular/interstitial (22%) and packed marrow (33%).[110] Patients with nodular aggregates of lymphocytes had significantly longer survival times.
CLL can also be divided according to the cellular criteria mentioned above (Fig. 3.24): small round (66%), notched (10%) and mixed (24%).[104,105,110,115] Both growth pattern and proliferative cell system reflect the aggressiveness of the disease and have clinical and prognostic relevance.

Evolution of disease
CLL is many-faceted and has considerable variations in its evolution. In early stages there is only a minimal interstitial infiltration, with or without nodular aggregates. With progression of disease the bone marrow is replaced by lymphoid cells, finally inducing bone marrow failure. The RAI staging system constitutes clinical staging according to the anatomical extent of disease, whilst bone marrow biopsies give information on the degree of bone marrow infiltration and the inherent 'malignancy' (growth pattern, cell type) of the disease. Terminal transformations of CLL into acute forms (e.g. Richter's syndrome) have been recognized in bone marrow biopsies in their early phases.[109]

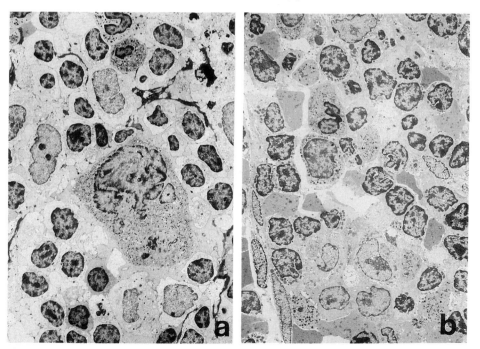

Fig. 3.24 Proliferative cell systems in CLL (Electron microscopy × 2500): (a) small round; (b) notched.

Diagnostic pitfalls

The morphological distinction between benign lymphoid nodules and early lymphomatous infiltration is not always possible.[116] In such cases, immunohistology on cryostat sections of the second biopsy half can be decisive.[117]

HAIRY CELL LEUKEMIA (HCL)

HCL has been assigned to the B-lymphocytic lineage on the basis of immunological, enzyme and electron microscopic studies.[114,118] Both clinical course and therapeutic response are variable, leading some observers to conclude that HCL represents a spectrum of conditions rather than a single disease entity.[118,119]

Bone marrow histology

Except in rare and early cases, bone marrow biopsy is diagnostic and presents a typical picture. There is patchy to complete infiltration of hairy cells (Fig. 3.25a).[120,121] The hairy cells have abundant cytoplasm with interdigitating extensions and many have rod-like cytoplasmic inclusions (Fig. 3.25b). The infiltration also contains plasma cells, lymphocytes, mast cells and erythrocytes within a network of reticulin fibers. At high magnification hairy cell nuclei exhibited a wide range of sizes and configurations. Islands of erythropoiesis with marked maturation inhibition were often found surrounded by hairy cells.

Histological subdivisions

Three subtypes of HCL based on nuclear configuration have been demonstrated in bone marrow histology (Fig. 3.26): ovoid (47%), convoluted (37%) and indented (16%).[121]

Evolution of disease

The hairy cell burden in the bone marrow correlates with the clinical course, and a rapid increase of tumor mass may indicate an unfavorable prognosis. Transformation of the ovoid into the indented type also signals a rapid progression.[121]

Diagnostic pitfalls

Hairy cells are easily recognized in plastic-embedded biopsies. However in some cases the differential diagnosis will include other malignant lymphomas and monocytic infiltrates.[121]

WALDENSTRÖM'S MACROGLOBULINEMIA

This disorder is a B-cell neoplasia of low grade malignancy, secreting monoclonal IgM.[122] The predominant cell type is a small lymphocyte with variable plasmacytoid differentiation, malignant lymphoma lymphoplasmacytoid/cytic (immunocytoma).[106]

Bone marrow histology

Bone marrow involvement was found in 80% of the patients studied and three distinct proliferation patterns are recognized:[123]

1. Nodular (42%) (Fig. 3.27a), with multiple lymphoid nodules in apposition to trabeculae and ectatic sinusoids, separated by fat cells from areas with hemopoiesis.
2. Interstitial/nodular (42%), in which nodules were dispersed within a loose interstitial infiltration.
3. Packed marrow (16%) with complete replacement of hemopoiesis and fat.

High power examination revealed a wide spectrum of lymphoid cells ranging from small lymphocytes to plasma cells. Electron microscopy and immunohistology often revealed the plasmacytoid nature of cells identified as lymphocytes in the light microscope.

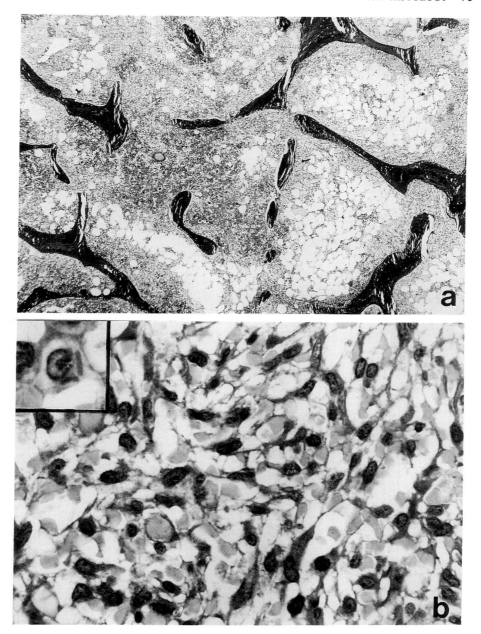

Fig. 3.25 HCL: (a) patchy infiltration. (Gomori × 60) (b) Infiltration of widely separated cells, within a network of fibers containing erythrocytes, plasma cells and mast cells; *upper left* rod-like intracytoplasmic inclusion. (× 600)

76 THE LEUKEMIC CELL

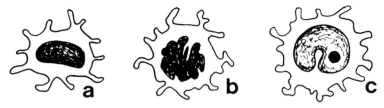

Fig. 3.26 The three hairy cell subtypes: (a) ovoid; (b) convoluted; (c) indented.

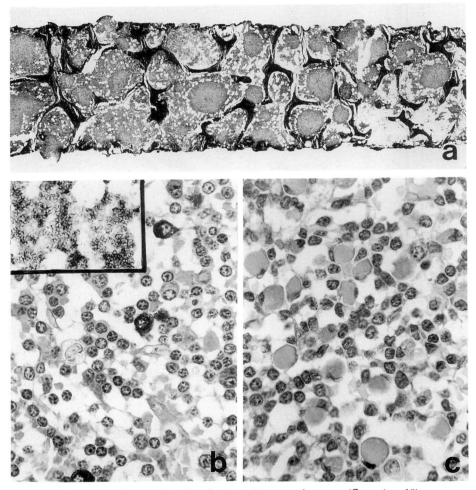

Fig. 3.27 Waldenström's macroglobulinemia: (a) nodular growth pattern (Gomori × 10)
(b) lymphoplasmacytic cell type, with lymphoplasmacytic cells, plasma cells, lymphocytes and mast cells; μ-chain positive cells in the cryostat section (PAP) (upper left). (Giemsa × 400)
(c) lymphoplasmacytoid cells with intracytoplasmic inclusions. (Giemsa × 400)

Histological subdivisions
Three main types of cell populations were discerned: lymphoplasmacytoid (47%), lymphoplasmacytic (42%) and polymorphous (11%). This classification was comparable with these subtypes in the lymph nodes (Fig. 3.27a and b). In addition, the three cell types were characterized by different growth patterns, clinical features, anatomic extent and median survival.[123]

Evolution of disease
Patients in each subtype were assigned to one of three stages according to the quantity of the lymphoid infiltration shown in the bone marrow biopsy. These stages correlated with the patient's history, the clinical progression and survival time. Conversion of an immunocytoma to an immunoblastic lymphoma has also been described.[124]

Diagnostic pitfalls
In the absence of PAS-positive intranuclear inclusions in the lymphoid cells, the histological picture resembles that of CLL; however, mast cells are more numerous in immunocytoma. Immunohistology can clarify such borderline cases. Nodular lymphoid hyperplasia can also be distinguished from lymphomatous infiltration by marker techniques (Fig. 3.27b).

OTHER NON-HODGKIN'S LYMPHOMAS

Malignant lymphoma, centrocytic
The frequency of bone marrow involvement is 70%. Most cases show a characteristic paratrabecular infiltration of small to medium-sized lymphoid cells with cleaved nuclei (Fig. 3.28a). A characteristic stromal pattern is formed by coarse fibers radiating out from the trabeculae (Fig. 3.28b). Nuclear size was used for subtyping: small cleaved (60%), large cleaved (25%) and polymorphous (15%). In biopsies with a packed marrow, the morphological distinction from CLL (B or T-cell types) or immunocytoma was often difficult. In these cases a definite diagnosis was achieved by immunological methods.

Malignant lymphoma, centroblastic/centrocytic
Bone marrow involvement was infrequent in our study (20%). Malignant lymphoma centroblastic/centrocytic has a nodular pattern in bone marrow, mostly follicles with germinal centers consisting of centrocytes, centroblasts and lymphocytes (Fig. 3.28c). The distinction of minimal lesions from immunocytoma, or from nodular lymphoid hyperplasia or lymphoid follicles in the bone marrow, was possible only by immunohistology.

Malignant lymphoma centroblastic and immunoblastic
All biopsies involved (20%) showed a packed marrow. The size of the cells, the basophilic cytoplasm and the typical aspect of the nuclei were diagnostic (Fig. 3.29).

MULTIPLE MYELOMA

There is a broad spectrum of initial presentations of plasma cell dyscrasias in multiple myeloma.[125-27] Patients with solitary, multifocal and sarcomatous plasmacytomas usually reveal no involvment in the iliac crest biopsy; however, most plasmacellular neoplasias show systemic spread from the start. It is astonishing that the morphological diagnosis of multiple myeloma, the most frequent lymphoproliferative disorder of the bone marrow, is still based on arbitrarily defined percentages of aspirated bone marrow cells, and that an accepted morphological classification has not yet been widely adopted.[128]

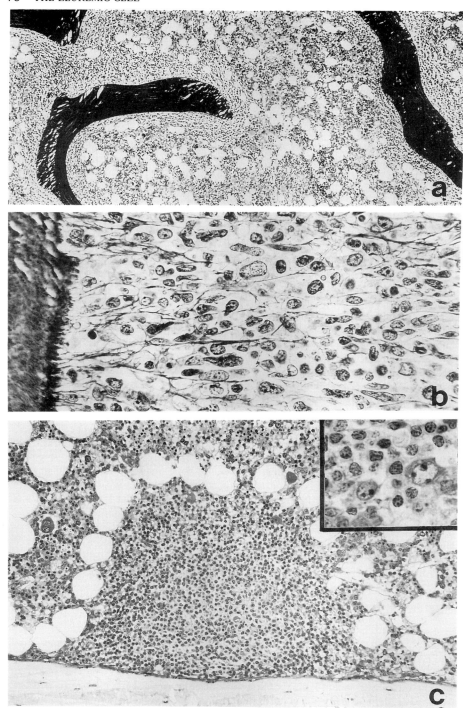

Fig. 3.28 Follicle center cell lymphomas: (a) paratrabecular growth pattern in malignant lymphoma (ML), centrocytic. (Gomori × 60) (b) Fibers radiating from the trabecular surface in ML centrocytic. (Gomori × 400) (c) Nodular infiltration in the paratrabecular region in ML centroblastic/centrocytic. (Giemsa × 100) Upper right: centroblasts and centrocytes. (Giemsa × 400)

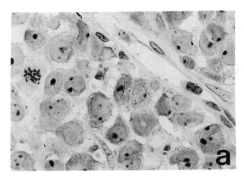 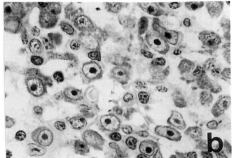

Fig. 3.29 Malignant lymphoma of high grade malignancy: (a) centroblastic; (b) immunoblastic. (Giemsa × 400)

Bone marrow histology

Initial bone marrow involvement was found in 90% of cases with multiple myeloma in the authors' study. The myeloma cells were usually dispersed in the interstitial spaces, in addition to small clusters or sheets in paratrabecular and perivascular regions. Only a few cases had a strictly nodular pattern. A thin fiber network was usually present, but coarse fibrosis was found in only about 10% of the cases. Lymphocytic nodules were observed in 10% of the bone marrow biopsies. Osteoclastic and osteoblastic remodeling were prominent and correlated with the plasma cell burden in the biopsy (Fig. 3.30a). Secondary amyloidosis was detected in 5% of our cases (Fig. 3.30b). High magnification revealed a wide spectrum of myeloma cells. Some nucleolated plasma cells were detected even in minimal infiltrations — a reliable diagnostic parameter for multiple myeloma.[129-31]

Histological subdivisions

Altogether six architectural patterns were observed in the bone marrow biopsies. (Fig. 3.31): interstitial (72%), interstitial/sheets (13%), interstitial/nodular (9%), nodular (4%), focal sarcomatous (1%) and packed marrow (15%). Two broad categories of myeloma cells were distinguished: the predominantly mature and the predominantly immature cell groups. However, when cellular size, cytoplasmic structure and nuclear configuration were all taken into consideration, the spectrum of myeloma cells could be divided into six classes:

1. Marschalko (59%).
2. Small cell (11%).
3. Cleaved (8%).
4. Polymorphous (9%).
5. Asynchronous (10%).
6. Blastic (2%).

These six types were subsequently combined into three prognostic grades: low (1,2), intermediate (3,4,5) and high malignancy (6), analogous to the malignant lymphomas.[131]

Evolution of disease

The clinical phases of multiple myeloma were investigated by sequential biopsies. In early cases the plasma cells were dispersed among hemopoietic and fat cells. In later stages the plasma cell clusters expanded to form 'multiple myelomas' and, finally, the packed marrow. Increase of plasma cell mass correlated with the osteoclastic index. Appearance of nodularity signaled progression. The quantity of plasma cell burden (vol%) in the biopsy proved to be a useful criterion for histological staging of multiple myeloma supplementing any clinical

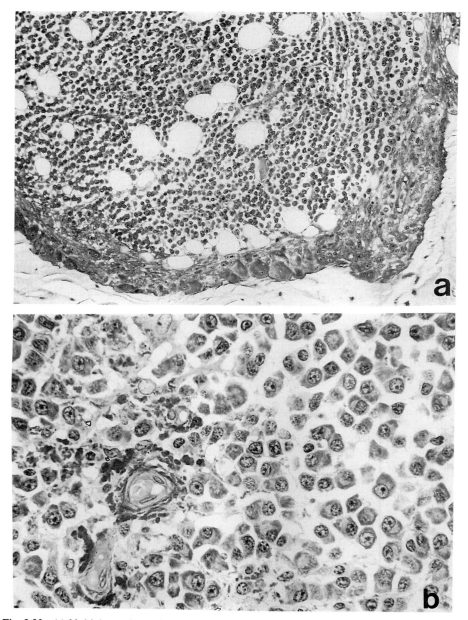

Fig. 3.30 (a) Multiple myeloma: dense plasmacytic infiltration with seams of active osteoclasts on the trabecular surface. (Giemsa × 100) (b) Secondary amyloidosis with homogeneous deposits around vessels. (Giemsa × 400)

staging system in use. Patients with very long survival times (smoldering myeloma) revealed a characteristic morphological picture: a minimal interstitial infiltration of predominantly mature plasma cells (Marschalko or small cell type).[131,132] Sequential biopsies can also be used to monitor the effect of treatment, especially to document residual infiltration, marrow atrophy or fibrosis (Fig. 3.32). Bone marrow biopsies may also indicate a stable phase in

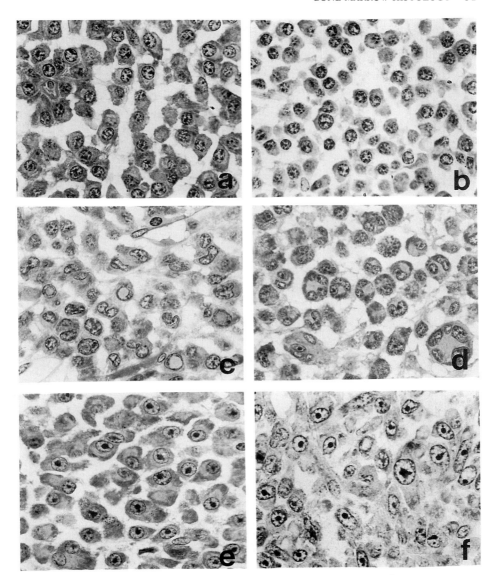

Fig. 3.31 Multiple myeloma cell types: (a) Marschalko; (b) small cell; (c) cleaved; (d) polymorphous; (e) asynchronous; (f) blastic. (Giemsa × 400)

which further treatment would be contraindicated. Transformation of multiple myelomas into other lymphoid neoplasias, MPDs or acute leukemia can be recognized in bone marrow biopsies at an early stage.

Diagnostic pitfalls
The histologic growth pattern together with the cellular morphology are reliable parameters for distinguishing between reactive and neoplastic plasmacytosis, and between benign and malignant monoclonal gammopathy.[129,133] Only in very early cases is immunohistology required to establish monoclonality.

82 THE LEUKEMIC CELL

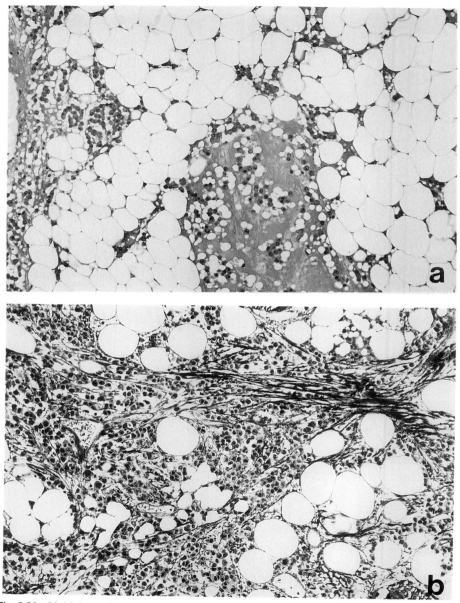

Fig. 3.32 Multiple myeloma: (a) Striking marrow atrophy after therapy, edema and residual plasmacytic infiltration, but no reconstitution of hemopoiesis. (Giemsa × 100) (b) Coarse fibrosis; this patient showed a striking resistance to chemotherapy. (Gomori × 100)

HODGKIN'S DISEASE

Accurate assessment of the extent of disease became mandatory when it was recognized that Hodgkin's disease has a contiguous spread and therefore might be cured by therapy to the involved sites. Since one of the criteria for systemic spread (stage IV) is involvement of the bone marrow, a bone marrow biopsy is an integral part of the initial investigation of patients with this disease.[134]

Bone marrow histology

In our recent re-evaluation, the overall incidence of Hodgkin's disease in the bone marrow of patients at initial presentation was 6%. Various factors may influence the rate of detection: the selection of patients, possibly giving rise to unequal proportions of the different lymph node histologies and clinical stages; biopsy technics and histological preparation; and differences in the interpretation of the histological findings.[135] Bone marrow involvement is extremely rare in stages I (1%) and II (2%), and in nodular sclerosis (4%). For initial diagnosis of Hodgkin's disease from the bone marrow biopsy, Reed–Sternberg cells within a characteristic stromal environment are obligatory. However, when the disease has already been diagnosed by other technics, mononuclear Hodgkin cells within an appropriate setting are considered evidence of involvement. The lesions observed in such biopsies ranged from small paratrabecular foci to large, patchy areas of lyphogranulomatous tissue (Fig. 3.33b).

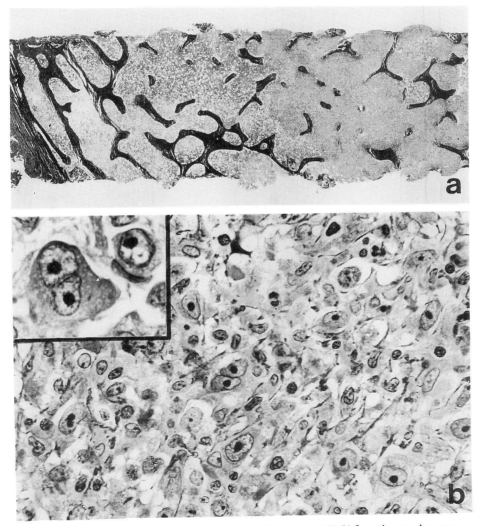

Fig. 3.33 Hodgkin's disease: (a) focal growth pattern. (Gomori × 10) (b) Lymphogranulomatous infiltration with low content of lymphocytes. (Gomori × 400) Reed–Sternberg and Hodgkin cells upper left. (Giemsa × 600)

Bone lesions ranged from osteolytic to osteosclerotic. Reed–Sternberg cells were found in 62% and Hodgkin cells in 100% of the involved cases (Fig. 3.33b *upper left*).[135-41]

Histological subdivisions
The degree of lymphocytic and epithelioid cell infiltrations constituted a significant prognostic factor and a reliable parameter for subtyping:[105,106]

1. Hodgkin's disease with low content of lymphocytes (58%) (Fig. 3.33b).
2. Hodgkin's disease with high content of lymphocytes (36%).
3. Hodgkin's disease with high content of epithelioid cells (6%).

Evolution of disease
Hodgkin's disease usually arises in a group of lymph nodes and spreads to adjacent nodes before metastasizing to other organs. Bone marrow involvement shows a multifocal pattern and by definition indicates stage IV. Hodgkin's lymphoma very rarely starts in the bone marrow. The presence of epithelioid-cell granulomas in negative bone marrow biopsies correlated with a favorable prognosis.[132,142] Bone marrow changes after chemotherapy with MOPP (mustine, vincristine, procarbazine and prednisolone) have been described by Myers et al[143] and others.[8] Twenty per cent of post-treatment patients showed hypocellularity, more pronounced in the posterior iliac crest and possibly a reaction to the radiotherapy; long-lasting megaloblastoid erythropoiesis is also frequently observed after multiagent chemotherapy.

ANGIOIMMUNOBLASTIC LYMPHADENOPATHY

Biopsies with involvement were detected in about 50% of cases diagnosed by lymph node histology. Multiple foci were observed with a heterogeneous cell population including immunoblasts, lymphocytes, centrocytes, plasma cells and eosiniophils. There were also arborizing capillaries, reticulin fibrosis and interstitial deposits of PAS positive material (Fig. 3.34).[144,145]

Diagnostic pitfalls
Similar focal 'lymphoid–histiocytic proliferations' have been found in the bone marrow biopsies of 38% of patients with AIDS (acquired immune deficiency syndrome).[146] Distinct morphological 'AIDS-patterns' in bone marrow biopsies have also been described recently.[147-149]

CONCLUDING REMARKS

Recent studies on bone marrow histology clearly demonstrate that four histologic parameters are of diagnostic relevance:

1. The proliferative cell system — the basis of all subdivisions.
2. The proliferation pattern, giving additional information for diagnosis and evolution of disease.
3. The tumor cell burden (vol%) — provides the basis for histological staging and supplements any clinical staging system.
4. The stromal reactions — influence the evolution and response to therapy of hematological neoplasias.

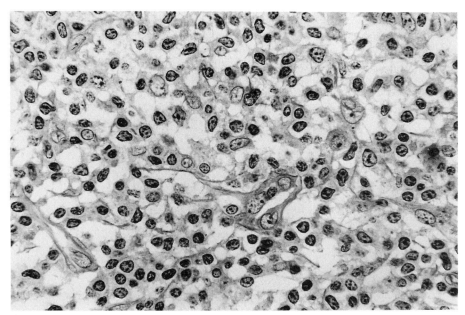

Fig. 3.34 Angioimmunoblastic lymphadenopathy with high content of capillaries and a heterogeneous lymphoid infiltration. (Giemsa × 400)

ACKNOWLEDGMENTS

The authors would like to express their gratitude to all colleagues who referred patients or sent biopsies specimens. The skilful assistance of the technical staff of the laboratories is gratefully acknowledged. The authors also would like to express their appreciation to Mrs H. Muthmann, Mrs H. Petry, Mrs G. Stark, Mrs I. Weltmeier and Mrs I. Werner for secretarial and technical assistance.

REFERENCES

1. Burkhardt R 1971 Bone marrow and bone tissue. In: Colour atlas of clinical Histopathology. Springer, Berlin
2. Duhamel G 1974 Histopathologie clinique de la moelle osseuse. Masson, Paris
3. Block M 1976 Text atlas of hematology. Lea and Febiger, Philadelphia
4. Rywlin A M 1976 Histopathology of the bone marrow. Little Brown, Boston
5. Krause J R 1981 Bone marrow biopsy. Churchill Livingstone, Edinburgh
6. Bartl R, Frisch B, Burkhardt R 1985 Bone marrow biopsies revisited. A new dimension for haematologic malignancies, 2nd edn. Karger, Basel
7. Wittels B 1985 Surgical pathology of bone marrow–core biopsy diagnosis. Saunders, Philadelphia
8. Frisch B, Lewis S M, Burkhardt R, Bartl R 1985 Biopsy pathology of bone and bone marrow. Chapman and Hall, London
9. Frisch B, Bartl R 1990 Atlas of bone marrow pathology. Kluwer Academic Publishers, London
10. Trentin J J 1971 Determination of bone marrow stem cell differentiation by stromal hemopoietic inductive microenvironments (HIM). American Journal of Pathology 65: 621
11. Singer J W, Keating A, Wight T N 1985 The human haematopoietic microenvironment. In: Hoffbrand (ed) Recent advances in haematology. Churchill Livingstone, Edinburgh, pp 1–24
12. Islam A, Catovsky D, Goldman J M, Galton D A G 1984 Studies on cellular interactions between stromal and haemopoietic stem cells in normal and leukemic bone marrows. Bibliotheca Haematologica 50: 17–30

13 Frisch B, Bartl R, Burkhardt R 1982 Bone marrow biopsy in clinical medicine: an overview. Haematologia, Budapest 3: 245–285
14 Burkhardt R, Frisch B, Bartl R 1982 Bone biopsy in haematological disorders. Journal of Clinical Pathology 35: 257–284
15 Rywlin A M 1976 Bone marrow histology, aspiration versus biopsy. American Journal of Clinical Pathology 66: 617–618
16 Frisch B, Bartl R 1984 Bone marrow biopsies updated. Bibliotheca Haematologica 50. Karger, Basel
17 Recker R R 1983 Bone histomorphometry: Techniques and interpretation. CRC Press, Boca Raton
18 Barer M, Jowsey J 1967 Bone formation and resorption in osteoporosis. Clinical Orthopaedics 52: 241–247
19 Capell D F, Hutchinson H E, Smith H G 1947 Marrow biopsy, preparation and use of parafin sections from sternal puncture material. British Medical Journal I: 403–404
20 Duncan H, Rao S D, Parfitt A M 1981 Complication of bone biopsy. In: Jee, Parfitt (eds) Bone histomorphometry. Société Nouvelle de Publications Médicales et Dentaires, Paris, pp 483–486
21 Malluche H H, Faugere M C 1986 Atlas of mineralized bone histology. Karger, Basel
22 Burkhalter J L, Patel B R 1983 Radionuclide bone scan as an aid in localizing lesion for bone biopsy. Skeletal Radiology 9: 246–247
23 Whitehouse W J 1977 Cancellous bone in the anterior part of the iliac crest. Calcified Tissue Research 26: 67–76
24 Burkhadt R, Kettner G, Boehm W et al 1987 Changes in trabecular bone, hematopoiesis and bone marrow vessels in aplastic anemia, primary osteoporosis, and old age: a comparative histomorphometric study. Bone 8: 157–164
25 Jamshidi K, Swaim W R 1971 Bone marrow biopsy with unaltered architecture – a new biopsy device. Journal of Laboratory and Clinical Medicine 77: 335–342
26 Ellis L D, Jensen W N, Westerman M P 1964 Needle biopsy of bone and marrow. Archives of Internal Medicine 114: 213–221
27 Westerman M P 1981 Bone marrow needle biopsy: an evaluation and critique. Seminars in Haematology 18: 293–300
28 Islam A 1982 Technical method. A new bone marrow biopsy needle with core securing device. Journal of Clinical Pathology 35: 359–364
29 Hodgson S F, Johnson K A, Muhs J M, Lufkin E G, McCarthy J T 1986 Out patient percutaneous biopsy of the iliac crest: methods, morbidity, and patient acceptance. Mayo Clinic Proceedings 61: 28–33
30 Bordier P, Matrajt H, Miravet L, Hioco D 1964 Mesure histologique de la masse et de la résorption des travées osseuses. Pathologie Biologie 12: 1238–1243
31 Lalor B, Freemont A, Carlile S 1986 An improved transilial crest bone biopsy drill for quantitative histomorphometry. Bone 7: 273–276
32 TeVelde J, Den Ottolander G J, Haak H L et al 1978 Iliac bone marrow trephine biopsy. Netherland Journal of Medicine 21: 221–228
33 Bartl R, Burkhardt R, Vondracek H, Sommerfeld W, Hagemeister E 1978 Rationelle Beckenkamm-Biopsie. Längsteilung der Proben zur Anwendung von mehreren Präparationsverfahren ohne Materialverlust. Klinische Wochenschrift 56: 545–550
34 Bartl R, Frisch B, Buchenrieder B et al 1984 Multiparameter studies on 650 bone marrow biopsy cores. Diagnostic value of combined utilisation of imprints, cryostat and plastic sections in medical practice. Bibliotheca Haematologica, 50: 1–16
35 Burkhardt R 1984 Histology of plastic embedded biopsies. In: Lennert K, Hübner K (eds) Pathology of the bone marrow. Fischer, Stuttgart, pp 10–14
36 TeVelde J, Burkhardt R, Kleiverda K, Leenheers-Binnendijk L, Sommerfeld W 1977 Methylmethacrylate as an embedding medium in histopathology. Histopathology 1: 319–330
37 Rowden G, Sacher R A, More N S 1982 Plastic embedded specimens for evaluation of bone marrow. In: Roath S (ed.) Topical reviews in haematology, vol II. Wright, Bristol
38 Islam A, Frisch B 1985 Plastic embedding in routine histology I: Preparation of semi-thin sections of undecalcified marrow cores. Histopathology 9: 1263–1274
39 Brinn N T 1979 Glycol methacrylate for routine, special stains, histochemistry, enzyme histochemistry and immunohistochemistry. A simplified method for surgical biopsy tissue. Journal of Histochemistry 3: 125–130
40 Block M H, Trenner L, Ruegg P, Karr M 1982 Glycol methacrylate embedding technique emphasizing cost containment, ultrarapid processing, and adaptability to a variety of staining techniques. Laboratory Medicine 13: 290–298
41 Beckstead J H 1986 The bone marrow biopsy. A diagnostic strategy. Archives of Pathology and Laboratory Medicine 110: 175–179

42 Beckstead J H, Halverson P S , Ries, C A, Bainton D F 1981 Enzyme histochemistry and immunohistochemistry on biopsy specimens of pathologic human bone marrow. Blood 57: 1088-1098
43 Falini B, Martelli M F, Tarallo D J et al 1984 Immunohistological analysis of human bone marrow trephine biopsies using monoclonal antibodies. British Journal of Haematology 56: 365-386
44 Chilosi M, Pizzolo G, Janossy G, Bofill M, Fiore-Donati L 1982 Enzyme histochemical analysis on cryostat sections of human bone marrow. Journal of Clinical Pathology 35: 1220-1226
45 Kerndrup G, Pallesen G, Melsen F, Mosekilde L 1980 Histomorphometrical determination of bone marrow cellularity in iliac crest biopsies. Scandinavian Journal of Haematology 24: 110-114
46 Revell P A 1983 Histomorphometry of bone. Journal of Clinical Pathology 36: 1323-1331
47 Robbins S L, Angell M 1971 Basic pathology. Saunders, Philadelphia pp 65-67
48 Jacobs A 1985 Myelodysplastic syndromes: pathogenesis, functional abnormalities, and clinical implications. Journal of Clinical Pathology 38: 1201-1217
49 Koeffler H P 1986 Myelodysplastic syndromes. Seminars in Hematology 23: 284-299
50 Block M, Jacobson L O, Bethard W F 1953 Preleukemic acute human leukemia. Journal of the American Medical Association 152: 1018-1028
51 Tricot G, Vlietinck R, Boogaerts M A et al 1985 Prognostic factors in the myelodysplastic syndromes: importance of initial data on peripheral blood counts, bone marrow cytology, trephine biopsy and chromosomal analysis. British Journal of Haematology 60: 19-32
52 Tricot G 1986 Annotation. Evolution of the myelodysplastic syndromes. British Journal of Haematology 63: 609-614
53 Frisch B, Bartl R, Chaichik S 1986 Therapy-induced myelodysplasia and secondary leukemia. Scandinavian Journal of Haematology (Suppl 45) 36: 38-47
54 Frisch B, Bartl R 1986 Bone marrow histology in myelodysplastic syndromes. Scandinavian Journal of Haematology (Suppl 45) 36: 21-37
55 Tricot G, deWolf Peeters C, Vlietinck R, Verwilghen R L The importance of bone marrow biopsy in myelodysplastic disorders. In: Frisch B, Bartl R (eds) Bone marrow biopsies updated. Bibliotheca Haematologica 50: 31-40
56 Bennett J M, Catovsky D, Daniel M T et al 1982 The French-American-British (FAB) Cooperative Group. Proposals for the classification of the myelodysplastic syndromes. British Journal of Haematology 51: 189-199
57 Galton D A G 1986 The myelodysplastic syndromes. Scandinavian Journal of Haematology (Suppl 45) 36: 11-20
58 Tricot G, Boogaerts M A, deWolfe-Peeters C, van den Berghe H, Verwilghen R L 1985 The myelodysplastic syndromes: different evolution patterns based on sequential morphological and cytogenetic investigations. British Journal of Haematology 59: 659-670
59 Sultan C, Sigaux F, Imbert M, Reyes F 1981 Acute myelodysplasia with myelofibrosis: a report of 8 cases. British Journal of Haematology 49: 11-16
60 Catovsky D, Tavares de Castro J 1983 The classification of acute leukaemia (AL) and its clinical significance. Schweizerische medizinische Wochenschrift 40: 1434-1437
61 Catovsky D, deCardullo L S, O'Brien M et al 1981 Cytochemical markers of differentiation in acute leukemia. Cancer Research 41: 4824
62 Foon K A, Todd R F 1986 Immunologic classification of leukemia and lymphoma. Blood 68: 1-31
63 Janossy G, Hoffbrand A V, Greaves M F et al 1980 Terminal transferase enzyme assay and immunological membrane markers in the diagnosis of leukaemia. A multiparameter analysis of 300 cases. British Journal of Haematology 44: 221
64 Rappaport H 1973 Histologic criteria for diagnosis and classification of acute leukemias. In: Mathé G, Pouillart P, Schwarzenberg L (eds) Recent results in cancer research, vol .43, Nomenclature, methodology and results of clinical trials in acute leukemias. Springer, Berlin, pp 35-42
65 Islam A, Catovsky D, Goldman J H, Galton D A G 1985 Bone marrow biopsy changes in acute myeloid leukemia, I: observations before chemotherapy. Histopathology 9: 930-957
66 Muretto P, Izzi T, Grianti C, Moretti L 1983 Histomorphologic study of bone marrow in acute leukemia following chemotherapy and autologous bone marrow transplantation. Tumori 69: 239-248
67 Bennett J M, Catovsky D, Daniel M T et al (FAB Co-operative Group) 1976 Proposals for the classification of the acute leukemias. British Journal of Haematology 33: 451
68 Bennett J M, Catovsky D, Daniel M T et al (FAB Co-operative Group) 1981 The morphological classification of acute lymphoblastic leukemia. Concordance among observers and clinical correlations. British Journal of Haematology 47: 553

69 Howe R B, Bloomfield C D, McKenna R W 1982 Hypocellular acute leukemia. American Journal of Medicine 72: 391
70 Maddox A M, Keating M J, Smith T L et al 1986 Prognostic factors for survival of 194 patients with low infiltrate leukemia. Leukemia Research 10: 995–1006
71 Manoharan A Horsley R, Pitney W R 1979 The reticulin content of bone marrow in acute leukemia in adults. British Journal of Haematology 43: 185–190
72 Truong L D, Saleem A, Schwarzt M R 1984 Acute myelofibrosis. A report of four cases and review of the literature. Medicine 63: 182
73 Dameshek W 1951 Some speculations on the myeloproliferative syndromes. Blood 6: 372–375
74 Gilbert H S 1973 The spectrum of myeloproliferative disorders. Medical Clinics of North America 57: 355–393
75 Spiers A S D 1984 Chronic granulocytic leukemia. Medical Clinics of North America 68: 713–727
76 Ellis J T, Peterson P 1979 The bone marrow in polycythemia vera. Pathology Annual 14: 383–403
77 Vykoupil K G, Thiele J, Stangel W, Krmpotic E, Georgii A 1980 Polycythaemia vera. I: Histopathology, ultrastructure and cytogenesis of the bone marrow in comparison with secondary polycythaemia. Virchows Archiv Pathologische Anatomie 389: 307–324
78 Lucie N P, Young G 1983 Marrow cellularity in the diagnosis of polycythaemia. Journal of Clinical Pathology 36: 180–183
79 Jäger K, Burkhardt R, Bartl R, Frisch B, Mahl G 1983 Lymphoid infiltrates in chronic myeloproliferative disorders (MPD). In: Lennert K, Hübner K (eds) Pathology of the bone marrow. Fischer, Stuttgart, pp 174–176
80 Frisch B, Bartl R, Burkhardt R, Jäger K, Pappenberger R 1984 Bone marrow histology in the chronic myeloproliferative disorders: criteria for recognition, classification and prognostic evaluation. A study of 3500 biopsies. Bibliotheca Haematologica 50: 57–80
81 Georgii A, Vykoupil K F, Thiele J 1984 Classification of chronic myeloproliferative diseases by bone marrow biopsies. Bibliotheca Haematologica 50: 41–56
82 Burkhardt R, Bartl R, Jäger K et al 1986 Working classification of chronic myeloproliferative disorders based on histological, haematological, and clinical findings. Journal of Clinical Pathology 39: 237–252
83 Ellis J T, Peterson P, Geller S A, Rappaport H 1986 Studies of the bone marrow in polycythemia vera and the evolution of myelofibrosis and second hematologic malignancies. Seminars in Hematology 23: 144–155
84 Murphy S, Iland H, Rosenthal D, Laszlo J 1986 Essential thrombocythemia: an interim report from the polycythemia vera study group. Seminars in Hematology 23: 177–182
85 Sedlacek S M, Curtis J L, Weintraub J, Levin J 1986 Essential thrombocythemia and leukemic transformation. Medicine 65: 353
86 Verhest A, Monsieur R 1983 Philadelphia chromosome-positive thrombocythemia with leukemic transformation. New England Journal of Medicine 308: 1603
87 Georgii A, Vykoupil K F, Thiele J 1980 Chronic megakaryocytic granulocytic myelosis-CMGM. A subtype of chronic myeloid leukemia. Virchows Archiv Pathologische Anatomie 389: 253–268
88 Lazzarino M, Morra E, Castello A et al 1986 Myelofibrosis in chronic granulocytic leukemia: clinicopathologic correlations and prognostic significance. British Journal of Haematology 64: 227–240
89 Islam A, Catovsky D, Goldman J M, Galton D A G 1981 Histological study of the bone marrow in blast transformation. II: Bone marrow fibre content before and after autografting. Histopathology 5: 491–498
90 Burkhardt R, Bartl R, Beil E et al 1975 Myelofibrosis-osteomyelosclerosis syndrome. Review of literature and histomorphology. In: Advances in the biosciences, vol 16. Pergamon Press, Oxford, pp 9–56
91 Frisch B, Bartl R 1985 Histology of myelofibrosis and osteomyelosclerosis. In: Lewis S M (ed.) Myelofibrosis, Pathophysiology and clinical management. Dekker, New York pp 51–86
92 Caligaris-Cappio F, Vigliani R, Novarino A, Camussi G, Campama D, Gavosto F 1981 Idiopathic myelofibrosis: a possible role for immune complexes in the pathogenesis of bone marrow fibrosis. British Journal of Haematology 49: 17–21
93 Hasselbalch H, Nielsen H, Berild D, Kappelgaard E 1985 Circulating immune complexes in myelofibrosis. Scandinavian Journal of Haematology 34: 177–180
94 Castro-Malaspina H, Moore M A S 1982 Pathophysiological mechanisms operating in the development of myelofibrosis: role of megakaryocytes. Nouvelles Revue Francaise d'Hématologie 24: 221–226
95 Moore M A S 1982 Pathogenesis of MF. In: Hoffbrand AV (ed) Recent advances in haematology. Churchill Livingstone, Edinburgh, pp 136–139

96 Burkhardt R, Bartl R, Jäger K et al 1984 Chronic myeloproliferative disorders (CMPD). Pathology Research and Practice 179: 131–186
97 Lewis S M, Szur L 1963 Malignant myelosclerosis. British Medical Journal II: 472–477
98 Bergsman K L, Van Slyck E J 1971 Acute myelofibrosis: an accelerated variant of agnogenic metaplasia. Annals of Internal Medicine 74: 232–235
99 Mahl G, Frisch B, Bartl R et al 1984 Acute myelofibrosis: only one extreme in the spectrum of 'idiopathic' myelofibrosis. Lenner K, Hübner K (eds) Pathology of the bone marrow. Fischer, Stuttgart pp 206–207
100 Thiele J, Krech R, Vykoupil K F, Georgii A 1984 Malignant (acute) myelosclerosis – a clinical and pathological study in 6 patients. Scandinavian Journal of Haematology 33: 95–109
101 Brunning R D, McKenna R W 1979 Bone marrow manifestations of malignant lymphoma and lymphoma-like conditions. In: Sommers S C, Rosen P P (eds) Pathology Annual, part 1. Appleton-Century-Crofts, New York, pp 1–59
102 Bartl R, Frisch B, Burkhardt R et al 1982 Assessment of bone marrow histology in the malignant lymphomas (non-Hodgkin's): correlation with clinical factors for diagnosis, prognosis, classification and staging. British Journal of Haematology 51: 511–530
103 Foucar K, McKenna R W, Frizzera G, Brunning R D 1982 Bone marrow and blood involvement by lymphoma in relationship to the Lukes-Collins classification. Cancer 49: 888–897
104 Bartl R, Frisch B, Burkhardt R, Jäger K, Pappenberger R, Hoffmann-Fezer G 1984 Lymphoproliferations in the bone marrow: identification and evolution, classification and staging. Journal of Clinical Pathology 37: 233–254
105 Bartl R, Frisch B, Kettner G et al 1984 Histologic classification of lymphoproliferative disorders in the bone marrow. Bibliotheca Haematologica 50: 98–127
106 Bartl R, Hausmann M-L, Frisch B et al 1988 Comparative histology of malignant lymphomas in lymph node and bone marrow. British Journal of Haematology 69: 229–237
107 Lipshutz M D, Mir R, Rai K R, Sawitsky A 1980 Bone marrow biopsy and clinical staging in chronic lymphocytic leukemia. Cancer 46: 1422–1427
108 Rozman C, Hernandez-Nieto L, Montserrat E, Brugger R 1981 Prognostic significance of bone-marrow patterns in chronic lymphocytic leukaemia. British Journal of Haematology 47: 529–537
109 Bartl R, Frisch B, Burkhardt R, Hoffmann-Fezer G, Demmler K, Sund M 1982 Assessment of marrow trephine in relation to staging in chronic lymphocytic leukemia. British Journal of Haematology 51: 1–15
110 Frisch B, Bartl R 1988 Histologic classification and staging of chronic lymphocyt leukemia. Acta Haematologica 79: 140–152
111 Rozman C, Montserrat E, Rodriguez-Fernandez J M et al 1984 Bone marrow histologic pattern – the best single prognostic parameter in chronic lymphocytic leukemia: a multivariate survival analysis of 329 cases. Blood 64: 642–648
112 Geisler C, Ralfkiaer E, Hansen M M, Jou-Jensen K, Larsen S O 1986 The bone marrow histological pattern has independent prognostic value in early stage chronic lymphocytic leukaemia. British Journal of Haematology 62: 47–54
113 Galton D A G, Goldman J M, Whiltshaw, E, Catovsky D, Henry K, Goldenberg G J 1974 Prolymphocytic leukaemia. British Journal of Haematology 27: 7–23
114 Catovsky D 1982 Prolymphocytic and hairy cell leukemias. Gunz F W, Henderson E S (eds) Leukemia 4th edn. Grune and Stratton, New York
115 Peterson L C, Bloomfield C D, Brunning R D 1980 Relationship of clinical staging and lymphocyte morphology to survival in chronic lymphocytic leukaemia. British Journal of Haematology 45: 563–567
116 Rywlin A M, Ortega R S, Dominguez G J 1974 Lymphoid nodules of bone marrow, normal and abnormal. Blood 43: 389–400
117 Pizzolo G, Chilosi M, Cetto G L, Fiore-Donati L, Janossy G 1982 Immuno-histological analysis of bone-marrow involvement in lymphoproliferative disorders. British Journal of Haematology 50: 95–100
118 Catovsky D, Pettit J E, Galletto J et al 1974 The B-lymphoctye nature of the 'hairy' cell of leukemic reticuloendotheliosis. British Journal of Haematology 26: 29–37
119 Cawley J C, Burns G F, Hayhoe F G J 1980 Hairy cell leukemia. Springer, Berlin
120 Burke J S 1978 The value of the bone-marrow biopsy in the diagnosis of hairy cell leukemia. American Journal of Clinical Pathology 70: 876–884
121 Bartl R, Frisch B, Hill W, Burkhardt R, Sommerfeld W, Sund M 1983 Bone marrow histology in hairy cell leukemia: identification of subtypes and their prognostic significance. American Journal of Clinical Pathology 79: 531–545
122 Mann R B, Jaffe E S, Berard C W 1979 Malignant lymphomas–a conceptual understanding of morphologic diversity. American Journal of Pathology 94: 105–157

123 Bartl R, Frisch B, Mahl G et al 1983 Bone marrow histology in Waldenström's macroglobulinaemia. Clinical relevance of subtype recognition. Scandinavian Journal of Haematology 31: 359–375
124 Emmerich B, Pemsl M, Wüst I et al 1983 Conversion of an IGM-secreting immunocytoma in a high grade malignant lymphoma of immunoblastic type. Blut 46: 81–84
125 Callihan T, Holbert J, Berard C 1983 Neoplasms of terminal B-cell differentiation. In: Sommer, Rosen (eds) Malignant lymphomas. Appleton-Century-Crofts, Norwalk, Conn. pp 169–268
126 Bergsagel D, Rider W 1985 Plasma cell neoplasma. In: DeVita, Hellmann, Rosenberg (eds) Cancer principles and practice of oncology, 2nd edn. Lippincott, Philadelphia
127 Oken M M 1984 Multiple myeloma. Medical Clinics of North America 3: 757–787
128 Greipp P R, Raymond N M, Kyle R A, O'Fallon W M 1985 Multiple myeloma: significance of plasmablastic subtype in morphological classification. Blood 65: 305–310
129 Bartl R, Frisch B, Burkhardt R et al 1982 Bone marrow histology in myeloma: its importance in diagnosis, prognosis, classifications and staging. British Journal of Haematology 51: 511–530
130 Canale D D, Collins R D 1974 Use of bone marrow particle sections in the diagnosis of multiple myeloma. American Journal of Clinical Pathology 61: 383–392
131 Bartl R, Frisch B, Faleh-Moghadam A et al 1987 Histological classification and staging of multiple myeloma. A retrospective and preoperative study of 674 cases. American Journal of Clinical Pathology 87: 342–355
132 Kyle R A, Greipp P R 1980 Smoldering multiple myeloma. New England Journal of Medicine 302: 1347–1349
133 Greipp P R, Kyle R A 1983 Clinical, morphological and cell kinetic differences among multiple myeloma, monoclonal gammopathy of undetermined significance and smoldering multiple myeloma. Blood 62: 166–171
134 Sutcliffe S B J, Timothy A R, Lister T A 1979 Staging in Hodgkin's disease. Clinics in Haematology 8: 593–609
135 Bartl R, Frisch B, Burkhardt R, Huhn D, Pappenberger R 1982 Assessment of bone marrow histology in Hodgkin's disease: correlation with clinical factors. British Journal of Haematology 51: 345–360
136 Bennet J M, Gralnick H R, DeVita V T 1968 Bone marrow biopsy in Hodgkin's disease. New England Journal of Medicine 278: 1179
137 TeVelde, Den Ottolander J G, Spaamder P J, van den Berg C, Hartgrink-Groeneveld C A 1978 The bone marrow in Hodgkin's disease: the non-involved marrow. Histopathology 2: 31–46
138 Webb D I, Ubogy G, Silver R T 1970 Importance of bone marrow biopsy in the clinical staging of Hodgkin's disease. Cancer 26: 313–317
139 Weiss R B, Brunning R D, Kennedy B J 1975 Hodgkin's disease in the bone marrow. Cancer 36: 2077–2083
140 Lee R E, Ellis L D 1976 Histopathologic and clinical findings in Hodgkin's disease of the bone marrow. American Journal of Clinical Pathology 65: 268
141 O'Caroll D I, McKenna R W, Brunning R D 1976 Bone marrow manifestations of Hodgkin's disease. Cancer 38: 1717–1728
142 Sacks E L, Donaldson S S, Gordon J, Dorfman R F 1978 Epithelioid granulomas associated with Hodgkin's disease. Clinical correlations in 55 previously untreated patients. Cancer 41: 562–567
143 Myers C E, Chabner R A, DeVita V T, Gralnick H R 1974 Bone marrow involvement in Hodgkin's disease, pathology and response to MOPP chemotherapy. Blood 44: 197–204
144 Pangalis G A, Moran E M, Rappaport H 1978 Blood and bone marrow findings in angioimmunoblastic lymphadenopathy. Blood 51: 71–83
145 Ghani A M, Krause J R 1985 Bone marrow biopsy findings in angioimmunoblastic lymphadenopathy. British Journal of Haematology 61: 203–213
146 Guarda L A, Butler J J 1983 Lymphoma versus AIDS. American Journal of Clinical Pathology 80: 547
147 Castella A, Croxson T S, Mildvan D, Witt D H, Zalusky R 1985 The bone marrow in AIDS. A histologic, hematologic, and microbiologic study. American Journal of Clinical Pathology 84: 425–432
148 Geller S A, Muller R, Greenberg M L, Siegal F P 1985 Acquired immunodeficiency syndrome. Archives of Pathology and Laboratory Medicine 109: 138–141
149 Shenoy C M, Liu J J 1986 Bone marrow findings in acquired immunodeficiency syndrome (AIDS). American Journal of the Medical Sciences 292: 372–375

4
Ultrastructure of the Leukemic Cell

J. Breton-Gorius

INTRODUCTION

For 100 years, histochemical reactions have been widely used in association with the Giemsa stain for the recognition of normal and leukemic hemopoietic cells. However, the study of films by light microscopic examination has some limitations.

As a consequence, hematologists have turned increasingly to electron microscopy for the analysis of the fine structure of cells and for determining the nature of some poorly differentiated cells. Over a period of 25 years, many papers have appeared on the ultrastructural aspect of leukemic cells and on the search for possible virus particles. The latter has been disappointing in the case of human leukemia. With the development of ultrastructural cytochemical methods, a new field of investigation was opened. More recently the membrane labeling of leukemic blasts by monoclonal antibodies (McAbs) using the immunogold method at electron microscopy provided new and useful information.

This chapter reviews the contribution of conventional transmission electron microscopy, cytochemical and immunogold methods to the knowledge of normal and leukemic cell differentiation; lymphoid differentiation is excluded and will be considered separately.

CONTRIBUTION OF CONVENTIONAL ELECTRON MICROSCOPY TO THE KNOWLEDGE OF LEUKEMIC CELLS

METHODS

The preparation of bone marrow cells
Bone marrow specimens are usually obtained by sternal aspiration of a suspension of marrow particles, contaminated by some blood; they are immediately immersed in a fixative solution. The sample is transferred to a Petri dish; the marrow particles can then be collected with a Pasteur pipette and resuspended in fresh fixative solution. Because no anticoagulant has been added, coagulation may occur in some cases; marrow fragments can be distinguished easily from clots as the latter look like cells that have been stained red.

In advanced myelofibrosis, or in aplasia in which the aspiration is unsuccessful, marrow biopsy can be performed; after prefixation, marrow particles may be separated from the bone marrow spicules under microscopic examination.

Collection of peripheral blood leukocytes
Twenty millilitres of venous blood are obtained in polyethylene syringes wetted with aqueous heparin. The buffy coat may be separated by several procedures.

When a normal or increased number of leukocytes is present, the usual procedure for concentrating the nucleated cells consists of sedimentation at room temperature in a tube slanted at 45° for 1 hour; the buffy coat is then removed with a thin Pasteur pipette and fixed. A good concentration of cells is also obtained by centrifugating in narrow Kaplow tubes[1] at 2000 revs./min for 10 min which increases the thickness of the buffy coat.

Separation of leukocytes from erythrocytes can also be enhanced by increasing the sedimentation in the presence of macromolecules. After sedimentation the white layer and supernatant platelet-rich plasma are collected and centrifugated for 5 min at 200 × g to concentrate the leukocytes with platelets remaining in suspension.[2] A mixture can also be prepared of 24 volumes of 9% Dextran T500 (Pharmacia, Sweden) in physiological saline with 10 volumes of 38% Radioselectan (Schering, France) in distilled water. One volume is transferred to a tube, and one volume of blood slowly added with a pipette. After 45 min of sedimentation, the supernatant contents leukocytes and platelets. The two categories of cells can be separated by centrifugation for 10 min at 100 × g. The pellet contains the leukocytes whilst the platelets remain in the supernatant.

Anderson's[3] method is a very good one when the leukocyte count is low or when the cells under study are rare. It is based on the fact that glutaraldehyde added to the buffy coat causes solidification of the plasma; subsequently, this zone may be cut into small blocks that will be oriented in the embedding material. In this procedure, the specimen is centrifuged giving layers of erythrocytes, leukocytes, platelets and plasma. The plasma is then removed and replaced with glutaraldehyde fixative. The buffy coat can be removed as a solid disk and cut into slices.

Leukemic blasts can also be separated by Ficoll–metrizoate gradient density centrifugation (Lymphoprep, Nyegaard, Oslo, density: 1.077).[4].

Fixation, dehydration and embedding
The marrow particles and the leukocyte suspension are prefixed by aldehyde solutions. The most commonly used aldehyde is 1.25% glutaraldehyde freshly prepared from distilled glutaraldehyde (TAAB Laboratories) in 0.1 mol/l phosphate buffer (pH 7.2) or in 0.1 mol/l cacodylate-HCl buffer (pH 7.4) with 1% sucrose.[5] Good results may also be obtained in a mixture of 1% freshly prepared paraformaldehyde and 3% glutaraldehyde in 0.1 mol/l sodium cacodylate buffer pH 7.4 with 0.5% $CaCl_2$.[6]

In order to preserve the integrity of microtubules, the fixation in aldehydes is made at room temperature for 30 min. Subsequently, marrow particles or leukocytes are washed three times in the same buffer – washing of a cell suspension involves centrifuging and resuspending the cell pellet obtained in buffer.

Subsequently, cells are postfixed in 1% osium tetroxide (OsO_4) in phosphate or cacodylate buffer for 30 min at 4°C, and are then rinsed in distilled water. The treatment with 1% uranyl acetate in distilled water for 60 min increases the density of DNA, ribosomes and all membranes; however, this procedure is not recommended for studying neutrophil leukocytes since the azurophil granules appear to be extracted. Cells in suspension are centrifuged at 10 000 × g in narrow tubes for 10 min. The pellet is then cut into pieces and treated as bone marrow fragments. Dehydration is accomplished at room temperature in graded ethanols (70°, 90° and absolute ethanol, two baths of 20 min for each). Most plastic embedding mixtures are not miscible with ethanol and, therefore, propylene oxide is used as the intermediate solvent; after two short passages, equal volumes of epon and propylene oxide left for 1 h facilitate the infiltration of the resin. The hardness of the final block can be adjusted by the ratio of two mixtures.

Solution A	Epikote (epon) 812	31 ml
	DDSA (Ciba Labs or Ladd Res. Indust.)	50 ml
Solution B	Epikote 812	100 ml
	Methyl nadic anhydride (MNA)	89 ml

Usually 7 ml of solution B and 3 ml of solution A are mixed with a final addition of six big drops of the activator DMP-30 (Ciba Labs or Ladd Res. Indust.). The mixture could also be prepared in advance and kept at −20°C in a 20-ml syringe. The mixture contains Epikote 48.8%, DDSA 16.5%, MNA 33.2%, DMP 1.5%. Each syringe is defrosted just prior to use.

Each marrow particle, or piece of pellet, is introduced into the bottom of a gelatin capsule; this is then filled with the final mixture of A, B and DMP. The polymerization is carried out at 60°C for 20 hours. Thin sections cut on an ultramicrotome are counterstained with alkaline lead citrate for 5 seconds preceded by uranyl acetate for 10 min (except when samples have been previously treated by uranyl acetate following the postfixation step).

For this purpose, the grids containing the sections are set on drops of solution in a plastic film. The counterstaining solutions are as follows:

1. Uranyl acetate: saturated aqueous uranyl acetate is filtered and diluted to half the concentration with distilled water.
2. Alkaline lead citrate (modified Reynolds'[7] method):
    lead nitrate 1 mol/l
    sodium citrate 1 mol/l
    sodium hydroxide 1 mol/l
    Mix 16 ml of water, 3 ml of sodium citrate and 2 ml of lead nitrate to form a precipitate. The solution is shaken and, after addition of 4 ml of sodium hydroxide, it clears. This solution is kept at 4°C in individual syringes.

After staining, the grids are washed with distilled water and dried on filter paper.

MAIN RESULTS

From morphological examination of leukemic cells an inventory of quantitative and qualitative alterations of the cell organelles has been devised. Numerous lesions or inclusions have been demonstrated which are not normally detectable by light microscopy. Abundant examples of ultrastructural contributions increasing knowledge about various leukemic cells can be found in several books.[8-10] All the abnormalities described in leukemic cells will not be reviewed, but Table 4.1 indicates the most frequent and striking features.

CONTRIBUTION OF CYTOCHEMICAL TECHNICS TO THE KNOWLEDGE OF NORMAL CELLS

METHODS

Peroxidases
Graham and Karnovsky[19] introduced a new substrate in 1966 – 3,3'diaminobenzidine (DAB). This substance, derived from benzidine, is oxidized by heme enzymes in the presence

Table 4.1 Some contributions of conventional electron microscopy to the study of leukemic cells

Types of leukemia	Abnormalities which may be present
Chronic lymphocytic leukemia	Crystalline inclusions in ER with IgM content[8,9,11]
Myeloma and Waldenström's disease	Nuclear inclusions[8,10,12]
Hairy cell leukemia	Ribosome–lamella complexes[13,14]
Acute myeloblastic leukemia	Fibrillar bodies[8]
	Abnormal granules[15]
	Asynchrony and anarchy of development of organelles[15]
	Periodicity array of dense lines in Auer bodies[9,15,16]
	Nuclear pockets[8,17]
	Intracytoplasmic crystalline inclusions[18]

of hydrogen peroxide. Oxidized DAB is an electron-dense insoluble polymer, whose density increases after osmium tetroxide postfixation. Myeloperoxidase (MPO), present in the monocyte and neutrophil series, and peroxidases from eosinophil and basophil series can easily be detected using the Graham–Karnovsky method after the usual glutaraldehyde prefixation. However, some other peroxidase or peroxidase-like enzymes can be inhibited; their demonstration requires special methods. Thus, the platelet peroxidase (PPO) present in the endoplasmic reticulum of megakaryocytes and platelets[20-22] and the peroxidase-like enzyme of hairy cells[23] are only revealed with good reproducibility by the method introduced by Roels[24] in which unfixed cells are directly incubated in buffered DAB medium. The cell morphology is not always well preserved but all the heme enzymes are revealed. PPO is also regularly demonstrated by Anderson's method[25] in which low concentrations of aldehydes are mixed with tannic acid. However, dependent on the batch of tannic acid, inconsistent results have been obtained in several countries. Using a newly proposed method,[22] PPO has been regularly detected (see below).

Graham and Karnovsky technic[19]
Bone marrow particles or buffy coat cells are fixed for 30 min at 4°C with 1.25% distilled glutaraldehyde in 0.1 mol/l phosphate buffer. The marrow particles and blood leukocytes are subsequently washed three times in 0.1 mol/l phosphate buffer. As DAB penetrates slowly into the bone marrow particles, 40 μm thick sections of bone marrow, cut on a Smith-Farquhar TC-2 tissue sectioner, are incubated in the DAB medium (see below). Marrow particles can also be pre-incubated for a long period (24 h) in DAB alone at 4°C in order to facilitate the penetration, before finally incubating in fresh DAB medium. Samples are incubated for 30 min at room temperature and in the dark, in DAB medium that has been prepared as follows: 0.05 mol/l Tris-HCl buffer pH 7.6 containing DAB, and 0.1 ml 1% H_2O_2 (freshly diluted from a 30% solution).

If free base DAB (K and K Laboratories, Plainview, New York) is used, a saturated solution is prepared by shaking 2–3 mg of DAB with 10 ml buffer. This solution is filtered before use.

DAB–tetra-HCl (Sigma Chemical Company, St Louis, Missouri) is more soluble: 5 mg are dissolved in 10 ml of buffer. The pH is adjusted to pH 7.6 with 1 mol/l sodium hydroxide.

The specificity of the reaction is determined by control incubations, in which either DAB or H_2O_2 has been omitted. All incubations are followed by two washes of the tissue or cells in 0.1 mol/l phosphate buffer and then by postfixation for 30 min in 1% osmium tetroxide solution. The cells are then processed as indicated previously. In order to evaluate the dense reaction product of oxidized DAB, sections are examined first without lead citrate counterstaining.

Roels technic[24]
Unfixed cells are incubated for 10 min to 1 h in a medium containing 20 mg DAB, 0.01 ml 3% H_2O_2 in 10 ml Ringer-Tris buffer pH 7.3. After washing in Ringer-Tris buffer, cells are fixed by glutaraldehyde followed by osmium tetroxide.

Anderson technic[25]
Prior to fixation, the buffy coat must be centrifuged at low speed for 10 min and then washed twice in Hanks' balanced salt solution in order to eliminate plasma proteins that would precipitate with the fixative. The bone marrow fragments obtained by aspiration in a heparinized syringe are washed several times in Hanks' solution. The fixative consists of 1% tannic acid (E. Merck, Darmstadt), 2% paraformaldehyde, and 0.5% distilled glutaraldehyde (25% biological grade, TAAB, England) in 0.1 mol/l phosphate buffer at pH 7.2. The fixative is prepared just prior to use, filtered and chilled at 4°C. Cells are fixed for 1 h at 4°C,

washed in phosphate buffer and are incubated in DAB medium, or can be stored at 4°C for prolonged periods before incubation in DAB medium; this medium contains 20 mg of DAB and 0.1 ml H_2O_2 at 1% in 10 ml 0.05 mol/l Tris-HCl buffer. The pH is readjusted to 7.6 with 1 mol/l sodium hydroxide. Incubation is carried out in a dark room at room temperature for 1 h. The cells are then rinsed in several changes of phosphate buffer (0.1 mol/l, pH 7.2) and postfixed for 30 min in a 1% solution of osmium tetroxide in phosphate buffer.

Fixation which preserves PPO activity[22]
In contrast to published views,[21,26] the high concentration of glutaraldehyde is not responsible for the inhibition of PPO activity. When the buffer used to dilute the glutaraldehyde was made isotonic by the addition of dextrose (Gey's basic salts) it was found that glutaraldehyde at a concentration greater than 1% did not abolish the PPO activity,[22] whilst the same concentration of fixative in 0.1 mol/l phosphate buffer caused inhibition.[22] In this complex Gey's medium, which also contained EGTA and $MgCl_2$, only the dextrose appeared to be essential. However, since the buffer preserves the polymerization of tubulin and maintains good morphology, only this method is currently used routinely in the author's laboratory for PPO detection.

To prepare Gey's buffer, *solution A* must be prepared with:

7 g	NaCl
0.37 g	KCl
0.225 g	$Na_2HPO_4 \cdot 7\ H_2O$
0.0237 g	KH_2PO_4
1 g	dextrose
5 mg	phenol red

in 100 ml H^2

This pink solution A must be kept at 4°C.

Solution stock:
10 ml solution A
83 ml H_2O
5 ml 0.1 mol/l tris (hydroxymethyl) aminomethane
2 ml 0.1 mol/l $MgCl_2$

Gey's buffer:
49 ml solution stock
1 ml 0.1 mol/l EGTA at pH 6.9

Gey's buffer must be adjusted to pH 7.2 and can be kept at 4°C. The cells were fixed in 1.25% glutaraldehyde in Gey's buffer for 10 min at room temperature. After three washes in Gey's buffer, cells were incubated in 2 mg/ml DAB medium[19] for 1 h. After three washes in Tris buffer, they were treated as above.

Catalase
The cytochemical methods using DAB media are not specific for peroxidases; several heme-containing molecules, including catalase, can oxidize DAB in the presence of hydrogen peroxide. In a number of cell types, catalase and hydrogen peroxide-generating oxidase have been found associated with particles, which can be sedimented, termed 'peroxisomes'. The peroxisomal catalase has been visualized cytochemically[27,28] in organelles with a nucleoid by modifications of the DAB technic. Incubation of fixed cells in DAB medium at a pH higher than the one used for staining peroxisomes facilitates identification of other smaller peroxisome-like particles which stain positively for catalase.[29] Their small size and close association with smooth endoplasmic reticulum have led Novikoff

et al[30] to introduce the term 'microperoxisome'. Microperoxisomes have been described in normal bone marrow cells: erythroblasts,[31] macrophages,[31] megakaryocytes and platelets,[32] and granulocytes.[33,34] The method is as follows:

Bone marrow particles and cells from the buffy coat are fixed for 30 min or longer at 4°C with 1.25% distilled glutaraldehyde in 0.1 mol/l phosphate buffer. The marrow particles and blood leukocytes are subsequently washed three times in 0.1 mol/l phosphate buffer. Incubation is carried out in alkaline DAB.[29] The medium contains 20 mg of DAB and 0.2 ml of 2.5% H_2O_2 (freshly diluted from a 30% solution) in 10 ml of 0.05 mol/l propanediol buffer pH 9.7. Incubation is carried out at 37°C for 3 h in a dark room. Following the incubation, the bone marrow fragments are rinsed in the buffer and postfixed in 1% osmium tetroxide at 4°C for 30 min. As controls, cells are incubated in the medium lacking either DAB or H_2O_2. In order to test the inhibitory effect of 3-amino-1,2,4-triazole (AMT) on catalase, the specimens are maintained in buffer containing 2×10^{-2} mol/l AMT for 30 min at 4°C prior to incubation, and are subsequently incubated in the appropriate medium to which 2×10^{-2} mol/l AMT has been added. In contrast, potassium cyanide, at a concentration of 1×10^{-2} mol/l, has no effect on microperoxisome staining.

Glycogen

Polysaccharides can be specifically stained by a reaction derived from that used for periodic acid-Schiff PAS. For electron microscopy, the Schiff is replaced by the thiosemicarbazide or the thiocarbohydrazide revealed by the silver proteinate.[35]

The sections of embedded material are treated by laying them on the surface of different reagents and transferring them from one to another using a platinum loop:

1. Treat sections with 1% periodic acid (in distilled water) for 20 min at room temperature.
2. Wash twice rapidly, then three times for 10 min each in distilled water.
3. Treat with 1% thiocarbohydrazide in 10% acetic acid for 30 min.
4. Wash with 10% acetic acid — two rapid washes then two washes of 15 min each, followed by three washes with distilled water.
5. Silver proteinate (1% in distilled water) for 30 min in a dark room.

SIMULTANEOUS DETECTION OF MEMBRANE MARKERS WITH MONOCLONAL ANTIBODIES AND ENZYME ACTIVITIES

The availability of McAbs has considerably improved knowledge of various steps in normal and leukemic hemopoiesis. The immunological analysis has now been introduced in routine clinical practice.

For immunoelectron microscopy (IEM), the membrane antigens can be detected by immunoferritin, immunoperoxidase and immunogold methods. Ferritin was first introduced by Singer[36] after conjugation to antibody by means of covalent bonds. Ferritin-coupled antibodies were used for the detection of lymphocyte surface antigens.[37,38]

Immunoperoxidase technics were developed independently by Avrameas[39] and Nakane.[40] It has been widely accepted since that horseradish peroxidase (HRP), which is the enzymatic marker coupled to antibody in these technics, was more suitable for IEM than ferritin.[41]

More recently, for IEM, electron-dense colloidal gold particles of various sizes have been coupled to antibodies of well-defined specificities.[42] The direct labeling of McAbs with colloidal gold permitted the detection of two surface antigens using gold particles of two different sizes;[42,43] gold-labeled lectins can also be used.[44–46] The combination of the cytochemical demonstration of various peroxidases, with the demonstration of acid phosphatases and membrane antigens by the immunogld method, has made it possible to determine precisely the concordance or discordance in the expression of surface antigens and cytochemical markers.[22,47]

METHOD

The isolated cells are washed twice and resuspended in phosphate-buffered saline (PBS) pH 7.3 with 1% bovine serum albumin (Sigma), 0.2% sodium azide (BDH Chemicals) at a concentration ranging from 25×10^6 to 1×10^7 cells/ml.

The cells are incubated at room temperature for 30 min with 200 µl of McAbs diluted in PBS at a concentration twice that used for immunofluorescence. After three washes in gold buffer (50 mmol/l Na_2HPO_4 plus 0.3 mg/ml Carbowax, PEG, mol.wt = 20 000 – Serva, Heidelberg, West Germany), the cells are incubated for 1 h with 200 µl of goat anti-mouse Ig coupled to 20 nm gold particles (Janssen, Pharmaceutica, Belgium), followed by three washes in the same buffer. Cells are fixed for 10 min in a solution of 1.25% glutaraldehyde in Gey's buffer, washed and incubated in DAB medium for the detection of MPO and PPO.[22] For acid phosphatase, the cells are fixed in 1.5% glutaraldehyde in 0.067 mol/l cacodylate buffer pH 7.4 at 4°C for 30 min, then washed three times in 0.1 mol/l cacodylate buffer containing 7.5% sucrose and incubated 1 h at 37°C in Gomori medium.[47]

Purified McAbs can also be conjugated directly to colloidal gold.[42]

CONTROLS

The specificity of labeling is checked by the following controls:

1. Omission of the first layer.
2. Replacement of McAbs by non-immune mouse ascites.
3. Prior incubation with aggregated human IgG to block the nonspecific binding by the Fc receptors[48] or use of monoclonal antibody Fab'$_2$

The cytochemical control includes the omission of the substrate.

The immunoperoxidase method

After the binding of monoclonal antibody and washing, the cells are incubated with 200 µl of goat anti-mouse Ig coupled to HRP (Institut Pasteur, Paris) diluted 1/25. After three washes, cells are fixed and incubated in DAB medium and processed as described above.

RESULTS

Localization of myeloperoxidase in the monocyte and neutrophil series and eosinophil and basophil peroxidases

As suggested by the peroxidase reaction seen by light microscopic examination, electron microscopic studies after incubation in Graham-Karnovsky medium have confirmed that MPO is located in granules. In addition, in promonocytes and neutrophil promyelocytes, the enzyme can be detected during its synthesis in the entire secretory apparatus: rough endoplasmic reticulum (RER), Golgi apparatus and its associated vesicles. This indicates that MPO is synthesized and packaged into granules by the same pathway which has been defined for other secretory proteins.[49] The promonocyte resembles the promyelocyte in that they are both defined by the presence of MPO in the RER, Golgi apparatus and all granules (Figs 4.1 and 4.2). Distinguishing features of the promonocyte are the irregular shape of the nucleus,

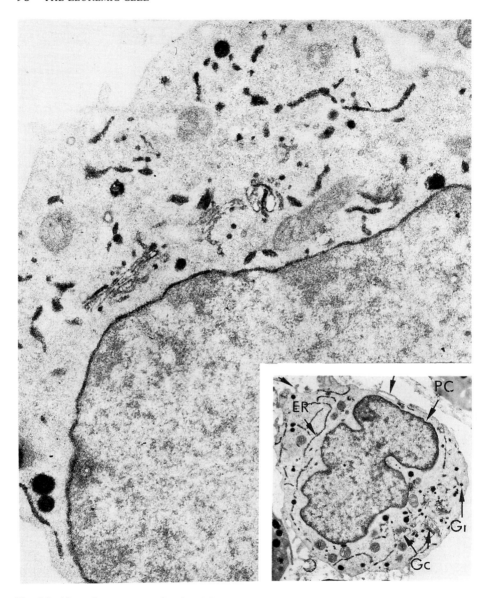

Fig. 4.1 Normal promonocyte incubated for the peroxidase reaction (Graham and Karnovsky method). **Inset**: as in the promyelocyte, the peroxidase reaction product is distributed in the perinuclear cisternae (PC), all segments of the endoplasmic reticulum (ER), the Golgi cisternae (Gc) and all cytoplasmic granules (Gr). Hence the promonocyte is sometimes difficult to distinguish from early neutrophil precursors. However, in promonocytes some characteristics are typical: granules are smaller, the nucleus is deeply indented and numerous microvillous extensions of the plasma membrane (arrows) can be seen related to the endocytosis capacity. (× 5700) **Enlargement of the Golgi zone**: all the cisternae and vesicles contain the dense reaction product. (× 20 000)

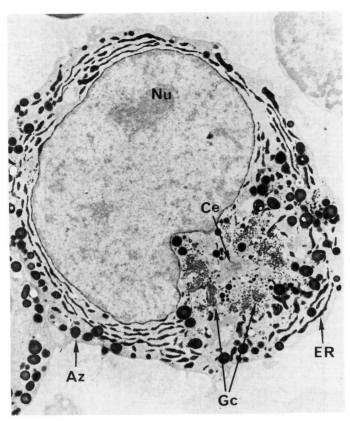

Fig. 4.2 Normal promyelocyte incubated for the demonstration of peroxidase (Graham and Karnovsky method). The cell with a nucleolus (Nu) exhibits a strong reaction product in the nuclear envelope, the endoplasmic reticulum (ER), the Golgi cisternae (Gc) and all azurophils (Az). The centriole (Ce) is located at the center of the Golgi zone. (× 7090)

membrane ruffling related to their capacity for ingestion, and the small size of their reactive granules.

After the arrest of MPO synthesis, the RER and Golgi apparatus of myelocytes become unreactive whilst the enzyme is detected only in azurophil granules, which are also called primary granules. A new category of granules (specific granules) is produced which have a different enzyme content.

When a low amount of hydrogen peroxide is used in the DAB medium, azurophil granules in neutrophil promyelocytes can be unreactive, whilst the RER and the Golgi apparatus are reactive. This was considered to be the result of the absence of MPO.[50] However, by increasing the concentration of hydrogen peroxide, these large granules became reactive.[51] This artefact was used to demonstrate a subpopulation of small azurophil granules that are reactive in this condition[51] (Fig. 4.3).

Eosinophils contain a peroxidase that is genetically and biochemically distinct from MPO. The Graham–Karnovsky technic reveals its presence in the RER and Golgi apparatus of developing eosinophils; the enzyme is seen in the granular matrix (Fig. 4.4), the crystal that appears in myelocytes being devoid of reaction.[49]

Basophil promyelocytes exhibit peroxidase activity in their granules and cisternal compartments. The granules can be recognized by their typical stippled appearance.

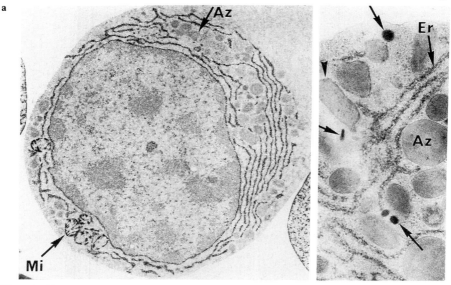

Fig. 4.3 Neutrophil promyelocyte from normal bone marrow which was incubated in Ringer's DAB before fixation. (a) Early promyelocyte: all azurophil granules (Az) are unreactive while peroxidase activity is present in the endoplasmic reticulum. The mitochondria (Mi) exhibit reaction in the cisternae due to cytochrome oxidase. (× 8100) (b) Mature promyelocyte: MPO is present in the endoplasmic reticulum (Er). Spherical azurophils (Az), as well as elongated azurophils, are unreactive whilst small granules which are round or elongated are reactive (arrows). (× 26 600) (Reproduced from Pryzwansky and Breton-Gorius[51] with permission.)

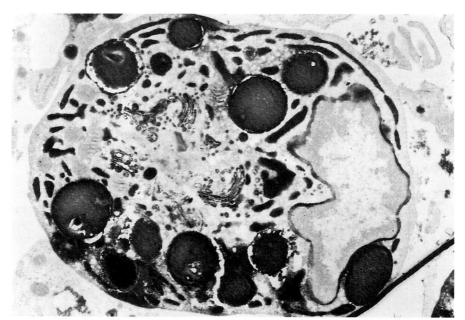

Fig. 4.4 Eosinophil promyelocyte incubated for the demonstration of peroxidase (Graham and Karnovsky method). A very strong activity is present in the endoplasmic reticulum, the Golgi apparatus and all large immature granules. (× 12 600)

Imperfect fixation of basophil granules with extraction makes detailed conclusions about granulogenesis difficult.[49]

The progenitors (myeloid colony-forming cells: CFU-C) cannot be recognized since they have not yet started synthesizing peroxidase. Several McAbs have been obtained which label CFU-C. Anti-My7 (CD13) appears to identify a fraction of CFU-C that is actively proliferating.[52] Using the immunogold method, the ultrastructural aspect of labeled cells can be observed (Fig. 4.5).

Localization of platelet peroxidase in the megakaryocyte lineage

Using the Roels[24] and Anderson technics,[25] PPO has been detected in the RER and smooth endoplasmic reticulum (SER) of megakaryocytes and platelets (Fig. 4.6). This technic also reveals granulocytic peroxidases (MPO). However, some distinctions can be made between

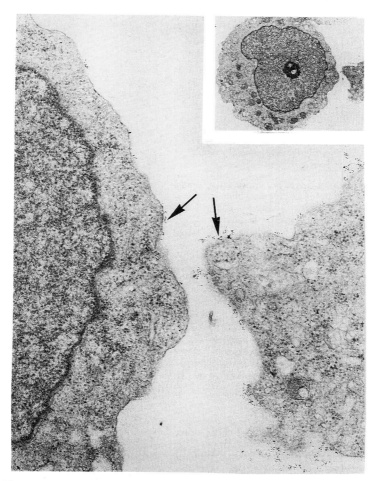

Fig. 4.5 Normal bone marrow cells incubated with the McAb anti-My7 (CD13) then with anti-IgG conjugated with gold particles, then fixed and incubated in DAB medium. **Inset:** at low magnification, the blast cell exhibits a nucleolus in the nucleus with euchromatin and no peroxidase activity. (× 3760) At higher magnification, the two cells without any MPO and granules have their cell membrane strongly labeled by the McAb anti-My7 (arrows). These cells are candidates for representing CFU-C. (× 23 800)

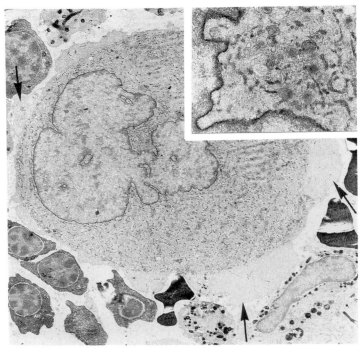

Fig. 4.6 Normal megakaryocyte reacted for platelet peroxidase (prefixation by the tannic acid–aldehyde mixture). The enzyme activity is seen in the nuclear envelope and small saccules of endoplasmic reticulum. The peripheral blebs (arrows) appear without organelle content. (× 1840)
Inset: Golgi cisternae and granules are unreactive, a positive reaction being present in the perinuclear space and in the endoplasmic reticulum cisternae. (× 10 840)

these two enzymes that have the same reactivity. The most important difference is that MPO is always located in the Golgi cisternae and granules of promonocytes and promyelocytes (see Fig. 4.2), whilst PPO is only detected in the RER and SER. The genes coding for MPO and PPO biosynthesis are different because PPO has been detected in platelets and megakaryocytes from patients with MPO deficiency.[33] The functions of MPO and PPO are also different: PPO is implicated in platelet prostaglandin biosynthesis, whilst the MPO-H_2O_2 system plays a role in bactericidal function. Finally, PPO is very sensitive to fixation with glutaraldehyde and its detection requires the use of special methods.[21,22,26] In contrast, MPO is very resistant. PPO can be detected in the RER of bone marrow cells with a blastic or lymphoid appearance.[49] These cells, which occur very infrequently, have a size similar to that of proerythroblasts and they should be considered as small precursors (2N or 4N) of megakaryocytes unrecognized by conventional methods (Figs 4.7 and 4.8). They do not possess any alpha-granules or demarcation membrane system characteristic of megakaryocytes. Their number is increased in the bone marrow of patients with thrombocytopenia. Since the term 'megakaryoblast' has been used to define the earliest precursor of megakaryocytes which can be identified by its large size, the small precursors recognized by the PPO reaction will be termed 'promegakaryoblasts'.

More recently, the simultaneous detection of membrane labeling by McAbs to platelet glycoproteins (GP) and PPO has confirmed the megakaryocyte nature of small PPO + cells.[22]

There was no peroxidase activity in normal B- and T-lymphocytes. However, when sensitive methods for peroxidase detection[22,24] were used, reactivity similar in its localization

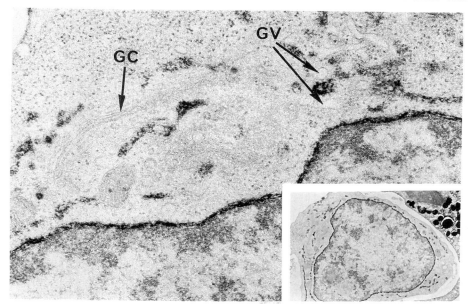

Fig. 4.7 Inset: low magnification of normal promegakaryoblast, tested for platelet peroxidase. A positive reaction is seen in the perinuclear space and endoplasmic reticulum. (× 3850) A higher magnification shows that the Golgi cisternae (GC) and Golgi vesicles (GV) are unreactive as is the case in more mature megakaryocytes. (× 25 300)

to PPO was observed in the RER from non-megakaryocytic cells. The peroxidase activities that are present exclusively in ER and undetectable at the light microscopic level are:

1. Monocytes activated by adherence and macrophages.[53–56]
2. Langerhans' and histiocytosis X cells.[57,58]
3. Mast cell precursors.[59]
4. Fibroblasts.[56]
5. Hairy cells.[23]
6. Normal and leukemic erythroid progenitors (CFU-E)[60]

Thus, to date, PPO cannot be considered as specific for the platelet–megakaryocyte lineage. For this reason, it was of interest to discover new early markers of megakaryocyte maturation.

Localization by IEM of platelet proteins during megakaryocyte maturation

Rabellino et al[61] have show that normal megakaryocytes and promegakaryoblasts were labeled by specific polyclonal antibodies recognizing different membrane platelet glycoproteins and several intracytoplasmic platelet proteins. Changes in the phenotypic profile of differentiating megakaryocytes can be recognized by the evolution in the labeling of cells with a panel of McAbs.[62] Similar studies[63,64] were performed in CFU-MK-derived megakaryocytes in vitro using McAbs to glycoproteins and monospecific antibodies to several proteins present in normal platelet α-granules.

Most promegakaryoblasts express glycoproteins IIb–IIIa at day 5 of culture. The glycoprotein Ib is detected later when, simultaneously, cytoplasmic proteins (von Willebrand's factor: vWF; thrombospondin: TSP; platelet factor 4: PF-4) appear. This labeling occurs in small cells with a round nucleus, and a diffuse pattern of staining. No α-granules are detected at the electron microscope level, at this stage of maturation. During the ensuing

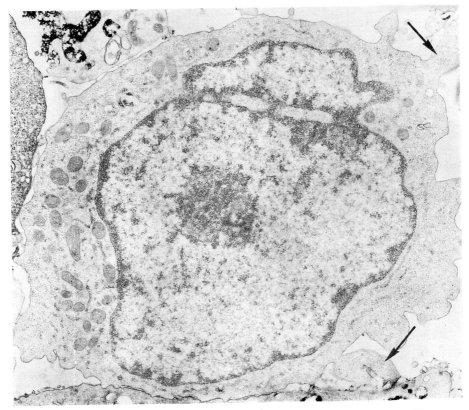

Fig. 4.8 Another aspect of a normal promegakaryoblast, tested for platelet peroxidase. The enzyme is localized in the perinuclear envelope and in all short segments of endoplasmic reticulum. Note the indented nucleus and cytoplasmic blebs (arrows). (× 9300)

period, cells increase their size; the intensity of membrane labeling enhances whereas cytoplasmic staining becomes granular, because of the packaging of different proteins in the α-granules.

Ultrastructural immunogold studies have confirmed the localization of vWF, PF-4, β-thromboglobulin, TSP, fibrinogen, fibronectin (see general review[65]), factor V[66] in all α-granules. Interestingly, vWF was detected in the α-granules with a specific eccentric distribution that coincided with the presence of tubular structures;[67] they closely resembled the tubular structures found in Weibel–Palade bodies which also contain vWF. The absence of immunolabeling for vWF and tubular structures in von Willebrand's disease strongly suggest that the tubular structures correspond to the vWF molecule itself.[68]

Characteristics of erythroid progenitors and precursors

The erythroid progenitors, burst-forming unit–erythroid (BFU-E) and colony-forming unit–erythroid (CFU-E), are defined by their capacity to form erythroid colonies in vitro in semisolid media. However, they cannot be identified by morphology. The first identifiable precursor is the proerythroblast. By electron microscopic examination, it can be seen that this cell, like the more mature erythroblasts, is organized forming an island, a central macrophage with closely associated maturing erythroblasts.[8] The examination of the proerythroblast periphery shows membrane invaginations, called rhopheocytosis, which permit the entrance of ferritin molecules into the cytoplasm.[8,49] These vesicles of rhopheocytosis represent an example of a coated vesicle which differs from pinocytosis in the presence of a specific receptor for some plasma proteins. In the Golgi zone, 3–12 granules also contain ferritin molecules.[69]

Recently, some antigens recognized by McAbs were identified on BFU-E, CFU-E, and not on other progenitors. One of them, Fa6-152,[70] has allowed the considerable enrichment of CFU-E from normal bone marrow by cell sorting or panning methods. Using a polyclonal anti-carbonic anhydrase I antibody, it was seen that this enzyme, which is restricted to erythroid lineage, was present in the cytoplasm of CFU-E, labeled by Fa6-152.[71] The ultrastructural and cytochemical methods on these presumptive CFU-E progenitors showed:

1. The blast with a big nucleolus and numerous polyribosomes has no rhopheocytosis.
2. In the Golgi zone, θ-granules previously described in blasts from some chronic myeloid leukemia (CML) blast crisis[72] were identified (Fig. 4.9). At high magnification, however, ferritin was present in the matrix (Fig. 4.10).
3. A proportion of CFU-E progenitors exhibits PPO-like activity[60] (Fig. 4.10).

Localization of catalase and glycogen

Catalase-containing particles have been identified early in the maturation of granulocytes,[33,34] erythroblasts[31] and megakaryocytes.[32] In promegakaryoblasts they are produced before the occurrence of α-granules.

Glycogen molecules can be revealed in cells treated for morphological examination and also in cells incubated in DAB media. In such cases, neutrophil promyelocytes which

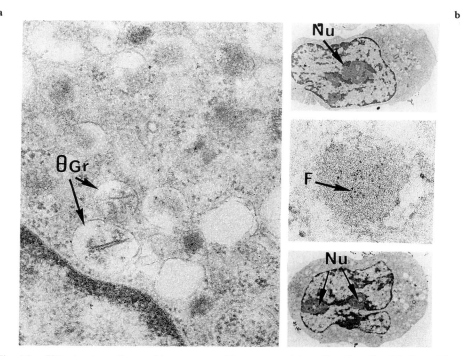

Fig. 4.9 Ultrastructure of normal bone marrow blasts separated by cell sorting after labeling with the McAb Fa6-152. (a) Enlargement of the Golgi zone of a blast. Several θ-granules (θ Gr) are bisected by membranes. (× 39 500) (b) view at low magnification of two blasts showing large nucleoli (Nu); in the cytoplasm several granules or vacuoles are seen in the Golgi zone. (× 2700) One of them is enlarged and contains ferritin (F) molecules. (× 60 000)

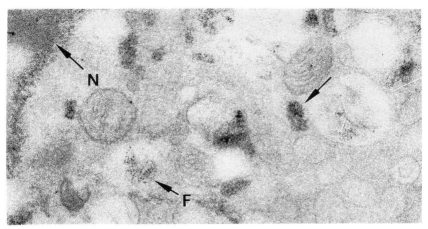

Fig. 4.10 Normal bone marrow blasts separated by panning using the McAb Fa6-152, fixed by glutaraldehyde in Gey's buffer and incubated in DAB medium. This unstained section shows θ-granules with ferritin (F). The cisterna surrounding the nucleus (N) and all endoplasmic reticulum cisternae contain PPO-like activity (arrows). ($\times$ 14 500)

synthesize MPO are seen to contain free glycogen molecules. During maturation their production increases and, in the neutrophil polymorphonuclear leukocytes, they are grouped in clusters; they disappear in red cells. In megakaryocytes their mumber increases with maturation, and in platelets they are present in aggregates.

CONTRIBUTION OF THE CYTOCHEMICAL DEMONSTRATION OF PEROXIDASES TO THE KNOWLEDGE OF LEUKEMIC CELLS

ACUTE MEGAKARYOBLASTIC LEUKEMIA

Until the introduction of McAbs against platelet proteins for identifying blasts as promegakaryoblasts, the demonstration of PPO was the only technic that permitted the diagnosis of acute megakaryoblastic leukemia (AMKL).[73-85]

In very rare cases, a partial PPO deficiency in platelets and promegakaryoblasts was reported.[86-88] Promegakaryoblasts with PPO activity may exhibit various morphological aspects (Figs 4.11-4.13). The abundant microfilaments (Fig. 4.13) represent vimentin intermediate filaments.[89]

Recently, AMKL was classified as M7 by the French-American-British (FAB) group when 30% or greater of promegakaryoblasts were recognized either by PPO or found by immunolabeling with antibodies against platelet glycoproteins and α-granule constituents.[90] The detection of both PPO and platelet markers is in good agreement in the majority of cases.[87,91-93] Very rarely (one in the author's series on 82 cases of AMKL), 95% of promegakaryoblasts exhibit platelet glycoproteins and are PPO-; after a brief liquid culture these blasts acquired PPO. Similarly PPO-blasts which were positive for the glycoprotein Ib were reported in a single case.[92] Figure 4.14 summarizes the different phenotypes of blasts found in AMKL and their frequency. Figures 4.15 and 4.16 illustrate the labeling and PPO localization of promegakaryoblasts type I and type III (Fig. 4.14).

Although McAbs which recognize an antigen present on normal CFU-MK, as judged by their cytotoxic effect have recently been reported[62] their specificity for megakaryocytes remains to be proven. Thus, at the present time, malignant blasts blocked in their maturation at a stage equivalent to CFU-MK cannot be recognized. The more immature phenotype (promegakaryoblast I) is identified only by the presence of PPO which constitutes the earliest

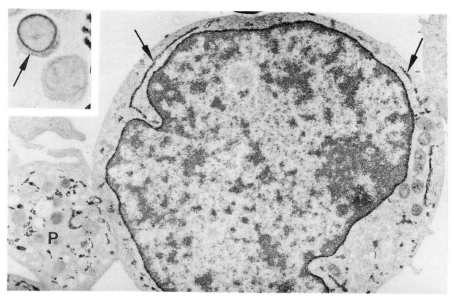

Fig. 4.11 Leukemic promegakaryoblasts fixed by glutaraldehyde in Gey's buffer and incubated in DAB medium. PPO is present in endoplasmic reticulum (arrows) in this blast with lymphoid morphology. The Golgi cisternae are unreactive. The intensity of the reaction is similar to that of a platelet (P). In the cytoplasm, there are mitochondria but no α- or θ-granules. (× 11 100) **Inset:** a thick section of the blasts shows a brown ring surrounding the nucleus of one cell (arrow) indicating that PPO in the nuclear cisterna could be visualized by light microscopic examination.

marker to date.[87,91,93] These blasts are HLA-DR + and possess acid phosphatase activity.[93] In contrast to blasts in acute early erythroblastic leukemia (AEL), they have no θ-granules with ferritin in the Golgi zone. In AEL, the blasts are HLA-DR − and are labeled by the McAb Fa6-152.[94]

The absence of the glycoprotein IIIa in PPO + blasts in the phenotype I is not due to an acquired glycoprotein IIIa deficiency since the platelets are strongly labeled by the

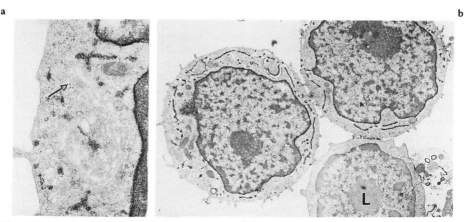

Fig. 4.12 Leukemic promegakaryoblasts treated as in Fig. 4.11 from another patient. (a) Enlargement of the Golgi apparatus showing that Golgi cisternae (arrow) are devoid of PPO. (× 18 870) (b) Two blasts with large nucleoli exhibit strong PPO reaction while a lymphocyte (L) has no activity. (× 4500)

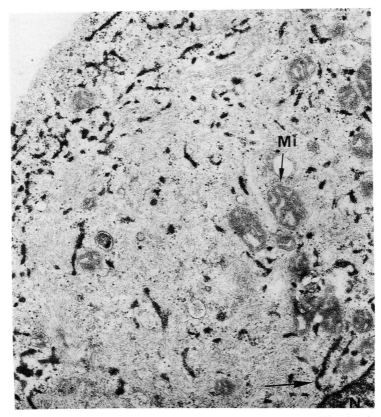

Fig. 4.13 Leukemic promegakaryoblast treated as in Fig. 4.11 from a baby. The abundant cytoplasm contains mitochondria (Mi). There is strong PPO in the endoplasmic reticulum (arrow) and numerous microfilaments which were characterized as vimentin intermediate filaments by immunolabeling. (× 21 900)

anti-glycoprotein III McAb (Fig. 4.14). The PPO + blasts without platelet glycoproteins may exhibit labeling with anti-My9 (CD33)[95] or McAb 80H5[96] which recognizes X hapten (3-fucosyl-N-acetyl-lactosamine); this carbohydrate is expressed on mature neutrophils but is not truly myeloid specific since it is expressed on all normal hemopoietic progenitors[97] and in non-granulocytic leukemias.[98]

The promegakaryoblast PMKB II is characterized by the presence of membrane glycoproteins IIb, IIIa and the complex IIb/IIIa whilst in PMKB III, there is, in addition, the glycoprotein Ib; with antibodies to vWF, PF-4 and TSP, PMKB III gives a weak diffuse fluorescence such as that from normal promegakaryoblasts and this is differentiated in culture from CFU-MK at day 5–6. In their phenotype, the more mature PMKB IV resembles cells at day 8 of culture: a granular labeling occurs with anti-vWF antibody. PMKB IV differs from micromegakaryocytes by the presence of immature α- granules in the zone of the Golgi apparatus.

Therefore PPO still appears to be the earliest marker of promegakaryoblast maturation.[87,91,93]

Due to the small series of patients reported, it is difficult to determine the frequency of AMKL among the acute leukemias. Various percentages were found from 3.6% to 12%.[84,99,100] In the author's group, 82 AMKLs were diagnosed in 6 years among acute

ULTRASTRUCTURE OF THE LEUKEMIC CELL 109

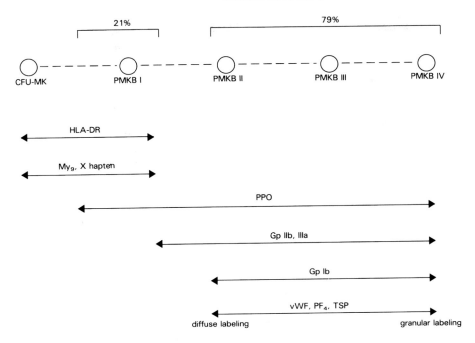

Fig. 4.14 Phenotypes of blasts in AMKL and their frequency.

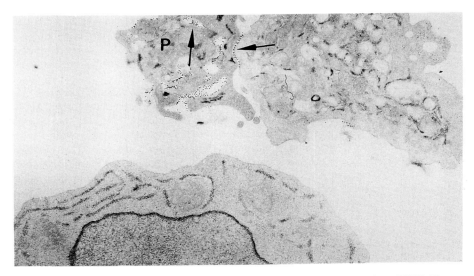

Fig. 4.15 Immunolabeling with the McAb C17 (anti-Gp IIIa) and then detection of PPO. Two platelets (P) with PPO exhibit gold particles indicating the presence of Gp IIIa on the membrane including in the open canalicular system. In contrast, the promegakaryoblast which is PPO+ has no membrane labeling. ($\times$ 13 800)

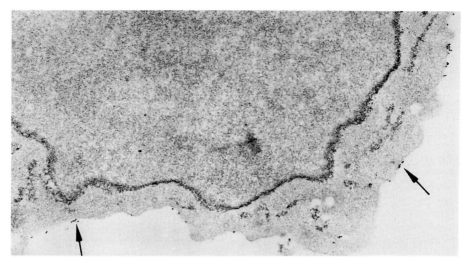

Fig. 4.16 Leukemic promegakaryoblast with phenotype III (see Fig. 4.14). The blasts were labeled with the McAb AN51 (anti-Gp Ib) and then fixed and incubated in DAB medium for the detection of PPO. This blast exhibits both membrane labeling (arrow) and PPO in the endoplasmic reticulum. (× 18 000)

leukemias in which the blasts were unclassifiable and without lymphoid markers. Megakaryocytes were considered malignant when the percentage of peripheral blood promegakaryoblasts exceeded 10%. Because the author is not involved in the routine diagnosis of acute leukemias and blasts are received from different hematology centers, the real frequency of AMKL cannot be determined.

Clinical and histopathological analysis confirmed the heterogeneity of AMKL.[83] A high percentage (46%) of AMKL represented CML in blast crisis as previously reported.[75,78,81,87,91,92,101,102] Fourteen per cent of the author's cases of AMKL were made up of patients who exhibited acute myelofibrosis[73,74,79,81,103-105] or the acute phase of myeloproliferative disorders.[106-108] Eleven per cent of cases of AMKL were observed in patients who had prior malignancies that were treated with alkylating agents and/or radiotherapy.[79,93,99,109,110]

AMKL occurring in Down's syndrome represented 8.5%. Because 11 children were studied by the author, the association of trisomy 21 and AMKL represents 30% of AMKL occurring in infancy. This assocation was previously emphasized.[77,83,85,111] Interestingly, promegakaryoblasts were also present in transient leukemia in neonates with Down's syndrome[112] and AMKL was reported in a child with a constitutional ring 21 chromosome defect.[113] Primitive acute leukemias without myelofibrosis represented 4.8% of the author's cases;[87,99] 2.4% of cases of AMKL were preceded by a preleukemic phase.[86] One patient with primary mediastinal germ cell tumors rapidly developed AMKL.[114]

The prognosis of AMKL is severe in spite of the treatments which have been proposed.[84,99,115] Some chronic and more benign forms have been reported.[116]

In half of the cases, promegakaryoblasts can be mixed with myeloblasts with small peroxidase-positive granules or basophil promyelocytes and/or with early erythroid blasts.

ACUTE EARLY ERYTHROBLASTIC LEUKEMIA

On the basis of conventional criteria, acute early erythroblastic leukemia (AEL) represents an uncommon disease; indeed some of these leukemias may not be true AELs since the marrow becomes progressively invaded by myeloblasts. In some of the acute leukemias considered as M6 in the FAB classification,[117] the erythroblasts may originate from residual normal cells. After the introduction of McAbs to glycophorin A, few cases of AEL have been recognized.[118-123] The ultrastructural detection of ferritin at the surface of blasts permitted the recognition of some cases of AEL.[81, 124] But the incidence of AEL remains very low. Using the McAb Fa6-152 and the anti-CA I antibody, nine cases of AEL have been diagnosed,[94] and ten additional cases of AEL have been recently identified. These cases were recognized among 120 acute leukemias which could not be classified by morphological and cytochemical criteria.

Five cases originated from CML blast crisis, four from Down's syndrome, two from therapy-related leukemia, and five cases represented a primary acute leukemia (four adults and one child); three represented leukemoid reaction in neonates with Down's syndrome.

Investigation with other erythroid markers helped the author to distinguish two main phenotypes for 19 patients: a phenotype 1 (14 patients) which related to that of normal CFU-E, a phenotype 3 (three patients) which corresponded to an immature erythroblast in which glycophorin A, spectrin, band 3 and hemoglobin were present, and an intermediate phenotype 2 (two patients) in which blasts are labeled by a polyclonal antibody but not with an McAb to glycophorin A. The erythroid origin of the leukemic cells with phenotype 1 was further sustained by the presence of the same karyotypic abnormalities in the blast cells and in the erythroid colonies which have acquired hemoglobin in culture in vitro. Ultrastructural investigation[60] on blasts from six patients with phenotype 1 and one patient with phenotype 2 revealed that the majority of blasts exhibit a weak PPO-like activity present in the perinuclear space, in the ER but not in the Golgi apparatus whilst the micromegakaryocytes have a strong PPO activity (Fig. 4.17). The Golgi zone contains θ-granules bisected by membrane. At higher magnification ferritin molecules are identified in θ-granules (Figs 4.18 and 4.19). These blasts are similar to normal CFU-E.

In phenotype 3, this PPO-like activity was not detected whilst the number of ferritin molecules increased (Fig. 4.20). In phenotype 1 and 2 both PPO-like positive and negative

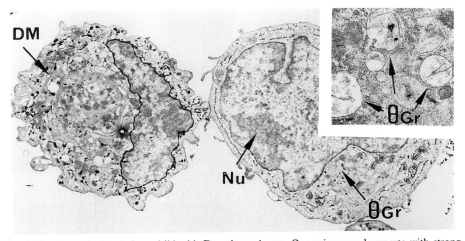

Fig. 4.17 Acute leukemia in a child with Down's syndrome. One micromegakaryocyte with strong PPO activity possesses demarcation membranes (DM) and α-granules. A larger blast with nucleolus (Nu) exhibits weaker PPO-like activity and θ-granules (θGr) clustered in the Golgi zone. (× 5625)
Inset: enlargement of θ-granules (θGr) showing the internal structure. (× 19 575)

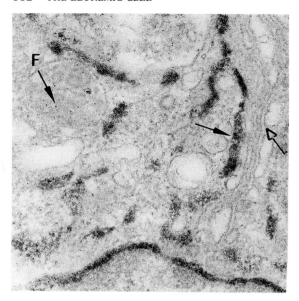

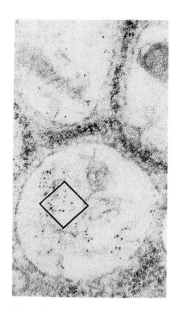

Fig. 4.18 Enlargement of the Golgi zone of a blast in AEL (blast crisis of CML) A strong PPO-like activity is present in the endoplasmic reticulum (black arrow) but not in the Golgi cisternae (white arrow). Dispersed ferritin molecules (F) are seen in granules. ($\times$ 57 500)

Fig. 4.19 Enlargement of θ-granules with complex internal structures. The molecules of ferritin in the square show their characteristic structure. ($\times$ 87 000)

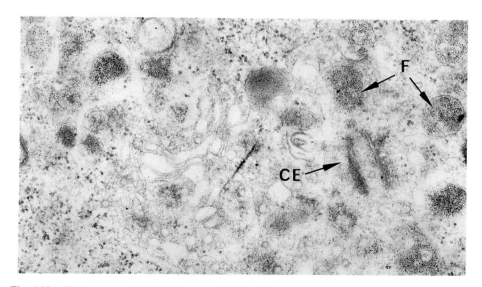

Fig. 4.20 Enlargement of the Golgi zone of a blast labeled by McAb anti-glycophorin A. In the more mature phenotype of AEL, no PPO-like activity is present; in the Golgi zone the granules with more dense matrix contain numerous ferritin molecules (F). A centriole (CE) is seen. ($\times$ 34 650)

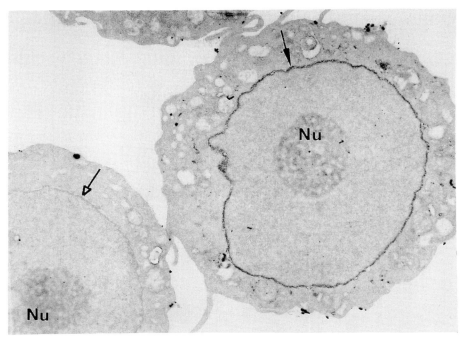

Fig. 4.21 Simultaneous immunogold labeling with the McAb Fa6-152, and PPO detection in blasts from AEL. Two blasts with a large nucleolus (Nu) have their membrane labeled by the McAb Fa6-152. One exhibits a PPO-like activity (black arrow) whilst the other has no activity (white arrow). (× 9750)

blasts were labeled by Fa6-152 (Fig. 4.21). In contrast promegakaryoblasts and micromegakaryocytes which exhibited glycoproteins IIb–IIIa have no θ-granules.

Acute myeloblastic leukemia

Granule formation is often abnormal in acute myeloblastic leukemia (AML).[125] First, an abnormal concentration and packaging of azurophil granules may occur resulting in the formation of Auer rods. The existence of periodicity in Auer rods was proved some 20 years ago. The arrangement of molecules constituting the crystalline material has been demonstrated with greater precision by means of the MPO reaction.[126] The dense reaction product has been used as a dark field to visualize the unreactive protein of Auer bodies, which may then be easily identified by its negative contrast. In four cases of AML, an identical pattern of protein associated in a regular linear arrangement with well-defined periodicity was identified. Secondly, numerous giant granules resembling those of the Chediak–Higashi syndrome may be present.[127,128] These giant granules are also formed by fusion of azurophil granules, as in the Chediak–Higashi syndrome; however, they appear different in that they contain numerous microcrystalline structures similar to those of Auer bodies.[128] However, the configuration, size and organization of the protein in the microcrystal are distinct (Fig. 4.22) from those seen in Auer bodies in AML.[126] These features suggest that the nature of the protein which crystallizes in Auer bodies may be heterogeneous.

Another anomaly concerns the granule production which may be absent[15] or a selective absence of MPO within the azurophil granule.[129,130]

Blasts which are peroxidase negative by light microscopic cytochemistry may exhibit a few small granules (0.02–0.3 μm) which contain MPO activity.[78,131–133] In the majority of cases,

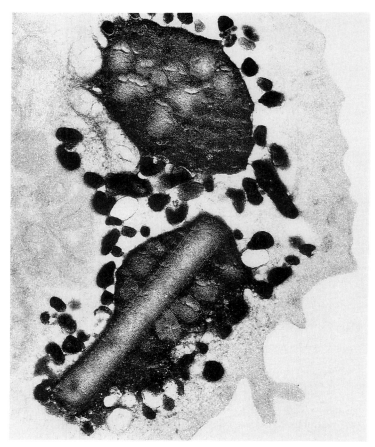

Fig. 4.22 Giant granules in a leukemic myeloblast treated to detect MPO. The giant granules result from a fusion of azurophil granules. The dense reaction product of MPO permits visualization of the unreactive proteins which appear in negative contrast. They are organized in microcrystals; the periodicity and the arrangement of the molecules in these micro-Auer bodies differ from Auer bodies found either in Auer rods of myeloblastic leukemia or promyelocytic leukemia. (× 33 600)

there is no MPO in the secretory apparatus. The morphological characteristics of these blasts are variable—they may resemble a lymphoid cell (Fig. 4.23) or a myeloblast (Fig. 4.24). On rare occasions, ribosome–lamella complexes, which are found in few cases of B-lymphocytic proliferations[134] and in hairy cells,[13,14] are present (Fig. 4.24). These acute leukemias may often be considered as lymphoblastic by routine methods.[133] The immunofluorescent method using an anti-MPO antibody appears to be more sensitive for detecting MPO than the cytochemical method. It is impossible to know if these blasts are related to neutrophils or to monocytes (non-specific esterases). In some of these cases, the peroxidase-positive blasts also expressed the cALLA antigen (CD10) on their membrane.[135] In 5 years, 50 cases of blasts with small peroxidase-positive granules have been identified, often mixed with promegakaryoblasts. The myeloid blasts are, on the whole, positive with My9 (CD33)[95] and/or My7 (CD13),[51] X hapten membrane antigens,[96] in the absence of lymphoid markers. However, few of them show the simultaneous expression of the lymphoid-associated antigen

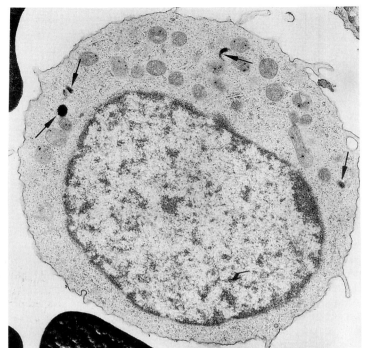

Fig. 4.23 Blast with small peroxidase granules. The low number and small size of the reactive granules (arrows) explain why the MPO cannot be detected by routine light microscope cytochemistry. Note the lymphoid morphology of the cell. (× 10 160)

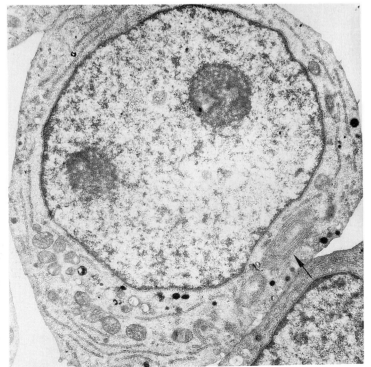

Fig. 4.24 Atypical myeloblast with two nucleoli has terminated MPO synthesis because the endoplasmic reticulum is unreactive. Several small peroxidase positive granules (not recognized by light microscopy) are seen. Two ribosome–lamella complexes (arrow) are identified. (× 7920)

116 THE LEUKEMIC CELL

Table 4.2 Unusual membrane phenotypes of blasts exhibiting small peroxidase positive granules

	J_5 (CD10) (%)	B_4 (CD19) (%)	My_7 (CD13) (%)	My_9 (CD33) (%)	HLA-DR (%)
Patient Fer...	74	70	0	0	79
Patient Tuc...	11	2.5	7.6	0	75

B4 (CD19)[136] and/or cALLA (CD10)[137] (Table 4.2 and Fig. 4.25). Since chromosome analysis was not performed some of these acute leukemias may correspond to the t(14;11) chromosome rearrangement in which small peroxidase-positive granules are also found[138,139] with the simultaneous expression of B4 and X hapten.[139] Light-chain immunoglobulin gene rearrangement was also reported in a few cases.[139] It is not known whether this phenomenon results from a leukemia affecting multipotential progenitor or from aberrant gene expression during differentiation.

Acute promyelocytic leukemia

In the hypergranular cells of acute promyleocytic leukemia (APL), 'bundles of firewood' of Auer bodies are seen. In all cases, Auer bodies reveal an identical substructure which consists of a hexagonal arrangement of tubes with a periodicity of 25 nm[16]. This has also been confirmed by examination after the cytochemical detection of MPO.[126]

A microgranular variant of APL,[140] in which the blasts exhibited the typical t(15;17) translocation,[141] was studied at ultrastructural level.[142]

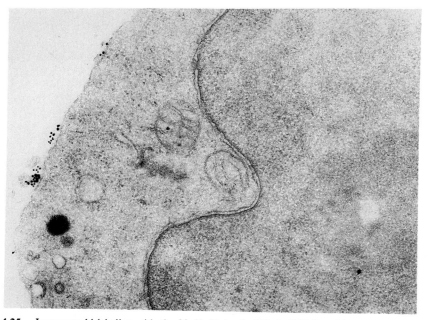

Fig. 4.25 Immunogold labeling with the McAb J5 (anti cALLA: CD10) and incubation in DAB medium of a blast from an atypical acute leukemia. This cell with a peroxidase-positive granule (myeloid marker) exhibits strong membrane labeling with J5 (lymphoid marker). (× 23 220)

Acute leukemia with proliferation of eosinophil and basophil precursors

The diagnosis of eosinophilic leukemia is based on the presence of immature eosinophil precursors in the blood with proliferation of these cells in different tissues. Examination by electron microscopy reveals large granules typical of immature eosinophils.

In M4Eo[143] with an inversion of chromosome 16, the eosinophil granules are abnormal, lacking their central crystalloids in mature cells; their cytochemical reactions are also distinct from normal eosinophils.[144] A mixture of eosinophil and basophil granules can be seen at light microscopy.[144] The prognosis of this subtype of acute myeloid leukemia appears to be favorable.[145] In cases of acute myeloblastic leukemia and CML in blast crisis, a simple blast may contain both eosinophil and basophil granules (Fig. 4.26). During the chronic phase of CML, an increased number of basophils can be seen. When the percentage reaches 50%, many authors use the term 'basophilic leukemia'.[8] The granules exhibit the characteristic metachromasia with toluidine blue stain.

During the blast crisis of CML, among vacuolated blasts that are negative with toluidine blue, the MPO reaction can reveal cells actively synthesizing peroxidase in the perinuclear envelope and RER. The vacuoles contain reactive punctate material in the center which resembles basophil granules. In the absence of fixation, the granular reaction is clear and no vacuoles are seen. The stippled appearance of the granules is identical to that of normal basophil granules. A possible explanation is that early basophil precursors do not acquire the characteristic metachromasia of more mature basophils and the soluble material of the granules is extracted during the fixation; in contrast, this solubility is circumvented by reacting the cells with DAB medium before the fixation, thus preventing the dissolution of

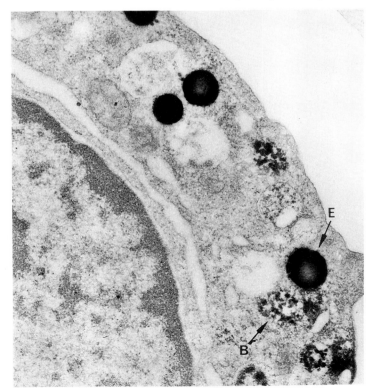

Fig. 4.26 Blast from a granulocytic crisis of CML which possesses peroxidase in both eosinophil (E) and basophil granules (B). (× 22 880)

the granular content.[78] Out of 12 cases of blast crisis of CML with peroxidase-negative blasts at light microscopy, 9 contained a variable percentage of such early basophil promyelocytes (from 5% to 75%) unidentified by usual methods, and detected by ultrastructural cytochemistry.[78] These precursors could also be detected by cultures in diffusion chambers. On day 30, 87% of the cells were mature basophils and all the metaphases contained the Philadelphia (Ph) chromosome. This demonstrates that, in the acute phase of CML, leukemic basophil precursors may grow and mature in vitro.[146]

It is also possible to detect a mixture of basophil granules and mast cell granules[72,81,147,148] or only mast cell granules[91] (Fig. 4.27). These forms are not recognized by light microscopy and may exhibit membrane cALLA (CD10) antigen.[149] Since it has been reported that the membrane glycoproteins of human mast cells and basophils are different,[150] it would be of interest to analyse the glycoproteins in the blasts with the two categories of granules. In Ph – acute leukemia a mixture of basophil precursors (Fig. 4.28) and early erythroid leukemia can also be found.

Acute monoblastic leukemia

As in AML, leukemic monocytic precursors may exhibit a complete absence of peroxidase in the cytoplasmic granules.[151] In other cases there is a discrepancy between positivity by

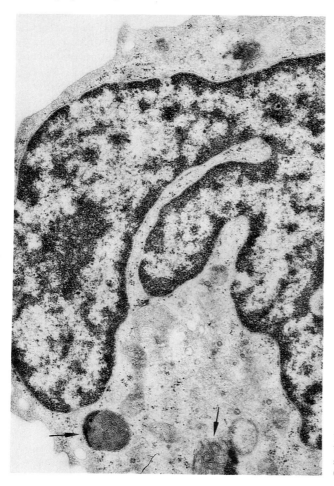

Fig. 4.27 Blast from a CML blast crisis with granules similar to those of mast cells (arrows). (× 19 440)

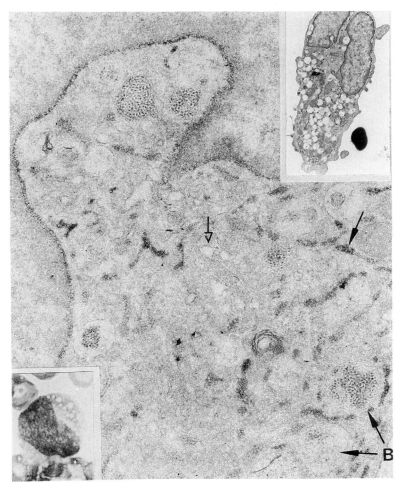

Fig. 4.28 Leukemic basophil promyelocyte. **Inset left**: stained film — the blast exhibits many vacuoles. **Inset right**: low magnification electron microscopy — the blast shows peroxidase activity in the endoplasmic reticulum. (× 4000) At higher magnification, it appears that the Golgi apparatus is unreactive (white arrow) as well as the granules with the stippled appearance of basophil granules (B), whilst the endoplasmic reticulum contains a dense peroxidase reaction product. (× 29 700)

electron microscopy and negativity at the light microscope; this could, however, be due to the small size and low number of cytoplasmic granules.[152,153]

REFERENCES

1 Kaplow L S 1969 Buffy coat preparatory tube. American Journal of Clinical Pathology 51: 806–807
2 Hirsch J G, Fedorko F 1968 Ultrastructure of human leukocytes after simultaneous fixation with glutaraldehyde and osmium tetroxide and post-fixation in uranyl acetate. Journal of Cell Biology 18: 615–627
3 Anderson D R 1966 Ultrastructure of normal and leukemic leucocytes in human peripheral blood. Journal of Ultrastructure Research Suppl. 9: 5–42
4 Boyum A 1968 Isolation of mononuclear cells and granulocytes from human blood. Scandinavian Journal of Clinical Investigation 21 (Suppl. 97): 77–89

5 Bainton D F, Ullyot J L, Farquhar M G 1971 The development of neutrophilic polymorphonuclear leukocytes in human bone marrow. Journal of Experimental Medicine 134: 907-934.
6 Karnovsky M J 1965 A formaldehyde-glutaraldehyde fixative of high osmolarity for use in electron microscopy. Journal of Cell Biology 27: 137A-138a (Abstract)
7 Reynolds E S 1963 The use of lead citrate at high pH, as an electron opaque stain in electron microscopy. Journal of Cell Biology 17: 208-212
8 Bessis M 1973 Living blood cells and their ultrastructure. Springer Verlag, Berlin
9 Cawley J C, Hayhoe F G J 1973 Ultrastructure of haemic cells. In: A cytological atlas of normal and leukemic blood and bone marrow. W B Saunders, London
10 Tanaka Y, Goodman J R 1972 Electron microscopy of human blood cells. Harper and Row, New York
11 Hurez D, Flandrin G, Preud'homme J L 1972 Unreleased intracellular monoclonal macroglobulin in chronic lymphocytic leukemia. Clinical and Experimental Immunology 10: 223-234
12 Bessis M, Breton-Gorius J, Binet J L 1963 Etude comparée du plasmocytome et du syndrome de Waldenström. Examen au microscope électronique. Nouvelle Revue Française d'Hématologie 3: 159-184
13 Katayama I, Schneider G B 1977 Further ultrastructural characterization of hairy cells of leukemic reticuloendotheliosis. American Journal of Pathology 86: 163-182
14 Daniel M T, Flandrin G 1974 Fine structure of abnormal cells in hairy cells (tricholeukocytic) leukemia, with special reference to their in vitro phagocytic capacity. Laboratory Investigation 30: 1-8
15 Bessis M, Breton-Gorius J 1969 Pathologie et asynchronisme de développement des organelles cellulaires au cours des leucémies aigües granulocytaires. Etude au microscope électronique. Nouvelle Revue Française d'Hématologie 9: 245-278
16 Breton-Gorius J, Houssay D 1973 Auer bodies in acute promyelocytic leukemia. Demonstration of their fine structure and peroxidase localization. Laboratory Investigation 28: 135-141
17 Bessho F, Fujiu M, Kinumaki H 1981 Acute non-lymphocytic leukemia showing abnormal nuclear lobulation. American Journal of Clinical Pathology 75: 684-692
18 Felman P, Morel D, Bryon P A, Espinouse D, Coeur P 1986 Intra-cytoplasmic crystalline inclusions in acute myeloid leukemia: a rare event. Scandinavian Journal of Haematology 36: 520-524
19 Graham R C, Karnovsky M J 1966 The early stages of absorption of injected horseradish peroxidase in the proximal tubules of mouse kidney: ultrastructural cytochemistry by a new technic. Journal of Histochemistry and Cytochemistry 14: 291-302
20 Breton-Gorius J, Guichard J 1972 Ultrastructural localization of peroxidase activity in human platelets and megakaryocytes. American Journal of Pathology 66: 277-286.
21 Breton-Gorius J, Guichard J 1976 Ameliorations techniques permettant de révéler la peroxydase plaquettaire. Nouvelle Revue Française d'Hématologie 16: 381-390
22 Breton-Gorius J, Van Haeke D, Pryzwansky K B et al 1984 Simultaneous detection of membrane markers with monoclonal antibodies and peroxidatic activities in leukemia: ultrastructural analysis using a new method of fixation preserving the platelet peroxidase. British Journal of Haematology 58: 447-458.
23 Reyes F, Gourdin M F, Farcet J P, Dreyfus B, Breton-Gorius J 1978 Synthesis of a peroxidase activity by cells of hairy cell leukemia: a study by ultrastructural cytochemistry. Blood 52: 537-550
24 Roels F, Wisse E, De Prest B, Van Der Meulen J 1975 Cytochemical discrimination between catalases and peroxidases using diamino benzidine. Histochemistry 41: 281-311
25 Anderson W A, Trantalis J, Kang Y H 1975 Ultrastructural localization of endogenous mammary gland peroxidase during lactogenesis in the rat. Results after tannic acid-formaldehyde glutaraldehyde fixation. Journal of Histochemistry and Cytochemistry 23: 295-302
26 Heynen M J, Tricot G, Verwilghen R L 1984 A reliable method with good cell preservation for the demonstration of peroxidase activity in human platelets and megakaryocytes. Histochemistry 80: 79-84
27 Fahimi H D 1969 Cytochemical localization of peroxidatic activity of catalase in rat hepatic microbodies (peroxisomes). Journal of Cell Biology 43: 275-288
28 Novikoff A B, Goldfischer S 1969 Visualization of peroxisomes (microbodies) and mitochondria with diaminobenzidine. Journal of Histochemistry and Cytochemistry 17: 675-680.
29 Novikoff A B, Novikoff P M, Davis C, Quintana N 1972 Studies on microperoxisomes. II A cytochemical method for light and electron microscopy. Journal of Histochemistry and Cytochemistry 20: 1006-1023

30. Novikoff A B, Novikoff P M, Davis C, Quintana N 1973 Studies on microperoxisomes. V. Are microperoxisomes ubiquitous in mammalian cells? Journal of Histochemistry and Cytochemistry 21: 737–755
31. Breton-Gorius J, Guichard J 1975 Fine structural and cytochemical identification of microperoxisomes in developing human erythrocytic cells. American Journal of Pathology 79: 523–536
32. Breton-Gorius J, Guichard J 1975 Two different types of granules in megakaryocytes and platelets as revealed by the diaminobenzidine method. Journal de Microscopie et de Biologie Cellulaire 23: 197–202
33. Breton-Gorius J, Coquin Y, Guichard J 1978 Cytochemical distinction between azurophils and catalase-containing granules in leukocytes. I Studies in developing neutrophils and monocytes from patients with myeloperoxidase deficiency: comparison with peroxidase-deficient chicken heterophils. Laboratory Investigation 38: 21–31
34. Breton-Gorius J, Guichard J 1978 Cytochemical distinction between azurophils and catalase-containing granules in leukocytes: distribution in human promyelocytes and promocytes. Journal of the Reticuloendothelial Society 24: 637–646
35. Thiery J P 1967 Mise en évidence des polysaccharides sur coupes fines en microscopie électronique. Journal de Microscopie 6: 987–1017
36. Singer S J 1959 Preparation of an electron-dense antibody conjugate. Nature 183: 1523–1525
37. Hammerling U, Rajewsky K 1971 Evidence for surface-associated immunoglobulin on T and B lymphocytes. European Journal of Immunology 1: 447–451
38. De Petris S, Raff M C 1973 Normal distribution, patching and capping of lymphocyte surface immunoglobulin studied by electron microscopy. Nature New Biology 241: 257–259
39. Avrameas S 1969 Coupling of enzymes to proteins with glutaraldehyde. Use of the conjugates for the detection of antigens and antibodies. Immunochemistry 6: 43–52
40. Nakane P K, Pierce G B 1966 Enzyme-labeled antibodies: preparation and application for the localization of antigens. Journal of Histochemistry and Cytochemistry 14: 929–931
41. Bretton R, Terninck T, Avrameas S, 1972 Comparison of peroxidase and ferritin labelling of cell surface antigen. Experimental Cell Research 71: 145–155
42. De Mey J 1983 Colloidal gold probes in immunocytochemistry. In: Polak J M, Van Norden S (eds) Immunocytochemistry: applications in pathology and biology. Wright, Bristol, pp 82–112
43. Breton-Gorius J, Lewis J C, Guichard J, Kieffer N, Vainchenker W 1987 Monoclonal antibodies specific for human platelet membrane glycoproteins bind to monocytes by focal absorption of platelet membrane fragments: an ultrastructural immunogold study. Leukemia 1: 131–141
44. Faulk W P, Taylor G M 1971 An immunocolloid method for the electron microscope. Immunochemistry 8: 1081–1083
45. Horisberger M, Rosset J 1977 Colloid gold, a useful marker for transmission and scanning electron microscopy. Journal of Histochemistry and Cytochemistry 25: 295–305
46. Tulliez M, Villeval J L, Lejeune F et al 1987 Expression of blood group A antigen during erythroid differentiation in A_1 and A_2 subjects. Leukemia 1: 44–51
47. Robinson D, Tavares de Castro J, Polli N, O'Brien M, Catovsky D 1984 Simultaneous demonstration of membrane antigens and cytochemistry at ultrastructural level: a study with the immunogold method, acid phosphatase and myeloperoxidase. British Journal of Haematology 56: 617–631
48. Lawlor E, Finn T, Blaney C, Temperley I J, McCann S R 1986 Monocytic differentiation in acute myeloid leukemia: a cause of Fc binding of monoclonal antibodies. British Journal of Haematology 64: 339–346
49. Breton-Gorius J, Reyes F 1976 Ultrastructure of human bone marrow cell maturation. International Review of Cytology 46: 251–321
50. Bredeeroo P, Van Der Meulen J, Daems W T H 1986 Ultrastructural localization of peroxidase activity in developing neutrophil granulocytes from human bone marrow. Histochemistry 84: 445–453
51. Pryzwansky K, Breton-Gorius J 1985 Identification of a subpopulation of primary granules in human neutrophils based upon maturation and distribution. Studies by transmission electron microscopy cytochemistry and high voltage electron microscopy of whole cell preparations. Laboratory Investigation 53: 664–671
52. Griffin J D, Ritz J, Beveridge R P, Lipton J M, Daley J F, Schlossman S F 1983 Expression of My 7 antigen on myeloid precursor cells. International Journal of Cell Cloning 1: 33–48
53. Bodel P T, Nichols B A, Bainton D F 1977 Appearance of peroxidase reactivity within the rough endoplasmic reticulum of blood monocytes after surface adherence. Journal of Experimental Medicine 145: 267–274

54 Beelen R H J, Van't Veer M B, Fluitsma D M, Hoefsmit E C M 1978 Identification of different peroxidatic activity patterns in human macrophages in vivo and in vitro. Journal of the Reticuloendothelial Society 24: 351–362
55 Breton-Gorius J, Guichard J, Vainchenker W, Vilde J L 1980 Ultrastructural and cytochemical changes induced by short and prolonged culture of human monocytes. Journal of the Reticuloendothelial Society 27: 289–301
56 Coulomb B, Dubertret L, Bell E et al 1983 Endogenous peroxidases in normal human dermis: a marker of fibroblast differentiation. Journal of Investigative Dermatology 81: 75–78
57 Dubertret L, Breton-Gorius J, Fosse M, Touraine R 1981 Peroxidatic activity in endoplasmic reticulum of normal human Langerhans cells. Journal of the Reticuloendothelial Society 30: 313–316
58 Soler P, Basset F, Mazin F, Grandsaigne M, Breton-Gorius J 1982 Peroxidatic activities of human alveolar macrophages in some pulmonary granulomatous disorders. Journal of the Reticuloendothelial Society 31: 511–521
59 Breton-Gorius J, Guichard J, Tabilio A, Vainchenker W, Vinci G, Henri A 1985 Ultrastructural cytology and cytochemistry of non-lymphocytic acute leukemias. In D Quagliano, F G J Hayhoe (eds) The cytobiology of leukaemias and lymphomas. Raven Press, New York, pp 178–199
60 Breton-Gorius J, Villeval J L, Mitjavila M T et al 1987 Ultrastructural and cytochemical characterization of blasts from early erythroblastic leukemias. Leukemia 1: 173–181
61 Rabellino E M, Levene R B, Leung L L K, Nachman R L 1981 Human megakaryocytes. II Expression of platelet proteins in early marrow megakaryocytes. Journal of Experimental Medicine. 154: 88–100
62 Levene R B, Lamaziere J M D, Broxmeyer H E, Rabellino E M 1985 Human megakaryocyte V. Changes in the phenotypic profile of differentiating megakaryocytes. Journal of Experimental Medicine 161: 457–474
63 Vainchenker W, Deschamps J F, Bastin J M et al 1982 Two monoclonal antiplatelet antibodies as markers of human megakaryocyte maturation: immunofluorescent staining and platelet peroxidase detection in megakaryocyte colonies and in vitro cells from normal and leukemic patients. Blood 59: 514–521
64 Vinci G, Tabilio A, Deschamps J F et al 1984 Immunological study of in vitro maturation of human megakaryocytes. British Journal of Haematology 56: 589–605
65 Breton-Gorius J, Vainchenker W 1986 Expression of platelet proteins during the in vitro and in vivo differentiation of megakaryocytes and morphological aspects of their maturation. Seminars in Hematology 23: 43–67
66 Wencel-Drake J D, Dahlback B, White J G, Ginsberg M H 1986 Ultrastructural localization of coagulation factor V in human platelets. Blood 68: 244–249
67 Cramer E M, Meyer D, Le Menn R, Breton-Gorius J 1985 Eccentric localization of von Willebrand factor in an internal structure of platelet α granules resembling that of Weibel–Palade bodies. Blood 66: 710–713
68 Cramer E, Caen J P, Drouet L, Breton-Gorius J 1986 Absence of tubular structures and immunolabeling for Willebrand factor in the platelet α-granules from porcine von Willebrand disease. Blood 68: 774–778
69 Bessis M, Breton-Gorius J 1961 Ultrastructure du pro-érythroblaste. Nouvelle Revue Française d'Hématologie 1: 529–533
70 Edelman P, Vinci G, Villeval J L et al 1986 A monoclonal antibody against an erythrocyte ontogenic antigen identifies fetal and adult erythroid progenitors. Blood 67: 56–63
71 Villeval J L, Testa U, Vinci G et al 1985 Carbonic anhydrase I is an early specific marker of normal human erythroid differentiation. Blood 66: 1162–1170
72 Parkin J, McKenna R W, Brunning R D 1980 Ultrastructural features of basophil and mast cell granulopoiesis in blastic phase Philadelphia chromosome-positive leukemia. Journal of the National Cancer Institute 65: 535–545
73 Breton-Gorius J, Daniel M T, Flandrin G, Kinet-Denoël C 1973 Fine structure and peroxidase activity of circulating micromegakaryoblasts and platelets in a case of acute myelofibrosis. British Journal of Haematology 25: 331–339
74 Breton-Gorius J, Reyes F, Duhamel G, Najman A, Gorin N C 1978 Megakaryoblastic acute leukemia: Identification by the ultrastrutural demonstration of platelet peroxidase. Blood 51: 45–60
75 Breton-Gorius J, Reyes F, Vernant J P, Tulliez M, Dreyfus B 1978 The blast crisis of chronic granulocytic leukemia: megakaryoblastic nature of cells as revealed by the presence of platelet peroxidase. A cytochemical ultrastructural study. British Journal of Haematology 39: 295–303
76 Breton-Gorius J, Bizet M, Reyes F et al 1982 Myelofibrosis and acute megakaryoblastic leukemia in a child. Topographic relationship between fibroblasts and megakaryocytes with an α-granule defect. Leukemia Research 6: 97–110

77 Cosson A, Despres P, Gazengel C, Breton-Gorius J, Prieur M, Josso F 1974 Syndrome leucémique singulier chez un nouveau-né trisomique 21: prolifération mégacaryocyto-plaquettaire; syndrome de coagulation intravasculaire diffuse. Nouvelle Revue Française d'Hématologie 14: 181–198
78 Marie J P, Vernant J P, Dreyfus B, Breton-Gorius J 1979 Ultrastructural localization of peroxidase in 'undifferentiated' blasts during the blast crisis of chronic granulocytic leukemia. British Journal of Haematology 43: 549–558
79 Bain B, Catovsky D, O'Brien M et al 1981 Megakaryoblastic leukemia presenting as acute myelofibrosis: A study of four cases with the platelet peroxidase reaction. Blood 58: 206–213
80 Michandani I, Palutke M 1983 Acute megakaryoblastic leukemia. Cancer 50: 2866–2872
81 Polli N, O'Brien M, Tavares de Castro J, Matutes E, San Miguel J F, Catovsky D 1985 Characterization of blast cells in chronic granulocytic leukemia in transformation, acute myelofibrosis and undifferentiated leukaemia. I Ultrastructural morphology and cytochemistry. British Journal of Haematology 59: 277–296
82 Sariban E, Oliver C, Corash L et al 1984 Acute megakaryoblastic leukemia in childhood. Cancer 54: 1423–1428
83 Bevan D, Rose M, Greaves M 1982 Leukemia of platelet precursors; diverse features in four cases. British Journal of Haematology 51: 147–164
84 Carney A E, Mc Kenna R, Arthur D C, Nesbit M E, Woods W G 1986 Acute megakaryoblastic leukemia in children. British Journal of Haematology 63: 541–554
85 Chan W C, Brynes P K, Kim T H et al 1983 Acute megakaryoblastic leukemia in early childhood. Blood 62: 92–98
86 Imbert M, Jarry M T, Tulliez M, Breton-Gorius J 1983 Platelet peroxidase deficiency in a case of myelodysplasic syndrome with myelofibrosis. Journal of Clinical Pathology 36: 1223–1228
87 Breton-Gorius J, Vainchenker W 1986 Immunological and cytochemical characterizations of megakaryocytic lineage leukemia. In: Megakaryocyte development and function. Alan R Liss, New York, pp 301–317
88 Woessner S, Lafuente R, Frorensa L 1986 Platelet peroxidase of circulating thrombocytes in acquired refractory anaemia. Scandinavian Journal of Haematology 36: 194–197
89 Dellagi K, Tabilio A, Portier M M et al 1985 Expression of vimentin intermediate filament cytoskeleton in acute nonlymphoblastic leukemias. Blood 65: 1444–1452
90 Bennett J M, Catovsky D, Daniel M T et al 1985 Criteria for the diagnosis of acute leukemia of megakaryocyte lineage (M_7). A report of the French–American–British cooperative group. Annals of Internal Medicine 103: 460–462
91 Tabilio A, Vainchenker W, Van Haeke D et al 1984 Immunological characterization of the leukemic megakaryocytic line at light and electron microscopic levels. Leukemia Research 8: 769–781
92 San Miguel J F, Tavares de Castro J, Matutes E et al 1985 Characterization of blast cells in chronic granulocytic leukemia in transformation, acute myelofibrosis and undifferentiated leukemia. British Journal of Haematology 59: 297–309
93 Koike T 1984 Megakaryoblastic leukemia: the characterization and identification of megakaryoblasts. Blood 64: 683–692
94 Villeval J L, Cramer P, Lemoine F et al 1986 Phenotype of early erythroblastic leukemias. Blood 68: 1162–1170
95 Griffin J D, Linch D, Sabbath K, Larcom P, Schlossman J F 1984 A monoclonal antibody reactive with normal and leukemic human myeloid progenitors cells. Leukemia Research 8: 521–534
96 Mannoni P, Janowska-Wieczorek A, Turner A R, McGann L, Turc J M 1982 Monoclonal antibodies against human granulocytes and myeloid differentiation antigens. Human Immunology 5: 309–323
97 Janowska-Wieczorek A, Mannoni P, Turner A R, McGann L, Shaw A R E, Turc J M 1984 Monoclonal antibody specific for granulocytic lineage cells and reactive with human pluripotent and committed haematopoietic progenitor cells. British Journal of Haematology 58: 159–168
98 Tabilio A, Del Canizo M C, Henri A et al 1984 Expression of SSEA-I antigen (3-fucosyl-N-acetyl-lactosamine) on normal and leukemic human haemopoietic cells: modulation by neuraminidase treatment. British Journal of Haematology 58: 697–710
99 Huang M J, Li C Y, Nichols W L, Young J H, Katzman N 1984 Acute leukemia with megakaryocytic differentiation: a study of 12 cases identified immunocytochemically. Blood 64: 427–439
100 Ruiz-Argüelles G J, Marin-Lopez A, Lobato-Mendizabal E, Ruiz-Argüelles A, Nichols W L, Katzman J A 1986 Acute megakaryoblastic leukemias: a prospective study of its identification and treatment. British Journal of Haematology 62: 55–63
101 Williams W C, Weiss G B 1982 Megakaryoblastic transformation of chronic myelogenous leukemia. Cancer 49: 921–926

102 Hanada T, Nakazawa M, Sakuma H, Takahashi M, Kondo I, Takita H 1984 Megakaryoblastic transformation of a chronic myelogenous leukemia in a child. Scandinavian Journal of Haematology 33: 476–481
103 Den Ottolander G J, Te Velde J, Brederoo P et al 1979 Megakaryoblastic leukemia (acute myelofibrosis): a report of three cases. British Journal of Haematology 42: 9–20
104 Marcus R E, Hibbin J A, Matutes E, Waterfield M D, Goldman J M 1986 Megakaryoblastic transformation of myelofibrosis with the expression of the C-sis oncogen. Scandinavian Journal of Haematology 36: 186–193
105 Dharmasena F, Catchpole M, Erber W, Mason D, Gordon-Smith E C 1986 Megakaryoblastic leukemia and myelofibrosis complicating Fanconi anaemia. Scandinavian Journal of Haematology 36: 309–313
106 Efrati P, Nir E, Yarri A, Berrebi A, Kaplan H, Dvilanski A 1979 Myeloproliferative disorders terminating in acute micromegakaryoblastic leukemia. British Journal of Haematology 43: 79–86
107 Egner J R, Aabo K, Dimitrov N 1982 Megakaryocytic leukaemia as a phase of myeloproliferative disorders. Scandinavian Journal of Haematology 28: 186–191
108 Jacobs P, Leroux I, Jacobs L 1984 Megakaryoblastic transformation in myeloproliferative disorders. Cancer 54: 297–302
109 Tabilio A, Herrera A, d'Agay M F et al 1984 Therapy-related leukemia associated with myelofibrosis. Blast cell characterization in six cases. Cancer 54: 1382–1391
110 Sultan C, Sigaux F, Imbert M, Reyes F 1981 Acute myelodysplasia with myelofibrosis: A report of eight cases. British Journal of Haematology 49: 11–16
111 Lewis D S, Thompson M, Hudson E, Liberman M M, Sampson D 1983 Down's syndrome and acute megakaryoblastic leukemia. Acta Haematologica 70: 236–242
112 Coulombel L, Derycke M, Villeval J L et al 1987 Characterization of the blast cell population in two neonates with Down's syndrome and transient myeloproliferative disorder. British Journal of Haematology 66: 69–76
113 Pui C H, William D L, Scaborough V, Jackson C W, Price R, Murphy S 1982 Acute megakaryoblastic leukemia associated with intrinsic platelet dysfunction and constitutional ring 21 chromosome in a young boy. British Journal of Haematology 50: 191–200
114 Nichols C R, Hoffman R, Einhor N L H, Williams S D, Wheeler L A, Garnier M P 1986 Hematologic malignancies associated with primary mediastinal germ-cell tumors. Annals of Internal Medicine 102: 603–609
115 Ninomiya H, Nakazawa M, Shibuya A, Aoki Y, Nagasawa T, Abe T 1986 Successful treatment of acute megakaryoblastic leukemia. Scandinavian Journal of Haematology 36: 147–153
116 Morishita K, Asano S, Takuwa N et al 1984 An atypical case of megakaryoblastic leukemia. Scandinavian Journal of Haematology 32: 442–451
117 Bennett J M, Catovsky D, Daniel M T et al 1976 Proposals for the classification of the acute leukemias. British Journal of Haematology 33: 451–458
118 Griffin J D, Todd R F, Ritz J et al 1983 Differentiation patterns in the blastic phase of chronic myeloid leukemia. Blood 61: 85–91
119 Andersson L C, Gahmberg C G, Teerenhovi L, Vuopio P 1979 Glycophorin A as a cell surface marker of early erythroid differentiation in acute leukemia. International Journal of Cancer 23: 717–720
120 Andersson L C, Wegelius R, Borgstrom G H, Gamberg C G 1980 Change in cellular phenotype from lymphoid to erythroid in a case of AL. Scandinavian Journal of Haematology 23: 115–121
121 Ekblom M, Borgstrom G, Von Willebrand E, Gahmberg C G, Vuopio P, Andersson L C 1983 Erythroid blast crisis in chronic myelogenous leukemia. Blood 62: 591–596
122 Greaves M F, Sieff C, Edwards P A W 1983 Monoclonal antiglycophorin as a probe for erythroleukemias. Blood 61: 645–651
123 Liszka K, Majdic O, Bettelheim P, Knapp W 1983 Glycophorin A expression in malignant hematopoiesis. American Journal of Hematology 15: 219–226
124 Reiffers J, Bernard P, Larrue J et al 1985 Acute erythroblastic leukemia presenting as acute indifferentiated leukemia: a report of two cases with ultrastructural features. Leukemia Research 9: 413–420
125 Bainton D F, Friedlander L M, Shohet S B 1977 Abnormalities in granule formation in acute myelogenous leukemia. Blood 49: 693–704
126 Tulliez M, Breton-Gorius J 1979 Three types of Auer bodies in acute leukemias. Visualization of their protein by negative contrast after peroxidase cytochemistry. Laboratory Investigation 47: 419–426
127 Mintz U, Djaldetti M, Rozenszajn L, Pinkhas J, De Vries A 1973 Giant lysosome-like structures in promyelocytic leukemia. Ultrastructural and cytochemical observations. Biomedicine 19: 426–430

128 Tulliez M, Vernant J P, Breton-Gorius J, Imbert M, Sultan C 1979 Pseudo Chediak–Higashi anomaly in a case of acute myeloid leukemia. Electron microscopic studies. Blood 54: 863–871
129 Bainton D F 1975 Abnormal neutrophils in acute myelogenous leukemia: identification of subpopulations based on analysis of azurophils and specific granules. Blood Cells 1: 191–199
130 Breton-Gorius J, Houssay D, Dreyfus B 1975 Partial myeloperoxidase deficiency in a case of preleukaemia. I. Studies of fine structure and peroxidase synthesis of promyelocytes. British Journal of Haematology 30: 273–278
131 Marie J P, Reiffers J, Brun B, Reyes F, Breton-Gorius J, Dreyfus B 1980 Chronic granulocytic aplasia with partial blastic bone marrow involvement. Demonstration of myeloid origin of the blast by ultrastructural detection of myeloperoxidase. A study of three cases. Leukemia Research 4: 399–407
132 Marie J P, Boucheix C, Zittoun J et al 1982 Determination of ultrastructural peroxidases and immunologic membrane markers in the diagnosis of acute leukemias. Blood 59: 270–276
133 Reiffers J, Darmendrail V, Larrue J et al 1981 Ultrastructural cytochemical prospective study of adult acute lymphoblastic leukemia: detection of peroxidase activity in patients failing to respond to treatment. Cancer 48: 927–931
134 Stefani S, Chandra S, Schrek R, Tonaki H, Knospe W H 1977 Endoplasmic reticulum-associated structures in lymphocytes from patients with chronic lymphocytic leukemia. Blood 50: 125–139
135 David B, Reiffers J, Vezon G et al 1985 ALL diagnosis remains uncertain or equivocal despite monoclonal antibodies and ultrastructural cytochemistry. In: Grignani F, Martelli M F, Mason D Y (eds) Monoclonal bodies in haematopathology. Raven Press, New York, pp 59–65
136 Nadler L M, Anderson K C, Marti G et al 1983 B_4, a human B lymphocyte-associated antigen expressed on normal, mitogen-activated and malignant B lymphocytes. Journal of Immunology 131: 244–250
137 Ritz J, Pesando J, Notis-McConart Y, Lazarus H, Schlossman S F 1980 A monoclonal antibody to human acute lymphoblastic leukemia antigen. Nature 283: 583–585
138 Parkin J L, Arthur D C, Abramson C S et al 1982 Acute leukemia associated with the t(4;11) chromosome rearrangement: ultrastructural and immunologic characteristics. Blood 60: 1321–1331
139 Mirro J, Kitchingman G, Williams D et al 1986 Clinical and laboratory characteristics of acute leukemia with the 4;11 translocation. Blood 67: 689–697
140 Bennett J M, Catovsky D, Daniel M T et al 1980 A variant form of hypergranular promyelocytic leukemia (M_3). British Journal of Haematology 44: 169–170
141 Berger R, Bernheim A, Daniel M T, Valensi F, Flandrin G 1981 Translocation in acute promyelocytic leukemia (M_3) and cytological M_3-variant. Nouvelle Revue Française d'Hématologie 23: 27–38
142 McKenna R W, Parkin J, Bloomfield C D, Sunberg R D, Brunning R D 1982 Acute promyelocytic leukemia: a study of 39 cases with identification of a hyperbasophilic microgranular variant. British Journal of Haematology 50: 201–214
143 Bennett J M, Catovsky D, Daniel M T et al 1985 Proposed revised criteria for the classification of acute myeloid leukemia. A report of the French–American–British Cooperative group. Annals of Internal Medicine 103: 620–625
144 Le Beaum M, Larson R A, Bitter M A, Vardiman J W, Golomb H, Rowley J 1983 Association of an inversion of chromosome 16 with abnormal marrow eosinophils in acute myelomonocytic leukemia. New England Journal of Medicine 309: 630–636
145 Larson R A, Williams S F, Le Beau M M, Bitterm M A, Vardiman J W, Rowley J 1986 Acute myelomonocytic leukemia with abnormal eosinophils and inv(16) or t(16;16) has a favorable prognosis. Blood 68: 1242–1249
146 Denegri J F, Naiman S C, Gillen J, Thomas J W 1978 In vitro growth of basophils containing the Philadelphia chromosome in the acute phase of chronic myelogenous leukaemia. British Journal of Haematology 40: 351–352
147 Parkin J L, McKenna R W, Brunning R D 1982 Philadelphia chromosome-positive blastic leukemia: ultrastructural and ultracytochemical evidence of basophil and mast cell differentiation. British Journal of Haematology 52: 663–667
148 Zucker-Franklin D 1980 Ultrastructural evidence for the common origin of human mast cells and basophils. Blood 56: 534–540
149 Lawlor E, McCann S R, Willoughby R, Dunne J, Temperley J 1983 Basophil differentiation in Ph-positive blast cell leukaemia. British Journal of Haematology 54: 157–160
150 Rimmer E F, Turberville C, Horton M A 1986 Cell membrane glycoproteins of human mast cells: a biochemical comparison with basophils. Experimental Hematology 14: 809–811
151 Bainton D F 1975 Ultrastructure and cytochemistry of monocytic leukemia. In: Mononuclear phagocytes in immunity, infection and pathology. Blackwell Scientific, Oxford, pp 83–93

152 Lambertenghi-Deliliers G, Pozzoli E, Zanon P, Maiolo A T 1978 Ultrastructural study of myeloperoxidase activity in acute leukemia cells. Journal of Submicroscopic Cytology 10: 239–247
153 O'Brien M, Catovsky D, Costello C 1980 Ultrastructural cytochemistry of leukemic cells. Characterization of the early small granules of monoblasts. British Journal of Haematology 45: 201–208

5
The Ultrastructure of Lymphoid Cells
Estela Matutes   Daniele Robinson

INTRODUCTION

Human lymphoproliferative malignancies include a broad spectrum of diseases which reflect the morphological and immunological heterogeneity of the lymphoid system. The classification and characterization of these disorders has greatly benefited from advances in immunological methods. Prior to the development of the hybridoma technic by Kohler and Milstein,[1] the markers available for the study of lymphoid cells included terminal deoxynucleotidyl transferase (TdT), heterologous anti-human B- and T-cell sera and rosetting tests: E-rosettes for T-lymphocytes and mouse red blood cell rosettes for B-lymphocytes.

In recent years, a wide panel of monoclonal antibodies (McAbs) detecting antigenic determinants on lymphocytes has made it possible to define more clearly the B and T lineages of differentiation. In addition, it has become apparent that a morphological analysis of neoplastic lymphoid cells at the ultrastructural level is important for the precise characterization of several disease entities. For instance, transmission electron microscopy (TEM) has been useful in recognizing cells from certain lymphoid malignancies such as Sézary syndrome (SS),[2,3] hairy cell leukemia (HCL)[4] and some cases of T-cell prolymphocytic leukaemia (T-PLL).[5]

More recently, immunolabeling technics, such as the immunogold method at the TEM level, have helped the characterization of normal and leukemic lymphocytes by allowing the simultaneous investigation of the fine structure of the cell and its membrane phenotype. The use of such technics in the study of normal blood has demonstrated a great morphological heterogeneity in human lymphocytes, and has disclosed the existence of distinct subsets that may represent the normal counterparts of some of the lymphoid leukemias.

This chapter will outline the main ultrastructural features which help to characterize the neoplastic cells from B and T lymphoproliferative disorders and will review the fine structure of normal peripheral blood lymphocytes defined according to their antigenic phenotype by means of McAbs and the immunogold method.

METHODS FOR THE ULTRASTRUCTURAL CHARACTERIZATION OF NORMAL AND NEOPLASTIC LYMPHOCYTES

PREPARATION OF SAMPLES

Bone marrow and peripheral blood
The mononuclear cell fractions from bone marrow (BM) and peripheral blood (PB) can be obtained by various methods that are based on the relative densities or sizes of the different cell types. In practice, the technic most widely applied is the one which uses Ficoll-Isopaque (Lymphoprep, Nyegaard, Oslo, density = 1.077 g/ml). Heparinized venous PB and BM aspirates are diluted volume to volume with phosphate-buffered saline (PBS)

(Oxoid, England) or Ca^{2+}/Mg^{2+} free Hanks' balanced salt solution (HBSS) (Gibco, Paisley, Scotland). Diluted peripheral blood or bone marrow (2 volumes) is then layered on Lymphoprep (1 volume) and centrifuged at 1800 rev/min for 30 min. The mononuclear fraction is then removed with a Pasteur pipette and washed three times in HBSS or PBS by centrifugation at 1200 rev/min each time for 10 min. The supernatant is removed and the cell pellet is resuspended in the fixative solution.

Lymphoid tissues: lymph nodes and spleen
Following surgical removal, a piece of spleen or lymph node is placed into a Petri dish containing medium RPMI-1640 (Gibco) with 20% fetal calf serum (Gibco). A fragment of the tissue is cut into small pieces (1 mm) and transferred to the fixative solution. The other fragment is carefully smashed with a spatula to free the cells into the medium which is collected into a tube and centrifuged at 1200 rev/min for 10 min. The cell pellet is then resuspended in the fixative solution. If the erythrocyte contamination is high, a preliminary separation on Lymphoprep is performed following the method described above for PB and BM specimens.

Skin
The skin fragment is placed into a Petri dish containing medium RPMI-1640 with 20% fetal calf serum and then cut into small pieces in a perpendicular direction to the layers of the skin.

FIXATION, DEHYDRATION, EMBEDDING AND STAINING

The tissue fragments and the cell pellets are fixed in a freshly prepared solution of 3% glutaraldehyde made from the 25% glutaraldehyde commercial reagent (TAAB) in 0.1 mol/l phosphate buffer pH 7.2 or in 0.1 mol/l sodium cacodylate buffer pH 7.4 (BHD Chemicals, Poole, England). The osmolarity of the fixative is adjusted by the addition of sucrose. The fixation is performed at room temperature for 30 to 120 min and, then, the specimens are washed three times in the same buffer as used in the fixative, either by changing the buffer (when using tissue fragments) or by centrifugation for 10 min at 1200 rev/min and resuspending the cell pellet each time in the buffer.

The aldehyde fixation is followed by a further fixation in 1% osmium tetroxide (JMC Platinum Group Chemicals, England) in Millonig's medium, pH 7.4–7.6 or in 0.1 mol/l sodium cacodylate pH 7.4, for 60 min at 4°C. Following this postfixation, the samples are washed twice in the buffer or in distilled water. Cells may then be stained en block by resuspending them in a solution of 4% aqueous uranyl acetate (BDH Chemicals) for 30 min at 4°C and are subsequently washed in distilled water. Uranyl acetate prestaining increases the density of all nucleic acids and proteins (DNA, RNA and all the cell membranes). The cells are pre-embedded in a warm (60°C) solution of 3% aqueous agar as follows: two or three drops of liquid agar are transferred to the dry cell pellet with a warm Pasteur pipette. The cells are resuspended in the agar which is then transferred to a glass slide, allowed to cool for a few minutes and cut into small pieces of approximately 1 mm which will be subsequently dehydrated.

Dehydration is carried out at room temperature by placing the tissue embedded in agar in a series of increasing concentrations of ethanol (70°, 90° and absolute). Each alcohol is changed twice and the fragments are incubated for 10 min in each one. Because most of the resins used for electron microscopy embedding are not miscible with ethanol, an extra step is included, using propylene oxide, which is an excellent solvent for resins. Thus, following the incubation in absolute ethanol, the tissue is placed for 5 min in propylene oxide and, in order to facilitate the penetration of the resin into the tissue, the fragments are placed for 10 min in a mixture of equal volumes of propylene oxide and the resin Araldite 1 (EMscope, Ashford, England). The Araldite is changed and the tissue is kept overnight or for 12 hours in Araldite 1 on a rotator. The Araldite 1 is then replaced by a freshly made Araldite 1 for 2 hours, and finally the tissue is kept for 3 hours at room temperature in a rotator in Araldite 2. The tissue fragments are embedded as follows: one or two drops of Araldite 2 are placed at the bottom of a plastic micromould (EMscope), shaped in the form of a pyramid, and then the pieces of tissue are transferred to the micromould and covered with Araldite 2. The micromoulds are kept at 60°C for 48 hours, which is the time required for complete polymerization of the resin. For skin samples, a flat micromould may be used in order to obtain the desired orientation of the tissue.

The resins Araldite 1 and 2 are prepared as follows:

Araldite 1 (EMscope):
Resin CY212	10	ml
Hardener DDSA	10	ml
Dibutylphthalate	0.25	ml

Araldite 2 (EMscope):
Araldite 1	20	ml
Benzyldimethylamine (BDMA)	0.4	ml

Araldite 1 and 2 are made by a thorough mixing of these compounds. The amount of the accelerator BDMA is critical for determining the rate of hardening and it is the most unstable component.

Semithin (thick) sections (0.5–2 μm) are cut on an ultramicrotome and transferred to a drop of water placed on a glass slide previously coated with poly-L-lysine (Sigma, Poole, England) and the sections are then allowed to dry. Counterstain may be performed with 1% toluidine blue in 1% borax or with Humphrey's stain which uses methylene blue–Azure II and basic fuchsin; the semithin sections are viewed by light microscopy.

Humphrey's stain is prepared as follows:

Stock solution A: methylene blue–Azure II
Methylene blue	0.13	g
Azure II	0.02	g
Glycerol	10	ml
Methanol	10	ml
Phosphate buffer*	30	ml
Distilled water	50	ml

*Phosphate buffer is prepared as follows:
$Na_2HPO_4 \cdot 2H_2O$	1.338	g
KH_2PO_4	0.908	g
Distilled water	100	ml

Mix all compounds and adjust pH to 6.9

Stock solution B: basic fuchsin
Basic fuchsin	0.100	g
Ethanol (50%)	10	ml

For the staining dissolve 3 ml of the stock solution in 57 ml of distilled water. The semithin sections are stained as follows:

1. Stain sections in solution A for 20 min at 60°C and wash twice in distilled water.
2. Stain sections with solution B at room temperature for 1 min and wash twice in distilled water.

The same block is then used to obtain ultrathin sections of 20–60 nm thickness to allow the integration of the light and electron microscopy findings. Ultrathin sections are collected on nickel or copper grids, and counterstained with 5% uranyl acetate in methanol for 10 min and with Reynold's lead citrate for 5 min.

Reynold's lead citrate is prepared as follows:

Lead nitrate (Sigma, Poole, England)	1.33 g
Sodium citrate (BDH, Poole, England)	1.76 g
Distilled water	30 ml

Place all the compounds in a clean 50 ml flask and shake vigorously for 1 min. Allow to stand for 30 min with some shaking. Add 8 ml of 1 mol/l NaOH and make up to 50 ml with distilled water. Mix by inversion. The solution is kept in small aliquots in Ependorf plastic tubes at 4°C.

CYTOCHEMICAL TECHNICS: ACID PHOSPHATASE

The method of Gomori modified by Barka and Anderson,[6] which uses β-glycerophosphate as a substrate and lead nitrate as a coupling agent, is the most commonly used method. The material is fixed in freshly made 1.5% glutaraldehyde in 67 mmol/l sodium cacodylate buffer pH 7.4 for 30 min at 4°C, and subsequently washed three times in 67 mmol/l sodium cacodylate buffer containing 7.5% sucrose.

The incubation medium of the reaction is prepared as follows:

Solution A: 1.25% sodium β-glycerophosphate (Sigma, St Louis, USA)
Solution B: 0.2 mol/l Tris–maleate buffer pH 5.0 (BDH Chemicals, England)
Solution C: 0.2% lead nitrate (Sigma, Poole, England)

The three solutions are made up with freshly boiled distilled water after it has cooled. Then, the following are mixed in clean glassware: 20 ml of solution A, 20 ml of solution B and 20 ml of distilled water; 40 ml of solution C are added dropwise, while stirring. A control medium is prepared as above in another flask but the substrate (solution A) is replaced by 20 ml of distilled water. The pH of both is adjusted to 5.0 using 1 mol/l HCl, maleic acid or Tris buffer. The mixture should be filtered if precipitates are formed.

The material is incubated for 45 min at 37°C and subsequently washed three times in Tris–maleate buffer with 7.5% sucrose. Postfixation, dehydration and embedding are performed as for ultrastructural morphology (see above) without the block-staining step with aqueous uranyl acetate.

Sections are viewed under the electron microscope unstained. The reaction is based on the hydrolysis of the substrate which produces phosphate ions that couple to the lead forming an electron-dense precipitate of lead phosphate; this is visible without the need for further staining.

IMMUNOELECTRON MICROSCOPY

Immunolabeling at the ultrastructural level allows the morphological analysis of cells which have been characterized by their reactivity with McAbs or polyclonal antibodies. In order to be successful, the technic should offer a high degree of labeling and, at the same time, should not interfere with the maintenance of a good preservation of the cell structures. In practice, these requirements appear to be mutually exclusive, since fixation of the cells or tissues in glutaraldehyde and, to some extent, in other fixatives tends to reduce the antigenicity, and hence the reactivity with relevant antibodies.[7]

A number of immunolabeling methods are available. These consist of marker molecules coupled either to the antibody whose reactivity is being tested (direct method) or to a second layer antibody (indirect method). The marker molecules, in order to be visualized at the ultrastructural level, must be electron dense, such as ferritin or colloidal gold particles, or have an electron-dense reaction product, for example enzymes such as horseradish peroxidase (HRP).

Immunoperoxidase

The immunoperoxidase method has been used successfully in the past for the localization of membrane antigens, in particular surface immunoglobulins (Ig).[8] Although this method has the advantage that the cells are fixed prior to the immunocytochemical technic and, therefore, the morphological preservation is optimal, prefixation may result in the loss of antigenicity.[9,10] This method has the disadvantage that the cells should be viewed in the absence of counterstain. This is because the immunocytochemical reaction, which is seen as an electron-dense deposit at the antigenic site, may be weak and obscured by uranyl acetate and lead citrate staining. Further, immunolabeling procedures involving a cytochemical reaction cannot easily be quantified and this may be a disadvantage in certain studies.

Cytoplasmic Ig can be identified in B-lymphocytes using a one-step immunoperoxidase technic which was originally developed for surface Ig.[8,11] However, these workers did suggest that the technic may not be adequate for the detection of small amounts of Ig. The method used in the authors' laboratory is a modification of that of Newell et al,[12] which includes a brief incubation in a detergent, saponin, which permeabilizes the membrane and facilitates the binding of the anti-Ig reagents to the Ig molecules located in the cytoplasm.[13] The cells are then fixed briefly for 15 min in 0.01% glutaraldehyde in PBS. They are subsequently incubated in 1% saponin (Sigma, Poole, England) solution in PBS which has been heated to 55°C. Although this procedure greatly increases the amount of immunolabeling obtained, the incubation of the cells in saponin significantly reduces the degree of morphological preservation and, futhermore, this loss of morphological detail is proportional to the length of incubation.

It may be necessary to perform a preliminary experiment to determine the optimal length of incubation in saponin that will give good immunolabeling whilst at the same time maintaining the best possible cellular morphology. For example, in B-prolymphocytes, which usually contain small amounts of cytoplasmic Ig, a 10–15 min incubation in saponin is often required with the result that cellular preservation is poor, whereas in plasma cell leukemia cells, in which the Ig is present in much greater amounts, a 5 min incubation in saponin may be sufficient. After washing, the cells are incubated for 60 min at room temperature with at least twice their volume of HRP-labeled anti-human Ig (Dako, High Wycombe, England) diluted 1:15 in PBS. The peroxidase is developed using the method of Graham and Karnovsky[14] and the section is viewed in the absence of counterstain.

Ferritin particles

The immunoferritin technic, as developed by Singer,[15,16] has been applied to a wide variety of biological systems. Early work investigating the expression of Ig on the surface of B-lymphocytes showed good morphology which could be better appreciated by counterstaining the sections.[17-19] Furthermore, ferritin, being particulate, lends itself to quantification, giving a measure of the extent of labeling. However, preparation of ferritin-labeled antibodies is both laborious and requires relatively large amounts of macromolecules for efficient coupling.[20] Moreover, there is usually loss of antibody activity following the coupling reaction, and the resultant heterogeneity of the product requires that the active ferritin–antibody conjugates be isolated before being introduced into the immunolabeling system.[7] Ferritin particles measure approximately 12 nm and, although they are easily visible at high magnifications, they are not apparent at low magnifications. In practice, however, it is less time consuming to screen rapidly a sample at low magnifications to assess the incidence of positive cells, and at these low magnifications it is not easy to visualize the ferritin particles.

Immunogold labeling of membrane antigens

Colloidal gold, which was first described as an immunocytochemical marker for TEM and scanning electron microscope,[21] offers many advantages as tracer for the localization of cell surface antigens at the ultrastructural level.[22,23] First, as a particulate marker with high electron density, it allows the distinctive localization of positive cells which can be detected easily at TEM level. Secondly, the sections may be counterstained, allowing good visualization of the fine structure of the labeled cells. Thirdly, colloidal gold particles can be prepared in a number of sizes from 5 nm to 150 nm, which permits the possibility of double labeling with antibodies coupled directly to gold particles of different diameters. Fourthly, cytochemical reactions for the localization of enzymes within the cell may be performed in combination with the membrane labeling.[24,25]

Originally, the immunolabeling with McAbs was performed on cells prefixed with a low concentration of 1% glutaraldehyde for 5 min.[26] Whilst this procedure works well for many antibodies and has the advantage of ensuring optimal morphological preservation, prefixation of the cells can greatly reduce the reactivity with some McAbs. The prefixation step was subsequently omitted but, in order to ensure good morphological preservation of the cells, the immunolabeling procedure should be performed quickly.[27] For this, all centrifugation steps after the incubation of the cells with the McAb or with the colloidal gold-labeled antibody are short (3 min) and at low speed (400 × g).

The principle involved in the immunogold labeling of cell surface antigens is represented schematically in Figure 5.1 and uses the following method:

200 µl of mononuclear cells (5 × 10^6) are incubated for 15 min at room temperature in 'gold buffer' (see below) which contains human AB serum. This preliminary step is to block any free Fc receptors on the cells and hence to reduce background labeling.[25] The cells are then incubated with the appropriate volume and dilution of McAb for 30 min at room temperature. The total volume of the incubation mixture should not be allowed to

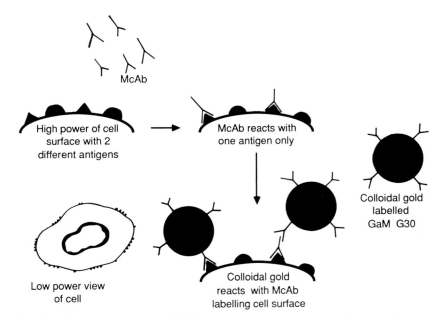

Fig. 5.1 Principles of the immunogold labeling technic at the ultrastructural level. GaM: goat anti-mouse second layer conjugated with 30 nm colloidal gold particles (G30).

exceed 250 µl. After the incubation, the cells are washed three times in the gold buffer and, after the final wash, care is taken to obtain a dry cell pellet. This is incubated for 60 min at room temperature with 40 µl of colloidal gold-labeled goat anti-mouse antibody (Janssen Life Sciences, Beerse, Belgium), which has been centrifuged for 15 min at 700 g before use to remove colloidal gold aggregates. The cells are then washed and fixed in 3% glutaraldehyde in PBS for 30 min at 4°C and subsequently processed as for TEM morphology (see above). Care must be taken not to dilute the cell pellet during the pre-embedding in liquid agar, and for this reason it is essential to obtain a dry cell pellet to which only one drop of agar is added.

Gold buffer
PBS (Oxoid, Basingstoke, England)
0.2% sodium azide (Sigma)
1% bovine serum albumin (Sigma)
2% human AB serum (decomplemented and heat inactivated)

The assessment of antigen expression using the above immunological technic may be combined with the detection of myeloperoxidase or acid phosphatase activity in the same cells.[25] Following the immunolabeling procedure, the cells are fixed in the fixative appropriate for the cytochemical reaction. Thus, 1.5% glutaraldehyde in 67 mmol/l cacodylate buffer for the acid phosphatase reaction and 3% glutaraldehyde in PBS for the myeloperoxidase reaction. Neither reaction affects the degree of immunolabeling and, conversely, the cytochemical reaction, which is performed on fixed cells is unaffected by the colloidal gold labeling.

The size of the colloidal gold particles used may affect the degree of immunolabeling. In general, the greater the diameter of the particle, the less efficient is the resultant labeling. However, very low diameters of less than 10 nm are difficult to distinguish at low magnifications. For this reason, the authors prefer the second layer antibody to be coupled to 30 nm colloidal gold particles, which represents a compromise between optimal labeling and the ready identification of the positive cells.

ULTRASTRUCTURAL FEATURES OF NORMAL LYMPHOCYTES

The existence of two major populations of human lymphocytes, B and T, which are characterized by a different origin, tissue distribution and functional capabilities, has long been recognized. Since the late 1970s, and concomitant with the development of immunological technics, it has been recognized that a great heterogeneity exists within the lymphoid cell populations. Nowadays, it is possible to distinguish by means of specific McAbs several B and T subsets that have distinct functions and can be found at different stages of maturation in the B and T differentiation pathways (Fig. 5.2).

Morphologically, lymphocytes are seen by light microscopy as round or ovoid cells with a nucleus containing clumped chromatin and a scanty cytoplasm. This may occasionally be more abundant and contain azurophil granules which are visible with Romanowsky's stains. Ultrastructural analysis shows that lymphocytes have a nucleus composed mainly of heterochromatin and a cytoplasm with organelles characteristic of eucaryotic cells such as mitochondria, ribosomes, lysosomes and a Golgi apparatus, although all these are, in general, poorly developed.

The application, at TEM level, of immunolabeling technics with McAbs against B and T antigenic determinants has allowed recognition of the morphological differences between the various lymphocyte subsets. The ultrastructural characteristics of normal B- and T-lymphoid subpopulations will be discussed here with particular emphasis on the identification of

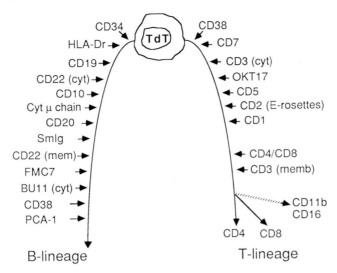

Fig. 5.2 B- and T-lymphoid differentiation pathway representing the sequential appearance of membrane (memb) and/or cytoplasmic (cyt) antigens recognized by McAbs grouped according to their cluster of differentiation (CD).

certain cell subtypes which are believed to be similar to the proliferating cells from some B and T lymphoproliferative disorders.

NORMAL B-LYMPHOCYTES

Four subpopulations of B-lymphocytes, identified primarily by their reactivities with McAbs against class II major histocompatibility antigens (HLA-DR), can be recognized in normal peripheral blood. Monocytes, which are also reactive with these antibodies, can be distinguished from B-lymphocytes by the presence of long cytoplasmic villi, an irregular nuclear outline and numerous small lysosomal granules which, using a combined method, have been shown to be myeloperoxidase positive.[25]

Within the whole population of B-lymphocytes (HLA-DR +), several subpopulations are distinguishable on morphological grounds (Fig. 5.3):

1. Forty per cent of cells have a high nucleo-/cytoplasmic (N:C) ratio, well-condensed chromatin, a centrally placed, often regular nucleus and little organelle development; nucleoli are not prominent (Fig. 5.4a).
2. In a further 40% of cells, the nucleolus is a prominent feature and is often seen accompanied by perinucleolar heterochromatin condensation. Usually these cells have a lower N:C ratio than those in (1) and have greater development of the endoplasmic reticulum (ER). A proportion of cells from this subpopulation resembles the prolymphocytes which are present in B-cell prolymphocytic leukemia (B-PLL) (Fig. 5.4b).
3. Ten per cent of cells have a highly villous outline, a low to medium N:C ratio and little heterochromatin condensation. Some of them display accumulations of ribosomes surrounding strands of parallel ER, but are without evidence of ribosome–lamella complex (RLC) (Fig. 5.4c).
4. A further 10% of normal HLA-DR + B-lymphocytes show features characteristic of lymphoplasmacytoid cells, as shown by a greater development of the ER. Within this

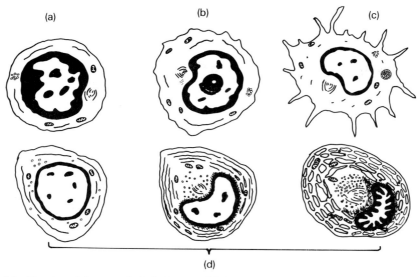

Fig. 5.3 Drawing of four morphological types of B-lymphocytes identified in normal peripheral blood: (a) non-nucleolated; (b) nucleolated (PLL-like); (c) villous (HCL like); (d) antibody-secreting cells, ranging from lymphoplasmacytoid to plasma cells.

subpopulation, certain cells have a few strands of parallel, undilated ER, whilst, in other cells, the ER development has become extensive and electron-dense material can be seen within the ER cisternae. The nuclear shape and the pattern of heterochromatin condensation parallel the increase in cellular maturity. Thus lymphoplasmacytoid cells (Fig. 5.5a) have a high N:C ratio, rounded nucleus and scanty heterochromatin, whereas in plasma cells (Fig. 5.5b) the chromatin is heavily condensed, the nucleus eccentrically located and is often kidney shaped.

In the last few years, the production of specific anti-B-cell McAbs has proved to be useful in the differential diagnosis of B-cell disorders (see Fig. 5.2). For example, the McAb FMC7[28] reacts mainly with hairy cells and B-PLL cells, whereas anti-HC1 and anti-HC2 have been shown to react specifically with hairy cells.[29-31] In addition, OKT10 (CD38), whose reactivity is primarily associated with thymic cells and activated T-lymphocytes, also reacts with cells at late stages of B-cell differentiation, such as lymphoplasmacytoid cells and plasma cells.[32,33]

Some of these McAbs also react with minority populations in normal peripheral blood. For example, 3–6% of lymphocytes are FMC7 +[28] and 2% react with anti-HC2.[30]

Two types of normal B-cell react with the McAb FMC7 (Fig. 5.6). One of these resembles morphologically the prolymphocytes from B-PLL and is characterized by a prominent nucleolus (Fig. 5.6a). The other B-cell type is characterized by a villous outline which resembles that of the cells from hairy cell leukemia (HCL) (Fig. 5.6b). In addition to their reactivity with FMC7, these normal villous lymphocytes react also with the two anti-hairy cell McAbs HC1 and HC2 (Fig. 5.7 a,b).

Although HLA-DR determinants are expressed on most B-cells, their expression on lymphoplasmacytoid cells is variable and is usually lost upon the acquisition of morphological features associated with mature plasma cells. In contrast, normal plasma cells, as well as those of Waldenström's macroglobulinaemia and multiple myeloma are positive with OKT10 (CD38) (Fig. 5.7c). Some of the villous cells seen in normal peripheral blood are also positive with OKT10 indicating a degree of B-cell activation.[25]

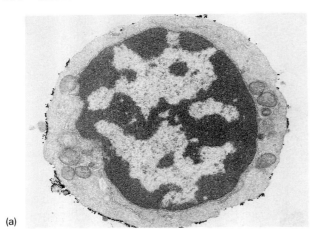

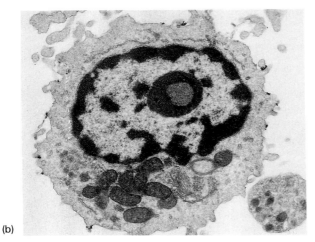

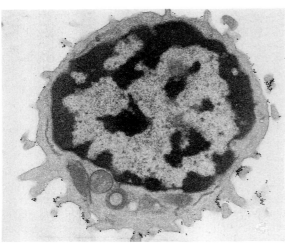

Fig. 5.4 Normal B-lymphocytes labeled with the McAb FMC4 (anti-class II MHC) by the immunogold method (GAM G30).
(a) Non-nucleolated lymphocyte with moderate N:C ratio, condensed nuclear chromatin and round, centrally placed nucleus; clusters of pale granules are seen in the cytoplasm. ($\times$ 12 000)
(b) Nucleolated B-cell. Note the large nucleolus and associated heterochromatin, and a prominent Golgi zone with a cluster of small pale granules. ($\times$ 9100)
(c) Normal villous lymphocyte, resembling cells of HCL or SLVL (splenic lymphoma with villous lymphocytes). ($\times$ 12 000)

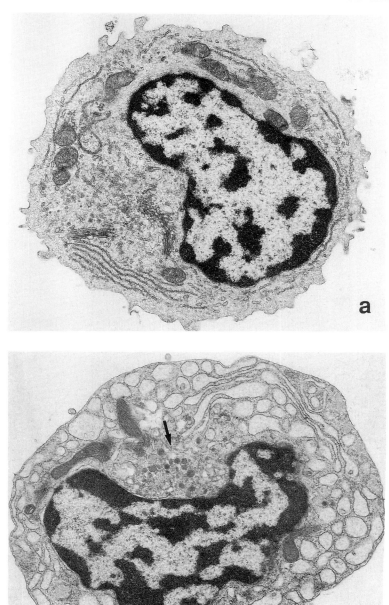

Fig. 5.5 Late B-cells from normal peripheral blood: (a) lymphoplasmacytoid cell showing long strands of ER and an active Golgi apparatus. (× 11 200) (b) Plasma cell with extensive development of dilated ER, Golgi-associated electron dense granules (arrow) and moderate to heavy condensation of the nuclear chromatin. (× 11 680)

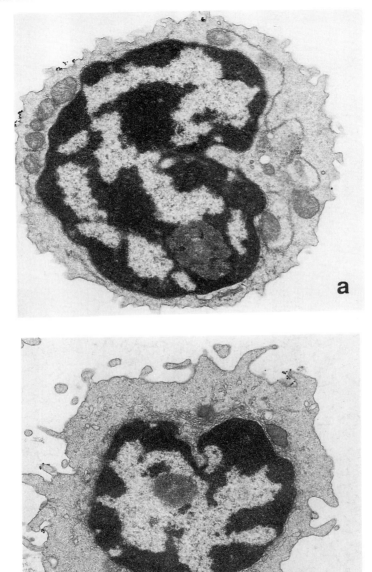

Fig. 5.6 B-lymphocytes labeled with the McAb FMC7: (a) nucleolated B-cell (GAM G30). (× 16 800) (b) Villous lymphocyte (GAM G20). (× 12 800)

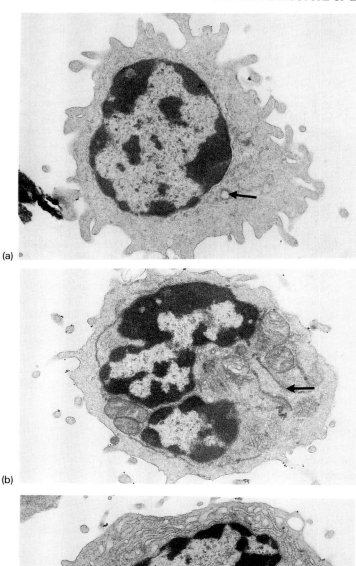

(a)

(b)

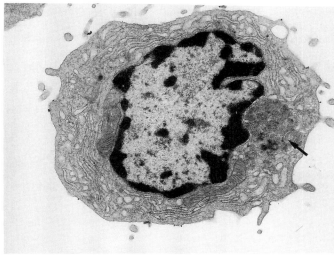

(c)

Fig. 5.7 (a) Villous lymphocyte weakly reactive with anti-HC1. This cell has numerous projections, free ribosomes and a fibrillar structure (arrow). ($\times$ 10 500) (b) Moderately villous cells reactive with anti-HC2, showing an active Golgi zone with pale granules and clusters of ribosome adjacent to two strands of ER (arrow). ($\times$ 11 250) (c) Cell with morphology of a plasma cell reactive with OKT10 (CD38). The numerous profiles of ER are dilated and numerous granules are seen in the Golgi region (arrow). ($\times$ 14 780)

140 THE LEUKEMIC CELL

Therefore, the morphological and immunological similarities of the nucleolated and villous normal subpopulations to those of B-cells leukemias (B-PLL and HCL respectively) indicated that they may represent the normal cell counterparts for these two diseases.

NORMAL T-LYMPHOCYTES

By the late 1970s Grossi et al[34] and Ferranini et al [35] had indicated the existence of two morphologically distinct normal blood T subpopulations: Tγ and Tμ, which could be characterized by having different membrane receptors, functional properties and morphology. By ultrastructural analysis, Tμ-lymphocytes have a high N:C ratio and fewer cytoplasmic organelles than Tγ-lymphocytes. In addition, other minor lymphoid populations have been recognized: the 'cerebriform' mononuclear cell[36,37] and the large granular lymphocyte (LGL) related to Tγ-cells[38–40] and associated with natural killer activity.[41]

The analysis of the ultrastructure of normal T-lymphocytes in relation to their antigenic phenotype is now more precise due to availability of anti-T-cell McAbs (see Fig. 5.2). These studies indicate that normal T-lymphocytes constitute a heterogeneous population when seen at the TEM level, and that there is a degree of correlation between the expression of some membrane antigens and ultrastructural features. For example, cells from the two major T-cell subsets CD8 + (OKT8) and CD4 + (OKT4) have a different morphology when viewed under TEM. CD8 + lymphocytes correspond mainly to the cells with abundant cytoplasm and numerous organelles which include the LGL (Fig. 5.8a).[26,42] In contrast, CD4 lymphocytes usually have a high N:C ratio and few cytoplasmic organelles (Fig. 5.8b); this population also included the cerebriform and convoluted lymphocytes.[27] The morphological distinction between the two major subsets is not always clearly defined since a proportion of CD8 + cells may show features more typical of CD4 + lymphocytes and, conversely, a minority population within the CD4 cells may have features of LGL.[42,43] Since LGL and convoluted T-cells constitute distinct morphological types, they will be considered below in detail.

Large granular lymphocytes
LGLs represent a minor population of lymphocytes of medium to large size with a relatively abundant cytoplasm and azurophil granules. At the TEM level, the most striking feature of LGLs is the marked development of cytoplasmic organelles and, in particular, of lysosomal granules (Fig. 5.9). These are of variable size and density and include characteristic lysosomal structures — the parallel tubular arrays (PTAs) which consist of bundles of packed microtubules in a parallel arrangement (Figs 5.8a and 5.9).

LGLs were first described as cells bearing Fcγ receptors[38,40,44] and more recently they have been associated with natural killer function.[41,45] When considering the antigenic repertoire of LGLs, the authors' observations indicate that they react with McAbs against natural killer (CD11b and CD16) and cytotoxic (CD8 and Leu-7) T-cells as well as with other McAbs (e.g. CD4).[42] LGL is the most common cell type within the Leu7 + cell population, whereas the proportion of LGL cells is variable within the CD8, CD11b(OKM1) and CD16(Leu–11) cell subsets. These findings are in agreement with the immunological information about these cells, namely:

1. A proportion of Tγ-cells (60%) express the antigen recognized by CD11b.[41]
2. The McAb CD16 possibly recognizes the Fcγ receptor.[45]
3. There is overlap in the expression of Leu-7, CD8 and CD3,[41] of Leu-7 and CD11b,[41] and of Leu-7 and CD16.[45]

Since Leu-7 recognizes a higher proportion of LGLs than the McAbs CD16 and CD11b, and the latter are known to react with the cell subset with the greatest natural killer

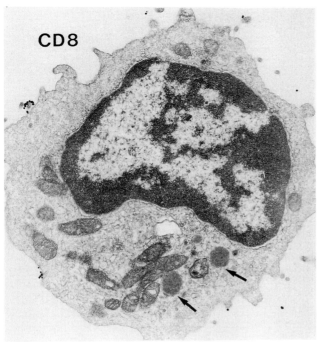

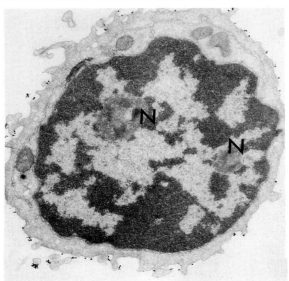

Fig. 5.8 Normal peripheral blood T-cells: (a) CD8+ lymphocyte showing an abundant cytoplasm with a well-developed Golgi zone, granules and parallel tubular arrays (arrows). (× 12 000) (b) Lymphocyte reactive with CD4 showing a high N:C ratio and two small nucleoli (N). (× 12 000).

activity,[41,45] it is possible that the natural killer activity is mediated only by the CD11b+, CD16+ cells with LGL features or, alternatively, that the two morphological cell types, granular and non-granular, are involved in this cytotoxic function.

Two other areas of interest concerning LGLs are:

1. There is a close morphological and phenotypic similarity between the normal blood LGL and the leukemic cells from T-chronic lymphocytic leukemia (T-CLL)

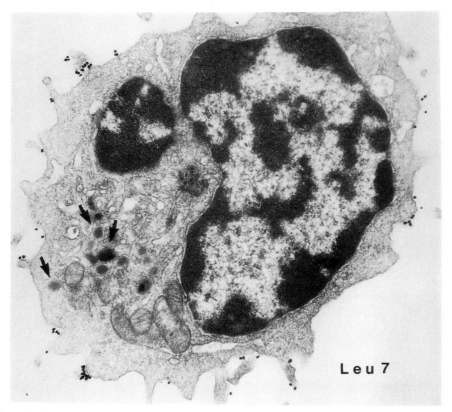

Fig. 5.9 Large granular lymphocyte reactive with the McAb Leu7 showing an eccentric nucleus and abundant cytoplasm with electron-dense granules and parallel tubular arrays (arrows). (× 16 200)

(see below). Cells from the authors' T-CLL patients show the characteristic TEM morphology of LGLs and often display the CD8+, Leu7+ markers. They rarely express CD11b and/or CD16, possibly reflecting the lower frequency of CD11b and CD16+ LGL in normal blood. It is possible that the LGL which displays a CD8+, Leu7+ phenotype may have a higher probability of leukemic transformation because it is the most common type of LGL found in normal blood.

2. There is also, within the CD4+ population, a minority of cells with LGL morphology;[42,43] in rare T-CLL cases this cell may represent the target for the leukemic transformation.[46] This CD4+ LGL subpopulation also expresses CD11b or CD16 and/or Leu-7. This is supported by unusual cases of T-CLL, one with a CD4+, CD11b+, CD16+ phenotype[46] and another whose cells displayed a CD4+, Leu7+ phenotype and had the typical features of LGLs including parallel tubular arrays.

Convoluted and cerebriform T-lymphocytes

In the late 1970s, a few reports described, in normal adult and cord blood[36,37] and in cultures of mitogen-stimulated lymphocytes,[47] the existence of a minority population of lymphocytes with a cerebriform nucleus similar to those of Sézary syndrome (SS). This cerebriform lymphocyte was also shown to form E-rosettes and to bear receptors for the Fc fragment of IgM (Tμ)[37] and, thus, a relationship with the characteristic cells from SS was suggested. The authors' studies, demonstrating that this normal T-cell has CD4, CD3 and OKT17 markers, confirm this view.[27] Furthermore, this lymphocyte, unlike 85% of normal blood T-lymphocytes but in common with the neoplastic cells from most cases of SS, lacks the p40 antigen recognized by McAbs of the CD7 group[27] such as 3A1.[48]

The authors' observations suggest that there are two minor populations of convoluted lymphocytes in normal blood which can be distinguished from each other on ultrastructural and phenotypic grounds. One is the cerebriform, Sézary-like lymphocyte and the other type has morphological similarities with the cells of adult T-cell leukemia/lymphoma (ATLL).[27] The cerebriform cells described by van der Loo et al[37] are characterized by a convoluted nucleus with narrow and deep indentations (Fig. 5.10a). The normal ATLL-like cells, like the leukemic ATLL cells (see below), have nuclear indentations which are broad and short or often appear to be multilobed (Fig. 5.10b).

The membrane phenotype of these two types of normal convoluted lymphocytes is very similar. Both express the pan-T antigens, OK17 and CD3, and are CD4+. Normal ATLL-like cells differ from leukemic cells in being CD7+.

In view of the etiological relationship between the human T-cell leukemia/lymphoma virus, HTLV-I, and ATLL,[49-51] it is interesting to note that healthy individuals of Caribbean descent who are serologically HTLV-I+ have an increased proportion of such polylobed lymphocytes in their peripheral blood. These cells, unlike those from the seronegative individuals and in common with leukemic ATLL cells, display receptors for interleukin 2 (IL-2) as demonstrated by the immunogold labeling with anti-Tac (CD25)[49] (Fig. 5.11a). Since lymphocytes from seropositive healthy individuals have been shown to release retrovirus particles in culture (Fig. 5.11b) and to react with McAbs against the HTLV-I core proteins p19 and p24,[49] it is likely that HTLV-I infects preferentially CD4+ polylobed lymphocytes which, following activation by the virus, express receptors for IL-2. It is possible too that the induction of IL-2 receptors by HTLV-I plays a role during the early stages of leukemogenesis by conferring a selective advantage on such lymphocytes to proliferate, and subsequently to undergo neoplastic changes following secondary events.

LYMPHOID LEUKEMIAS OF B-CELL TYPE

The B-cell leukemias are a heterogeneous group of disorders in terms of morphology, membrane phenotype, clinical presentation and prognosis.

CHRONIC LYMPHOCYTIC LEUKEMIA (B-CLL)

This is the most common type of B-cell leukemia. B-cell lymphocytes are characterized at the TEM level by their small size (diameter of approximately 5 μm) with a rounded cell outline, moderately scanty cytoplasm and a high N:C ratio; cytoplasmic organelles are poorly developed. The nucleus is usually centrally placed and contains heavy condensation of heterochromatin, both at its periphery and in large clumps throughout the nuclear matrix. A cartwheel pattern of heterochromatin condensation is frequently seen in those cells. Nucleoli are not usually seen or, when apparent, they are small and inconspicuous in less than 30% of the cells (Fig. 5.12a). Large nucleoli may be seen in less than 10% of cells from CLL patients. These nucleolated cells, which may be distinguished further from the small CLL cells by their large size, lower N:C ratio, greater development of cytoplasmic organelles and reduced heterochromatin condensation, represent the small subpopulation of prolymphocytoid cells seen in CLL.[52,53] Intracytoplasmic inclusions, which may be globular[54,55] or crystalline[56,57] in appearance, may be seen in cells from 5–10% of CLL cases. These are composed of the Ig molecule κ-chains or λ-chains, respectively, which have precipitated into the cytoplasm (Fig. 5.12b, c).

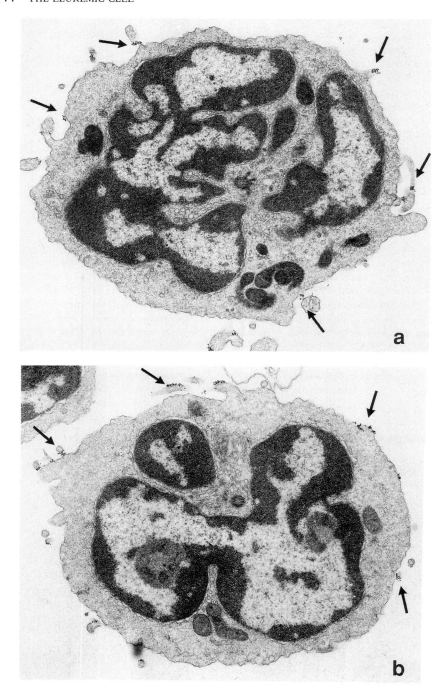

Fig. 5.10 Two types of normal blood T-lymphocytes with irregular or convoluted nucleus. (a) Sézary-like lymphocyte reactive with CD3 (arrows) showing marked nuclear irregularities. (× 16 500) (b) Lymphocyte reactive with CD4 (arrows). The cell shows a polylobed nucleus which resembles cells from ATLL. (× 16 500)

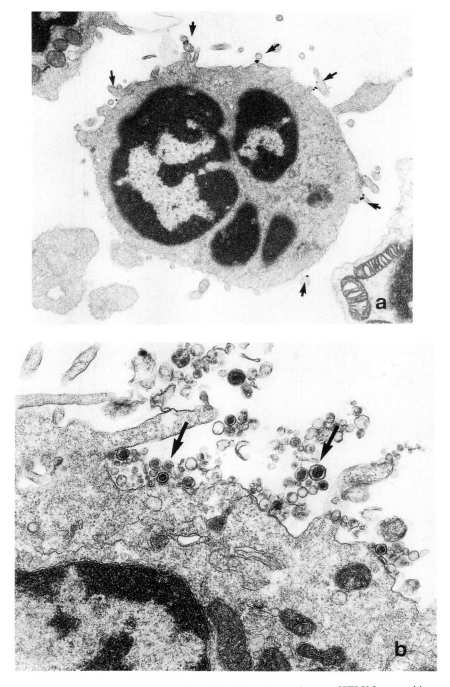

Fig. 5.11 Effects of HTLV-I infection: (a) polylobed lymphocyte from an HTLV-I seropositive normal donor showing reactivity with anti-Tac (CD25) (arrows). (× 9000) (b) Release of retroviral particles (arrows) from a cultured cell from a HTLV-I seropositive individual. (× 36 000)

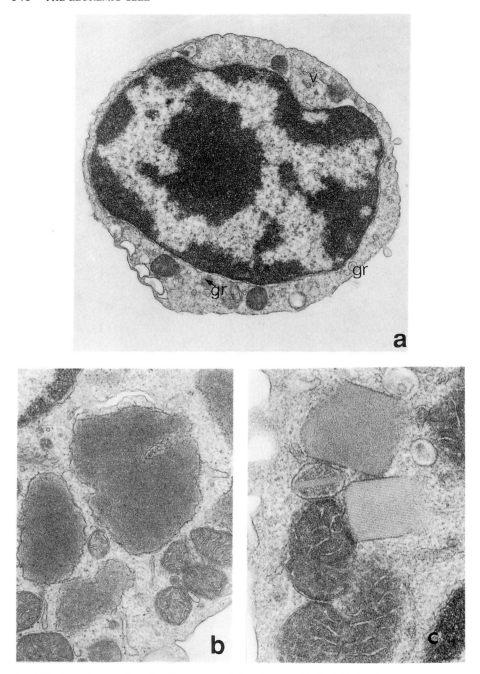

Fig. 5.12 Lymphocytes from B-CLL: (a) typical lymphocyte with high N:C ratio, condensed chromatin and small number of lysosomal granules (gr) in the cytoplasm. (× 17 550) (b) Globular inclusions (infrequent) lack periodicity and are bound by their own membrane; (c) cytoplasmic inclusions with periodicity of 7–10 mm (more frequent). (× 38 250)

PROLYMPHOCYTIC LEUKEMIA (B-PLL)

B-PLL was first described as a distinct variant of CLL in 1974.[58] Phenotypically, prolymphocytes can be distinguished from B-CLL cells by the high expression of membrane Ig, lack of receptors for mouse RBC and strong reactivity with the McAb FMC7.[59] B-prolymphocytes may be distinguished from CLL cells by their larger size (6.5–7.5 μm), lower N:C ratio, and by the large vesicular nucleolus which is characteristic of these cells. At the ultrastructural level (Fig. 5.13), the nucleolus can be seen surrounded by a halo of heterochromatin.[60–62] The nuclear outline is slightly irregular and the nucleus slightly displaced from the center. Prolymphocytes have a variable degree of heterochromatin condensation but this is invariably less marked than in the small lymphocyte of CLL. Most cells have a few profiles of long or medium length ER, usually not dilated; the Golgi region is not prominent. Many cells have a small number of localized lysosomal granules which vary from 0.1 μm to 0.25 μm in diameter and have a range of electron densities. These are often localized to one area of the cell, frequently opposite the Golgi region. The cell outline is generally smooth, although occasionally a villous outline may be seen.

Intracytoplasmic inclusions have been described in 10–15% of B-PLL cases. Some resemble the inclusions seen in CLL cells which contain Ig of the λ-chain type, whereas others are long and needle-like, display periodicity and may be associated with lysosomal granules.[63] In one case from the authors' laboratory, distinct inclusions were seen. These were small, multiple, within the cell, electron dense and lacked discernible periodicity. Immunoperoxidase staining at light microscopic level suggested that they were composed of IgM κ molecules and immunocytochemical reactions at the TEM level confirmed the Ig nature of these unusual inclusions.[13]

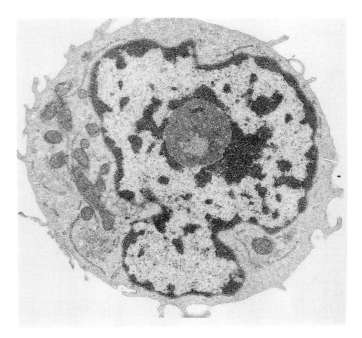

Fig. 5.13 Prolymphocyte from a case of B-PLL with a slightly irregular nucleus, moderate chromatin condensation mainly in the periphery of the nucleus, and a prominent nucleolus with associated heterochromatin. (× 12 240)

CLL WITH MORE THAN 10% PROLYMPHOCYTES (CLL/PL)

Originally, this term was used to describe a change seen during the evolution of CLL and defined by the gradual appearance of cells with the morphology of prolymphocytes.[52] Because in most cases the cells retained the phenotypic characteristics of CLL cells, the term 'prolymphocytoid' was used to signify that these cells were not true prolymphocytes. More recently, this condition was designated CLL/PL and was defined by the presence in the peripheral blood of between 11% and 55% prolymphocytes.[64] Two morphologically distinct subpopulations may be identified within the mononuclear cell fraction from CLL/PL cases (Fig. 5.14):

1. *The small cell component*: these cells have features in common with the small lymphocytes of CLL, the only difference being that the cells in CLL/PL have a lower N:C ratio and a more irregular nuclear outline.
2. *The prolymphocytic component*: these cells may be distinguished from the small lymphocyte of CLL/PL by their larger size, reduced heterochromatin condensation and large nucleolus. When compared to the prolymphocytes of B-PLL, CLL/PL prolymphocytes are pleomorphic in terms of heterochromatin condensation, cell size and nuclear outline (Fig. 5.14).

HAIRY CELL LEUKEMIA

Hairy cell leukemia (HCL), first described as leukemic reticuloendotheliosis by Bouroncle et al,[65] is now a well-defined clinicopathological entity. The B-cell nature of this disorder has been well documented by immunological analysis and by molecular approaches.[66]

Hairy cells have a strong expression of surface Ig, are positive with the McAb FMC7[59] and with either or both of the two anti-hairy cell antibodies anti-HC1 and anti-HC2.[29] They also display IL-2 receptors (Tac+ or CD25+).

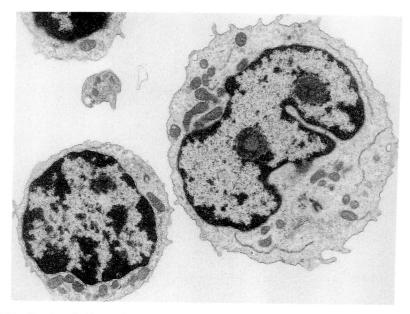

Fig. 5.14 Two lymphoid cells from a case of CLL/PL, illustrating the differences in size, chromatin condensation, N:C ratio and organelle development between the prolymphocytoid (nucleolated) cell component and the small lymphocyte population. (× 8000)

THE ULTRASTRUCTURE OF LYMPHOID CELLS 149

At light microscopy, the cells have an abundant cytoplasm, a villous outline and a strong tartrate-resistant acid phosphatase (TRAP) activity.[67] The villous outline can be best appreciated at the ultrastructural level (Fig. 5.15a).[4,68-70] The length of the villi is highly variable, not only between different cells but also within the same cell. Most cells are round and have a low N:C ratio. The nucleus is slightly eccentrically placed and is often irregular

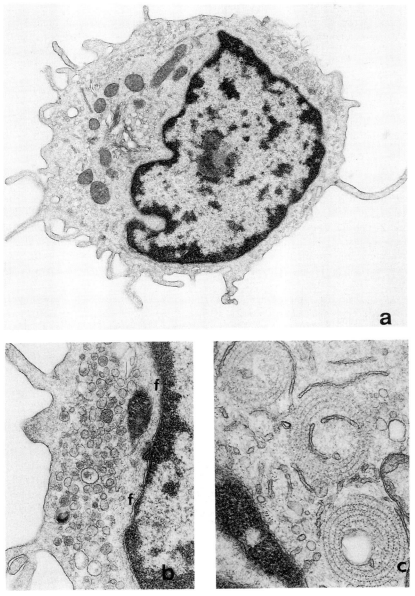

Fig. 5.15 Hairy cells from HCL: (a) typical cell with numerous villi and an active Golgi region with many associated vesicles. (× 12 800) (b) Numerous lysosomal granules of moderate electron density in an area of the cytoplasm of a hairy cell; perinuclear fibrils (f) are seen. (× 25 440) (c) Ribosome–lamella complexes in the cytoplasm of a hairy cell. (× 40 000)

in outline or kidney shaped, the heterochromatin tends to be scanty and small nucleoli may be seen in 25–30% of cells. The ER is usually abundant and is present as short, randomly scattered strands; the Golgi region is well developed and contains a large number of associated vesicles. Hairy cells frequently contain an extensive meshwork of perinuclear fibrils which are randomly orientated and often extend into the Golgi region. Numerous medium-sized lysosomal granules of variable electron density may be seen opposite the Golgi region (Fig. 5.15b).

Cells from approximately 50% of cases of HCL have intracytoplasmic inclusions called ribosome–lamella complexes (RLCs).[4] RLCs have recently been documented in cells from other B-[71] and T-cell[72] malignancies and in cells from several non-hematological conditions such as insulinoma,[73] although their incidence is much greater in HCL cells. RLCs consist of a central core surrounded by a variable number of lamellae with free ribosomes between them (Fig. 5.15c). The function and significance of the RLCs is unclear, although a viral sign was originally postulated.[74] Some workers have recently suggested that RLC may be associated with an increased rate of protein synthesis induced either by the neoplastic transformation or by a change in the microenvironment of non-neoplastic cells.[75]

HAIRY CELL VARIANT

This condition was first described in 1980.[76] More recently a few other cases have been reported and it has been suggested that the hairy cell variant (HCL-variant) represents an intermediate entity between PLL and HCL based on clinical, immunological and morphological data.[77] HCL-variant cells have strong surface Ig, weak expression of mouse RBC receptors, and positivity with FMC7; however, in contrast to HCL cells, they lack reactivity with the anti-hairy cell antibodies anti-HC1 and anti-HC2[77,78] and with anti-Tac (CD25).

The variant cells, like typical hairy cells, are large, highly villous, have a prominent Golgi region with numerous associated vesicles, a large meshwork of perinuclear fibrils and small to medium-sized, moderately electron-dense lysosomal granules localized to one area of the cytoplasm (Fig. 5.16). The majority of cells have, as prolymphocytes, a centrally located round or slightly irregular nucleus and a prominent nucleolus. The ER tends to be in long parallel strands and the heterochromatin condensation is low; a cartwheel pattern of chromatin distribution is common.

SPLENIC LYMPHOMA WITH CIRCULATING VILLOUS LYMPHOCYTES (SLVL)

This term refers to a disease which, although documented under several different names in the past[79-82] remains ill defined. Phenotypically, SLVL cells have strong surface Ig and weak expression of mouse RBC receptors and are FMC7+ but anti-HC2− and Tac− (CD25−).[83] In the past, this disease has often been misdiagnosed as CLL, PLL or HCL. SLVL cells can be distinguished from hairy cells by their smaller size and higher N:C ratio. Furthermore, the nucleus is centrally located and there is heavy heterochromatin condensation — a cartwheel pattern of chromatin distribution is common; 40% of SLVL cells have a large nucleolus which is accompanied by perinucleolar heterochromatin condensation. Few lysosomal granules are seen in these cells.

Based primarily on the type of villi, two subpopulations of cells can be recognized:

1. Cells with numerous short villi (Fig. 5.17a).
2. Cells with few long villi (Fig. 5.17b).

In both types the villi are preferentially located to one pole of the cell.

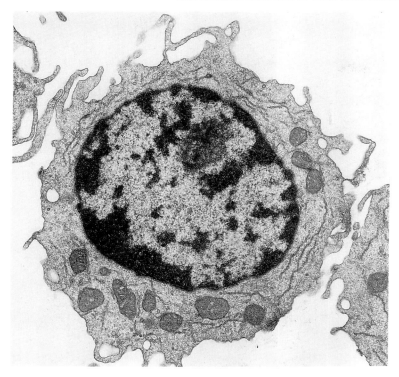

Fig. 5.16 Cell from a case of HCL-variant with a highly villous outline, nucleolus in a centrally placed nucleus and abundant ER. (× 12 000)

PLASMA CELL LEUKEMIA

This is a rare form of B-cell disease. Accepted criteria for diagnosis are the presence of more than $2 \times 10^9/l$ of plasma cells in the blood and evidence of other clinical and laboratory features of plasmacytic dycrasia.[84,85] In contrast to B-lymphocytes, circulated plasma cells do not express membrane Ig or other B-cell antigens (e.g. CD19, CD20). HLA-DR expression is weak but they are almost always CD38 (OKT10) and cytoplasmic Ig positive.

Although there is some variability in morphology, all cells show some evidence of plasma cell differentiation. For example, in some patients, the cells are mainly lymphoblastoid in appearance with a large, often centrally placed, nucleus, little heterochromatin and few parallel strands of ER. In other patients, the majority of cells appear as mature plasma cells with an eccentrically located nucleus, heavily condensed chromatin and extensive and dilated ER. In many cells, this forms sacs and bundles which contain moderately electron-dense material (Fig. 5.18); in other patients, the cell population may show features intermediate between the above two types with morphologies ranging from lymphoplasmacytoid (Fig. 5.18a) to plasma cells (Fig. 5.18b). In rare cases the cells have a blastic appearance but the parallel strands of ER confirm the plasma cell nature, which is suggested also by the immunological markers.[86]

Some morphological features are common to all cases of plasma cell leukemia. For example, most cells have an accumulation of fibrils which surrounds the nucleus and often occupies large areas of the cytoplasm.[86-89] These fibrils measure 9–11 nm in diameter and

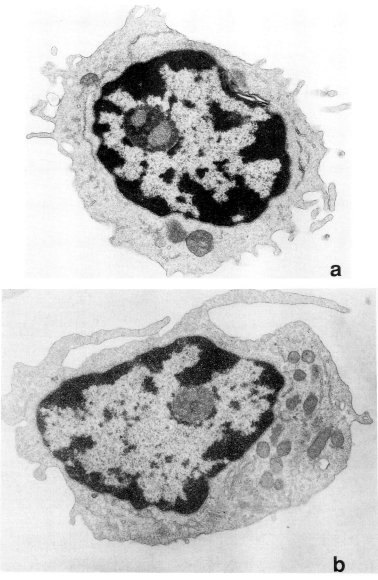

Fig. 5.17 Two types of villous lymphocytes from SLVL: (a) cell with short villi polarized in two areas of the cytoplasm. (× 12 000) (b) cell with fewer and longer, broader-based villi than seen in (a) (× 11 200)

are arranged randomly to give a criss-cross meshwork; their prominence does not appear to be related to any nuclear indentation. The mitochondria of the cells are often morphologically bizarre;[89] many are elongated or expanded and the substructure of the cristae is distorted, resulting in an apparent vacuolation of the mitochondria.[89] Finally, cytoplasmic blebs or protusions of unknown significance can be seen in a proportion of plasma cells. These are often large and contain strands of ER or other cytoplasmic elements.

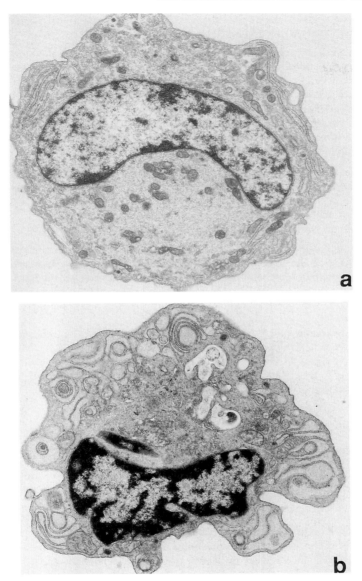

Fig. 5.18 Cells from plasma cell leukemia: (a) lymphoplasmacytoid cell with excentrically located nucleus, scanty chromatin condensation and parallel strands of non-dilated ER; note a large meshwork of fibrils (f). (× 9200) (b) Mature plasma cell with extensive and dilated sacs and bundles of ER; the nuclear chromatin is condensed and the cytoplasm has a typically irregular outline. (× 9300)

T-CELL LEUKEMIAS

T-cell leukemias constitute a heterogeneous group of diseases which possibly reflect the phenotypic, morphological and functional diversity of normal T-cells. According to the expression of T-cell differentiation antigens and the enzyme terminal deoxynucleotidyl transferase (TdT), the T-cell malignancies can be divided into two main groups:

1. Thymic (immature) (TdT +, CD7 +, CD1a + / −, CD2 + / −, CD5 +, CD3 − / +).
2. Post-thymic (mature) (TdT −, CD1a −, CD2 +, CD3 +, CD5 − / +, CD7 − / +).

These two groups can also be distinguished by their biological, clinical and morphological features. Thymic-derived leukemias affect children and young adults and have an acute clinical course whereas post-thymic leukemias affect mainly adults and have a subacute or chronic clinical course. The morphology of the leukemic cells corresponds to lymphoblasts in the thymic conditions and to mature lymphoid cells in the post-thymic malignancies.

The main ultrastructural characteristics of the mature post-thymic T-cell leukemias are outlined here. These conditions constitute a spectrum of entities whose precise classification requires the following information:

1. Clinical features and epidemiology including HTLV-I status.
2. Cell morphology by light and electron microscopy.
3. Membrane phenotype.
4. Cytogenetic analysis.
5. Molecular analysis using probes for the T-cell receptor β-, γ- and δ-chain genes.

The immunophenotype and the molecular analysis are needed to demonstrate the T-cell origin of the disease and sometimes to establish monoclonality. These approaches alone are not sufficient to allow a precise characterization of the various disease entities. For example, various T-cell leukemias, T-PLL, SS and ATLL, all express similar CD4 +, CD8 − membrane markers on their leukemic T-cells, but each has distinct clinical and morphological features.

Four types of post-thymic T-cell leukemia can be recognized by morphological examination: T-PLL, in which the prolymphocyte is the main cell type; T-CLL, a disease of large granular lymphocytes; SS with cerebriform cells; and ATLL with polylobed lymphocytes. The identification of these four cell types is possible by light microscopy, but often the precise characterization requires ultrastructural analysis.

T-PROLYMPHOCYTIC LEUKEMIA (T-PLL)

PLL was first described[58] as a B-cell-derived disease. However, the advent of lymphoid markers allowed the recognition of T-cell PLL which represents 20% of all PLL cases in the authors' institution.[90] Most T-PLL cases correspond to CD4 +, CD8 − proliferations and more rarely co-express CD4 and CD8 or are CD4 −, CD8 +. A consistent feature which distinguishes T-PLL from other post-thymic T-cell diseases is the strong expression of the p40 (CD7) antigen.[5]

The identification of the prolymphocyte by light microscopy constitutes a key diagnostic feature. T-prolymphocytes appear as medium-sized cells with clumped nuclear chromatin and a single prominent vesicular nucleolus; the cytoplasm is often deeply basophilic and devoid of granules. Ultrastructural analysis has disclosed the existence of some T-PLL cases which could be easily misdiagnosed by light microscopic examination only. Because TEM studies have not been widely performed, such cases have often been referred to as T-CLL or T-cell leukemia with knobby cells.[91-94]

Under TEM, T-prolymphocytes are seen as medium sized with a relatively high N:C ratio. The nuclear heterochromatin is preferentially marginated at the periphery and is often arranged in a few intranuclear patches. A single large nucleolus is identified in over 70% of the cells from all cases (Fig. 5.19). Two morphological types of T-prolymphocytes have been recognized which are found with similar frequency. Regular T-prolymphocytes show a round, regular nuclear outline and are, in fact, similar to B-prolymphocytes (Fig. 5.19a). Irregular T-prolymphocytes are characterized by one or more short and broad nuclear indentations which only rarely are long and narrow (Fig. 5.19b).

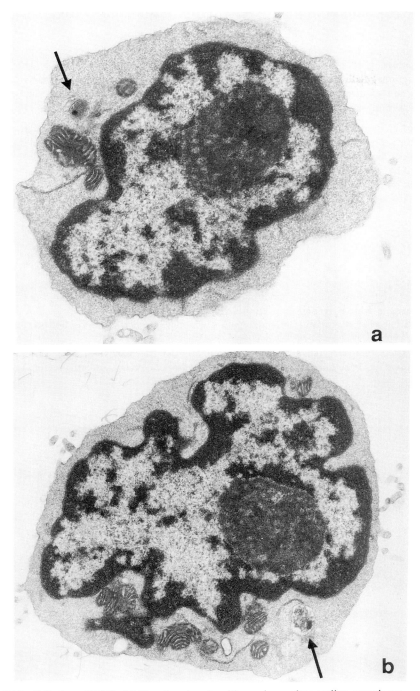

Fig. 5.19 Cells from T-PLL: (a) T-prolymphocyte with regular nuclear outline, prominent nucleolus, scattered ribosomes and localized cytoplasmic granules (arrow). (× 13 500) (b) Irregular cell with short nuclear indentations, a prominent nucleolus and few localized granular structures. (× 13 500)

The main cytoplasmic features of T-prolymphocytes are:

1. Long and/or circular profiles of ER associated with clusters of ribosomes which account for the cytoplasmic basophilia of these cells when examined by light microscopy.
2. Large- to medium-sized dense granules clustered in one or two areas of the cytoplasm. These structures are not visible by light microscopy but are always present in a proportion of cells from all cases (Fig. 5.19).

TEM analysis has allowed the recognition of a small cell variant of T-PLL which consists of small prolymphocytes with a regular or irregular nucleus[5] (Fig. 5.20). The clinical and laboratory features of this group of patients are identical to those of the more typical T-PLL cases. The recent observation that T–PLL cells have a characteristic cytogenetic abnormality, inv(14)(q11; q32),[95] which appears to be unique to this disease, supports the classification of T-PLL as a separate, distinct entity.

T-CLL OR LARGE GRANULAR LYMPHOCYTE LEUKEMIA

T-CLL with granular lymphocytes was first described in 1975.[96] A number of other T-cell malignancies have also been described under the term 'T-CLL' but this term has been restricted to cases of a well-defined clinical syndrome which is characterized cytologically by the expansion of mature-looking lymphocytes with abundant cytoplasm containing azurophil granules and which are designated as LGLs.

T-CLL cases present with splenomegaly, cytopenia(s) and a moderate but persistent PB lymphocytosis ($> 5 \times 10^9/1$). With a few exceptions, the clinical course is chronic when compared to the other T-cell disorders. For this reason, the reactive or neoplastic nature of this disease has been questioned.[97] The demonstration of clonality by cytogenetic analysis in

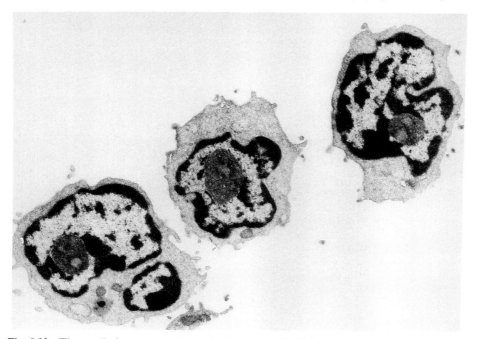

Fig. 5.20 Three cells from a case of a small cell variant of T-PLL showing a single central nucleolus. (× 7700)

some cases[98-101] and, more recently, by molecular analysis of the T-cell receptor β-, γ- and δ-chain gene rearrangement[102-105] (see also Chapter 13) in many of these cases supports the view that the T-cell proliferation is monoclonal in nature.

Phenotypically, T-CLL lymphocytes display a mature post-thymic T-cell phenotype. Most cases (common phenotype) are expansions of LGLs recognized by Leu7.[41] Membrane antigens linked to natural killer activity and recognized by the McAbs CD11b (OKM1) and CD16 (Leu11) are rarely expressed in this common form of T-CLL. Some T-CLL cases display unusual T-cell phenotypes: CD4+, CD8−, Leu7+/−, CD11b+, CD16+[46] or CD4+, CD8−, Leu7+, CD11b−, CD16−, or CD4+, CD8+, Leu7+, CD11b+, CD16−.

The authors' data, based on a series of 22 T-CLL patients, indicate that, in contrast to this degree of heterogeneity in membrane phenotype, there is homogeneity in the cytological features of T-CLL when examined by light microscopy, in that cells from all of these patients had the morphology of LGLs. LGLs are seen by TEM as mature lymphocytes with a low N:C ratio and an eccentrically placed nucleus with relatively abundant heterochromatin; a small nucleolus may occasionally be identified. The main cytoplasmic features of LGL, however, are lysosomal granules and a highly developed Golgi region as indicated by the presence of multiple microvesicles, microtubules and centrioles. The granular structures are identified as:

1. Round granules of different size and density scattered throughout the cytoplasm.
2. Parallel tubular arrays (PTAs) which correspond to granular structures composed of bundles of packed microtubules arranged in a parallel fashion. PTAs are not unique to T-CLL cells but are also found in a proportion of normal blood T-lymphocytes (see above). These structures may be free in the cytoplasm or more often are membrane bound and are usually multiple in T-CLL cells (1–9/cell section—Fig. 5.21a, b). PTAs have been consistently identified in all the T-CLL cases studied by the authors except in one case with an uncommon phenotype.[46]
3. Cells from a few patients may also have a peculiar type of granule that characteristically contains material arranged in an orderly fashion in scrolls resembling the granular content of mast cells.

The authors' findings suggest that lymphocytes from T-CLL, regardless of the benign or aggressive clinical course and of the membrane phenotype (common and uncommon), have the overall ultrastructural morphology of LGLs. Subtle differences may be identified, however, by TEM and these relate mainly to nuclear characteristics. Thus irregular nuclei, prominent nucleoli, less mature nuclear chromatin and the presence of atypical granules resembling those of mast cells, are seen mainly in cells from T-CLL patients with an aggressive clinical course and whose cells have uncommon phenotypes.

There is a striking similarity between the phenotypic and ultrastructural features of T-CLL cells and those of the LGL subpopulation from normal blood. The only morphological difference observed between the T-CLL cells and normal LGLs is in the number and size of the PTAs which are seen significantly more frequently in T-CLL.

SÉZARY SYNDROME

Sézary syndrome (SS) is a well-defined clinicopathological entity characterized by skin involvement and the presence in the peripheral blood of a neoplastic cell with a distinct cerebriform nucleus known as the Sézary cell.[106] SS is included within the spectrum of the cutaneous T-cell lymphomas, a term applied to a group of T-cell malignancies with predominant or primary skin infiltration and variable peripheral blood involvement.

Sézary cells were first considered to be of non-lymphoid origin, but in the mid-1970s, the T-cell nature of the Sézary cell was demonstrated.[107-109] The phenotypic characteristics of

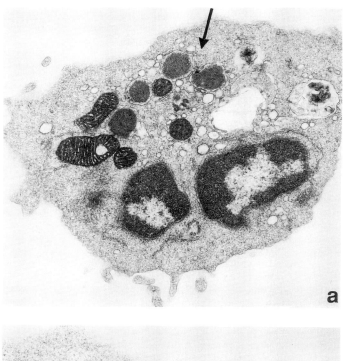

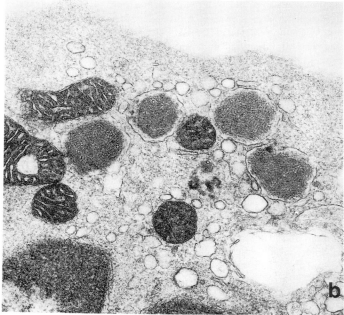

Fig. 5.21 Granular lymphocytes from T-CLL: (a) cell with a low N:C ratio and a nucleus with abundant heterochromatin. The cytoplasm contains several large parallel tubular arrays (arrow). ($\times$ 7500) (b) High magnification of (a) showing the disposition of the microtubules from the parallel tubular arrays. ($\times$ 28 500)

Sézary cells have been defined more precisely by anti-T-cell McAbs; in most cases, the disease results from the expansion of CD4 +, CD8 – lymphocytes which are, as a rule, CD7 –.[48] In rare cases, Sézary cells may be CD8 –, CD4 – or may react with Leu7[110] or, more rarely, are CD4 –, CD8 +. In one exceptional case of SS from the authors' series, the Sézary cells displayed a very unusual phenotype as revealed by their reactivity with McAbs against natural killer and cytotoxic cells (CD11b +, CD16 +). It is of interest that the putative cellular counterpart for SS in normal blood, identified by the immunogold technic (see above), displays an identical phenotype — CD3 +, CD4 +, OKT17 +, CD7 – — to that of the Sézary cells from the majority of cases of SS.

The role of the TEM for the diagnosis of SS has been recognized for many years. Lutzner and Jordan[111] first described the ultrastructural features of the Sézary cell and confirmed the light microscopy findings which showed a highly serpentine nucleus that corresponded on ultrathin sections to a cerebriform aspect if viewed on a three-dimensional scale. Sézary cells, when examined by TEM, have a convoluted nucleus with at least two long and narrow indentations and often one or two independent nuclear lobes. When considering the ratio between the length of the longest nuclear indentation and that of the maximal nuclear diameter (I/N), this is usually equal to or over 0.66 in one-third of the circulating Sézary cells (Fig. 5.22). A small or medium-sized nucleolus may be seen and the cytoplasm may contain localized large granular structures and multivesicular bodies.

The typical Sézary cell was described as a large cell measuring 12–18 µm in diameter. In the mid-1970s, however, a small cell variant with similar nuclear configuration, but with the size of a normal lymphocyte, was recognized.[21] Many cases of small cell SS have been

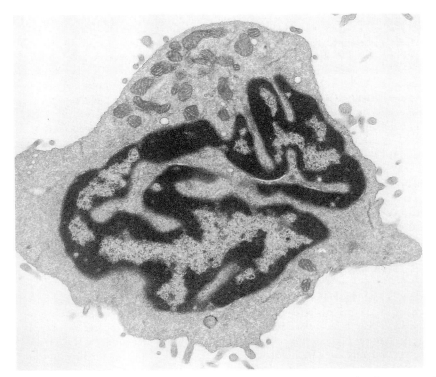

Fig. 5.22 Lymphoid cell from a case of small cell variant of Sézary syndrome showing a serpentine nucleus with several long and narrow indentations characteristic of Sézary cells. (× 12 000)

reported since,[109,112,113] and it would indeed appear that it is the most common of the two cell types.

Ultrastructural analysis of blood samples in SS seems particularly useful in cases in which the nuclear convolutions may only be suspected by light microscopic examination. The relevance of morphometry for the early diagnosis of SS and differential diagnosis with reactive dermatoses has also been documented.[114-115] The difficulty in recognizing Sézary cells by light microscopy is due to the overlap of the nuclear foldings and the narrow nature of the indentations. TEM analysis is also useful to distinguish Sézary cells from convoluted cells of other post-thymic T-cell malignancies, chiefly ATLL and the irregular type of T-PLL. Unlike those of Sézary cells, the nuclear indentations of ATLL cells are shorter and broader and the nucleus multilobed and not cerebriform. T-prolymphocytes are recognized by their prominent nucleolus, the pattern of chromatin distribution and the less pronounced nuclear indentations.

A few cases of T-cell leukemia have been documented in which the neoplastic cells were morphologically similar to the Sézary cells but without the patient having obvious skin involvement. Morphologically, the cells from one of these cases were identical to small Sézary cells; another case had a mixture of typical Sézary cells and T-prolymphocytes and a third case had large SS cells coexisting with multilobed large cells with a blastic appearance. Cells from all these cases expressed an uncommon membrane phenotype: CD8 +, CD4 −[116], or CD8 +, CD4 +, or CD8 −, CD4 −. Thus, it is likely that the target cell for these diseases is different from that of classical SS.

ADULT T-CELL LEUKEMIA LYMPHOMA

Adult T-cell leukemia lymphoma (ATLL) is a distinct post-thymic T-cell leukemia, etiologically related to the retrovirus HTLV-I.[50,117] The pathogenic role of HTLV-I in ATLL has been well supported by seroepidemiological studies,[118] the release of virus particles from ATLL cells when grown in culture[119,120] and by molecular studies which have demonstrated the monoclonal integration of HTLV-I proviral DNA sequences into the leukemic cells.[121]

ATLL cells display a mature T-cell phenotype often corresponding to CD4 +, CD8 − cells and, in common with Sézary cells, rarely expressing the p40 antigen recognized by McAbs of the CD7 group.[122] The expression of IL-2 receptors, as assessed by the reactivity of the cells with the McAb anti-Tac,[123] is a consistent finding but not exclusive to ATLL lymphocytes since IL-2 receptors may also be present in cells from a minority of T-PLL and SS cases.[101]

ATLL cells are morphologically heterogeneous with respect to cell size, degree of chromatin condensation and nuclear shape. The predominant cell type is a 'polylobed' lymphocyte characterized by having several nuclear foldings resembling the petals of flowers; the presence of 5-10% immunoblast-like cells is a frequent finding in peripheral blood samples. TEM analysis shows that the nucleus of ATLL cells is composed of several independent segments and/or a single nuclear lobe with indentations which are short and wide (Fig. 5.23a). Immunoblasts are consistently identified (Fig. 5.23b). A semiquantitative assessment of the nuclear irregularities obtained by measuring the I/N ratio is useful to distinguish ATLL cells from Sézary cells. Although there is a degree of overlap in the cytological features of these two cell types, ATLL cells display lower I/N ratios than SS cells and more frequently have multiple nuclear lobes. Some of these differences in the nuclear configuration of ATLL and Sézary cells can be suspected by light microscopic analysis but TEM offers more objective criteria for the identification of both cell types.

Cells from 3 out of 17 ATLL cases studied by the authors contained PTAs in the cytoplasm. This lysosomal structure, which is characteristic of T-CLL cells and normal

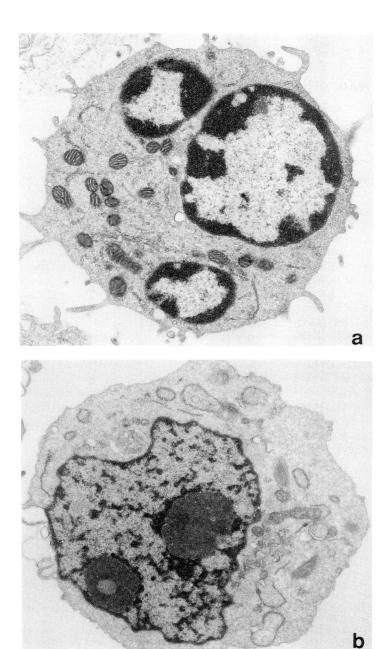

Fig. 5.23 Circulating lymphocytes from ATLL: (a) cell with a polylobed nucleus and smooth nuclear outline. (× 9000) (b) Immunoblast from another case of ATLL showing a nucleus with little heterochromatin, two prominent nucleoli scatter ribosomes and circular profiles of rough ER. (× 11 250)

blood LGLs has not been identified in cells from the other T-cell leukemias. It has been suggested that lysosomal granules play a role in the process of cytotoxicity but it is not known whether they may also be involved in the suppressor function displayed by LGLs of some T-CLL cases[124,125] as well as by ATLL cells. Cells from the majority of ATLL patients have a suppressor function (see Chapter 9) and normally this function is mediated through normal CD8 + cells.[126] It is possible that PTAs are characteristic of a CD4 + lymphocyte inducer of the CD8 + suppressor subset, or alternatively, that they characterize a CD4 + suppressor subset.

SUMMARY

Detailed morphological, immunological and molecular studies have allowed a more precise characterization of the human lymphoproliferative disorders. The immunological analysis is essential to establish the B- and T-lymphoid nature of the disease as well as the stage of differentiation of the neoplastic cells. The molecular and cytogenetic studies are necessary to demonstrate clonality. The clinical and morphological aspects are relevant for the identification of the various disease entities. Ultrastructural analysis represents a useful tool because it allows a more objective and accurate estimation of the cytological features which characterize the various lymphoid disorders. In some circumstances, it may also be critical for the precise recognition of certain neoplastic cells such as the Sézary cell and the small T-prolymphocyte. Ultrastructural analysis also makes possible the distinction between cells from different, but sometimes closely related, B-cell leukemias which have been diagnosed by other clinical or laboratory studies. For example, it is sometimes difficult at the light microscopic level to distinguish SLVL cells from HCL cells, or HCL-variant cells from those of either PLL or HCL. The application of the immunogold method with specific anti-B and anti-T McAbs has provided evidence for the existence in normal blood of cell counterparts for certain B- and T-lymphoid leukemias which resemble phenotypically and morphologically the corresponding neoplastic lymphoid cells.

REFERENCES

1 Kohler G, Milstein C 1975 Continuous cultures of fused cells secreting antibody of predefined specificity. Nature 256: 495–497
2 Lutzner M A, Emerit I, Durepaire R, Flandrin G, Grupper Ch, Prunieras M 1973 Cytogenetic, cytophotometric and ultrastructural study of large cerebriform cells of the Sézary syndrome and description of a small cell variant. Journal of the National Cancer Institute 50: 1145–1162
3 Zucker-Franklin D 1974 Properties of the Sézary lymphoid cell. An ultrastructural analysis. Mayo Clinical Proceedings 49: 567–574
4 Katayama I, Li C Y, Yam L T 1972 Ultrastructural characteristics of the "hairy cells" of leukemic reticuloendotheliosis. American Journal of Pathology 67: 361–370
5 Matutes E, Garcia Talavera J, O'Brien M, Catovsky D 1986 The morphological spectrum of T-prolymphocytic leukaemia. British Journal of Haematology 64: 111–124
6 Barka T, Anderson P J 1962 Histochemical methods for acid phosphatase using hexazonium pararosanilin as coupler. Journal of Histochemistry and Cytochemistry 10: 741–753
7 Horisberger M 1984 Electron-opaque markers; a review. In: Polak J M, Varndell I M (eds) Immunolabelling for electron microscopy. Amsterdam, Elsevier, pp 17–28.
8 Reyes F, Lejonc J L, Gourdin M F, Mannoni P, Dreyfus B 1975 The surface morphology of human B-lymphocytes as revealed by immunoelectron microscopy. Journal of Experimental Medicine 141: 392–410
9 Leduc E H, Scott G B, Avrameas S 1969 Ultrastructural localisation of intracellular immunoglobulins in plasma cells and lymphoblasts by enzyme-labelled antibodies. Journal of Histochemistry and Cytochemistry 17: 211–224

10 Kuhlman W D, Avrameas S, Ternynck T 1974 A comparative study for ultrastructural localization of intracellular immunoglobulins using peroxidase conjugates. Journal of Immunological Methods 5: 33–48
11 Gourdin M F, Farcet J P, Reyes F 1982 The ultrastructural localisation of immunoglobulins in human B cells of immunoproliferative diseases. Blood 59: 1132–1140
12 Newell D G, Bohane C, Payne S, Smith J L 1980 The intracellular localisation of immunoglobulin in human lymphoid cells and haematopoietic cell lines by immunoperoxidase electron microscopy. Journal of Immunological Methods 37: 275–286
13 Robinson D S F, Melo J V, Andrews C A, Schey S A, Catovsky D 1985 Intracytoplasmic inclusions in B prolymphocytic leukaemia: ultrastructural, cytochemical and immunological studies. Journal of Clinical Pathology 38: 897–903
14 Graham R C, Karnovsky M J 1966 The early stages of absorption of injected horse radish peroxidase in the proximal tubules of mouse kidney: ultrastructural cytochemistry by a new technique. Journal of Histochemistry and Cytochemistry 14: 291–302
15 Singer S J 1959 Preparation of an electron-dense antibody conjugate. Nature 183: 1523–1524
16 Singer S J, Schick A F 1961 The properties of specific stains for electron microscopy prepared by the conjugation of antibody molecules with ferritin. Journal of Biophysical and Biochemical Cytology 9: 519–537
17 Biberfeld P, Biberfeld G, Perimann P 1971 Surface immunoglobulin light chain determinants on normal and PHA stimulated human blood lymphocytes studied by immunofluorescence and electron microscopy. Experimental Cell Research 66: 177–189
18 de Petris S, Raff M C 1972 Distribution of immunoglobulin on the surface of mouse lymphoid cells as determined by immunoferritin electron microscopy. Antibody-induced, temperature-dependent redistribution and its implications for membrane structure. European Journal of Immunology 2: 523–535
19 de Petris S, Raff M C 1973 Normal distribution, patching and capping of lymphocyte surface immunoglobulin studied by electron microscopy. Nature New Biology 241: 257–259
20 Horisberger M, Rosset J 1977 Colloidal gold, a useful marker for transmission and scanning electron microscopy. Journal of Histochemistry and Cytochemistry 25: 295–305
21 Faulk W P, Taylor G H 1971 An immunocolloid method for the electron microscope. Immunochemistry 8: 1081–1083
22 Horisberger M, Rosset J, Bauer H 1975 Colloidal gold granules as markers for cell surface receptors in the scanning electron microscope. Experientia 31: 1147–1149
23 Romano E L, Romano M 1984 Historical aspects. In: Polak J M, Varndell I M (eds) Immunolabelling for electron microscopy. Amsterdam, Elsevier, pp 3–16
24 de Waele M 1984 Haematological electron microscopy. In: Polak J M, Varndell I M (eds) Immunolabelling for electron microscopy. Amsterdam, Elsevier pp 267–288
25 Robinson D, Tavares de Castro J, Polli N, O'Brien M, Catovsky D 1984 Simultaneous demonstration of membrane antigens and cytochemistry at ultrastructural level: a study with the immunogold method, acid phosphatase and myeloperoxidase. British Journal of Haematology 56: 617–623
26 Matutes E, Catovsky D 1982 The fine structure of normal lymphocyte subpopulations – a study with monoclonal antibodies and the immunogold technique. Clinical and Experimental Immunology 50: 416–425
27 Matutes E, Robinson D, O'Brien M, Haynes B F, Zola H, Catovsky D 1983 Candidate counterparts of Sézary cells and adult T-cell lymphoma-leukaemia cells in normal peripheral blood: an ultrastructural study with the immunogold method and monoclonal antibodies. Leukemia Research 7: 787–801
28 Brooks D A, Beckman I G R, Bradley J, McNamara P J, Thomas M E, Zola H 1981 Human lymphocyte markers defined by antibodies derived from somatic cell hybrids IV. A monoclonal reacting specifically with a subpopulation of human B-lymphocytes. Journal of Immunology 126: 1373–1377
29 Posnett D N, Chiorazzi N, Kunkel H G 1982 Monoclonal antibodies with specificity for hairy cell leukemia cells. Journal of Clinical Investigation 70: 254–261
30 Posnett D N, Marboe C C 1984 Differentiation antigens associated with hairy cell leukemia. Seminars in Oncology 11: 413–415
31 Posnett D N, Wang C-Y, Chiorazzi N, Crow M K, Kunkel H G 1984 An antigen characteristic of hairy cells is expressed on certain activated B cells. Journal of Immunology 133: 1635–1640
32 Stashenko P, Nadler L M, Hardy R, Shlossman S F 1981 Expression of cell surface markers following human B lymphocyte activation. Proceedings of the National Academy of Sciences of the USA 78: 3848–3852

33. van Camp I, Reynaert P, Broodaerts L 1981 Studies on the origin of the precursor cells in multiple myeloma, Waldenström's macroglobulinaemia and benign monoclonal gammopathy. 1 Cytoplasmic isotype and idiotype distribution in peripheral blood and bone marrow. Clinical and Experimental Immunology 44: 82–89
34. Grossi D E, Webb S R, Zicca a, Lydyard F M, Moretta L, Mingari M C, Cooper M D 1978 Morphological and histochemical analyses of two human T-cell subpopulations bearing receptors for IgM or IgG. Journal of Experimental Medicine 147: 1405–1417
35. Ferranini M, Cadoni A, Franzi A T, Ghiglioti C, Leprini A, Zicca A, Grossi C E 1980 Ultrastructure and cytochemistry of human peripheral blood lymphocytes. Similarities between the cells of the third population and Tg lymphocytes. European Journal of Immunology 10: 562–570
36. Meijer C J L M, van Leeuwen A W F M, van der Loo E M, van de Putte L B A, van Vloten W A 1977 Cerebriform (Sézary-like) mononuclear cells in healthy individuals: a morphologically distinct population of T cells. Virchows Archives B (Cell Pathology) 25: 95–104
37. van der Loo E M, Cnossen J, Meijer C J L M 1981 Morphological aspects of T cell subpopulations in human blood: characterization of the cerebriform mononuclear cells in healthy individuals. Clinical and Experimental Immunology 43: 506–516
38. Huhn D, Andreewa P, Rodt H, Thiel E, Eulitz M 1978 Demonstration of the Fc receptor of blood cells by soluble peroxidase anti-peroxidase (PAP) complexes. Blut 36: 263–273
39. Grossi C E, Cadoni A, Zicca A, Leprini A, Ferranini M 1982 Large granular lymphocytes in human peripheral blood: ultrastructural and cytochemical characterisation of the granules. Blood 59: 277–283
40. Payne C M, Glasser L 1981 Evaluation of surface markers on normal human lymphocytes containing parallel tubular arrays: a quantitative ultrastructural study. Blood 57: 567–573
41. Abo T, Balch C M 1982 Characterization of HNK-1+ (Leu-7) human lymphocytes. II. Distinguishing phenotypic and functional properties of natural killer cells from activated NK-like cells. Journal of Immunology 129: 1758–1761
42. Polli N, Matutes E, Robinson D, Catovsky D 1987 Morphological heterogeneity of Leu-7, Leu-11 and OKM1 positive lymphocyte subsets: an ultrastructural study with the immunogold method. Clinical and Experimental Immunology 68: 331–339
43. Velardi A, Grossi C E, Cooper M D 1985 A large subpopulation of lymphocytes with T helper phenotype (Leu-3a/T4+) exhibits the property of binding to NK cell targets and granular lymphocyte morphology. Journal of Immunology 134: 58–64
44. Hiraoka A, Machii T, Konishi I, Kanayama Y, Yonezawa T, Kitani T 1978 Parallel tubular arrays in lymphocytes. Journal of Clinical Electron Microscopy 11: 535–536
45. Lanier L L, Le A M, Phillips J H, Warner N L, Babcock G F 1983 Subpopulations of human natural killer cells defined by expression of the Leu-7 (HNK-1) and Leu-11 (NK-15) antigens. Journal of Immunology 131: 1789–1796
46. Moss V E, Miedema F, Matutes E, Terpstra F, Brownell A, Brozovic M, Catovsky D 1986 An unusual variant of T-CLL: evidence of a hitherto unrecognised T cell subset. Clinical and Experimental Immunology 63: 303–311
47. Yeckley J A, Weston W L, Thorne E G, Krueger G G 1975 Production of Sézary like cells from normal human lymphocytes. Archives of Dermatology 111: 29–32
48. Haynes B F, Bunn P, Mann D, Thomas C, Eisenbarth G, Minna J, Fauci A S 1981 Cell surface antigens of the malignant T cell in Sézary syndrome and mycosis fungoides. Journal of Clinical Investigation 67: 523–530
49. Matutes E, Dalgleish A G, Weiss R A, Joseph A P, Catovsky D 1986 Studies in healthy human T-cell leukemia lymphoma virus (HTLV-I) carriers from the Caribbean. International Journal of Cancer 38: 41–45
50. Gallo R C, Essex M E, Gross L (eds) 1984 Human T-cell leukemia/lymphoma virus. Cold Spring Harbor Laboratory, New York
51. Weiss R, Teich N, Varmus H, Coffin J 1985 Molecular biology of tumor viruses. RNA tumor viruses, 2nd edn, Cold Spring Harbor Laboratory, New York
52. Enno A, Catovsky D, O.Brien M, Cherchi M, Kumaran T O, Galton D A G 1979 "Prolymphocytoid" transformation of chronic lymphocytic leukaemia. British Journal of Haematology 41: 9–18
53. Melo J V, Catovsky D, Galton D A G 1986 The relationship between chronic lymphocytic leukaemia and prolymphocytic leukaemia. II Patterns of evolution of 'prolymphocytoid' transformation. British Journal of Haematology 64: 77–86
54. Hurez D, Flandrin G, Preud'homme J L, Seligmann M 1972 Unreleased intracellular monoclonal macroglobulin in chronic lymphocytic leukaemia. Clinical and Experimental Immunology 10: 223–234

55 Guglielmi P, Preud 'homme J L, Gourdin M-F, Reyes F, Daniel M-T 1982 Unusual intracytoplasmic immunoglobulin inclusions in chronic lymphocyte leukaemia. British Journal of Haematology 50: 123-134
56 Cawley J C, Barker C R, Britchford R D, Smith J L 1973 Intracellular IgA λ immunoglobulin crystals in chronic lymphocytic leukaemia. Clinical and Experimental Immunology 13: 407-416
57 Peters O, Thielemans C, Steenssens L, de Waele M, Hijmans W, van Camp B 1984 Intracellular inclusions bodies in 14 patients with B cell lymphoproliferative disorders. Journal of Clinical Pathology 37: 45-50
58 Galton D A G, Goldman J M, Wiltshaw J, Catovsky D, Henry K, Goldenberg G J 1974 Prolymphocytic leukaemia. British Journal of Haematology 27: 7-23
59 Catovsky D, Cherchi M, Brooks D, Bradley, J, Zola H 1981 Heterogeneity of B-cell leukemias demonstrated by the monoclonal antibody FMC7. Blood 58: 406-408
60 Costello C, Catovsky D, O'Brien M, Galton D A G 1980 Prolymphocytic leukaemia: an ultrastructural study of 22 cases. British Journal of Haematology 44: 389-394
61 Katayama I, Aiba M, Pechet L, Sullivan J L, Roberts P, Humphreys R E 1980 B-lineage prolymphocytic leukemia as a distinct clinicopathological entity. American Journal of Pathology 99: 399-412
62 Kjeldsberg C R, Bearman R M, Rappaport H 1980 Prolymphocytic leukemia: an ultrastructural study. American Journal of Clinical Pathology 73: 150-159
63 Costello C, Catovsky D, O'Brien M 1981 Cytoplasmic inclusions in a case of prolymphocytic leukemia. American Journal of Clinical Pathology 76: 499-501
64 Melo J V, Catovsky D, Galton D A G 1986 The relationship between chronic lymphocytic leukaemia and prolymphocytic leukaemia I. Clinical and laboratory features of 300 patients and characterisation of an intermediate group. British Journal of Haematology 63: 377-387
65 Bouroncle B A, Wiseman B K, Doan C A 1958 Leukemic reticuloendotheliosis. Blood 13: 609-630
66 Korsmeyer S J, Greene W C, Cossman J et al 1983 Rearrangement and expression of immunoglobulin genes and expression of Tac antigen in hairy cell leukemia. Proceedings of the National Academy of Sciences of the USA 80: 4522-4526
67 Yam L T, Li C Y, Lam K W 1971 Tartrate-resistant acid phosphatase isoenzyme in the reticulum cells of leukemic reticuloendotheliosis. New England Journal of Medicine 284: 357-360
68 Flandrin G, Daniel M T, Fourcade M, Chelloul 1973 Leucémie a "tricholeucocyte" (hairy-cell leukemia), étude clinique cytologique de 55 observations. Nouvelle Révue Française d' Hématologie 13: 609-640
69 Daniel M T, Flandrin G 1974 Fine structure of abnormal cells in hairy cell (tricholeukocytic) leukemia, with special reference to their *in vitro* phagocytic capacity. Laboratory Investigation 30: 1-8
70 Cawley J C, Burns G F, Hayhoe F G J 1980 Hairy cell leukaemia. Recent results in cancer research 72. Berlin, Springer-Verlag
71 Brunning R D, Parkin J 1975 Ribosome-lamella complexes in neoplastic hematopoietic cells. American Journal of Pathology 79: 565-578
72 Sebahoun G, Bayle J, Muratore R, Carcassonne Y 1979 Ribosome lamella complex in neoplastic cells of a Sézary's syndrome. Journal of Clinical Pathology 32: 1041-1044
73 Perez-Atayde A, Hartman A S, Seiler M W 1982 Ribosome lamellae complexes in a symptomatic insulinoma. Archives of Pathology and Laboratory Medicine 106: 221-223
74 Zucker-Franklin D 1963 Virus-like particles in the lymphocytes of a patient with chronic lymphocytic leukemia. Blood 21: 509-512
75 Zimmerman K G, Payne C M, Nagle R B 1984 Ribosome-lamellae complexes in benign plasma cells accompanying neoplastic infiltrates. American Journal of Clinical Pathology 81: 364-367
76 Cawley J C, Burns G F, Hayhoe F G J 1980 A chronic lymphoproliferative disorder with distinctive features: a distinct variant of hairy cell leukaemia. Leukemia Research 4: 547-559
77 Catovsky D, O'Brien M, Melo J V, Wardle J, Brozovic M 1984 Hairy cell leukemia (HCL) variant: an intermediate disease between HCL and B-prolymphocytic leukemia. Seminars in Oncology 11: 362-369
78 Melo J V, San Miguel J F, Moss V E, Catovsky D 1984 The membrane phenotype of hairy cell leukaemia: a study with monoclonal antibodies. Seminars in Oncology 11: 381-385
79 Neiman R S, Sullivan A L, Jaffe R 1979 Malignant lymphoma simulating leukemic reticuloendotheliosis. Cancer 43: 329-342

80 Fohlmeister I, Schaefer H E, Modder B, Hellriegel K-P, Fischer R 1981 Chronische lymphoproliferative Erkrankung unter dem Bild einer Haarzell-leukamie. Blut 42: 367–377
81 Palutke M, Tabaczka P, Mirchandani I, Goldfarb S 1981 Lymphocytic lymphoma simulating hairy cell leukemia: a consideration of reliable and unreliable diagnostic features. Cancer 48: 2047–2055
82 Spriano P, Barosi G, Invernizzi R, Ippoliti G, Fortunato A, Rosso R, Magrini U 1986 Splenomegalic immunocytoma with circulating hairy cells. Report of eight cases and revision of the literature. Haematologica 71: 25–33
83 Melo J V, Robinson D S F, Gregory C, Catovsky D 1987 Splenic B-cell lymphoma with "villous" lymphocytes in the peripheral blood: a disorder distinct from hairy cell leukaemia. Leukemia 1: 294–299
84 Kyle R A, Maldonado J E, Bayrd E C 1974 Plasma cell leukemia: report on 17 cases. Archives Internal of Medicine 133: 813–818
85 Zawadski Z A, Kapadia S, Barnes A E 1978 Leukemic myelomatosis (Plasma cell leukemia). American Journal of Clinical Pathology 70: 605–611
86 Parreira A, Robinson D S F, Melo J V et al 1985 Primary plasma cell leukaemia: immunological and ultrastructural studies in 6 cases. Scandinavian Journal of Haematology 35: 570–578
87 Jean G, Lambertenghi-Deliliers G, Ranzi T, Polli E 1971 Ultrastructural aspects of bone marrow and peripheral blood cells in a case of plasma cell leukaemia. Acta Haematologica 45: 36–49
88 Beltran G, Stuckey W J 1972 Nuclear lobulation and cytoplasmic fibrils in leukemic plasma cells. American Journal of Clinical Pathology 58: 159–164
89 Djaldetti M 1984 Plasma cell leukemia: ultrastructural aspects in diagnosis. In: Polliack A (ed) Human leukemias: cytochemical and ultrastructural techniques in diagnosis and research. Boston, Martinus Nijhoff Publishing, pp 309–327
90 Catovsky D, Linch D C, Beverley P C L 1982 T-cell disorders in haematological diseases. Clinics in Haematology 11: 661–695
91 Levine A M, Meyer P R, Lukes R J, Feinstein D I 1981 Clinical and morphological heterogeneity of T-cell chronic lymphocytic leukemia (T-CLL). Blood 58, (Supplement) p. 144a
92 Geisler C, Ralfkaer E, Astrup L et al 1983 Chronic lymphocytic leukaemia of T-cell origin. Clinical variation possibly due to involvement of different T lymphocyte subpopulatons. Scandinavian Journal of Haematology 31: 109–121
93 Witzig T E, Phyliky R L, Li C-Y, Homburger H A, Dewald G W, Handwerger R S 1986 T-cell chronic lymphocytic leukemia with a helper/inducer membrane phenotype: a distinct clinicopathologic subtype with a poor prognosis. American Journal of Hematology 21: 139–155
94 Simpkins H, Kiprov D D, Davis J L, Morand P, Puri S, Grahn E P 1985 T-cell chronic lymphocytic leukemia with lymphocytes of unusual immunologic phenotype and function. Blood 65: 127–133
95 Brito-Babapulle V, Pomfret M, Matutes E, Catovsky D 1987 Cytogenetic studies on prolymphocytic leukemia. II. T-cell prolymphocytic leukemia. Blood 70: 926–931
96 Brouet J C, Flandrin G, Sasportes M, Preud'homme J L, Seligmann M 1975 Chronic lymphocytic leukaemia of T cell origin. Immunological and clinical evaluation in eleven patients. Lancet 2: 890–893
97 Matutes E, Brito-Babapulle V, Foroni L, Catovsky D 1986 The nature of T-chronic lymphocytic leukaemia. British Journal of Haematology 62: 402–403
98 Brody J I, Burningham R A, Nowell P C, Rowlands D T, Freiburg P, Daniele R P 1975 Persistent lymphocytosis with chromosomal evidence of malignancy. American Journal of Medicine 58: 547–552
99 Siegal F P, Rambotti P, Siegal M et al 1982 Helper cell function of leukemic Leu-2a +, histamine receptor + T gamma lymphocytes. Journal of Immunology 129: 1775–1781
100 Loughran T P, Kadin M E, Starkebaum G et al 1985 Leukemia of large granular lymphocytes; association with clonal chromosomal abnormalities and autoimmune neutropenia, thrombocytopenia and hemolytic anemia. Annals of Internal Medicine 102: 169–175
101 Brito-Babapulle V, Matutes E, Parreira L, Catovsky D 1986 Abnormalities of chromosome 7q and Tac expression in T cell leukemias. Blood 67: 516–521
102 Knowles D M, Dalla-Favera R, Pelicci P G 1985 T-cell β chain gene rearrangements. Lancet 2: 159–160
103 Foa R, Pelici P G, Migone N et al 1986 Analysis of T-cell receptor beta chain (Tβ) gene rearrangements demonstrates the monoclonal nature of T-cell chronic lymphoproliferative disorders. Blood 67: 247–250

104 Berliner N, Duby A D, Linch D C et al 1986 T-cell receptor gene rearrangement defines a monoclonal T-cell population in patients with T-cell lymphocytosis and cytopenia. Blood 67: 914–918
105 Foroni L, Matutes E, Foldi J, Morilla R, Rabbitts T H, Luzzatto L, Catovsky D 1988 T cell leukemias with rearrangement of the λ but not β T cell receptor genes. Blood: 71: 356–362
106 Sézary A M M, Bouvrain Y 1938 Erythrodermie avec présence de cellules monstrueuses dans la derme et le sang circulant. Bullétin Société de Dermatologie et de Syphilographie: 254–260
107 Brouet J C, Flandrin G, Seligmann M 1973 Indications of the thymus derived nature of the proliferating cells in six patients with Sézary's syndrome. New England Journal of Medicine 289: 341–344
108 Broome J D, Zucker-Franklin D, Weiner M S, Bianco C, Nussenzweig V 1973 Leukemic cells with membrane properties of thymus derived (T) lymphocytes in a case of Sézary's syndrome: morphologic and immunologic studies. Clinical Immunology and Immunopathology 1: 319–329
109 Zucker-Franklin D, Melton J W, Quagliata F 1973 Variants of chronic lymphocytic leukemia with cells having surface properties of T lymphocytes. Journal of Clinical Investigation 52: 92a–93a (abstract)
110 Feller A C, Ziegler A, Sterry W, Good M, Parwaresch M R 1983 Phenotypic heterogeneity of leukemic Sézary cells. Blut 47: 333–341
111 Lutzner N A, Jordan H W 1968 Ultrastructure of an abnormal cell in Sézary's syndrome. Blood 31: 719–726
112 Edelson R L, Lutzner M A, Kirkpatrick C H, Shevach E M, Green I 1974 Morphologic and functional properties of the atypical T lymphocytes of the Sézary syndrome. Mayo Clinic Proceedings 49: 558–567
113 Nowell P C, Finan J B 1977 Isochromosome 17 in atypical myeloproliferative and lymphoproliferative disorders. Journal of the National Cancer Institute 59: 329–331
114 Meijer C J L M, van der Loo E M, van Vloten W A, van der Velde E A, Scheffer E, Cornelisse C J 1980 Early diagnosis of mycosis fungoides and Sézary's syndrome by morphometric analysis of lymphoid cells in the skin. Cancer 45: 2864–2871
115 van der Loo E M, van Vloten W A, Cornelisse D J, Scheffer E, Meijer C J L M 1981 The relevance of morphometry in the differential diagnosis of cutaneous T cell lymphomas. British Journal of Dermatology 104: 257–269
116 Matutes E, Keeling D M, Newland A C et al 1990 Sézary cell-like leukemia: a distinct type of mature T-cell malignancy. Leukemia 4: 262–266
117 Gallo R C, Kalyanaraman V S, Sarngadharan M G et al 1983 Association of the human type C retrovirus with a subset of adult T-cell cancers. Cancer Research 43: 3892–3899
118 Blattner W A, Gibbs W N, Saxinger C et al 1983 Human T-cell leukaemia/lymphoma virus-associated lymphoreticular neoplasia in Jamaica. Lancet 2: 61–64
119 Miyoshi I, Taguchi H, Kubonishi I et al 1982 Type C virus producing cell lines derived from adult T cell leukemia. In: Hanaoka M, Takatsuki K and Shimoyama M (eds) Adult T cell leukemia and related diseases, Plenum Press, New York, pp 219–228
120 Matutes E, Carrington D, Hegde U, Catovsky D 1983 C-type particles in cells from T-cell lymphoma/leukaemia after 5–7 days' culture. Lancet 2: 335–337
121 Yoshida M, Seiki M, Yamaguchi K, Takatsuki K 1984 Monoclonal integration of human T-cell leukemia provirus in all primary tumors of adult-T-cell leukemia suggests causative role of human T-cell virus in the disease. Proceedings of the National Academy of Sciences of the USA 81: 2534–2537
122 Matutes E, Brito-Babapulle V, Catovsky D 1985 Clinical, immunological, ultrastructural and cytogenetic studies in black patients with adult-T-cell leukaemia–lymphoma. In: Miwa M et al (eds) Retroviruses in human lymphoma–leukemia. Japan Scientific Society Press, Tokyo, pp 59–70
123 Uchiyama T, Broder S, Waldmann T A 1981 A monoclonal antibody (anti-Tac) reactive with activated and functionally mature human T cells. I. Production of anti-Tac monoclonal antibody and distribution of Tac (+) cells. Journal of Immunology 126: 1393–1397
124 Thien S L, Catovsky D, Oscier D et al 1982 T-chronic lymphocytic leukaemia presenting as primary hypogammaglobulinaemia–evidence of a proliferation of T-suppressor cells. Clinical and Experimental Immunology 47: 670–676
125 Hofman F M, Smith D, Hocking W 1982 T-cell chronic lymphocytic leukaemia with suppressor phenotype. Clinical and Experimental Immunology 49: 401–409
126 Morimoto C, Letvin N L, Distaso J A, Aldrich W R, Schlossman S F 1985 The isolation and characterization of the human suppressor inducer T cell subset. Journal of Immunology 134: 1508–1515

6
Monoclonal Antibodies in the Diagnosis of Acute Leukemia

G. Janossy   D. Campana

INTRODUCTION

During the last 15 years, the exciting advances in cellular immunology have influenced a number of clinically oriented disciplines, including hematology. A new discipline, cellular immunohematology, has developed which is making strides by applying two major technical advances as part of its routine: the use of monoclonal antibodies (McAbs) and flow cytometry. These developments have already been highlighted in the previous volume of *The Leukemic Cell* in 1981[1] and also summarized in a more recent book edited by P.C.L. Beverley on *Monoclonal Antibodies* in 1984.[2] The latter also included a chapter by M. Loken on the state of art in cell sorting and analysis with fluorescence activated cell analysers.[3] This chapter therefore takes these major developments for granted and focuses on the latest ventures which will be expanding the boundaries of these fields in two rapidly changing and interconnected areas: detecting minimal residual disease and determining the uniquely aberrant features of leukemic cells. These areas have been put into the context of prior technological achievements and five stages of development that have evolved in last 10 years have been tentatively identified.

First, during 1975–80 the origin of leukemias was mapped with the then novel use of a few well-characterized antisera prepared by the conventional methods of immunization and extensive absorptions.[4-7] These included antisera to T-cells, B-cells, immunoglobulin (Ig) heavy and light chains, common-ALL antigen[4] and terminal deoxynucleotidyl transferase (TdT),[8] complemented by two carefully chosen methods for rosetting with sheep and mouse erythrocytes.[9] With these technics, reviewed in the previous edition,[10] it has been established that the blast cells in common-ALL reflect features of normal bone marrow precursors[11] and those in T-ALL reflect the characteristics of thymic cells.[12-14] The heterogeneity of B-cell malignancies[9] has also been traced to their origin from different sets of normal B-cells: those with strong expression of surface Ig (SmIg +) accumulate in the lymphocyte corona within lympoid organs and mirror the features of B-prolymphocytic leukemia,[9] whilst a peculiar B-cell seen mostly in fetal lymph node, spleen and peritoneum[15] is the candidate for the role of the normal equivalent of chronic lymphocytic leukemia (B-CLL).[16] Some of these reagents still form part of the current diagnostic panels.

Second, the monoclonal antibody revolution has dramatically expanded the volume of results, provided further confirmation about leukemic origin and yielded additional precise tools for study. Nevertheless, during the 'introductory' years the primary aim has been two-fold: to characterize leukemia, and also to investigate the reactivity pattern of a wide range of reagents, leading to the apparent over-complication of diagnostic panels. The immunologists have, however, rapidly realized the need for standardization and, in 1982, an international committee was formed in order to define McAbs which recognize the same differentiation antigens. As a result of the Workshops organized in Paris,[17] Boston[18] and Oxford, and Vienna,[19a] 45 clusters of differentation (CD) have so far been accepted, with additional subdivision of reactivity in the CD1, CD11 and CD45 groups (Table 6.1). This classification is based upon the identification of antigens with known molecular weights and,

Table 6.1 The panel of monoclonal antibodies arranged according to clusters of differentiation (CD)

Cluster	Example	Mol.wt (kDa)	Main distribution	Other reactivity on normal	Reactivity on leukemia/lymphoma
CD1a	NA1/34	49	Thymocytes	Langerhans' cells	A few T-ALL and histiocytosis X
CD1b	NU-T2	45			
CD1c	M241	43			
CD2[a]	T11	50	Pan-T-cell	SRBC receptor	all T-ALL
CD3[a]	T3	28,22,20	Pan-T-cell	TCR complex	cCD3: reliable T-ALL marker[b]
CD4	T4	60	T-helper subset	Macrophage subset	Some T-ALL and 'helper' T malignancies (Sézary)
CD5	T1	67	Pan-T-cell	B-CLL-like rare B-cells	B-CLL and T-ALL
CD6	OKT17	120	Pan-T-cell	B-CLL-like rare B-cells	B-CLL and some peripheral T lymphoma/leukemia
CD7[a]	T2	40	Pan-T-cell	Strong on immature, weak on memory T-cells	Reliable marker for T-ALL (and a subset of AML)
CD8	T8	32,30	T-suppressor cell	Nerves, splenic sinusoid	Some T-ALL and T-PLL
CD9	BA-2	24	Pre-B-cells	Monocytes, platelets	Common-ALL
CD10[a]	J5	100	Pre-B, Common-ALL	Kidney, intestine	Common-ALL antigen in ALL, some B lymphomas
CD11a	LFA-1	180 (95)	Leukocytes	Share β-chain CD18	
CD11b	Mac 1	160 (95)	Monocytes, PMN		
CD11c	3.9	150 (95)	Monocytes, PMN		AMML, AMoL and hairy cell leukemia
CD13a	MY7	150	Monocytes, PMN	Skin, kidney + others	AML, AMML
CD14a	UCHM1	55	Monocytes (PMN)	FDC	AMML, AMoL
CD15	Leu M1		PMN (monocytes)	X-hapten, granulocytes	Granulocytic differentiation in APL, CGL
CD16	MG38	50–60	PMN	FcR-low	NK cells
CD17	(G)035		PMN, monocytes, platelets	Lactoceramide	
CD18	60.3	95	Leukocytes	Common β-chain of CD11	
CD19[a]	B4	90	B-cells	FDC	Reliable marker for common- and 'null'-ALL and B
CD20[a]	B1	35	B-cells	FDC	Pre-B-ALL, B-cell malignancies
CD21	B2	180	B-cells	FDC, C3dR	Some lymphomas
CD22[a]	HD39	135	B-cells	Nil	cCD22: reliable marker for common- and 'null'-ALL[b]

Table 6.1 The panel of monoclonal antibodies arranged according to clusters of differentiation (CD) (*Continued*)

Cluster	Example	Mol.wt (kDa)	Main distribution	Other reactivity on normal	Reactivity on leukemia/lymphoma
CD23	MHM6	45	Activated B-cell	FDC	B lymphomas
CD24	BA-1	45,55,65	B-cells, PMN		Common-ALL
CD25	Tac	55	T-cells, B-cells	Macrophages	Peripheral T-cell malignancies such as HTL
CDw26	TI19-4-7	130	Activated T-cells		
CD27	VIT14	120–55	T-cells, plasma cells		
CD28	9.3	44	T-cytotoxic subset		
CD29	4B4	135	T-helper inducer	PMN, B-cells	
CD30	Ki — 1		Activated T and B-cells		Hodgkin's and Reed-Sternberg cell
CD31	SG134	130–140	Monocytes, PMN, platelets	gpIIa	
CD32	2E1	40	Monocytes, PMN, platelets	FcR-high	
CD33[a]	MY9	67	Myeloid precursor		AML
CD34[a]	MY10	115	Myeloid stem cells		AML and common-ALL (only 70% of cases)
CD35	TO5	220	PMN, monocytes, FDC	CR1 — kidney	
CD36	4C7	85	Monocytes, platelets	gpIV	
CD37	BL14 RFB7	40–45	Pan-B-cells	FDC	
CD38		45	Multiple lineages		
CD39	G28-10	80	B-cells, macrophages	Blood vessels	
CD40	G28.5	50	B-cells, IDC	Carcinomas	
CD41	J15		Platelets	gpIIb/IIIa	Megakaryocytic leukemia
CD42	HPL14		Platelets	gpIb	
CD43	G10-2	95	Leukocytes	Brain	
CD44	F10-44-2	65–85	Leukocytes	Brain	
CD45	T200	220,205,190	Leukocytes	LCA	
CD45RA	2H4	220,205	Leukocyte subsets	LCA on virgin T-cells	
CD45RO	UCHL1	180	Leukocyte subsets	LCA on memory T-cells	Most T-cell lymphomas

Compiled from 3rd International Workshop on Human Leukocyte Differentiation Antigens, Oxford, 1986. The Vienna Conference,[19a] standardized 33 additional clusters but few of these are used in leukemia diagnosis.

a Markers used in the microplate assay for acute leukemia diagnosis.
b cytoplasmic staining and also reacts with peripheral malignancies when the antigen is expressed on the surface.

Abbreviations: SRBC — sheep red blood cell receptor; TCR — T-cell receptor; B-CLL — chronic lymphocytic leukemia; AML acute myeloid leukemia; ALL — acute lymphoblastic leukemia; FDC — follicular dendritic cell; X-hapten — α-lacto-N-fucose pentosyl; FcR-low — low affinity Fc receptor; C3dR — C3d receptor; PMN — granulocytes; FcR-high — high affinity Fc receptor; CR1 — complement receptor type 1; LCA — leukocyte common antigen; gp — glycoprotein.

frequently, with known physiological function. The McAbs within each CD (sub) group can then be used interchangeably as diagnostic tools.

Third, during these studies a virtually complete agreement has been reached between the immunodiagnostic laboratories about the most useful panel of such reagents.[20-22] These sets of reagents can be applied in a microplate assay in order to introduce both uniformity and economy.[20] In this chapter we describe the set of McAbs routinely used in such assay. An additional important requirement is, however, the flexibility for both more detailed diagnostic work and research. In order to accommodate this, it is suggested that after the use of a first set of 12 reagents, second sets of further McAbs are applied according to the investigator's choice. The ease and speed of the microplate assay renders the performance of two rounds of assays on the same leukemic sample feasible, even on the same day, and the reagents for the second run can be selected, for maximum information, on the basis of the first diagnostic results.

Fourth, the current knowledge about the most crucial B- and T-cell differentiation antigens has been greatly expanded by identifying the monomorphic molecules which promote adherence or cell activation during crucial interactions with antigen presenting cells. These are the CD22 antigens[23,24] on B-lineage cells and CD3 group of antigens[25-27] on T-lineage cells. The crucial issue about these molecules is that, within a given lineage, i.e. B or T, the CD22 or CD3 moieties are expressed first in the cytoplasm of immature cells (cCD22 and cCD3). Subsequently, the cytoplasmic expression of Ig heavy chain (cμ) in pre-B cells and the TCRβ in thymocytes appears and finally these moieties are inserted into the membrane, as a functional membrane-bound, antigen-specific receptor complex.[23-27] It will be indicated below that the biologically important cCD3 and cCD22 molecules also represent one of the most reliable leukemia markers for T-ALL and common-ALL, respectively, together with the nuclear TdT- a sign of lymphoid immaturity.[8,11-13] Therefore, with the application of carefully selected McAbs to leukemia diagnosis there is very little uncertainty left about the exact classification of acute leukemias. When appropriate McAbs are applied in conjunction with the study of gene rearrangements, even peculiar cases of undifferentiated and mixed leukemias can be identified with great precision. It is therefore to be expected that the aims of research are now changing towards more ambitious goals.

Fifth, it has come to be appreciated that leukemic cells express normal differentiation antigens which may frequently appear in aberrant combinations not seen among normal cells.[28-29] These aberrant combinations, referred to as asynchronous development, are often unique to individual cases and need to be identified at presentation. These combinations can later be exploited to identify residual leukemia and be used to assess both the efficacy of treatment and the occurrence of early relapse. Additional investigations of the biology of leukemic cells are permitted by the application of phenotypic markers in conjunction with cell cycle studies and gene analysis. An introductory step in this direction is the use of McAbs with markers of cellular proliferative activity, in order to investigate the phenotype and proportions of leukemic cells in the proliferative cycle.[30] A further development will be immunological phenotyping combined with in situ hybridization.[31] To conclude this introduction it should be emphasized that all these approaches are based on simple technics for combination staining at single cell level, and such methods of double and triple marker combinations will be described below.

METHOD 1

MEMBRANE IMMUNOFLUORESCENCE (IF) STAINING (MICROPLATE METHOD)

Principle
The microplate method allows processing of multiple samples and staining with multiple McAbs. Four elements contribute to its economy:[20]

1. Microplates with U-wells provide a vehicle for simultaneously staining and washing 96 samples.
2. Antibody panels are constructed as multiples of six tests, and Titertek multipipettes are employed to handle six reagents and six samples simultaneously. These samples are transferred onto slides, for viewing, in a prearranged pattern of 2 x 6;
3. Twelve-well multitest slides receive the 12 droplets of cells which are fixed in formalin vapor and viewed on a standard microscope under a coverslip. Bright 63 x Phaco objectives with numerical apertures of 1.4 are used without compromising optical quality.
4. Depending on the results, it is possible either to re-stain the residual cells left in the microplate wells using directly labeled second antibodies; or to prepare cytospins from selected microwells and stain these for cytoplasmic or nuclear antigens (see Method 2); or to analyse cells from selected microwells on the cell sorter.

Reagents and materials

1. McAbs for investigating acute leukemia (Table 6.2) together with normal control serum (from the same species). Goat anti-mouse Ig labeled with fluorescein isothiocyanate (FITC; Sigma Cat. No. F1010, Seralab Cat. No. FAES-084, or Kallestad Cat. No. 147)
2. PBS (phosphate-buffered saline) containing 0.2% bovine serum albumin and 0.2% azide (PBSAA).
3. Microplates with U-bottomed wells (Sterilin; Cat. No. M24A).
4. Adhesive microplate cover (Flow Labs. Cat. No. 77-400-05).
5. Plastic stoppers for individual wells (e.g. from Pierce & Warriner Ltd).
6. Microplates with V-bottomed wells (stock plates of reagent panel).
7. PTFE-coated multispot slides with 12 wells (Cat. No. PH001, Headley, Essex, UK) and 22 x 64 mm coverslips (Raymond Lamb, London Cat. No.E/23).
8. Formalin vapor (40% formaldehyde in a moist chamber).
9. Semipermanent mountant: 20 g polyvinylalcohol in 80 ml PBS + 40 ml glycerol containing 3 g diazo-bicyclooctane (DABCO) pH 8.6, or temporary mountant: PBS and glycerol in 1:1 ratio.

Equipment

1. Beckman TJ-6 with plate carriers (Cat. No. 340509) or MSE Centaur 2 (Cat. No. 41132-3657) with plate carriers (Cat. No. 43121-116).
2. Microscope with epi-illumination, filter sets for FITC and tetramethyl-isothiocyanate (TRITC), phase contrast condenser and objective 63 Phaco NA = 1.3-1.4.
3. Plate shaker (Dynatech; Cat. No. AM69).
4. Titertek 8-fold multi-pipettes: 5-50 µl (Cat. No. 77-858-00); Titertek 12-fold multipipette: 50-250 µl (Cat. No. 77-969-00; both from Flow Labs), together with trays for solutions; also tips in unlimited quantity, changed after each operation. Note that only six out of the eight channels of the smaller volume Titertek pipettes are used.
5. 50 µl automatic pipette (e.g. Ependorf; Cat. No. 3135-0000-0000).

Microplate method

1. Twelve (2 x 6) McAbs (Tables 6.1 and 6.2), kept in a V-bottomed plate as a row of concentrated stock solution and diluted with PBSA prior to use, are transferred in 50 µl volumes onto the cells with a Titertek multipipette (using six of the eight available channels).

Table 6.2 Diagnostic reagents in leukemia ('acute leukemia' panel)

McAb	Function or role	Mol.wt. (kDa)	Frequently used example	Ref.
1. Membrane markers in the microplate				
Thymocyte and T-lymphoid associated[a]				
CD7	thymocyte + T-cell	40	3A1, WT1, Leu9, RFT2	32
CD2	thymocytes, T-cells + NK	50	(OK) T11, Leu5, RFT11	17
Myeloid associated[b]				
CD13	myeloblasts, granulocytes and monocytes	150	My7, MCS2, WM15	33
CD33	myeloblasts		My9, WM54	33
CD14	monocytes		UCHM1	34
Common-ALL and B lymphoid associated[c]				
CD19	pre-B + B	95	B4, Leu12, SB4, RFB9	35
CD10	pre-pre-B and cALL	100	J5, VILA1, RFAL1	37
CD20	B-cells	35	B1, Leu16	38
IgM	B-cells	75 IgM	Goat anti-human-IgM	6
Stem cell associated[b,c]				
CD34	lymphoid + myeloid precursors		BI-3C5, My10	39,40
Class-II	lymphoid + myeloid precursors + B-cells	28,35	Anti-HLA-DR	7
Normal mouse serum				
2. Intracellular markers in cytocentrifuge preparations				
TdT	Immaturity marker in ALL and some 20% of AML		Rabbit anti-TdT McAb anti-TdT	8
cCD3[d]	T-lineage commitment in T-ALL[a,e]	19,20,25	UCHT1, Leu4	25–27
cCD22[d]	B-lineage commitment in common-ALL, 'null'- and pre-B-ALL[c]	135	RFB4, To15, Leu14	23,24
cμ[d]	Cytoplasmic IgM in pre-B-ALL[c]	75	Goat anti-human-IgM	11
cTCRβ[d]	Cytoplasmic T-cell receptor β-chain in 'pre-T'-ALL[a,e]	44	βF1	56

a = Fig. 6.4; b = Fig. 6.5; c = Fig. 6.3; d = cytoplasmic; e = Fig. 6.6.

2. 1–2 × 10^5 cells in 50 μl aliquots are placed into each U-bottomed well of a 12-well row using automatic pipette.
3. The individual wells on the whole plate are covered with an adhesive sheet and occasionally agitated while incubating for 10 min at 20°C.
4. The wells are spun in a centrifuge at maximum acceleration until it reaches 2000 rev/min and then braked to a standstill. The supernatant is flicked out of the plate.
5. The cells are suspended on a plate shaker, 150 μl PBSAA added and steps (4) and (5) repeated four times.
6. Cells are then incubated for 10 min with diluted goat anti-mouse-Ig-FITC (30 μl), after which they are washed as in steps (4) and (5).
7. After the last wash, 5–6 μl PBSAA is added to each of the small cell pellets using a smaller Titertek multipipette, and 3 μl of resuspended cells are transferred, as two rows of six samples, onto a PTFE-coated multispot slide.

8. One slide (12 samples) for each patient is placed into formalin vapor for 10 min, air-dried at 20°C and covered with glycerol:PBS (1:1) and a coverslip.

Comments
It is important to adhere to the washing procedure (resuspension and number of washes). Residual traces of the first antibody in the supernatant can form soluble complexes with the second antibody and bind to Fc receptors on irrelevant cells. Slides should be mounted as soon as they are dry in order to avoid the deposition of intercellular crystals.

Interpretation
Many laboratories use a fairly uniform primary panel of McAbs in the microplate assay for acute leukemias. These are: (1) T-lineage related, (2) myeloid associated, (3) common-ALL and B-lineage associated and (4) markers of immaturity; these descriptions are only convenient approximations for the predominant reactivity of these McAbs (Fig. 6.1).

T-cell associated markers
The T-cell associated markers include CD7 and CD2: *CD7* reagents, detect a 40-kilodalton (kDa) antigen, strongly react with T blasts and are positive in virtually all cases of T-ALL, including those which are negative with sheep erythrocyte rosetting, and the corresponding T11-like *CD2* antibodies. Although common-ALL blasts are CD7 −, this marker shows reactivity with some acute myeloid leukemias (AMLs)[32] and therefore is not as specific for T-ALL as cytoplasmic staining for CD3 (cCD3; see below).

Myeloid associated
Three types of myeloid antibodies are included in the first screening range. The first two react with most myeloid leukemias − these are *CD13* including My7 or MSC-2 and *CD33* including My9. The highest percentage of AML reactivity has been recorded with CD13, although the staining intensity in some AMLs can be low and the proportion of positive blasts is variable.[33] The third McAb is used to detect malignancies with a monocytic component such as acute myeloid monocytic leukemia (AMML) and acute monocytic leukemia (AMoL). As yet there is no general agreement as to which CD group is optimal for this purpose, and the two best candidates are the CD14 group (such as UCHM1)[34] and the CD11c group (also referred to as p150/95; see Table 6.1). These reagents bind strongly to normal and malignant monocytes but show additional reactivity with non-monocytic cells. For example, CD14 reagents label B-cells when used on smears and CD11c reagents are also strongly positive on hairy cell leukemia.

Common-ALL and B-cell associated
There are four groups of McAbs within the common-ALL-B-cell-associated category. The widest cover, from early precursors through cALL + ,TdT + cells to B-lymphocytes, is given by CD19 reagents such as B4 and Leu-12[35] which recognize an antigen of 95kDa expressed both on common-ALL and 'null'-ALL, but absent on T-ALL and AML. This marker is extremely reliable and gives the same results as cytoplasmic CD22 in more than 95% of common-ALL cases (see below), with the exception of unconfirmed reports of CD19 reactivity in AMML.[36] The CD10 McAbs react with the common-ALL antigen (cALL; 100 kDa), present on 80-90% of ALL cases.[37] The next reagent, CD20, strongly reacts with an antigen of 35 kDa on B-cells[38] and most mature B-cell malignancies without labeling the majority of cALL + cells. An alternative is CD37 (RFB7) antibody. The conventional B-cell marker, anti-IgM, completes this range.

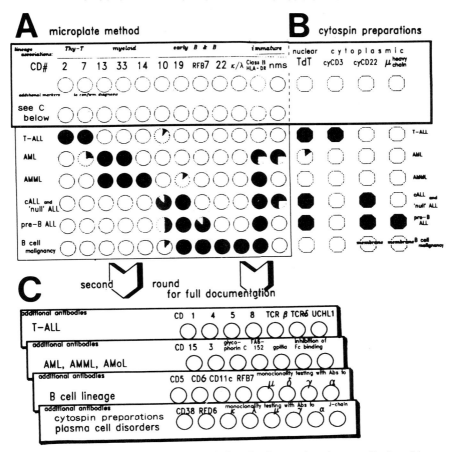

Fig. 6.1 The principle of the microplate method. Samples from each patient are distributed into a row of 12 microwells and labeled with the 'first round' of reagents shown followed by FITC-labeled goat anti-mouse-Ig second layer (with the exception of the testing for monoclonality where a mix of anti-κ-FITC and anti-λ-TRITC is used: (A). Following the evaluation of the first results, cytospin preparations are made from the rest of cells taken from the positively stained wells. These are labeled for nuclear TdT and cytoplasmic antigens as shown (B). Second rounds of additional McAb are investigated in order to fully document the phenotypic features (C). This method is suitable to characterize the leukemic cells when present in low proportions, and to identify asynchronous and aberrant phenotypes. In order to demonstrate the reactivity pattern of the various acute leukemias, the positive reactions are indicated by shaded circles. The white segments show that not all cases of the given leukemia type are positive. On cytospin preparations, the shaded areas depict intracellular labeling but some membrane staining may also be detected. A suggestion for the selection of the 'second round' of McAb is shown in (C).

Markers of maturity

The stem-cell-related McAbs, such as CD34 (including BI-3C5[39] and My10[40]) and anti-class-II, are found on immature cells without discriminating between acute myeloid (AML) and common acute lymphoid leukemias (cALL). The CD34 McAb may be used instead of one of the myeloid reagents or the class II McAbs (Fig. 6.1). Large numbers of CD34 + cells in a sample immediately indicate a preponderance of 'immature' leukemic cells, but not all cases of ALL and AML are positive. Anti-class II (usually anti-HLA-DR)

176　THE LEUKEMIC CELL

is also reactive with B-cell disorders. The vast majority of T-ALL cases are, however, class II − (HLA-DR) and CD34 − .

As the reactivity pattern with the first antibodies emerges, further tests might be required. These are largely dependent upon the location of the laboratory (i.e. leukemia center, general hospital or pediatric oncology group, etc.). An immediate task is double staining for TdT and for cytoplasmic antigens such as CD3 (cCD3), cCD22 and cμ heavy chain in cytocentrifuge preparations (see Method 3 and Fig. 6.1). The 'second round' reagents include additional erythroid (glycophorin C) and megakaryocytic (glycoprotein IIIa) reagents as well as anti-Ig heavy chain antibodies (anti-IgM, IgG, IgA; heavy chain specific) for B-cell malignancies (Fig. 6.1) or CD34 if it has not yet been used in the first round. For further useful antibodies and their CD numbers see Table 6.1.

METHOD 2

TWO-COLOUR IMMUNOFLUORESCENCE METHOD

Principle
Double IF staining can be performed simultaneously with non-cross-reacting reagents directly labeled with different fluorochromes such as FITC and TRITC, or phycoerythrin (PE). The direct method is recommemded when there is the need to investigate the absolute amounts of antigens expressed on the cells. The single layer antibodies are used at saturating conditions in such experiments. Commercial companies supply such labeled McAbs of high quality. The disadvantage of this system is that relatively large amounts of reagents are required. The advantages of indirect IF are three-fold:

1. The second layer amplifies the intensity of labeling, and gives good results with antigen expressed in low density.
2. It is economical with the first layer McAbs.
3. The same fluorochrome-labeled second antibody can be used with a wide variety of first layers.

When the first layer McAbs are of different (sub)classes such as IgM and IgG1 or IgG2, these are identified with specific goat anti-mouse IgM and IgG conjugated with different fluorochromes. With the standardization of CD clusters it is easy to find McAbs of the same specificity but belonging to different classes. An equally successful method is to conjugate McAbs with haptens such as biotin[41] or arsanilic acid and use avidin (or streptavidin) and goat anti-arsanilic antibodies, respectively, as fluorochrome-conjugated second layers.[42]

Reagents

1. For establishing the monoclonality of B-cell malignancies use goat anti-human κ-TRITC together with goat anti-human λ-FITC, available from various companies including Southern Biotechnology Associates (SBA; Birmingham, Ala, Cat. Nos. 2060–03 and 2070–02).
2. For the simultaneous labeling of CD5 (T1; p67) antigen and surface immunoglobulin use CD5 + goat anti-mouse Ig-TRITC together with directly labeled goat anti-human IgM−FITC (μ heavy chain specific SBA; Cat. No. 2020–02) or rabbit anti-human IgM-FITC F(ab)$_2$ (Kallestad, Cat. No. 140).
3. In order to perform indirect two-colour immunofluorescence with McAbs of different class goat anti-mouse-IgM-TRITC and anti-mouse-IgG-FITC, class-specific, column-purified second layers are available from SBA (Cat. Nos. 1020–03 and 1030–02,

respectively). The alternative colour combination (IgM-FITC with IgG-TRITC) is also available (Cat. Nos. 1020-02 and 1030-03). The UK distributors for SBA are Seralab Ltd, Crawley Down, Sussex.
4. Other directly conjugated secondary antibodies are available from Coulter Immunology (Hialeah, FI, USA) or Coulter Ltd (Luton, UK and from Becton Dickinson, USA).
5. Mouse serum used at 1:10 dilution, or mouse myeloma proteins of different (sub)classes with no anti-human reactivity in appropriate amounts.

For equipment see Method 1.

Method

1. As the 'lymphocyte' microplate is performed (see Table 6.2 and Fig. 6.1) a mixture of goat anti-human-κ-TRITC and goat anti-human-λ-FITC is placed into the tenth well. After washing four times, FITC and TRITC positive cells can be counted by microscopy with separate filters.
2. When B-cell malignancies are studied McAbs of CD5 (T1-type) are labeled with goat anti-mouse-Ig-FITC and used in combination with goat anti-human-IgM-TRITC. After washing four times and mounting on slides, cells are examined to see if CD5 + (T) cells and IgM + (B) cells represent separate normal populations or, alternatively, whether they co-express CD5 and IgM as seen in B-CLL and some centrocytic lymphomas.
3. The samples may contain low proportions of leukemic cells admixed with normal myeloerythropoietic cells and T-lymphocytes. The cells remaining in the microplate wells can still be used for further staining: 20 µl mouse serum is added for 5 min in order to block goat anti-mouse-Ig activity and the plate is washed once. Now the cells can be incubated with another McAb, directly conjugated with TRITC, washed four times, and the heterogeneity of the leukemia assessed.

Comments and interpretation

In samples labeled for κ and λ, the microscopic analysis of normal blood shows that 10–15% of lymphocytes form caps and patches on the membrane in a 2:1 ratio of κ/λ. Occasionally, some cells are doubly stained despite acetate washing indicating passively absorbed Ig. In leukemia/lymphoma the diagnosis of B-cell malignancy is made if the κ/λ ratio is more than 10:1 or less than 1:5[43] When the sample is not severely involved, a two-color combination is necessary for accurate diagnosis. The percentage positivity with anti-Ig reagents has to be interpreted in the light of positivity with other B-cell markers, such as CD19 and CD20, because some B-cell malignancies express low or undetectable amounts of sIg, and may express Ig in cytoplasm and/or show the monoclonal rearrangements of their Ig genes.

METHOD 3

INVESTIGATION OF CELLS IN CYTOCENTRIFUGE PREPARATIONS AND SMEARS

Principle
The analysis of immunofluorescence in cytospins has three purposes:

1. Once the membrane antigens on viable cells are labeled in cell suspension, cells can be viewed on a slide, and stored in the dark at 4°C without loss of fluorescence for longer than 1 month.

2. Slides are prepared from *unstained* cells and labeled with antibodies *after fixation*.[44] Under these conditions the labeling of cytoplasmic and nuclear antigens dominates. Strongly expressed membrane antigens are also stained, but the pattern of labeling is different from that seen in suspension. A typical example is the analysis of plasma cell disorders.[45,46]
3. Following *membrane staining* of cells in suspension with FITC-labeled McAbs, cytospins are made and restained for *cytoplasmic* or *nuclear* antigens with McAbs labeled with TRITC. The typical example of this method is the further analysis of cells studied in the microplate for the expression of nuclear TdT and cCD3, cCD22 and cμ (Fig. 6.1).

Materials

Fixatives

1. Pure methanol to fix cells for nuclear TdT.
2. If anti-TdT staining is combined with staining for cCD3, cCD22 or cμ a 1:1 mixture of acetone:methanol is used.
3. Glacial acetic acid 5% in 95% ethanol to fix plasma cells for labeling with anti-Ig reagents.
4. In addition, acetone and formalin vapor might be tried for staining with McAbs which may give weak staining following methanol fixation.

Reagents

1. Rabbit antibody to calf TdT[8] (rabbit-anti-TdT, affinity purified; Cat. No. 004, Supertech, Bethesda, MD, USA) and goat anti-rabbit-Ig-TRITC (SBA Cat. No. 4010-03) or swine anti-rabbit-Ig-TRITC second layer (Dakopatt, Copenhagen, DK; Cat. No. R156). Alternatively, goat anti-rabbit-Ig-FITC second layer (Supertech, Bethesda, MD; Cat. No. 008). McAbs to TdT are also available from the same sources.
2. Selected CD3 McAbs suitable for cCD3 labeling:[47] UCHT1 or Leu4 (Cat. No. 7340, Becton-Dickinson) with goat anti-mouse-Ig-TRITC (e.g. from SBA, Cat. No. 1010-03) as well as similar directly conjugated CD3-FITC (Cat. No. 92-0001 or 770 310 respectively).
3. CD22 McAb (To15, Dakopatt or anti-Leu14; Becton-Dickinson; Cat. No. 7570).
4. Goat anti-mouse-Ig-FITC or TRITC from a reliable commercial source (such as SBA, Kallestad, Tago, Meloy, Nordic, etc.). If mouse McAbs of different class are used in combination, goat antisera to mouse IgG and IgM are also needed (see above).
5. Goat anti-human-IgM-TRITC (Cat. No. 2020-03, SBA).

Other

1. Microscope slides, absorbent cytospin paper, coverslips and mounting media for permanent storage as in Method 3.
2. Glass micropipettes (2, 5 and 10 μl volume) for adding antibodies to smeared cells.
3. Mouse serum 10%.

Equipment

1. Bench centrifuge for Ficoll–Hypaque separation (see Ch. 2).
2. Cytocentrifuge (Cytospin-2; Shandon, Runcorn, UK, Cat. No. 59900101).
3. Moisture chamber, to prevent the evaporation of reagents from cytospins.

Method

1. Place microscope slides with absorbent paper into the cytocentrifuge.
2. Adjust cell concentration of unfixed viable cells to $5-7 \times 10^5$/ml. You may choose to use fresh cell populations, or to use cells from selected microwells of a microplate, already labeled for membrane antigen and FITC-second layer. Add 1-2 drops (100 µl) into the plastic well of the cytocentrifuge and spin at 500 rev/min for 5 min. Air-dry the deposits rapidly, and check for optimal cell density (40-50 cells per high power field).
3. Fix slides for 30 min in cold methanol at 4°C for TdT staining, and for 15 min in ethanol with 5% acetic acid for cytoplasmic Ig staining in plasma cells. Use other fixatives, if required, after careful standardization with individual McAbs. Wash slides in PBS.
4. If necessary draw a circle with diamond needle around the cytospin. While leaving the cytospin fully covered with PBS (approximately 20 µl), wipe the moisture off the rest of the slide. Add reagent diluted in 10 µl PBS to the droplet covering the cells and mix fluid gently with the micropipette.
5. Incubate at 20°C for 30 min, wash in three successive batches of PBS. If indirect immunofluorescence is performed, leave 20 µl fluid on the smear and add 10 µl pretested second layer antibody. After incubation (30 min) wash three times and mount the preparations in PBS:glycerol (1:1 mixture with 2% formalin).

Controls

1. Cytospins from known cases of acute lymphoblastic (TdT +) and acute myeloid leukemia (TdT −).
2. Cytospins of normal lymphoid cells from blood as well as from suspension of tonsil lymphocytes and/or phytohemagglutinin-stimulated T blasts.

Not all commercial sources scrutinize their batches of anti-TdT with the same care and some commercial anti-TdT reagents may show extra non-specific activity against nuclear antigens in normal or activated lymphocytes/blasts.[47] These reagents are very dangerous because their use can lead to misleading diagnosis of 'ALL' rather than to the correct diagnosis of lymphocytosis.[48] Thus a new batch of anti-TdT needs to be tested with tonsil or phytohemagglutinin (PHA) blast cells.

Comments

In a recent study the reliability of leukemia diagnosis using tests for membrane and cytoplasmic antigens has been compared.[49] The design of the investigation was to make a provisional diagnosis on the basis of the membrane staining seen in the microplate assay (Method 1) together with TdT staining[20] and then to re-analyse the expression of CD22 and CD3 in the cytoplasm of the same cells (Method 3). First the reliability of cCD22 in the diagnosis of B-lineage ALL, including common-ALL, 'null'-ALL and pre-B-ALL, has been established by confirming previous studies;[50,51] of the 50 cases, 48 (96%) showed cCD22 positivity in the cytocentrifuge preparations, and one of the two cCD22 − cases became cCD22 + in relapse. None of the 83 non-B malignancies showed false positivity (Table 6.3). It can be concluded that cCD22, together with CD19, are the most reliable markers of early B-lineage commitment in acute leukemias. CD19 has performed equally well in the same group of diseases with only one case being CD19 − (98% positivity) and only 6% of non-B cases exhibiting false positivity. When these two McAbs are used in the same diagnostic panel, they represent a virtually 100% reliable approach for B-lineage detection.

Next the reliability of cCD3 was tested in T-ALL on the basis of previous studies.[25-27,47] Of the 36 cases of T-ALL studied with UCHT1 (CD3 reagent detecting the ε-chain), all

180   THE LEUKEMIC CELL

Table 6.3 CD3 and CD22 expression on the surface and in the cytoplasm of acute leukemia blasts[a]

	cCD22	sCD22	cCD3	sCD3
Common-ALL	29/31[b,c]	5/31	0/31	0/31
'Null'	6/6	0/6	0/6	0/6
Pre-B-ALL	11/11	0/11	0/11	0/11
B-ALL	2/2	1/2	0/2	0/2
T-ALL	0/36	0/36	36/36[d]	7/36
AML	0/32	0/32	0/32	0/32
AML CD7+	0/1	0/1	0/1	0/1
AML TdT+	0/5	0/5	0/5	0/5
AML CD7+, TdT+	0/2	0/2	0/2	0/2
Erythroleukemia	0/1	0/1	0/1	0/1
Undifferentiated[e]	0/5	0/5	0/5	0/5

a = When positive CD22 (RFB4) was expressed in 40% to >98% of blasts and CD3 (UCHT1) was expressed in >80% blasts.
b = One of the two cCD22− cases was cCD22+ in relapse.
c = One of the cCD22+ cases was CD10+, TdT+ but CD19−.
d = One case was CD3a+ (UCHT1+) but CD3c− (OKT3−).
e = Three cases were class II+, TdT+, CD34+. One case was CD7+, TdT−, cCD3− and one case was CD7+, CD34+, TdT−, cCD3−. CD13, CD33 and Sudan black staining were negative in all five cases.

were cCD3+, TdT+ (100% positivity) and another reagent OKT3 (cCD3) showed negativity in one case (97% positivity). An independent study has also shown that UCHT1 is one of the few optimal CD3 McAbs for cCD3 antigen detection.[47] No false positivity was found in 132 cases of non-T malignancies (Table 6.3). The same 36 cases of T-ALL also expressed CD7 antigen (100% positivity) but 7 of the 32 cases of AML (CD13+, CD33+) were also CD7+ indicating 22% false positivity within the AML group. These results are illustrated in Fig. 6.2 where only T-ALL is cCD3+ and in other cases only residual normal TdT− T-cells are positive. It can be concluded that cCD3 is a fully reliable marker of T-ALL. Finally it must be emphasized that 5 out of the total 132 leukemias (3.8%) were classified as 'undifferentiated' because they lacked signs of lymphoid differentiation, showed no Ig or TCR β-gene rearrangements and were negative with myeloid markers (see footnotes to Table 6.3).

Interpretation

The surprisingly uniform expression of some characteristics in leukemia require explanation. This is given by a comparative analysis of leukemia phenotypes with those of the most immature normal precursor cells (Figs. 6.3–6.5). The first point to emphasize is that the population analysis of B-cell precursors in the bone marrow (Fig. 6.3) and that of T-cell precursors in the thymus (Fig. 6.4) has been carried out by the technics shown above, demonstrating their suitability for studying minute cell populations. The second important notion is that during the last 4 years a unified view was obtained about the development of B- and T-lineages.[23,26,27] This view is based upon the discovery of the murine and human T-cell receptors (TCR), and on the understanding of the similarities of the Ig heavy (μ) and light (κ or λ) chain genes as well as the TCR β- and α-chain genes.

This unified view has now been reinforced by two additional sets of facts. First, it well known that the monomorphic part of the T-cell receptor is the CD3 complex.[52,53] It has been suggested, on the basis of experimental evidence[54] and the pattern of expression during development (see Fig. 6.2), that CD22 antigens also play a very important role: in helping interactions of B-cells and monocytes.[55] Secondly, it has recently been

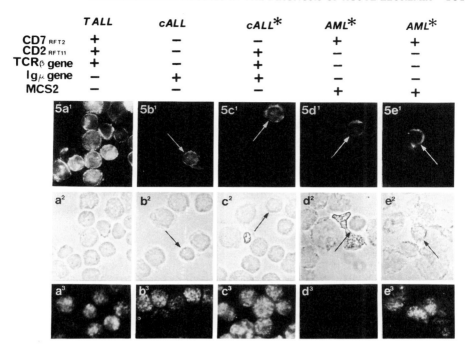

Fig. 6.2 The expression of cCD3 and TdT in leukemia. The same fields were photographed with filters for FITC (CD3 in a^1-e^1), TRITC (TdT in a^3-e^3) and phase contrast (a^2-e^2). The diagnoses are as follows: (a) typical T-ALL, mCD3 −, cCD3 +, TdT +; (b) typical common-ALL; cCD3 −, TdT +: (c–e) a selection of unusual cases. The common-ALL in (c) has an unusual reactivity with anti-CD2 and rearranged TCR β-gene, and CD10 +, HLA-DR +, CD7 − and cCD3 −. In (d) a case of AML is shown with CD7 positivity and otherwise typical features (CD33 +, cCD3 − and TdT −). In (e) a peculiar case of AML is depicted: CD7 +, TdT +, CD33 + and the blasts are cCD3 −. Arrows in (b–e) point to residual CD3 + normal T-lymphocytes (TdT −). (From Campana et al[27] with permission of the Journal of Immunology.)

documented that the successive steps of differentiation within the early stages of B-cell development (see Fig. 6.3) and those of T-cell development (see Fig. 6.4) are virtually identical.[55,56] The lineage commitments in both lineages appear to coincide with the cytoplasmic expression of important functional antigens: cCD22 in B and cCD3 in T, respectively. This is the first step of differentiation. At the same time the cellular expression of TdT is at its highest level. This enzyme inserts extra nucleotides (N region) into the heavy chain μ and the TCRβ in the respective B and T precursors.[57] Obviously, while these rearrangements of μ-genes and β-genes occur the precursors do not, as yet, synthesize μ and β. These early B precursors express on their membrane CD10 and CD19 antigens[11,31] (see Fig. 6.3) and the T-cell precursors express CD7 and, variably, CD2 (see Fig. 6.4).

As has been emphasized elsewhere,[30,58] the most immature characteristics of the *earliest* committed precursors of the B- or T-lineage, are faithfully preserved in the corresponding acute leukemias. This concept explains the fidelity of cCD22, TdT, CD10 and CD19 in common-ALL, and the fidelity of cCD3, TdT, CD7 and CD2 in T-ALL (see Table 6.3). These are the immunological markers of choice for ALL diagnosis.

During the second stage of development the TdT enzyme is still retained, although at a lower level, and the first traces of heavy chains (μ or β in B or T, respectively) appear in the cytoplasm. This population is extremely rare in the normal bone marrow where less than

182 THE LEUKEMIC CELL

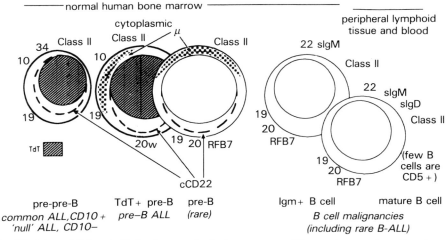

Fig. 6.3 Normal B lymphoid development in the bone marrow. The numbers on the cells refer to CD numbers of McAb (see Table 6.1). CD19 is present on all B-cell types. The early B-lymphoid precursors (pre-pre-B-cells) contain nuclear TdT, cytoplasmic CD22 (cCD22) and membrane CD10 (cALL antigen). A stem cell-associated marker CD34 is also present. The corresponding leukemia is referred to as common-ALL; a variant 'null'-ALL is CD10 –. The TdT +, cμ + pre-B-cells are a rare transit population, but a corresponding leukemia exists (pre-B-ALL: TdT +, cμ +). Proper pre-B-cells have no TdT but are cμ +, CD19 +, CD20 +, RFB7 + and cCD22 +. The immature B-lymphocytes express sIgM, whilst recirculating B-lymphocytes are sIgM +, sIgD +.

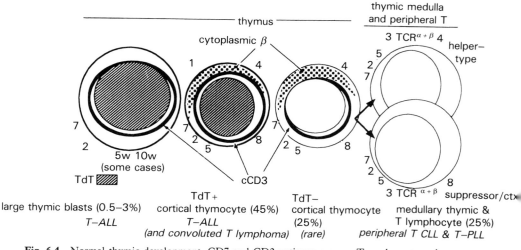

Fig. 6.4 Normal thymic development. CD7 and CD2 antigens are pan-T markers strongly expressed on large thymic blasts, a minority population of thymocytes (0.5–3%). These are also strongly TdT +, contain cytoplasmic CD3 (cCD3 +), but are CD1 –, CD4 – and CD8 –. These antigens appear on small cortical thymocytes (70% of thymocytes). The β-chain of the T-cell receptor (TCR) is first seen in the cytoplasm at the cortical thymocyte stage and is inserted into the membrane with CD3 and TCR α-chain at the mature stage (mCD3 +). Thus a functional TCR (α + β) and mCD3 is exhibited. These cells are heterogeneous in respect of CD4 and CD8 expression (2:1 ratio).

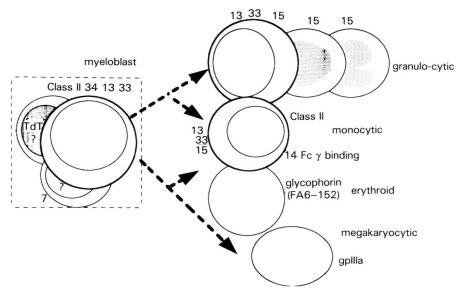

Fig. 6.5 Myeloid development. Myeloblasts express class II antigens, a stem cell-associated CD34 antigen and myeloid/monocytic markers CD13 and CD33. On myeloid/granulocyte cells additional CD15 antigens are expressed; CD14 signifies monocytic differentiation. Monoblasts/monocytes may show strong non-specific binding of IgG to their avid Fcγ receptor; this can be blocked by preincubation with rabbit serum. Glycophorin C and Fa6–152 are McAbs to erythroid precursors: anti-GpIIIa is a megakaryocytic marker. In AML frequently only subsets of blast cells are positive with any given marker. An intriguing finding is that 20% of AML cases are also TdT + or CD7 + and occasionally express both (see Fig. 6.4). The normal counterparts of these blasts are not known (?).

0.1% of B-cell precursors are TdT +, cμ + (see Fig. 6.3),[55] but is a sizeable one in the thymus where 30–40% of cells are TdT +, β + cortical thymocytes (see Fig. 6.4). These cells' features correspond to those of the pre-B-ALL (TdT +, cμ +) and a subgroup of T-ALL with β-chain expression (see below and the literature[55]). These cases of ALL with a residual capacity for differentiation also express an array of unusual features and asynchronous patterns of development (see below). Finally, it is clear from Figures 6.3 and 6.4 that during the successfully completed normal B or T differentiation, TdT synthesis is switched off in an organized manner before the last molecules of the antigen receptor, the light chains κ or λ of Ig and the α-chain of TCR, appear. The fully assembled functional antigen-specific receptor is inserted into the membrane. The mCD22 +, SmIg + B-cell and mCD3 +, βα + T-cells are virgin mature lymphocytes. These cells are rarely represented among acute leukemias.

The emphasis on the fidelity of early differentiation signs may, at first glance, be at variance with the apparently 'promiscuous' patterns of gene rearrangements in common-ALL and T-ALL.[59–64] Nevertheless, as the blast cells are 'arrested' at an early developmental stage characterized by a high TdT and recombinase activity, the rearrangments of illegitimate genes are not surprising. In contrast, the transcriptional and translational events appear to be partially controlled even in leukemia where the irrevocable decision to commit the malignant population towards the T or B direction is signified by the presence of *either* cCD3 or cCD22.

The twin concept of *fidelity* for exhibiting early signs of differentiation, and an accompanied *maturation block* seems to be valid not only for ALL but also for AML. The

184 THE LEUKEMIC CELL

interpretation of phenotypic features in AML is, however, more difficult. The population structure of normal immature hemopoietic precursors, based on phenotypic features, is less well understood than those of the B- and T-lineages (Fig. 6.5) for two reasons:

1. There is no single specific positive marker for hemopoietic 'immaturity' such as TdT for lymphoid immaturity. The marker which comes closest to this criterion, CD34, is expressed on subgroups of both AML and B-pre-ALL (but curiously not in T-ALL)[39,40]
2. The hemopoietic precursors include a whole array of related cell types with their variable differentiation commitments. This is reflected in the fact that even the best markers such as CD13 and CD33 are likely to pick up only part of the relevant precursor cell populations, and only parts of the leukemic pool. In spite of this, the correspondence between the normal precursor development and the leukemia groups is obvious,[33] and well demonstrated in the reciprocal expression of class II, and signs of granulocytic or erythroid differentiation such as CD15 or glycophorin both in normal cells and in many cases of leukemias.

The intriguing unexplained question is the presence of TdT or CD7, and occasionally both, in 15–20% of myeloid malignancies which also express CD13 and CD33 without signs of Ig or TCR β-gene rearrangements.[59–61] These features are compatible with very early precursor cells, and some of these cells may indeed be uncommitted (Fig. 6.6). It is relevant that the corresponding cases of AML are the most primitive forms that have been tentatively placed into the M0 and M1 categories[61] The authors believe that among these normal

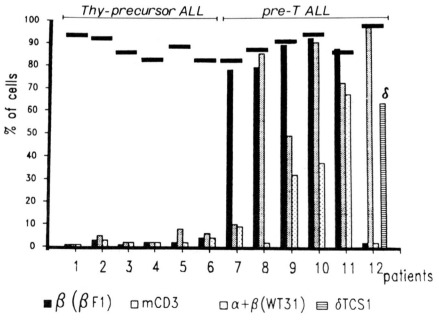

Fig. 6.6 Heterogeneity and asynchronous expression of TCR-associated antigens in T-ALL. In 12 cases of T-ALL the large (>80%) proportion of TdT+, CD7+, cCD3+ blast cells are shown by horizontal bars. The cytoplasmic staining for TCR β-chain (■) reveals heterogeneity. Cases 1–6 are TCRβ− when tested with βF1 McAb whilst cases 7–11 are TCRβ+ and case 12 has TCRδ. Cases 8–12 express mCD3 (▨) with a proportion of blasts also WT31+ (TCRβα; ▨). CD1+ blasts were seen in cases 8–10 and 12. CD4+ blasts were detected in cases 9,10 and 12, and CD8+ blasts were present in cases 8–11. (Reproduced from Janossy et al,[49] with permission of the publishers).

precursors and malignancies the representatives and aberrant variants of pluripotential stem cells 'hide'. Finally, 3.8% of acute leukemias can be regarded as undifferentiated because they lack not only cCD3, cCD22, CD19 and Ig- and TCR gene rearrangements, but also myeloid markers such as CD13 and CD33 (see Table 6.3).

METHOD 4

DETECTION OF ABERRANT LEUKEMIC FEATURES

Principle
The principle here is not a new technical venture: the necessary methods have been covered in Methods 1–3. The concept has also been documented years ago; microscopic observations of malignant cells have clearly shown asynchronous morphological maturation of the nucleus and the cytoplasm. 'Modern' markers (i.e. differentiation antigens defined by McAbs) are merely convenient tools used in order to freshly document this old concept at a molecular level.[62] The concept is not in conflict with the principle of lineage fidelity because it has been demonstrated in Method 3 that fidelity is observed with selected differentiation antigens that signify early lineage commitments, while it will be demonstrated below that asynchrony is more frequently observed with another set of differentiation antigens which appear at somewhat later stages of normal development.

Observations and comment
Twelve cases of T-ALL were investigated for the expression of TCR-associated molecules and CD antigens. All cases were TdT +, CD7 + and cCD3 + but there has been a marked heterogeneity in terms of cytoplasmic TCRβ expression: cases 1–6 were TCRβ −, cases 7–11 were TCRβ + and case 12 had TCRδ rather than TCRβ. The important observation is that in the TCRβ + and δ + group TdT + blast cells frequently expressed mCD3 as well as membrane TCRβ + α (see Fig. 6.6). Furthermore, more cases expressed CD1, CD4 and CD8 antigens in the TCRβ + group than in the TCRβ − T-ALL; the patterns of CD1, CD4 and CD8 expression were different from those of normal thymocytes shown in Figure 6.4. These findings indicate that there are two groups of T-ALL, and these are tentatively referred to as 'T-precursor-ALL' with virtually no evidence of differentiating capacity, and 'pre-T-ALL' exhibiting a limited asynchronous differentiation (see Fig. 6.6).

A similar phenomenon can be observed among B-lineage ALL, where the majority of cases show no additional differentiation beyond the expression of cCD22, CD10 and CD19 antigens. Some cases, however, express mCD22 (Table 6.4) and/or exhibit cμ in various combinations. The latter group is referred to as pre-B-ALL.[63] The degree of maturity represented by the CD10 − variant 'null'-ALL is controversial. On the one hand, the configuration of the mRNA transcripts of the IgH DJ region would suggest immaturity,[64] and on the other, the relatively low occurrence of 'aberrant' TCR rearrangements[65] would be in agreement with a more mature, B-cell-committed normal counterpart.

Interpretation
Asynchrony, defined as an unusual combination of reactivity with McAbs, is a feature seen in a subgroup of ALL, and the pattern is different from case to case. Examples of such asynchrony are represented by the expression of markers of maturity such as mCD22 on TdT + B-lineage ALL blasts. Furthermore, normal TdT +, cμ pre-B-cells are also extremely rare in the normal bone marrow (<0.1%),[11] and for that reason the phenotype of pre-B-ALL is also operationally leukemia associated. In parallel, some TdT + T-ALLs express mCD3 and even membrane TCRβ.[55,66] In addition, the normal TdT +, cCD3 +

Table 6.4 Acute lymphoblastic leukemia samples expressing combinations of antigens absent or extremely rare in normal bone marrow

	No. of cases studied	No. of cases with features absent in bone marrow	Combination of positivity not seen in normal bone marrow
Common- and 'null'-ALL	70	7[a]	CD13+, CD33+, TdT+
		4[a]	mCD22+, TdT+
		3[a]	RFB7+, TdT+
		3[a]	CD2+, TdT+
		1	CD10+, CD19−, TdT+
Pre-B-ALL	15	14[b]	cμ+, TdT− (4/15 were CD13+, cμ+)
B-ALL	4	1[a]	sIg+, TdT+
T-ALL	18	18[a]	CD7+, cCD3+, TdT+
Total	107	51 (47.8%)	

a = In these cases it is possible to identify 10^{-4} leukemic blasts.
b = In these cases it is possible to identify 10^{-3} leukemic blasts.

thymic cells do not leave this central lymphoid organ at their early stages of development unless they are leukemic. Thus TdT+, cCD3+ cells are totally absent in normal bone marrow, peripheral lymphoid tissues and blood ($<10^{-4}$). This combination again detects leukemia.

In the microplate assay described above two independent reliable markers are used to identify each line of differentiation. For the B-lineage these are cCD22 and CD19. For T-ALL, cCD3 and CD7 plus CD2 are used. For myeloid precursors CD13 and CD33 are applied. If a single marker fails, this sign becomes a useful 'sign of aberration' because the rest of the panel still secures a safe diagnosis. Haphazard deviations from the norm are invariably picked up by these multiple assays: these are either 'failures' such as the absence of cCD22 or CD19 in common-ALL, or 'additions' that would normally appear on other cell types, e.g. the display of CD13 and CD33 (myeloid) antigens in common-ALL.

In a recent study of 107 cases of ALL, sensitive double immunofluorescence assays were found to distinguish leukemic blasts from normal cells in 51 cases (47.8% of cases; see Table 6.4). These assays can be utilized to monitor patients during therapy and to identify early relapse from the same odd clone of malignant cells. Finally, these assays should be utilized as control tests for the standardization of gene probes, such as polymerase chain reactions. These methods have a great potential in terms of increased sensitivity but can also introduce artefacts and should therefore be adequately controlled by immunological technics which are capable of identifying 10^{-4} leukemic cells.[67,68]

METHOD 5

IMMUNOLOGICAL STAINING WITH COLLOIDAL GOLD

Principle
Conjugating separate antibodies with different sized colloidal gold particles allows multiple antigens to be detected during immunoelectron microscopy. On the light microscope the immunogold (IG) particles of 30–40 nm are visualized by silver enhancement. On the microscope they can be seen using epi-illumination and polarized light.[69] This labeling is not affected by other dyes so that the cells can be stained with May–Grünwald-Giemsa. This

combination of immunology and conventional hematology[69] gives optimal morphology that is superior to phase contrast used with immunofluorescence or to immunohistochemical technics such as immunoperoxidase or APAAP. One advantage of this method is that it can be combined with FITC and TRITC or PE.[70] A multiplicity of questions can be answered with this technology; van Dongen et al[71] inquired whether rare TdT+ cells of CD7+, class-II+ phenotype are present in normal bone marrow. A modification of this method is described.

Materials

1. Microscope (Nikon, Zeiss or Leitz) with epifluorescence attachment, containing a polarization filter combination (polarizer, beam-splitter and analyser,[69] as well as a FITC non-selective filter set for the simultaneous viewing of FITC and TRITC (see Method 2).
2. 63 × objective, NA = 1.4, Planapo without Phase.
3. Rabbit anti-TdT and second layer-FITC as in Method 3; anti-HLA-DR directly labeled with TRITC (Seralab, Cat. No. RMAS206p).
4. CD7 McAb and the second layer goat anti-mouse-Ig-IG (conjugated with G40 gold particles, Cat. No. 818040; Janssen Pharmaceutica, Beerse, Belgium).
5. Normal mouse serum in 1:10 dilution (NMS).

Triple-labeling method

1. Take normal or regenerating bone marrow and incubate at 20°C for 10–15 min with pre-titrated amounts of CD7 antibody, wash three times and incubate with G40–IG for another 10 min; wash twice.
2. Incubate cells with NMS, wash once and incubate with pre-titrated anti-HLA-DR-TRITC for 10 min. Wash three times and prepare cytospins.
3. Label nuclear TdT with FITC as described in Method 3.
4. Count CD7+, TdT− cells (peripheral T-cells); these are mostly HLA-DR−.

Investigate the proportion of CD7+ and CD7− cells within the TdT+/HLA-DR+ cells (pre-B precursors).

Comments and interpretation

With this method a minor population of TdT+, HLA-DR+, CD7+ cells was demonstrated (1–5% of TdT+ cells) mainly in bone marrow samples taken from patients during maintenance chemotherapy for non-T-ALL.[71] These cells are almost certainly cCD3−[29] and their physiological role is unknown. It has been suggested that these cells might be prothymocytes or a close relative to undifferentiated precursors (see Fig. 6.5); their phenotype corresponds to some of the 'undifferentiated' leukemias described in the footnotes to Table 6.3.

This sensitive method has been recently applied to investigate a third parameter — the proliferative capacity of acute leukemias — and the results were compared with that of the normal counterparts.[36,72] The parameters measured are the DNA synthetic activity detected by uptake of bromodeoxyuridine (BrdU) and anti-BrdU McAb,[73] or the visualization of cells that entered the proliferative cell cycle by labeling for a nuclear antigen detected by the McAb Ki67.[74] Three important observations were made. First, it was demonstrated that the DNA synthetic activity and Ki67 positivity in the normal B-cell precursor cells of the bone marrow is higher than that seen in common-ALL and pre-B-ALL. Secondly, the DNA synthetic activity of large thymic blast cells in the thymus is also higher than in T-ALL. Thirdly, the normal cells stop their DNA synthetic activity and return to the G_0 phase as soon as they exhibit their antigen-specific receptors on the membrane. Their proliferative activity is subsequently reinitiated after an antigen stimulation.[75] These observations confirm previous studies on AML and myeloid precursors[76] and support the hypothesis[58] which states that the essential defect in acute leukemias is not their proliferation advantage but their inability to differentiate into mature non-dividing (resting) populations.

Similarly, combination of labeling for immunological markers and probes for RNA and DNA using in situ hybridization are being developed.[31] These additional parameters might require triple labeling methods and the efforts of careful standardization as well as the evaluation of results with triple colour flow cytometry[3] and image analysers will be rewarded by the wealth of information gained by analysing, at single cell level, rare precursor cell populations.

METHOD 6

ANALYSIS OF NUCLEAR TDT BY FLOW CYTOMETRY

Principle

In the last decade the precision and simplicity of operating the flow cytometers has greatly increased. The most recent analysers such as the FACScan and the EPICS PROFILE routinely perform double labeling analysis with FITC and phycoerythrin (PE).[3] The two most novel developments are (1) the successful efforts to reproducibly detect intracellular antigens such as nuclear TdT[77] and c-myc protein[78] in leukemias and (2) the addition of the third immunofluorescent colour, DuoCHROME (DC) to the arsenal of triple immunofluorescent analyses with a single laser system. These two new developments, together with the help of the quantitative documentation of the asynchronous expression of normal antigens in leukemia, contribute to the definition of malignancy-associated phenotypes in individual patients. The specificity and sensitivity of TdT staining by flow cytometry is shown below.

Materials

1. FACScan (Becton Dickinson, Mountain View, California, USA).
2. Monoclonal anti-human TdT antibody (cocktail referred to as H-TdT; Cat. No. 5100, Supertech Inc. Bethesda, MD, USA).
3. Goat anti-mouse Ig-FITC, e.g. from Southern Biotechnology Associates (Birmingham, AL, USA, Cat. No. 1030-02).
4. Medium for immunofluorescence assay (IFA medium) containing 10 mmol/l HEPES buffer pH 7.4, 150 mmol/l NaCl and 4% heat inactivated newborn calf serum.
5. Buffered formalin–acetone fixative[77] referred to as BFA (pH 6.8) containing 0.2 mg $Na_2HPO_4/2$ ml H_2O, 1 mg KH_2PO_4/ml, 9.25% (vol/vol) formaldehyde (all from BDH, Poole, UK), 45% (vol/vol) acetone and 45.75% distilled water. Alternatively, 1% paraformaldehyde fixative in PBS is used[78] containing 10 parts EM grade formalin (methanol free), 10 parts 10 × PBS and 80 parts water.
6. 1% Triton X-100 (Sigma, UK) in IFA medium.
7. Falcon 2052 polystyrene tubes with round bottom (Becton Dickinson).

Method

1. Mononuclear cells (10^6 cells in 50 µl) are washed twice in PBS or IFA medium in Falcon tubes. Six tubes are prepared containing common-ALL blasts (tubes A and B), B-CLL cells (tubes C and D) and normal peripheral lymphocytes from blood or from tonsil (tubes E and F).

2. The two alternative procedures for the fixation and permeabilization of cells are as follows:
   (a) cells are spun and the supernatant is decanted; the pellet is rapidly resuspended in 25–50 µl BFA by vigorous tapping; after 2 seconds the tube is filled with chilled PBSAA and the cells are washed twice;[77]
   (b) cells are gently agitated in 2 ml 1% paraformaldehyde for 15 minutes at 4°C; after spinning and decanting the fixative the cells are permeabilized in 2 ml 0.1% Triton for 3 min at 4°C and then spun;[78] the supernatant is discarded; during such permeabilization the cells shrink and centrifugation at 460 × g for 10 min will be required to pellet.
3. The fixed cells are resuspended in 50 µl PBSAA and H-TdT is added to tubes A, C and E, whilst 1% normal mouse serum is added to tubes B, D and F. The optimal H-TdT concentration has to be titrated: it is in the range of 5–10 ng/50 µl.
4. After incubation for 30–60 min at 4°C with occasional agitation, the cells are washed twice in PBSAA (after having used fixation (a)) or in 0.1% Triton (after fixation (b)).
5. The second layer reagent is added to all tubes and incubated for 30–60 min at 4°C and step (4) is repeated. The cells are resuspended in PBSAA and analysed on the FACScan (Fig. 6.7).

Comments and interpretation

The positive TdT staining in the case of common-ALL shown (95% in A — Fig. 6.7) corresponds to the proportion of blast cells in this peripheral blood sample (5% residual normal cells). However, the signal in both the CLL (C in Fig. 6.7) and normal blood or tonsil (not shown) following the incubation with the H-TdT is low (<0.1%) and similar to the values of the negative controls (B and D in Fig. 6.7). Mixing experiments adding known

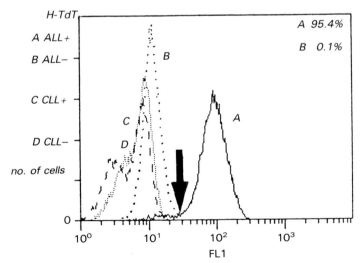

Fig. 6.7 Staining of nuclear TdT in suspension for flow cytometry with monoclonal anti-TdT. H-TdT antibodies were obtained from Supertech Inc. TdT + common-ALL blasts (95% positives; A and B) and TdT − B-CLL cells (<0.1% in C and D) were labeled with TdT (A and C) or incubated with 1% normal mouse serum (B and D). The discrimination between the positive and negative results is excellent (see large arrow) and the observations agree with the findings seen in cytocentrifuge preparations on the microscope. The cells in tonsil are also negative (<0.1% positivity) but normal bone marrow and thymus contain, as expected, TdT + cells in the range of 1–5% and 50–70%, respectively (not shown). In artificial mixtures of known TdT + and TdT − cells, this method detects more than 0.2% positive cells.

numbers of TdT + leukemic blasts in varying proportions to normal mononuclear cells, obtained from blood or tonsil tissues, have also been performed. The sensitivity of the flow cytometric method for TdT detection has been confirmed: the malignant TdT + population becomes detectable at the level of less than 0.5% (D. Campana and E. Coustan-Smith, unpublished observations). In the normal bone marrow and thymus 1–5% and 50–72% TdT + cells are detected, respectively, corresponding to the findings of intranuclear staining observed in the cytocentrifuge preparations of the same samples.

METHOD 7

TRIPLE IMMUNOFLUORESCENCE USING FLOW CYTOMETRY

Principle
Here the attention is focused on Figure 6.5 again where it has been emphasized that some cases of AML express CD13, class II and CD7 antigen simultaneously (see box and legend to Fig. 6.5). The triple marker analysis of such cases can be documented with flow cytometry as a clear example of leukemic cells expressing normal differentiation antigens in an asynchronous manner.

Materials

1. FACScan (Becton Dickinson, Mountain View, California, USA).
2. PBSA.
3. Falcon 2052 tubes as in Method 6.
4. CD13 antibody of IgG1 class (e.g. WM15) with goat anti-mouse IgG1–FITC (subclass specific from SBA, Cat. No. 1070-02) for labeling myeloid-associated antigen.
5. Anti-HLA-DR antibody of IgM class (e.g. RFDR2) with goat anti-mouse IgM–PE (class specific from SBA, Cat. No. 2020-09) for detecting class II antigen.
6. Biotinated CD7 antibody of IgG_{2a} class (e.g. RFT2) with streptavidin DuoCHROME (Becton Dickinson, Cat. No. 9026) in order to document CD7, a T-cell-associated marker also present on some immature cells.[79]

Method

1. Mononuclear cells (10^6) in 50 µl PBSA are distributed into Falcon tubes. Tubes A and B contain normal bone marrow cells, tubes C and D contain AML blasts (>80%) with a leukemia-associated phenotype. Additional tubes can be prepared containing bone marrow and AML cells admixed in various proportions (e.g. bone marrow cells with 50%, 10%, 1%, 0.1%, 0.01% blasts). Two tubes should be ready for each mixture.
2. Add CD13, anti-HLA-DR and CD7–biotin McAbs to tubes A, C and to one of the two tubes containing the different mixtures. Add 1% mouse serum into the remaining tubes. Incubate at 20°C for 10 minutes.
3. Wash twice in PBSA.
4. Add the second layer reagents and incubate at 20°C for 10 minutes.
5. Wash twice in PBSA and read the results in the FACScan (Fig. 6.8). It is essential that an accurate compensation setting is adjusted on the flow cytometer (see manufacturer's instructions).

Comments and interpretations
After staining the cells can be fixed in 2–4% formaldehyde or 1% paraformaldehyde and stored at 4°C for days. The evaluation of triple colour investigations is most frequently

MONOCLONAL ANTIBODIES IN THE DIAGNOSIS OF ACUTE LEUKEMIA   191

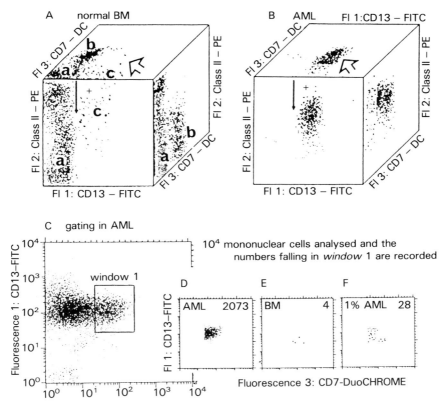

Fig. 6.8 Five parameter analysis of normal bone marrow (BM: A) and AML (B) on the FACScan. Two parameters, the 90° scatter and the forward angle scatter, are used for gating on lymphoid and blast cell populations and to exclude cells with granular cytoplasm (e.g. maturing myeloid cells; not shown). The remaining three fluorescence channels are CD13 (fluorescence 1: FITC), class II (fluorescence 2: PE) and CD7 (fluorescence 3: DC). In the normal bone marrow (A) triple labeled cells are virtually absent but in this particular AML sample (B) 20–30% of myeloblasts carry all three markers (see large arrows in A and B). In the normal bone marrow the unlabeled cells are mostly erythroid ('a'), and T-lymphocytes ('b') and myeloblasts ('c') are also present; populations 'a' and 'b' are rare in the AML sample. In the next phase of the analysis live gates are drawn around the cells with aberrant phenotypes (CD13+, CD7+ window 1 in C). These parameters are stored for each patient analysed at presentation. Large proportions of AML cases show aberrant asynchrony not seen in the normal bone marrow but these are different for each case.[82] When the original AML (D), normal bone marrow (E) and mixtures of AML and normal bone marrow (F: 1% AML) are studied by counting a constant number of cells (e.g. 10^4) then the recorded events within window 1 are 2073, 4 and 28, respectively, indicating that leukemic cells are detected at 1% level above the normal values seen for this reagent combination.

carried out with the Paint-a-Gate program which uses various colours to depict the different populations.[80] The illustrative analysis is shown here in black and white (Fig. 6.8) which is less informative than the Paint-a-Gate program but still adequately demonstrates several populations. In this study, with the help of the forward angle and 90° scatters (not shown), the lymphoid and blast cell populations were selected for analysis and cells with high granularity, e.g. maturing myeloid cells, were excluded from the study. Among the positively gated population in the normal bone marrow (Fig. 6.8A) the unlabeled cells ('a') mostly correspond to erythroid forms while the CD7+, class II−, CD13− cells are T-lymphocytes ('b'). In the normal bone marrow CD13+, class II+ myeloblasts ('c') are also seen. The important point for comparisons in leukemia is however, that triple labeled cells are virtually absent (see empty areas marked with large arrow).

The same setting has been used to analyse AML (Fig. 6.8B). The erythroid and T-lymphoid cells are absent and 70% CD13+, class II+ cells can be seen: these are phenotypically similar to myeloblasts. However, 27% of cells are triple labeled unique cells (large arrows). Other investigators[81,82] also emphasized that large proportions of AML cases show substantial deviations from normal myeloblasts when investigated with triple marker technology. It will be feasible to establish the peculiar 'leukemia-associated' asynchronous features of many patients at the presentation of the leukemia, and these parameters can be stored in the powerful microcomputers. When bone marrow samples of the same patients are analysed after chemotherapy in hematological remission, the absence or presence of cells with the 'leukemia-associated' phenotypes should give clinically relevant information about the probable absence of disease or the emergence of a relapse.

REFERENCES

1 Catovsky D (ed) 1981 The leukemic cell. Churchill Livingstone, Edinburgh
2 Beverley P C L (ed) 1986 Methods in hematology: monoclonal antibodies. Churchill Livingstone, Edinburgh
3 Loken M R 1986 Cell surface antigen and morphological characterization of leukocyte populations by flow cytometry. In: Beverley P C L (ed) Methods in hematology: monoclonal antibodies. Churchill Livingstone, Edinburgh, pp. 132-144
4 Greaves M F, Brown G, Rapson N T, Lister T A 1975 Antiserum to acute lymphoblastic leukaemia cells. Clinical Immunology and Immunopathology 4: 67-77
5 Preud'homme J L, Seligmann M 1972 Surface bound immunoglobulins as a cell marker in human lymphoproliferative diseases. Blood 40: 777-785
6 Catovsky D, Frisch B, Van Noorden S 1975 B, T and null cell leukaemias. Electron microscopy and surface morphology. Blood Cells 1: 115-117
7 Schlossman S F, Chess L, Humphreys R E, Strominger J L 1976 Distribution of Ia-like molecules on the surface of normal and leukemic human cells. Proceedings of the National Academy of Sciences of the USA 73: 288-1296
8 Bollum F J 1975 Antibody to terminal deoxynucleotidyl transferase. Proceedings of the National Academy of Sciences of the USA 72: 4119-4122
9 Catovsky D, Pittman S, O'Brien M et al 1979 Multiparameter studies in lymphoid leukemias. American Journal of Clinical Pathology 72: 736
10 Janossy G 1981 Membrane markers in leukemia. In: Catovsky D (ed) Methods in haematology: the leukemic cell. Churchill Livingstone, Edinburgh, pp. 129-183
11 Janossy G, Bollum F, Bradstock K F, Ashley J 1980 Cellular phenotypes of normal and leukemic haemopoietic cells determined by analysis with selected antibody combinations. Blood 56: 430-441
12 Janossy G, Thomas J A, Bollum F J et al 1980 The human thymic microenvironment: and immunohistologic study. Journal of Immunology 125: 202-212
13 Bradstock K F, Janossy G, Pizzolo G et al 1980 Subpopulations of normal and leukemic human thymocytes: an analysis using monoclonal antibodies. Journal of the National Career Institute 65: 33-41
14 Greaves M F, Rao J, Hariri G et al 1981 Phenotypic heterogeneity and cellular origins of T-cell malignancies. Leukemia Research 5: 281-299
15 Bofill M, Janossy G, Janossa M et al 1985 Human B cell development. II. Subpopulations in the human fetus. Journal of Immunology 134: 1530-1537
16 Caligaris-Cappio F, Janossy G 1985 Surface markers in chronic lymphoid leukemias of B cell type. Seminars in Hematology 22: 1-12
17 Bernard A, Boumsell L, Dausset J, Milstein C, Schlossman S F (eds) 1984 Leucocyte Typing I. Springer Verlag, Berlin
18 Reinherz E L, Haynes B F, Nadler L M, Bernstein I D (eds) 1986 Leukocyte Typing II. Springer Verlag, New York
19 McMichael A (ed) 1987 Leucocyte typing III. Oxford University Press, Oxford
19a Knapp W (ed) 1989 Leucocyte typing IV. Oxford University Press, Oxford
20 Campana D, Janossy G 1986 Leukaemia diagnosis and testing of complement fixing antibodies for bone marrow purging in ALL. Blood 68: 1264-1271

21 Harden E A, Haynes B F 1985 Phenotypic and functional characterization of human malignant T-cells. Seminars in Hematology 22: 13–26
22 Chan L C, Pegram S M, Greaves M F 1985 Contributation of immunophenotype to the classification and differential diagnosis of acute leukaemia. Lancet 1: 475–479
23 Campana D, Janossy G, Bofill M et al 1985 Human B cell development. I. Phenotypic differences of B lymphocytes in the bone marrow and peripheral lymphoid tissue. Journal of Immunology 134: 1524–1529
24 Dorken B, Moldenhauer G, Pezzutto A, Schwartz R, Feller A, Kiesel S et al 1986 HD39 (B3), a B lineage restricted antigen whose cell surface expression is limited to resting and activated human B lymphocytes. Journal of Immunology 136: 4470–4478
25 Link M P, Stewart S J, Warnke R A, Levy R 1985 Discordance between surface and cytoplasmic expression of Leu 4 (T3) antigen in thymocytes and in blast cells from childhood T lymphoblastic malignancies. Journal of Clinical Investigation 76: 248–255
26 Furley A J, Mizutani S, Weilbaecher K et al 1986 Developmentally regulated rearrangement and expression of genes encoding the T cell receptor-T3 complex. Cell 46: 75–87
27 Campana D, Thompson J S, Amlot P, Brown S, Janossy G 1987 The cytoplasmic expression of CD3 antigens in normal and malignant cells of the T lymphoid lineage. Journal of Immunology 138: 648–655
28 Hurwitz C A, Loken M R, Graham M L et al 1988 Asynchronous antigen expression in B lineage acute lymphoblastic leukemia. Blood 72: 299–307
29 Greaves M F, Chan L C, Furley A J W, Watt S M, Molgaard H V 1986 Lineage promiscuity in hemopoietic differentiation and leukemia. Blood 67: 1–11
30 Campana D, Janossy G 1988 Proliferation of normal and malignant human immature lymphoid cells. Blood 71: 1201–1210
31 Brahic M, Haase A T, Cash E 1984 Simultaneous in situ detection of viral RNA and antigens. Proceedings of the National Academy of Sciences of the USA 81: 5445–5448
32 Vodinelich L, Tax W, Yan B, Pegram S, Capel P, Greaves M F 1982 A monoclonal antibody WT1 for detecting leukemias of T cell precursors. Blood 60: 742–752
33 Drexler H G, Sagawa K, Menon M, Minowada J 1986 Reactivity pattern of myeloid monoclonal antibodies with emphasis on MCS-2. Leukemia Research 10: 17–23
34 Linch D C, Allen C, Beverley P C L, Bynoe A G, Scott C S, Hogg N 1984 Monoclonal antibodies differentiating between monocytic and non-monocytic variants of AML. Blood 63: 566–573
35 Nadler L M, Anderson K C, Marti G et al 1983 B4, a human B lymphocyte-associated antigen expressed on normal, mitogen-activated, and malignant B lymphocytes. Journal of Immunology 131: 244–250
36 Campos L, Guyotat D, Gentilhomme O, Treille D, Fiere D, Germain D 1987 Expression of CD19 on ANLL cells. In: McMichael A J et al (eds) Leucocyte typing III. Oxford University Press, Oxford, pp 470–473
37 Greaves M F, Hariri G, Newman R A, Sutherland D R, Ritter M A, Ritz J 1983 Selective expression of the common acute lymphoblastic leukemic (gp100) antigen on immature lymphoid cells and their malignant counterparts. Blood 61: 628–638
38 Stashenko P, Nadler L M, Hardy R, Schlossman S F 1980 Characterization of a human B-lymphocyte specific antigen. Journal of Immunology 125: 1678–1685
39 Tindle R W, Nichols R A B, Chan L, Campana D, Catovsky D, Birnie G D 1985 A novel monoclonal antibody BI-3C5 recognizes myeloblasts and non-B non-T lymphoblasts in acute leukaemias and CGL blast crisis, and reacts with immature cells in normal bone marrow. Leukemia Research 9: 1–9
40 Civin C I, Strauss L C, Brovall C, Feckler M J, Schwartz J F, Shaper J H 1984 Antigenic analysis of hematopoiesis. III. A hematopoietic progenitor cell surface antigen defined by a monoclonal antibody raised against KG-1a cells. Journal of Immunology 133: 1–10
41 Guesdon J L, Ternyuck T, Avrameas S 1979 The use of avidin-biotin interaction in immunoenzymatic techniques. Journal of Histochemistry and Cytochemistry 27: 1131–1139
42 Simmonds R G, Smith W, Marsden H 1982 3-Phenylazo-4-hydroxyphenylisothiocyanate: versatile reagent for the efficient haptenation of Ig and other carrier molecules. Journal of Immunological Methods 54: 23–30
43 Galton D A G, MacLennan I C M 1982 Clinical patterns in B lymphoid malignancy. In: Clinics in haematology 11, WB Saunders, London
44 Moir D J, Gosh A K, Abdulaziz Z, Knight P M, Mason D Y 1983 Immunoenzymatic staining of haematological samples with monoclonal antibodies. British Journal of Haematology 55: 395–405
45 Bast E J E G, Van Camp B, Boom S E, Jaspers F C A, Ballieux R E 1981 Differentiation between benign and malignant monoclonal gammopathy by the presence of the J chain. Clinical and Experimental Immunology 44: 375–382

46 Caligaris-Cappio F, Bergui L, Tesio L et al 1985 Identification of malignant plasma cell precursors in the bone marrow of multiple myeloma. Journal of Clinical Investigation 76: 1243-1251
47 Van Dongen J J M, Krissansen G W, Wolvers-Tettero I L M et al 1988 Cytoplasmic expression of the CD3 antigen as a diagnostic marker for immature T-cell malignancies. Blood 71: 603-612
48 Barr R D, Koekebakker M, Mahony P 1984 Demonstration of TdT in single cells by indirect immunofluorescence. II. An examination of specificity. Leukemia Research 8: 429-434
49 Janossy G, Coustan-Smith E, Campana D 1989 The reliability of cytoplasmic CD3 and CD22 antigen expression in the immunodiagnosis of acute leukaemia — a study of 500 cases. Leukemia (in press) 3: 170-181
50 Mason D Y, Stein H, Gerdes J et al 1987 Value of monoclonal anti-CD22 (p. 135) antibodies for the detection of normal and neoplastic B lymphoid cells. Blood 69: 836-840
51 Chen Z, Sigaux F, Miglierina R, Valensi F, Daniel M, Ochoa-Noguera M, Flandrin G 1986 Immunological typing of acute lymphoblastic leukaemia: concurrent analysis by flow cytofluorometry and immunocytology. Leukemia Research 10: 1411-1417
52 Brenner M B, Trowbridge I S, Strominger J L 1985 Cross linking of human T cell receptor proteins: association between the T cell idiotype subunit and the T3 glycoprotein heavy subunit. Cell 40: 183-196
53 O'Flynn K, Beverley P C L, Linch D C 1985 The influence of anti-T cell monoclonal antibodies on calcium mobilization. Springer Verlag, New York, pp. 205-212
54 Pezzutto A, Dorken B, Moldenhauer G, Clark E A 1987 Amplification of human B cell activation by a McAb to the B cell specific antigen CD22, BP 130/140. Journal of Immunology 138: 98-103
55 Janossy G, Campana D 1989 Ontogeny of the human T cell receptors — single cell studies. In: Kendall M D, Ritter M (eds) Thymus update. Vol. II, T lymphocyte differentiation in human thymus Harwood Academic Publishers, London, pp. 39-58
56 Campana D, Janossy G, Coustan-Smith E, Tian W T, Ip S, Wong L, Amlot P L 1988 The expression of T cell receptor-associated proteins during T cell ontogeny in man. Journal of Immunology 142: 57-66
57 Desiderio S V, Yancopoulos G D, Paskind M et al 1984 Insertions of N regions into heavy chains genes is correlated with expression of terminal deoxytransferase in B cells. Nature 311: 752-755
58 Greaves M F 1986 Differentiation-linked leukemogenesis in lymphocytes. Science 234: 697-704
59 Tawa A, Hozumi N, Minden M, Mak T W, Gelfrand E W 1985 Rearrangement of the T cell receptor beta chain gene in non-T cell, non-B cell acute lymphoblastic leukemia of childhood. New England Journal of Medicine 313: 1033-1037
60 Sangster R N, Minowada J, Sucio-Fuca N, Minden M, Mak T W 1986 Rearrangement and expression of the α, β and δ chain T cell genes in human thymic leukemia cells and functional T cells. Journal of Experimental Medicine 163: 1491-1508
61 Cheng G Y, Minden M D, Toyonaga B, Mak T W, McCulloch E A 1986 T cell receptor and immunoglobulin gene rearrangements in acute myeloblastic leukemia. Journal of Experimental Medicine 163: 414-424
62 Greenberg J M, Quertermous T, Seidman J G, Kersey J H 1986 Human T cell γ chain gene rearrangements in acute lymphoid and non-lymphoid leukemia: comparison with the T cell receptor β chain gene. Journal of Immunology 137: 2043-2049
63 Vogler L B, Crist W M, Bockman D E 1978 Pre-B leukemia: a new phenotype of childhood lymphoblastic leukemia. New England Journal of Medicine 298: 872-877
64 Mizutani S, Ford A M, Wiedemann et al 1986 Rearrangement of immunoglobulin heavy chain genes in human T leukaemic cells shows preferential utilization of the D segment (DQ52) nearest to the J region. EMBO Journal 5: 3467-3473
65 Goorha R, Bunin N, Mirro J et al 1987 Provocative pattern of rearrangements of the genes for the γ and β chains of the T-cell receptor in human leukemias. Proceedings of the National Academy of Sciences of the USA 84: 4547-4551
66 Spits H, Borst J, Tax W, Capel P J A, Terhorst C, Devries J E 1985 Characterization of a monoclonal antibody (WT31) that recognizes a common epitope on the human T-cell receptor for antigen. Journal of Immunology 135: 1922-1935
67 Van Dongen J J M, Hooijkaas H, Hahlen K et al 1984 Detection of minimal residual disease in TdT positive T-cell malignancies by double immunofluorescence staining. In: Lowenberg P, Hagenbeck J (eds) Minimal residual disease in acute leukaemia. Martinus Amsterdam, Nijhoff, pp. 67-76

68 De Mey J, Hacker G W, De Waele M, Springall D R 1986 Gold probes in light microscopy. In: Van Noorden S, Polak J (eds) Immunocytochemistry, 2nd edn, Wright, Bristol, pp. 71–88
69 Janossy G, Campana D, Burnett A et al 1988 Autologous bone marrow transplantation in acute lymphoblastic leukemia — preclinical studies. Leukemia 2: 485–495
70 Van Dongen J J M, Hooijkaas H, Comans-Bitter W M, Benne K, Van Os T M, De Jong J D J 1985 Triple immunological staining with colloidal gold, fluorescein and rhodamine as labels. Journal of Immunological Methods 80: 1–10
71 Van Dongen J J M, Hooijkaas H, Comans-Bitter M et al 1985 Human bone marrow cells positive for terminal deoxynucleotidyl transferase, HLA-DR, and a T-cell marker may represent prothymocytes. Journal of Immunology 135: 3144–3150
72 Campana D, Coustan-Smith E, Janossy G 1987 Double and triple staining methods for studying the proliferative activity of human B and T lymphoid cells. Journal of Immunological Methods 107: 79–80
73 Gratzner H G 1982 Monoclonal antibody to 5-bromo- and 5-iododeoxyuridine: a new reagent for detection of DNA replication. Science 218: 474–475
74 Gerdes J, Lemke H, Baisch H, Wacker H H, Schwab U, Stein H 1984 Cell cycle analysis of a cell proliferation-associated human nuclear antigen defined by the monoclonal antibody Ki-67. Journal of Immunology 133: 1710–1715
75 Nossal G J V 1987 Immunology: the basic components of the immune system. New England Journal of Medicine 316: 1320–1325
76 Gavosto F, Pileri A, Bachi C, Pegoraro L 1964 Proliferation and maturation defect in acute leukaemia cells. Nature 203: 92–97
77 Slaper-Cortenbach I C M, Admiraal L G, Kerr J M, van Leeuwen E F, von dem Borne A E G, Tetteroo P A T 1988 Flow cytometric detection of terminal transferase and other intracellular antigens in combination with membrane antigens in acute lymphatic leukemias. Blood 72: 1639–1646
78 Kastan M B, Slamon D J, Civin C I 1988 Proto-oncogene c-myb is expressed in normal human hematopoietic progenitor cells. Experimental Hematology 16: 507
79 Haynes B F, Martin M E, Kay H H, Kurtzberg J 1988 Early events in human T-cell ontogeny. Phenotypic characterization and immunohistologic localization of T-cell precursors in early human fetal tissues. Journal of Experimental Medicine 168: 1061–1074
80 Loken M R, Shah V O, Hollander Z, Civin C I 1988 Flow cytometric analysis of normal B lymphoid development. Pathology Immunopathology Research 7: 357–379
81 Terstappen L W M, Loken M R 1988 Five dimensional flow cytometry as a new approach for blood and bone marrow differentials. Cytometry 9: 548–556
82 Loken M R, Shah V O, Terstappen L W M 1989 Multicolor analysis of myeloid antigens of normal human bone marrow. Leucocyte Typing 4: 859–862

7
Immunocytochemical Labeling of Leukemia Samples with Monoclonal Antibodies by the APAAP Procedure

David Y. Mason   Wendy N. Erber

INTRODUCTION

When antibodies against white cell-associated antigens were first used for immunophenotyping leukemia samples, these studies were performed by immunological laboratories as a direct extension of their research activities. Since immunofluorescent labeling of cells in suspension is the most widely used technic for immunological characterization of cell populations, this procedure was the obvious one to adopt in these early studies of hematological neoplasms.

Although immunofluorescent technics are widely used and reliable, they suffer from several practical disadvantages from the viewpoint of the diagnostic hematologist. For one thing, immunofluoresence is often not routinely practised in hematology laboratories and setting up the procedure may require the purchase of new equipment and the acquisition of new technical skills. Secondly, the requirement to work with living cells often represents a major inconvenience for the routine laboratory (being better suited to the research laboratory where experiments can be planned in advance). Finally, the results have to be assessed by fluorescence microscopy or flow cytometry, so that the hematologist is deprived of the ability to correlate morphological detail with antigen expression.

DEVELOPMENT OF CELL SMEAR LABELING TECHNICS

For the above reasons, there has been interest in several laboratories in developing technics which will allow anti-white cell antibodies to be used for cell phenotyping by a procedure which is convenient and informative for the hematologist, while offering the same degree of sensitivity and specificity as conventional immunofluorescence.

The first step in this direction dates back to the mid-1970s and followed from an earlier study by one of the authors in which the immunoperoxidase staining reactions of blood smears using antibodies against cytoplasmic constituents were explored.[1] One of the antibodies evaluated at this time, a polyclonal rabbit antibody against IgM, was found to stain, in addition to intracytoplasmic IgM in plasma cells, a small number of lymphoid cells in smears of peripheral blood cells.[2] The reaction was quite different in its appearance from the staining of intracellular immunoglobulin seen in plasma cells, being strongest around the cell periphery and often having a villous pattern (Fig. 7.1). This suggested that the antibody might be detecting IgM present on the surface membrane of B-lymphocytes, but this interpretation conflicted with the generally held belief that surface antigens could only be detected on cells stained in the living state. Cell smears, it was thought, were suitable for staining cytoplasmic antigens but inappropriate (because of antigenic denaturation during cell smearing and drying) for the detection of surface antigens.

Further investigation showed, however, that the ring-like labeling of these cells did indeed represent surface immunoglobulin staining, since capping (i.e. redistribution of surface IgM

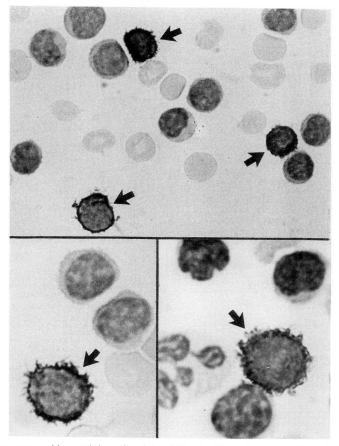

Fig. 7.1 Immunoperoxidase staining of peripheral blood white cell smears with polyclonal anti-IgM. Strongly stained lymphoid cells (arrowed) showing a ring-like pattern of labeling, with villous projections on many cells. These studies, performed in the mid-1970s, gave an early hint that white cell membrane antigens could be detected in air-dried cell smears.[2]

by incubating cells in suspension with anti-IgM) abolished this staining pattern.[2] Since the morphology of the cells in these preparations was as well preserved as in routinely processed blood smears, the exciting possibility was offered of being able to label cell surface markers and at the same time to visualize the morphology of individual cells.

Subsequently this approach was extended to the study of neoplastic lymphoid cells (Fig. 7.2) and it was shown that IgM of κ or λ type could be detected on neoplastic B-cells by staining them in cell smears.[3] However, it was not possible to take this approach any further owing to the very restricted number of antisera against human white cell surface antigens that had been produced at that time and the limited availability of these reagents. Monoclonal antibodies (McAbs) changed this position radically when they first began to appear in the late 1970s and offered the dual advantage of minimizing problems due to contaminating antibodies of unwanted specificity, and of being more widely available.

The author's initial attempts to stain surface antigens on smeared cells with McAbs were reported in 1979, the antibodies used being two of the earliest monoclonal anti-human antibodies to be reported, i.e. W6/32 (anti-HLA class I) and NA1/34 (anti-CD1).[4,5] These

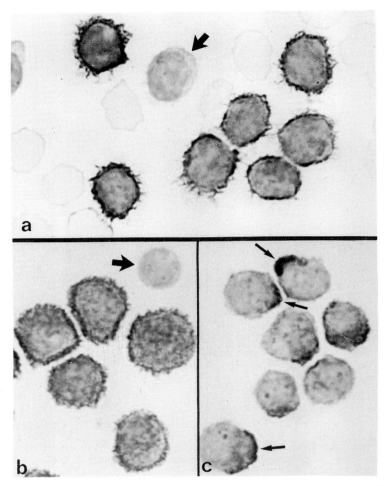

Fig. 7.2 The demonstration of smeared surface IgM on normal human white cells (see Fig. 7.1) was followed by similar studies on neoplastic B-cells. (a) Surface IgM is seen on smeared prolymphocytic leukemia cells. An unstained normal cell is arrowed. (b) A film of hairy cell leukemia cells stained for κ light chains showing their characteristic feathery surface appearance. An unstained normal lymphocyte is arrowed. (c) Pre-incubation of the cells from this patient with anti-κ antibody prior to smearing and staining dramatically modified the staining pattern: with the formation of polarized caps (arrowed). This proved that much of the staining seen in (b) represented surface membrane immunoglobulin. (Reproduced, with permission, from Mason et al.[3])

studies showed that each of these antigens survived cell smearing, and gave an indication of the potentially broad application of the procedure in the future. However, it was also evident that use of an immunoperoxidase technic left much to be desired for the diagnostic hematologist since many cells in blood and marrow smears (e.g. myeloid cells, red cells, etc.) contain endogenous peroxidase activity which can obscure specific staining. The development at that time of a procedure (the alkaline phosphatase–anti-alkaline phosphatase or APAAP technic) for staining antigens, using alkaline phosphatase rather than peroxidase as antibody label, was thus an important advance because the endogenous enzyme present in white cells can easily be inhibited (by adding the selective inhibitor levamisole to the substrate) without causing any antigenic denaturation.[6]

It may be noted in passing that the problem of endogenous enzymes is not an absolute obstacle to the staining of hematological samples. The substrate conditions for horseradish peroxidase differ from those which are optimal for molecules such as myeloperoxidase or hemoglobin, and the fixatives usually employed when immunostaining cell smears are also not optimal for endogenous peroxidase activity. For these reasons, endogenous peroxidase does not always interfere seriously with interpretation of antigen labeling in cell smears, and this is reflected by the number of laboratories which have used immunoperoxidase methods successfully for staining antigens in hematological films.[7-14] However, in the authors' experience, alkaline phosphatase is a clearly preferable label, as much because of the greater visibility of the reaction product as because of the avoidance of endogenous enzyme activity. Li and his colleagues, whose laboratory has made extensive use of immunoenzymatic cell smear labeling technics, compared six different staining procedures, and concluded that the specificity of immunoperoxidase methods 'is low because of inadequate inhibition of endogenous peroxidase'.[15] They therefore now favoured immunoalkaline phosphatase procedures for staining cells in films, and noted that of the three major methods based on this enzyme label 'APAAP gave the best results'.

Having established that human leukocyte antigens could be demonstrated by immunoenzymatic labeling of cell smears, the next step was to see how many McAbs were suitable for use by this technic, and to assess whether it was suitable for typing leukemic samples and whether it gave satisfactory results on the type of specimens most frequently evaluated by the hematologist (i.e. routine blood and bone marrow films, often several days old). In a study by Moir et al[16] it was shown that at least 16 different antigens, (including T- and B-cell markers and CD10(CALLA), could be stained in cell smears, and also that the procedure could be used to distinguish between common and T-cell acute lymphoblastic leukemia. In two subsequent papers from the authors' laboratory, it was shown that routine blood and bone marrow smears can also be stained in this way, and the fact that the smeared cells lie in a film of dried serum proteins does not interfere with the detection of cell surface antigens.[17,18] The second of these papers further lengthened the list of antigens that could be demonstrated in cell smears, and was based on the study of a total of more than 250 cases of hematological neoplasia.[18]

Similar studies were reported from a number of other laboratories and these are summarized, together with work from the authors' laboratory, in Table 7.1. One of the earliest was a technic reported by Bross et al[19] which continues to be used by that author and his colleagues.[23] This method differs from the cell smear technic described in the present chapter in that it involves allowing separated mononuclear cells to adhere to polylysine-coated slides, the cells then being fixed in glutaraldehyde. Although it gives good antigen preservation, the cell preparation technic is clearly less convenient than simply using routine blood and marrow films, and the morphological appearance of the cells, which are not smeared but fixed in the adherent state, is very different from that seen in routine blood and marrow preparations.

Papers from other laboratories, of which the first was a publication by Fishleder et al in 1984,[9] have confirmed the value of phenotyping cell smears, and at least two studies have compared the results with those obtained by flow cytometry, finding a good correlation.[8,9] A variety of labeling technics have been used in these studies (e.g. APAAP, ABC:peroxidase, indirect immunoalkaline phosphatase) as detailed in Table 7.1.

It may be noted in passing that immunoenzymatic staining of cell smears is of diagnostic value, not only for the hematologist, but also in the field of cytology. In the authors' laboratory a number of such studies were carried out by Dr Anna Ghosh in collaboration with Dr Arthur Spriggs, in which APAAP staining was performed on routinely processed

Table 7.1 Immunoenzymatic staining of surface membrane antigens in cell smear and cytocentrifuge preparations

Author (year)	Ref.	Fixative(s)	Technic(s)	Antibodies	Samples stained	Comments
Mason et al (1977)	2	Buffered formol acetone	PAP	Polyclonal anti-Ig	White cell smears	Surface IgM on normal B-cells demonstrated
Bross et al (1978)	19	None	PAP	Human anti-HLA sera	Mononuclear cells adherent to polylysine-coated slides	Technic proposed as an alternative to lymphocytotoxicity testing
Mason et al (1980)	3	Buffered formol acetone	PAP	Polyclonal anti-Ig	White cell smears	Technic used to detect surface Ig in B-cell lymphoproliferative disorders
Moir et al (1983)	16	Buffered formol acetone	APAAP	16 McAbs	Blood and marrow cytospins	Double labeling performed by combining APAAP technic with rosetting or immunoperoxidase
Erber et al (1984)	17	Buffered formol acetone	APAAP	5 McAbs	Blood films	Technic used to detect T- and B-cell populations
Fishleder et al (1984)	9	Acetone	ABC:peroxidase	4 McAbs	Cytospins of marrow	Good correlation with flow cytometry
Huang et al (1984)	20	Buffered formol acetone	Indirect immunoalkaline phosphatase	Monoclonal anti-platelet gp IIb/IIIa	Blood and marrow films	Technic used in the diagnosis of acute megakaryoblastic leukemia
Hui and Joyce (1984)	10	Buffered formol acetone	Indirect immunoperoxidase	5 McAbs	Cytospins of blood or marrow	
Hui and Lawton (1984)	11	Buffered formol acetone	Indirect immunoperoxidase	Monoclonal anti-CD2 and anti-CD20	Cytospins of blood	
Koike (1984)	21	Buffered formol acetone	Indirect immunoalkaline phosphatase	Monoclonal anti-platelet gp IIb/IIIa	Blood films or cytospins	Technic used in the diagnosis of megakaryoblastic leukemia

Table 7.1 Immunoenzymatic staining of surface membrane antigens in cell smear and cytocentrifuge preparations (*Continued*)

Author (year)	Ref.	Fixative(s)	Technic(s)	Antibodies	Samples stained	Comments
Li et al (1984)	22	Buffered formol acetone (other fixatives evaluated)	Indirect immunoalkaline phosphatase	14 McAbs	Blood and marrow films	Immunostaining combined with peroxidase and esterase cytochemistry
Sandhaus et al (1984)	14	Acetone	ABC:peroxidase	5 McAbs	Blood and marrow films	
Frickhofen et al (1985)	23	Glutaraldehyde	ABC:peroxidase or PAP plus ABC:alkaline phosphatase	10 McAbs	Mononuclear cells adherent to polylysine-coated smears	Double immunoenzymatic labeling performed
Bodewalt et al (1986)	7	Not stated	Indirect immunoperoxidase or immunoalkaline phosphatase	10 McAbs	Blood and marrow films and cytospins	Technic used to phenotype 40 cases of AML
Chen et al (1986)	8	Buffered formol acetone (methanol formalin for CALLA)	ABC:peroxidase	18 McAbs	Cytospin of blood and marrow cells	Good correlation with flow cytometry results
Erber et al (1986)	18	Buffered formol acetone or acetone methanol + formalin	APAAP	28 McAbs polyclonal anti-TdT and myeloperoxidase	Blood and marrow films and cytospins	Technic used to analyse 259 cases of hematological neoplasia
Koller et al (1986)	12	Buffered formol acetone or glutaraldehyde	Indirect immunoperoxidase	13 McAbs	Blood and marrow films and cytospins	New technic for endogenous peroxidase inhibition described
Markey et al (1986)	13	Baker's formol calcium	Indirect immunoperoxidase	Monoclonal anti-CD4 and anti-CD8	Mononuclear cell cytospins	Technic used to determine CD4/CD8 ratios in 54 cases of CLL
Neumann et al (1986)	24	Acetone or formalin/acetone	APAAP	9 McAbs	Blood and marrow films and cytospins	Technic used to phenotype 15 Ph positive blastic leukemias
Chen et al (1987)	25	Acetone	APAAP and indirect immunoperoxidase	10 McAbs 2 polyclonal antisera	Blood mononuclear cell cytospins	Optimization of two-colour double-staining technic described

Table 7.1 Immunoenzymatic staining of surface membrane antigens in cell smear and cytocentrifuge preparations (*Continued*)

Author (year)	Ref.	Fixative(s)	Technic(s)	Antibodies	Samples stained	Comments
Davey et al (1987)	26	Acetone/methanol/formalin	APAAP	7 McAbs polyclonal antilactoferrin	Blood and marrow films and cytospins	Technic used to phenotype 29 cases of AML
Erber et al (1987)	27	Acetone/methanol/formalin	APAAP	14 McAbs polyclonal anti-TdT	Bone marrow and blood films and cytospins	Technic used to phenotype cases of megakaryoblastic leukemia
Erber et al (1987)	28	Acetone/methanol/formalin	APAAP	2 anti-platelet glycoprotein McAbs	Blood films	Technic used in 67 cases of myelodysplasia to detect circulating micromegakaryocytes
Erber and Mason (1987)	29	Variety of fixatives evaluated	APAAP	Polyclonal and monoclonal anti-TdT	Blood and marrow films and cytospins	Terminal transferase expression analysed in leukemic cells
Hanson et al (1987)	30	Formalin:acetone	APAAP	23 McAbs	Blood and marrow films	Technic used to phenotype 58 cases of acute leukemia
Choate et al (1988)	31	Not specified	Indirect immunoalkaline phosphatase	Monoclonal anti-platelet gp Ib and IIb/IIIa; polyclonal anti-factor VIII	Blood films	Technic used to diagnose megakaryoblastic leukemia
Erber and Mason (1988)	32	Acetone:methanol	APAAP	2 anti-CD25 (Tac) McAbs	Blood and marrow films and cytospins	Interleukin-2 receptor (CD25/Tac) expression in hematological neoplasia analysed

ABC = avidin biotin technic.
APAAP = alkaline phosphatase:anti-alkaline phosphatase technic.
McAbs = monoclonal antibodies.
PAP = peroxidase–anti-peroxidase technic.
TdT = terminal deoxynucleotidyl transferase.

smears from serous effusions (in which there are often many necrotic cells and debris). It was possible not only to demonstrate intracytoplasmic markers of potential value for the demonstration of metastatic malignant cells (e.g. cytokeratin), but also surface markers on lymphoid cells.[33-35] This was of particular value given the unsuitability of many routine cytological specimens for analysis by conventional surface immunofluorescence. Subsequently, a number of other papers have pointed out the value of labeling cell smears from cytological samples by immunoenzymatic technics.[15,36-38]

The experience gained in investigating cytological samples for carcinoma cells proved applicable to detection of these cells in marrow smears, and it was shown that this approach can be of diagnostic value in cases of suspected metastatic marrow infiltration.[39]

PRACTICAL ADVANTAGES OF APAAP LABELING

Before describing practical aspects of the APAAP procedure for staining cell smears, its advantages over conventional technics may be described in more detail. These are as follows:

1. Compatibility with light microscopy.
2. Visualization of intracellular antigens.
3. Storage of slides prior to staining.
4. Permanence of APAAP stained preparations.
5. Detection of rare cells.
6. Suitability for small samples.

Compatability with light microscopy

Cells stained by the APAAP technic retain much of their morphological detail, with the consequence that fine distinctions, based upon simultaneous visualization of antigen expression and cytological features, can be made. This is useful when morphologically abnormal cells in a blood or bone marrow film differ only subtly from normal cells, particularly so if they are present in relatively low numbers. In the latter situation, it is often difficult to identify the abnormal cells in a preparation stained by surface immunofluorescence, and immunological typing results, which are quoted simply as percentages of nucleated cells labeled by different antibodies may be difficult to interpret. In contrast, it is usually possible to identify the abnormal cells in APAAP-stained films and thus to assess whether or not they carry any individual antigen.

It may be added that there is something of a trade-off between morphology and antigen preservation. Leukocyte antigens differ in their susceptibility to denaturation by fixation (one of the most susceptible being CD10(CALLA) and it may sometimes be advisable to use a fixative which does not preserve cell morphology optimally, but which retains antigen activity. In these circumstances subtle morphological detail may not be as readily appreciated. A variety of different fixatives may be used (as detailed in the Technical Appendix) but generally speaking the 'softest' fixative (i.e. the one which is best for antigen preservation and worst for morphological preservation) is pure acetone, whilst the 'hardest' fixatives are mixtures containing formalin, since these give excellent morphological detail but may also reduce the reactivity of some antigens.

Visualization of intracellular antigens

Since cells are air dried and fixed before the APAAP technic is performed, not only can surface membrane antigens be visualized, but also molecules within the cells. Examples of intracellular antigens of interest in neoplastic white cells are terminal transferase and immunoglobulin. More recently, as more information has been gathered concerning the sequence of expression of antigens during T- and B-cell maturation, it has become evident that there are at least two molecules in these lineages which are expressed as surface antigens in the mature cell, but which are found only in the cytoplasm at earlier maturation stages. One of these antigens CD3 (T3) appears as an intracytoplasmic constituent in immature (cortical) thymocytes, and then subsequently emerges on the cell surface at about the time that the cells acquire the phenotype of medullary thymocytes. The practical significance is that T-cell acute lymphoblastic leukemia (T-ALL) is usually unreactive with anti-CD3 antibodies when tested in cell suspension, but positive in the majority of cases when tested in cell smears (or tissue sections) by a technic such as the APAAP procedure.[40] The other antigen which behaves in a similar fashion is CD22, a pan-B marker which is first expressed as a cytoplasmic constituent early in B-cell maturation (at the pre-B-cell stage).[41,42] With the consequence that many cases of common- and pre-B-cell ALL are positive when tested by the APAAP technic, but negative by surface immunofluorescence for CD22. This phenomenon of intracellular expression preceding cell surface expression is also seen in the case of Ig μ heavy chains.

Storage of slides prior to staining

Antigens in cell smears prepared from hematological samples are stable on storage, offering the advantage for the diagnostic laboratory that slides can be stored for a period of time until staining is performed. The authors' experience, and that of other laboratories, is that antigens are undiminished in their reactivity if slides have been stored unfixed at room temperature for at least a week. Storage for longer periods (i.e. for one or more years), without loss of antigenic reactivity, is easily achieved by keeping slides at $-20°C$.

This aspect of the technic not only facilitates the study of samples which arrive at inconvenient times, but also means that cell smears known to contain cells positive for a particular antibody, e.g. leukemia blasts which express CD10 (CALLA), can be stored and a single slide stained as a positive control each time the antibody is used. The stability of the antigens in air-dried films also enables the slides to be sent by post to another laboratory for APAAP staining.

Permanence of APAAP-stained preparations

Once stained and mounted, the APAAP reaction product does not fade, with the consequence that slides can be reviewed if required on numerous occasions and several observers can examine the same slide. This is particularly useful both for demonstrating the technic and also when there is difficulty over the interpretation of a staining reaction.

Detection of rare cells

As noted above, cells labeled by the APAAP reaction product stand out particularly clearly against the background of unstained cells. In consequence it is usually possible to identify antigen-positive cells which are only present at low frequency (e.g. a few dozen cells in a flm containing more than a million cells). This level of detection is possible because of the absence of non-specific reactivity in optimally stained APAAP preparations, and is difficult to achieve, because of background noise, by flow cytometry. Slides can be rapidly scanned at low magnification to look for rare cells, something which is usually not possible when using immunofluorescent technics.

This aspect of the APAAP procedure has proved useful in the authors' hands when staining smears of bone marrow or serous effusion samples in which only very rare carcinoma cells are present,[34,39] and also for detecting circulating micromegakaryocytes.[28] The latter cells can be found, by staining for platelet glycoprotein IIIa, in some cases of acute myeloid leukemia and myelodysplasia, but their numbers are often low, so that staining of buffy coat smears by the APAAP procedure offers an optimal approach to their detection. Recently

Wang and Zipursky have provided further confirmation of the ability of immunoalkaline phosphatase labeling to pick out infrequent cells in a report on the detection of maternal red cells in the fetal circulation, which gave an estimated sensitivity of one positive cell per 50 000 (i.e. 0.002%).[43]

Suitability for small samples

APAAP staining of films and cytocentrifuge preparations is economical in terms of the number of cells needed, making it the method of choice when only small samples are available. Practical instances in which this aspect may be of value include heel prick samples and CSF samples.[44]

APPLICATIONS OF THE APAAP TECHNIC

ACUTE LEUKEMIA

The staining reactions by the APAAP procedure characteristic of acute leukemia are summarized in Table 7.2 and illustrated in Plates 25-32. Confirmation of a diagnosis of ALL is usually readily made by this means and T-ALL easily distinguished from common or pre-B-ALL. There are a number of McAbs which react with cases of acute myeloid leukemia (AML), as summarized in Table 7.2. These include both surface molecules and also those which are expressed within the cell cytoplasm (myeloperoxidase and elastase).[26,45]

Interest has focused in a number of laboratories on the possibility of correlating immunological phenotype with the French–American–British (FAB) subdivision of AML. Such studies have been performed both by cell surface labeling and by the APAAP procedure. The consensus view at present appears to be that, although there is some tendency for antigenic profiles to correlate with the different subcategories of the FAB classification, the association is not sufficiently close that FAB classification could be performed by immunophenotype alone. However, an exception is acute megakaryoblastic leukemia, which was added in 1985 to the FAB classification of AML, as M7.[46] This type of acute leukemia can be readily detected using McAbs against platelet glycoproteins.[20,21,27,31] Furthermore, the authors have found that an antibody (Y1/82A) which shows a high degree of specificity in normal tissues for macrophages and monocytes, will react preferentially with leukemias showing monocytic differentiation (AML types M4 and M5).[47,48] It may thus be worth including an antibody of this sort in a panel to confirm an impression that a leukemia shows monocytic features.[7]

Terminal transferase is readily demonstrated in leukemic cells by the APAAP technic. The only anti-TdT antibody that has been found in the past to give specific labeling for this molecule is the polyclonal affinity purified rabbit antibody produced by Dr F. Bollum. A modification of the APAAP technic was, therefore, employed by the authors in which monoclonal mouse anti-rabbit Ig was used as a second stage reagent (see Technical Appendix). Since this technic is a multistage procedure, it may be expected to be of relatively high sensitivity, and this may account for the fact that the authors have found a higher percentage of AML expressing this molecule than is usually quoted in the literature.[29] However, it is of interest that previously published reports of TdT expression in AML have shown a wide variation from laboratory to laboratory, and also a clear absence in many series of an obvious cut-off between positive and negative cases (e.g. the number of 'positive' cases depends on the investigators' arbitrary choice of threshold values). Biochemical analysis of TdT + AML cases reveals a continuum from values below the detection threshold up to levels, in a few cases, equal to those seen in lymphoblastic leukemia,[29] further suggesting that the percentage of cases classified as TdT + is influenced by the sensitivity of the detection system. From a diagnostic point of view, the important point is therefore that the absence of

Table 7.2 Pattern of antigen expression seen in acute leukemia samples stained by the APAAP technic

	B-cell-associated antigens				T-cell-associated antigens					Myeloid-associated antigens			Miscellaneous		
	CyIgM	CD10 (CALLA)	CD19 (B4)	CD22	CD1 (T6)	CD2 (T11)	CD3 (T3)	CD5 (T1)	CD7	p150,95 (CD11c)	Myelo-PX/ elastase	Macrophage antigens	HLA-DR	TdT	Platelet gp IIIa
'Common' lymphoblastic	-/+	+	+/-	+/-	-	-	-	-	-	-	-	-	+	+	-
T-cell lymphoblastic	-	-/+	-	-	-/+	+/-	+/-	+/-	+	-	-	-	-	+	-
Myeloblastic	-	-	-	-	-	-/+	-	-	-/+	+/-	+	-	+/-	-/+	-
Myelomono-monocytic	-	-	-	-	-	-	-	-	-	+	+/-	+	+	-/+	-
Megakaryo-blastic	-	-	-	-	-	-/+	-	-	-	-/+	-	-	+	-/+	+

+ = all cases positive with no, or only occasional, exceptions.
- = all cases negative with no, or only occasional, exceptions.
+/- = majority of cases positive.
-/+ = majority of cases negative.
CyIgM = intracytoplasmic μ heavy chain.
Myelo-PX = myeloperoxidase.

TdT is significant, since it makes a diagnosis of lymphoblastic leukemia very unlikely, whereas the presence of TdT is much less informative and does not exclude a diagnosis of AML.

CHRONIC LEUKEMIAS (Plates 27, 28, 31)

The APAAP technic provides a convenient means of distinguishing between chronic lymphocytic leukemia of T- and B-cell type. It may also be of value on occasion for the investigation of patients in whom the differential diagnosis lies between early chronic lymphocytic leukemia and a reactive (polyclonal) lymphocytosis. Table 7.3 summarizes the reaction patterns seen in these two situations.

Hairy cell leukemia also has a characteristic reaction pattern when stained by the APAAP technic.[49] Of particular value is the fact that these cells consistently express high levels of the p150,95 antigen (CD11c), a two-chain molecule belonging to the LFA/MAC1 'family' of antigens. Expression of this antigen at high level, together with strong expression of B-cell antigens (e.g. CD19, CD22), is diagnostic of hairy cell leukemia, and may on occasion be of practical value (e.g. in patients in whom circulating hairy cells are only present in low numbers). (Plate 31.)

MULTIPLE MYELOMA

Although this disease is usually easy to diagnose by conventional clinical and cytological criteria, cases are occasionally encountered in which the nature of the neoplastic cells is not certain. In these circumstances APAAP labeling can provide valuable diagnostic information, since myeloma cells have a very characteristic pattern of antigen expression (as illustrated in Plate 32).

Non-hemopoietic neoplasms

As noted previously, the APAAP technic may, on occasion, be of value for the detection of metastatic carcinoma cells in bone marrow aspirates when they are only present in low numbers.[36] McAbs directed against cytokeratin, epithelial membrane antigen (although this may also be seen on some plasma cells) and carcinoembryonic antigen are of value for this purpose. Occasionally bone marrow samples are encountered showing heavy infiltration with non-hemopoietic malignant cells which are morphologically difficult to distinguish from leukemic cells. APAAP staining can resolve problems of this sort since classic hemopoietic

Table 7.3 Comparison between the immunocytochemical staining reactions of chronic lymphocytic leukemia and reactive lymphocytosis

	Anti-HLA-DR	Anti-B-cell	Anti-T-cell (CD2 or 3)	Anti-T-cell subsets (CD4 and CD8)
B-CLL	Positive	Positive	Negative	Negative
T-CLL	Negative	Negative	Positive	Positive for one or other antigen
Reactive lymphocytosis	Positive	Negative	Positive	Positive for both antigens–often CD8 exceeding CD4

The reactions refer to the abnormal cell population. A minority of cells showing the opposite reaction will always be present, e.g. normal T-lymphocytes in B-CLL, etc.

markers (and also leukocyte common antigen) will be absent, but other tissue markers may be detectable. The dramatic appearance of a rhabdomyosarcoma identified in this way using monoclonal anti-desmin has been illustrated by Ghosh et al.[39]

CONCLUSION

From this review of the APAAP procedure for staining cell smears, it should be evident that it has much to offer the diagnostic hematologist (and the clinical cytologist) as an alternative to more traditional means of detecting cellular antigens. If it has a disadvantage, it is that the technic requires some degree of experience (e.g. in ensuring that reagents are applied to the appropriate area of the slide, and that they do not dry during incubation) and that it takes several hours to complete. However, when compared to surface immunofluorescence procedures, there is probably little difference in terms of operator-skill and time required. Furthermore, in the last few years a semi-automated procedure for performing the APAAP procedure has been in routine use in the authors' laboratory[50] and this innovation has substantially reduced the manual work entailed in the technic, and also ensured a high degree of consistency in terms of staining quality. It is hoped that wider use will be made of such semi-automated procedures in the future, thereby further increasing the attractiveness of the APAAP procedure for the routine laboratory.

TECHNICAL APPENDIX

PRINCIPLE OF TECHNIC

The APAAP immunoalkaline phosphatase labeling comprises a three layer sequence of reagents (Fig. 7.3). The primary monoclonal antibody which recognizes the cellular antigen is in turn recognized by anti-mouse Ig in the second incubation stage. Use of the latter antibody in excess ensures that only one antigen binding site is occupied, leaving the other site free to bind the immune complexes of alkaline phosphatase and monoclonal anti-alkaline phosphatase (APAAP complexes) which constitute the third stage in the 'sandwich'.

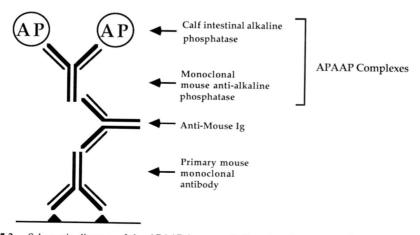

Fig. 7.3 Schematic diagram of the APAAP immunoalkaline phosphatase procedure.

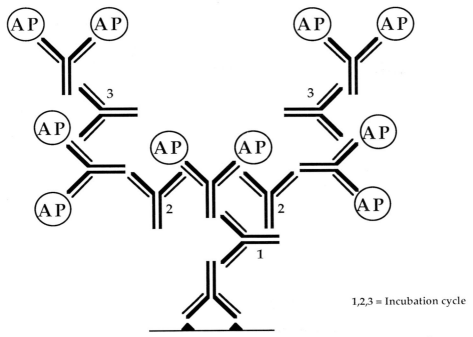

Fig. 7.4 Diagramatic representation of how the intensity of labeling by the APAAP procedure may be enhanced by repeating the second and third incubation stages (anti-mouse Ig and APAAP complexes) one or more times.

Repetition of the 'bridging' anti-mouse Ig and the APAAP stage produces considerable enhancement in the amount of alkaline phosphatase bound, and hence an increase in the intensity of the final reaction. The consequence of these additional incubations is shown schematically in Fig. 7.4. The alkaline phosphatase enzyme reaction is developed using an azo-dye cytochemical substrate in which Fast Red is the diazonium salt. This yields a vivid red reaction product, which contrasts well with hematoxylin counterstaining and is easily seen under the light microscope. Although the APAAP technic is most widely used for detecting antigens recognized by monoclonal antibodies, it can also be used, by a simple modification, in conjunction with rabbit antisera (e.g. antibody to terminal transferase). This is shown schematically in Fig. 7.5.

SAMPLES

Preparation of cell smears

Air-dried smears of blood or bone marrow are prepared by conventional methods on routine microscope slides. They should be dried at room temperature for a least 1 hour before staining. However, drying for up to 48 hours at room temperature will give equally good antigenic preservation and usually offers better morphological results. Cytocentrifuged cell preparations should be handled in the same way as blood and bone marrow smears. If staining for surface immunoglobulin, cells should be washed before cytocentrifugation to remove serum immunoglobulin.

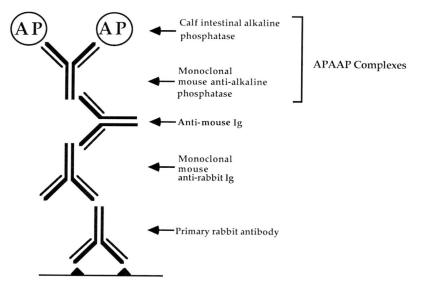

Fig. 7.5 Schematic representation of how the monoclonal APAAP technic may be performed when the primary antibody is of rabbit origin (e.g. anti-terminal transferase).

Storage

If smears are to be stored for longer than a week before staining, they should be wrapped in aluminium foil and kept at −20°C. Cellular antigens are preserved without detectable loss under these conditions for long periods (i.e. at least one year). The foil wrapping should be removed only after the slides have been out of the freezer for a few minutes (and have hence warmed to room temperature), because otherwise condensation will form on the slides and give poor morphological results.

REAGENTS

Antibodies

Suitable monoclonal antibodies for APAAP staining of hematological samples are now obtainable from numerous sources, and the great majority will be found suitable for use in this procedure. Rabbit anti-mouse immunoglobulin, APAAP immune complexes and monoclonal anti-rabbit Ig are all obtainable from Dakopatts.

Buffers

Tris-buffered saline (TBS)
Prepare a stock solution of 0.5 mol/l Tris-HCl pH 7.6. Prepare the working buffer by diluting the stock solution 1/10 in 0.15 mol/l isotonic saline.

Substrate buffer
Prepare a stock solution of 0.01 mol/l Tris pH 8.2.

Fixatives

A variety of fixatives is suitable for fixing cell smears prior to APAAP staining. The acetone:methanol mixture is recommended for general use. If optimal preservation of cell morphology is important, formaldehyde may be added to give a final concentration of 2% (i.e. one part in 20 of a 40% solution).

Acetone:methanol	Acetone	1 part
	Methanol	1 part

Substrate

Naphthol AS-MX phosphate (Sigma Catalogue no. N4875)	2 mg
Dimethylformamide	0.2 ml
Tris buffer 0.1 M, pH 8.2	9.8 ml
Levamisole (1M)	10 µl
Fast Red TR salt (Sigma Catalogue no. F1500)	10 mg

Prepare this solution by dissolving the naphthol AS-MX phosphate in dimethylformamide in a glass tube. Dilute to 10 ml with Tris buffer pH 8.2 and add the levamisole (to block endogenous alkaline phosphatase activity). This solution can be stored if necessary at 4°C for several weeks (and for longer at $-20°C$). Immediately before applying the substrate (i.e. at the completion of the APAAP sandwich–see below) dissolve the Fast Red salt in the substrate solution and filter directly onto the slides.

METHOD

Fixation

1. Fix smears in acetone:methanol or acetone:methanol:formalin for 90 s. When staining cells for common-ALL antigen (CD10) fixation in acetone (10 min) alone will usually give better results. Fixation for terminal transferase detection should be for 15 min at 4°C in methanol.
2. Transfer directly to TBS. (Do not allow the slides to dry at any stage after fixation.)
3. Leave for 1–5 min.

Staining

After fixation and washing, take slides from TBS and remove excess buffer.

1. Add primary monoclonal antibody and incubate in a moist chamber for 30 min at room temperature (RT).
2. Wash for 1–2 min in TBS.
3. Add anti-mouse immunoglobulin (at 1/25 dilution) and incubate in a moist chamber for 30 min at RT.
4. Wash for 1–2 min in TBS.
5. Add APAAP complex (1/25 dilution) and incubate in a moist chamber for 30 min at RT.
6. Wash for 1–2 min in TBS.

The intensity of final staining can be greatly enhanced at this point by repeating steps 3–6 inclusive. When carrying out this repeat cycle the incubation time for steps 3 and 5 should be reduced to 10 min.

7. Add alkaline phosphatase substrate (see above) and incubate for 15–20 min at RT.
8. Wash in TBS and then tap water. Counterstain with hematoxylin and mount in a suitable aqueous mounting medium (e.g. Apathy's medium).

REFERENCES

1. Mason D Y, Farrell C, Taylor C R 1975 The detection of intracellular antigens in human leucocytes by immunoperoxidase staining. British Journal of Hematology 31: 361–370
2. Mason D Y, Labaume S, Preud'homme J-L 1977 The detection of membrane and cytoplasmic immunoglobulins in human leucocytes by immunoperoxidase staining. Clinical and Experimental Immunology 29: 413–421
3. Mason D Y, Leonard R C F, Laurent G, Gourdin M-F 1980 Immunoperoxidase staining of surface and intracellular immunoglobulin in human neoplastic lymphoid cells. Journal of Clinical Pathology 33: 609–616
4. Brown G, Biberfeld P, Christensson B, Mason D Y 1979 The distribution of HLA on human lymphoid, bone marrow and peripheral blood cells. European Journal of Immunology 9: 272–275
5. McMichael A J, Pilch J R, Galfré G, Mason D Y, Fabre J W, Milstein C 1979 A human thymocyte antigen defined by a hybrid myeloma monoclonal antibody. European Journal of Immunology 9: 205–210
6. Cordell J L, Falini B, Erber W N et al 1984 Immunoenzymatic labelling of monoclonal antibodies using immune complexes of alkaline phosphatase and monoclonal anti-alkaline phosphatase (APAAP complexes). Journal of Histochemistry and Cytochemistry 32: 219–229
7. Bodewadt S, Radzun H J, Feller A C, Parwaresch M R 1986 Immunophenotyping of acute non-lymphoblastic leukaemias. Virchows Archiv Abteilung B Zellpathologie (Cell Pathology) 51: 79–88
8. Chen Z, Sigaux F, Miglierina R et al 1986 Immunological typing of acute lymphoblastic leukaemia: concurrent analysis by flow cytofluorometry and immunocytology. Leukemia Research 10: 1411–1417
9. Fishleder A J, Tubb R R, Savage R A et al 1984 Immunophenotypic characterization of acute leukaemia by immunocytology. American Journal of Clinical Pathology 81: 611–617
10. Hui P-K, Joyce R 1984 Simple immunocytochemical staining procedure for lymphoid cell surface markers done on cell smears. Journal of Clinical Pathology 37: 708–712
11. Hui P-K Lawton J W M 1984 Immunoperoxidase detection of T and B cells in blood compared with conventional methods. Journal of Clinical Pathology 37: 1343–1346
12. Koller U, Stockinger H, Majdic O, Bettelheim P, Knapp W 1986 A rapid and simple immunoperoxidase staining procedure for blood and bone marrow samples. Journal of Immunological Methods 86: 75–81
13. Markey G M, Alexander H D, Agnew A N D et al 1986 Enumeration of absolute numbers of T lymphocyte subsets in B-chronic lymphocytic leukaemia using an immunoperoxidase technique: Relation to clinical stage. British Journal of Haematology 62: 257–273
14. Sandhaus L M, Gajl-Peczalska K J, Brunning R D 1984 Immunophenotyping of leukaemia: an immunoperoxidase method using air-dried smears. British Journal of Haematology 56: 131–138
15. Li C-Y, Lazcano-Villareal O, Pierre R V, Yam L T 1987 Immunocytochemical identification of cells in serous effusions. American Journal of Clinical Pathology 88: 696–706
16. Moir D J, Ghosh A K, Abdulaziz Z, Knight P M, Mason D Y 1983 Immunoenzymatic staining of haematological samples with monoclonal antibodies. British Journal of Haematology 55: 395–410
17. Erber W N, Pinching A J, Mason D Y 1984 Immunocytochemical detection of T and B cell populations in routine blood smears. Lancet i: 1042–1045
18. Erber W N, Mynheer L C, Mason D Y 1986 APAAP labelling of blood and bone-marrow samples for phenotyping leukaemia. Lancet i: 761–765
19. Bross K J, Pangalis G A, Staatz C G, Blume K G 1978 Demonstration of cell surface antigens and their antibodies by the peroxidase–antiperoxidase method. Transplantation 25: 331–334
20. Huang M-J, Li C-Y, Nichols W L, Young J-H, Katzmann J A 1984 Acute leukaemia with megakaryocytic differentiation: a study of 12 cases identified immunocytochemically. Blood 64: 427–439
21. Koike T 1984 Megakaryocytic leukaemia: the characterization and identification of megakaryoblasts. Blood 64: 683–692
22. Li C-Y, Ziesmer S C, Yam L T, English M C, Janckila A J 1984 Practical immunocytochemical identification of human blood cells. American Journal of Clinical Pathology 81: 204–212
23. Frickhofen N, Bross K J, Heimpel H 1985 Modified immunocytochemical slide technique for demonstrating surface antigens on viable cells. Journal of Clinical Pathology 38: 671–676
24. Neumann M P, De Solas I, Parkin J L et at 1986 Monoclonal antibody study of Philadelphia chromosome-positive blastic leukemias using the alkaline phosphatase anti-alkaline phosphatase (APAAP) technic. American Journal of Clinical Pathology 85: 564–572

25 Chen K, Demetris A J, Van Thiel D H, Whiteside T L 1987 Methods in laboratory investigation: double immunoenzyme staining method for analysis of tissue and blood lymphocyte subsets with monoclonal antibodies. Laboratory Investigation 56: 114–119
26 Davey F R, Erber W N, Gatter K C, Mason D Y 1987 Immunophenotyping of acute myeloid leukemia by immuno-alkaline phosphatase (APAAP) labeling with a panel of antibodies. American Journal of Hematology 26: 157–166
27 Erber W N, Breton-Gorius J, Villeval J L, Oscier D G, Bai Y, Mason D Y 1987 Detection of cells of megakaryocyte lineage in haematological malignancies by immuno-alkaline phosphatase labelling cell smears with a panel of monoclonal antibodies. British Journal of Haematology 65: 87–94
28 Erber W N, Jacobs A, Oscier D G, O'Hea A-M, Mason D Y 1987 Circulating micromegakaryocytes in myelodysplasia. Journal of Clinical Pathology 40: 1349–1352
29 Erber W N, Mason D Y 1987 Immunoalkaline phosphatase labeling of terminal transferase in hematologic samples. American Journal of Clinical Pathology 88: 43–50
30 Hanson C A, Gajl-Peczalska K J, Parkin J L, Brunning R D 1987 Immunophenotyping of acute myeloid leukaemia using monoclonal antibodies and the alkaline phosphatase-antialkaline phosphatase technique. Blood 70: 83–89
31 Choate J J, Domenico D R, McGraw T P, Freed J, Molnar Z, Schumacher H R 1988 Diagnosis of acute megakaryoblastic leukemia by flow cytometry and immunoalkaline phosphatase techniques. American Journal of Clinical Pathology 89: 247–253
32 Erber W N, Mason D Y 1988 Expression of the interleukin-2 receptor (Tac antigen/CD25) in hematologic neoplasms. American Journal of Clinical Pathology 89: 645–648
33 Ghosh A K, Spriggs A I, Taylor-Papadimitriou J, Mason D Y 1983 Immunocytochemical staining of cells in pleural and peritoneal effusions. Journal of Clinical Pathology 36: 1154–1164
34 Ghosh A K, Mason D Y, Spriggs A I 1983 Immunocytochemical staining with monoclonal antibodies in cytologically 'negative' serous effusions from patients with malignant disease. Journal of Clinical Pathology 36: 1150–1153
35 Ghosh A K, Spriggs A I, Mason D Y 1985 Immunocytochemical staining of T and B lymphocytes in serous effusions. Journal of Clinical Pathology 38: 608–612
36 Martin S E, Zhang H-Z, Magyarosy E, Jaffe E S, Hsu S-M, Chu E W 1984 Immunologic methods in cytology: definitive diagnosis of non-Hodgkin's lymphomas using immunologic markers for T- and B-cells. American Journal of Clinical Pathology 82: 666–673
37 Janckila A J, Yam L T, Li C-Y 1985 Immunocytochemical diagnosis of acute leukaemia with pleural involvement. Acta Cytologica 29: 67–72
38 Yam L T, Lin D G, Janckila A J, Li C-Y 1985 Immunocytochemical diagnosis of lymphoma in serous effusions. Acta Cytologica 29: 833–841
39 Ghosh A K, Erber W N, Hatton C S R et al 1985 Detection of metastatic tumour cells in routine bone marrow smears by immuno-alkaline phosphatase labelling with monoclonal antibodies. British Journal of Haematology 61: 21–30
40 Link M P, Stewart S J, Warnke R A, Levy R 1985 Discordance between surface and cytoplasmic expression of the Leu 4 (T3) antigen in thymocytes and in blast cells from childhood T-lymphoblastic malignancies. Journal of Clinical Investigation 76: 248–253
41 Mason D Y, Stein H, Gerdes J et al 1987 Value of monoclonal anti-CD22 (p135) antibodies for the detection of normal and neoplastic B lymphoid cells. Blood 69: 836–840
42 Campana D, Janossy G, Bofill M et al 1985 Human B cell development. I. Phenotypic differences of B lymphocytes in the bone marrow and peripheral lymphoid tissue. Journal of Immunology 134: 1524–1530
43 Wang X-H and Zipursky A 1987 Maternal erythrocytes in the fetal circulation. The immunocytochemical identification of minor populations of erythrocytes. American Journal of Clinical Pathology 88: 346–348
44 Li C-Y, Witzig T E, Phyliky R L, Ziesmer S C, Yam L T 1986 Diagnosis of B-cell non-Hodgkin's lymphoma of the central nervous system by immunocytochemical analysis of cerebrospinal fluid by lymphocytes. Cancer 57: 737–744
45 Pulford K A F, Erber W N, Crick J A et al 1988 Use of monoclonal antibody against human neutrophil elastase in normal and leukaemic myeloid cells. Journal of Clinical Pathology 41: 853–860
46 Bennett J M, Catovsky D, Daniel M-T et al 1985 Criteria for the diagnosis of acute leukemia of megakaryocyte lineage (M7). Annals of Internal Medicine 103: 460–462
47 Davey F R, Cordell J L, Erber W N, Pulford K A F, Gatter K C, Mason D Y 1988 Monoclonal antibody (Y1/82A) with specificity towards peripheral blood monocytes and tissue macrophages. Journal of Clinical Pathology 41: 753–758

48 Davey F R, Erber W N, Gatter K C, Mason D Y 1988 The use of monoclonal antibody Y1/82A in the identification of acute myeloblastic and monocytic leukemias. American Journal of Clinical Pathology 89: 76–80
49 Falini B, Schwarting R, Erber W et al 1985 The differential diagnosis of hairy cell leukemia with a panel of monoclonal antibodies. American Journal of Clinical Pathology 83: 289–300
50 Stross W P, Jones M, Mason D Y 1989 Automation of APAAP immunocytochemical technique. Journal of Clinical Pathology 42: 106–112

8
Terminal Deoxynucleotidyl Transferase, Adenosine Deaminase and Purine Nucleoside Phosphorylase: diagnostic tools and chemotherapeutic targets

Mary Sue Coleman   Lela K. Riley   Jennifer K. Morrow

INTRODUCTION

Human lymphoid leukemias and lymphomas constitute a group of phenotypically heterogeneous diseases that represent clonal populations of cells arrested at different stages of lymphoid ontogeny. The composite cellular phenotypes of leukemic cells have been determined through the use of monoclonal antibodies that define cell surface antigens,[1,2] through the use of selected biochemical markers[3,4] and through the use of nucleic acid probes that identify rearranged immunoglobulin and T-cell receptor genes.[5-9] The subclassification of acute leukemias and the various lymphomas has continued to be refined as more specific diagnostic tools have become available. The lineage designation of acute lymphoblastic leukemia (ALL) is the most clearly understood.[2] The largest class of ALL has been designated non-T-ALL (70% of cases). Most non-T-ALLs undergo clonal rearrangements of immunoglobulin genes and are malignancies of B-cell origin. Within this group, six subtypes exist, representing early to late differentiation stages. The precise classification of these diseases is still in transition since a significant proportion has also been reported to have rearrangements in the T-cell receptor (Tβ) gene.[10]

Approximately 25% of ALL cases have been designated as T-ALL, based on monoclonal antibody analysis and rearrangement of the T-cell receptor genes. Further subclassification of T-ALL is still controversial, but a general scheme suggests that at least three subtypes exist.[2] Individual patients have also been shown to exhibit phenotypic shifts in the predominant malignant cell population throughout disease progression.[11]

ALL phenotypes can also be transiently expressed in non-lymphoid leukemias. In blast crisis, approximately one-third of Philadelphia chromosome positive chronic myelogenous leukemia (CML) patients have leukemic cells with lymphoid features. A small but significant proportion of patients with acute undifferentiated leukemia (AUL) express ALL phenotypes. In acute myelogenous leukemia (AML), a minority of patients has cellular phenotypes related to ALL.[12-16] In these types of leukemias, distinction between lymphoid and myeloid phenotypes may be important because patients with the lymphoid phenotype may respond to chemotherapy with two lymphoid-specific drugs, vincristine and prednisone.[17,18]

Three enzymes, terminal deoxynucleotidyl transferase (TdT), adenosine deaminase (ADA) and purine nucleoside phosphorylase (PNP) are proposed to have integral relationships with the development of normal immune function in humans. TdT is a unique DNA polymerase that catalyzes the polymerization of deoxynucleoside triphosphates without a template.[19] The expression of this enzyme is normally restricted to cortical thymocytes[20] and lymphoid precursors in marrow.[21] In the mid-1970s, TdT activity was first detected in lymphoblastic leukemia cells.[21,22] Since then, TdT has been used as a biochemical marker of lymphoid progenitor cells in the differential diagnosis of leukemia.

The template independence of TdT coupled with its expression in lymphoid progenitor cells fueled hypotheses that implicated TdT in the generation of immunological diversity.[23,24] Most recently, experimental evidence has linked the expression of TdT with the putative insertion of extra random nucleotides between variable (V), diversity (D) or joining (J) regions during the rearrangement of immunoglobulin heavy chain genes or T-cell receptor β-genes during lymphoid ontogeny. These added sequences have been designated as N regions and are thought to contribute to the potential diversity of the antigen receptors encoded by these genes.[25,26]

ADA and PNP are purine salvage pathway enzymes which, unlike TdT, are present in a variety of different cell types. Both PNP and ADA are elevated at specific stages of lymphoid development and the enzyme activities have been shown to vary inversely with respect to each other during T-cell differentiation.[27] Since the normal levels of ADA and PNP are relatively high in all blood cells, delineation of abnormal enzyme activities is not simple. Repeated assays of ADA activity have shown limited usefulness in monitoring the transition of CML from stable to accelerated disease phase,[18] whilst monitoring of PNP activity has not shown promise in the management of leukemia. Nevertheless, these two enzymes seem to have a special relationship to a functional immune system since inherited deficiency of either is associated with severe lymphopenia.[28,29] In ADA deficiency, both T- and B-cells are affected, whereas in PNP deficiency only T-cell lymphopenia is observed. The mechanisms by which these hereditary enzyme deficiencies might cause selective destruction of lymphoid cells have been suggested with the discovery of distinctive biochemical abnormalities in tissues from these patients. When ADA is absent in lymphocytes and erythrocytes, large quantities of dATP accumulate[30-32] and, when PNP is absent, dGTP accumulates.[33] Increased levels of dATP and dGTP have been postulated to result in cytotoxicity by inhibiting ribonucleotide reductase, by interfering with the function of TdT or by depleting cells of essential deoxynucleoside triphosphates.[30,34] Deoxyadenosine, a substrate for ADA, has also been shown to be a potent inactivator of S-adenosylhomocysteine hydrolase which could result in an accumulation of S-adenosylhomocysteine and inhibition of essential methylation.[35] Whilst the underlying mechanisms of cytotoxicity are still a subject of active investigation, the observation that inhibition of either of these enzymes is correlated with selective killing of lymphoid cells is exciting from a chemotherapeutic viewpoint. Both ADA and PNP hold promise as target enzymes for the treatment of selected leukemias.

BIOCHEMICAL PARAMETERS

TERMINAL DEOXYNUCLEOTIDYL TRANSFERASE

The TdT protein has been purified to homogeneity from a variety of different leukemias.[36] It is translated as a 58 kDa protein which is sequentially degraded to 45 kDa and to a two subunit form of 30 kDa and 12 kDa. All forms of the enzyme have virtually identical catalytic activities. Recently, human, mouse and calf cDNAs have been cloned,[37,38] and the predicted amino acid sequences compared. High degrees of homology (>90%) exist for the enzyme from these three sources. Extensive protein sequencing information is also now available for TdT from calf thymus.[39] The human gene coding for TdT has recently been isolated in the authors' laboratory from genomic libraries constructed from fetal liver and leukocyte DNA sequences. The gene was isolated as a series of overlapping DNA fragments which span approximately 35 000 base pairs. The structure of the TdT gene has been analyzed by Southern blot and nucleotide sequence analysis (Fig. 8.1). The protein coding region is organized into 11 exon and 10 intron regions. An interesting feature of this gene is that the exon sequences are very asymmetrically distributed. The intracellular abundance of TdT mRNA is extremely low and its expression is tissue specific. The precise mechanism(s) responsible for the regulation of TdT mRNA transcription has not been established.

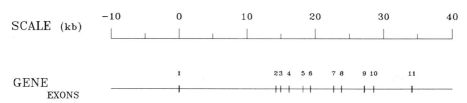

Fig. 8.1 Map of the human TdT gene. The positions and sizes of the exons are represented by solid boxes.

Knowledge of the structure and organization of the TdT gene will provide a framework for comparative studies of TdT regulation in normal and neoplastic cells.

ADENOSINE DEAMINASE

ADA has been isolated from human erythrocytes as a single polypeptide of molecular weight of 36 000.[40] The enzyme isolated from leukemic cells and thymus has an apparent mol. wt of 44 000.[41] The protein can bind to a large 'complexing protein' (mol. wt = 298 000) in lung and kidney, but the function of the complex is unknown. Human ADA cDNAs have been cloned and the nucleotide sequence determined.[42,43] Recently, the entire gene coding for human ADA has been cloned and sequenced.[44] The gene was isolated in a series of overlapping λ-phage clones containing human germline DNA. The gene, including the 5'- and 3'-flanking regions, encompasses about 37 000 base pairs and contains 12 exons separated by 11 introns. The apparent promoter region of the gene lacks the 'TATA' and 'CAAT' consensus sequences often found in eucaryotic promoters and is extremely G/C rich. Within the 5'-flanking region are areas homologous to other G/C-rich promoters. The availability of the entire gene sequence should be beneficial in studies aimed at understanding regulation of ADA expression in normal as well as in leukemic cells.

The variation in ADA enzyme activity in leukemic cells probably reflects abnormal regulation of enzyme expression since ADA purified from normal and leukemic cells exhibited no differences in K_m, temperature stability, electrophoretic mobility, immunological reactivity or specific activity.[40,41] This hypothesis was supported by preliminary studies in the authors' laboratory in which the levels of ADA activity, antigen and mRNA in normal cells and in a series of leukemic cells were examined. The results revealed at least three general categories of abnormal expression of ADA activity: (1) 'superactive' ADA enzyme, (2) elevated levels of ADA mRNA, (3) elevated levels of ADA protein. Definition of the precise control mechanisms underlying the complex array of abnormal phenotypes of ADA activity expression in these leukemias awaits detailed comparative studies of normal and neoplastic cells.

PURINE NUCLEOSIDE PHOSPHORYLASE

PNP has been purified from a number of sources, including human leukemic cells.[45] The human enzyme has a trimer subunit structure with electrophoretically identical subunits of molecular weight 33 000. The refined crystal structure of PNP has recently been determined and parameters obtained have been critical in suggesting strategies for the design of potent enzyme inhibitors.[46] Human cDNAs have been cloned and the entire nucleotide sequence of the PNP coding region determined.[47] Several genomic clones have been isolated and characterized.[47] Exon-containing sequences span a region of approximately 9000 base pairs with a minimum of four intervening sequences. Whilst PNP can be detected in all tissues,

218 THE LEUKEMIC CELL

the levels of enzyme activity vary.[48] As yet no information is available concerning regulation of expression of this enzyme in normal or leukemic cells.

CLINICAL CORRELATES

TDT IN LEUKEMIA

High levels of TdT are present in malignant cells from certain patients with acute leukemia and lymphoma, and detection of this enzyme is useful for differential diagnosis. Tumor cells from any source (such as peripheral blood, bone marrow, pleural fluid, bulk tumor) are satisfactory for determination of TdT level. Several methods of detection are available and are described in a later section. A summary of the large clinical studies of TdT in leukemia is presented in Table 8.1.

TDT IN ACUTE LYMPHOBLASTIC LEUKEMIA

Eighty-eight per cent of the 2516 ALL patients tested displayed high amounts of TdT activity or antigen. Examination of the data entries from each institution revealed that, although a variety of methods and reagents was employed in the various assays, the percentage of TdT positive cases within each study was remarkably similar to the aggregate average. Consistent with the previous report,[57] a significant correlation between TdT activity in peripheral lymphoblasts and activity in the bone marrow was apparent in the studies represented by Table 8.1.

The level of TdT varies with leukemic subtype. The average TdT activity is significantly lower in T-marked lymphoblasts than in non-T (B-lineage) lymphoblasts.[3] There are two ALL variants in which TdT activity in blasts may be virtually absent: B-cell ALL where blasts bear immunoglobulin on their surface[3] and blasts with cytoplasmic IgM, but without surface immunoglobulin.[83] During normal differentiation of lymphocytes, TdT activity first appears after differentiation of stem cells, rises during gene rearrangement and declines as lymphocytes are firmly committed to B- or T-cell lineages. As indicated earlier, the various leukemias appear to be clonal populations arrested at different stages of differentiation. The variations in TdT levels observed in these leukemias may parallel the normal differentiation-specific levels of this enzyme.

TDT AS A PROGNOSTIC FACTOR IN ALL

Several investigators have analyzed disease progression in large populations of ALL patients who had a TdT determination at diagnosis. Most agree that the absence of TdT in ALL indicates a poor prognosis.[84-86] In a very large clinical study that entered patients ($n = 169$) over a 6-year period with prolonged follow-up, the authors' laboratory measured the effect of a number of variables determined at diagnosis on the prognosis of children with ALL.[86] As a quantitative variable, TdT activity in cells from blood or marrow was not a predicting factor in those ALL patients. When the data were analyzed in a different way, by coding TdT activity as a dichotomous variable, high or low, a weak effect of TdT was observed; low TdT activity at diagnosis was associated with a longer duration of complete remission than high TdT activity ($P = 0.05$). However, the TdT variable was less important than mediastinal mass, treatment group or the absence of sheep cell receptor. Analyzed by this method, TdT activity at diagnosis did not affect survival.[86]

TdT as a Predictor of Relapse in ALL
Of great interest has been whether TdT levels increase in marrow or blood prior to frank clinical relapse. Several laboratories have reported that ALL patients, prior to relapse, had

Table 8.1 Presence of elevated TdT in hematologic diseases

Institution	Fraction of patients with elevated TdT before treatment[a]				Lymphomas and lymphoma leukemias tested[b]
	Acute myelogenous leukemia	Acute lymphoblastic leukemia	Chronic myelogenous leukemia		
			Stable	Blastic	
Imperial Cancer Research Fund[49,50,51]	28/310[c]	594/780	0/7	53/196	No
Memorial Sloan-Kettering Cancer Center[52-56]	61/379	290/306	0/14	44/125	Yes[52,53]
University of Kentucky[57-60]	32/344	408/455	0/14	2/6	Yes[57-59]
Boston University[61,62]	3/70	472/476	0/20	70/210	No
Stritch School of Medicine[63]	12/92	111/128	0/17	10/28	Yes[63]
Japan[64-67]	12/60	67/70	0/22	42/107	Yes[64]
Italy[68,69]	7/78	50/58	—	24/65	Yes[69]
National Institutes of Health[70,71]	7/52	28/28	0/30	12/30	No
University of Pennsylvania[72]	4/36	41/49	—	3/5	No
A. Roswell Park Memorial Institute[73,74]	9/45	43/43	—[d]	—[d]	Yes[74]
Germany[75,76]	2/34	31/41	0/6	0/8	No
Spain[77]	8/71	—	—	—	No
Sweden[78]	24/52	—	—	—	No
City of Hope National Medical Center[73]	0/8	26/27	0/1	6/9	Yes[79]
University of California, San Francisco[80]	1/4	20/21	—	2/8	No
SUNY Upstate Medical Center[81]	1/5	18/19	—	3/9	No
University of Minnesota Medical School[82]	—[e]	15/15	—	—[e]	No

[a]TdT was detected by a variety of different methods. Values were classified as 'high' by individual authors using a variety of criteria. Studies were included that had more than 30 cases in which patient numbers could be evaluated. The number of patients with specimens having high TdT is recorded as the numerator with total patients as the denominator. Acute myelogenous leukemia = all variants of AML excluding CML in blast crisis; acute lymphoblastic leukemia = all variants of ALL, excluding lymphoid leukemia which occurs in patients with lymphoma. Patients were excluded unless malignant cells were studied before treatment of the leukemia.
[b]The histological classification of lymphomas is complex. The tissues assayed for TdT varied from lymph nodes to pleural fluid. In the interests of clarity, whether investigators studied patients with lymphoma is noted, but original papers should be consulted.
[c]The authors originally classified 45 patients as AML in Jani et al.[49] However, only 28 were available for detailed follow-up.
[d]Patient numbers were not evaluable in Srivastava et al.[74]
[e]Patient numbers were not evaluable in Yasmineh et al.[82]

a progressive increase in TdT + cells or TdT activity.[87,88] In contrast, other detailed studies of relatively short duration have shown that TdT determinations, by activity or antigen, did not consistently predict relapse of ALL.[89-91] In the authors' 6-year clinical study, this question was examined by measuring TdT activity in blood or marrow multiple times while patients were in remission and relapse.[86] It was demonstrated by statistical analyses of serial TdT determinations that at the time of frank morphologic relapse at any site (including testis or central nervous system), TdT activity was significantly elevated at some time during remission in 64% of patients. Patients who relapsed in the testis or the central nervous system rarely had concurrent elevated TdT in blood or marrow cells. It was also found that, during remission, those patients who would eventually relapse did not exhibit significant sustained increases in TdT activity in blood or bone marrow cells. In fact, dramatic fluctuations in TdT levels occurred during remission in response to unknown biological signals. Therefore, repeated measurements of TdT activity or antigen alone do not seem to be of value in the management of childhood ALL.[86]

TdT in Acute Myelogenous Leukemia

Patients with cytochemically confirmed acute myeloblastic and myelomonocytic leukemia are grouped as acute myelogenous leukemia (AML) in Table 8.1. Terminal transferase is generally absent in AML cells or in the low control range and is much lower than in ALL cells. However, selected AML patients exhibit high levels of TdT activity. A number of laboratories have now reported on the incidence of above normal TdT levels in AML using a variety of enzyme assay and antigen detection technics. Of 1640 AML patients, 211 (or 13%) had positive TdT values (Table 8.1).

In contrast to ALL, where frequency of TdT positivity is highly consistent between laboratories, frequency of TdT positivity in AML is highly variable. The frequency of positive TdT levels in large AML populations varies from about 5%[49] to greater than 40%.[78] The reason for this variance is not known. There is also some controversy concerning the prognosis of TdT + AML patients. Some investigators find TdT positivity to indicate poor prognosis regardless of whether patients are treated with AML regimens or in combination with ALL-specific drugs.[49,58,72] Other investigators report significantly higher remission rates in TdT + AML than in TdT − AML patients.[78] The precise lineage designation of TdT + 'myeloid' cell leukemias is still not understood. These leukemic cells are clearly different from lymphoid blasts of CML (cALL +, TdT +, myeloid enzyme-negative) that are clinically responsive to ALL regimens. TdT + AMLs are difficult to treat effectively and will require extensive investigation including development of new drug regimens.

TdT in Chronic Myelogenous leukemia

Chronic myelogenous leukemia (CML) in the stable phase is not associated with elevated TdT levels. Of the 131 patients reported (see Table 8.1), none had above normal TdT. In the accelerated phase of CML (blast crisis), 34% of patients have elevated levels of TdT (271 of 806 patients). At least three independent studies have demonstrated that patients with high TdT in blast crisis respond more favorably to treatments with vincristine and prednisone than do patients with low levels of TdT.[50,64,65] These data suggest that patients in blast crisis with TdT-containing blasts should be identified prospectively and treated with drugs effective in lymphoid leukemia. Thus, TdT measurements may be useful in routine monitoring of CML patients.

TdT in Lymphomas

Known B-cell-derived lymphomas of the follicular center-cell type are uniformly negative for TdT. However, certain cases of non-Hodgkin's lymphoma have malignant cells with high levels of TdT. This includes cells from diverse sites such as bone marrow, peripheral blood, pleural fluid, lymph nodes and testicle. Studies of TdT in lymphoma are referred to in Table 8.1. It appears that TdT is elevated in lymphoblastic lymphoma and the assay of TdT may serve as a diagnostic tool. This group of patients is generally young, has a poor prognosis and behaves clinically like patients with ALL. The recognition of their relation to ALL and the institution of appropriate therapies have vastly improved prognosis in this disease.

Recommended Applications of TdT Assays

Based upon information presently available, measurements of TdT can be helpful in specimens from patients with:

1. Undifferentiated leukemias where blasts do not react with standard cytochemical stains. Cases of ALL may be identified.
2. Blast crisis of CML initially and at relapse. High levels of terminal transferase in blasts are associated with 'lymphoid' crisis.
3. Leukemias with unusual morphologic features, particularly where mixed proliferations of myeloid and lymphoid cells are suspected or the response to treatment is not as expected.
4. Diffuse non-Hodgkin's lymphoma where lymphoblastic lymphoma is possible. Lymphoblastic lymphoma may respond best to treatment regimens appropriate for ALL.

ADA IN LEUKEMIA

Investigations of ADA in leukemic cells have shown that assay of ADA activity has limited use as a complementary diagnostic marker for subclassification of human leukemias.[18,93] A summary of ADA activities in peripheral blood or bone marrow samples from leukemia patients is presented in Table 8.2. The majority of the patients with CML and chronic myelogenous leukemia in blast crisis (CML/BC) display elevated levels of ADA activity. In contrast, ADA activity is normal or low in chronic lymphocytic leukemia (CLL). ADA levels are substantially higher in T-cell CLL compared with B-cell variants. In acute leukemia

Table 8.2 Activity of ADA in leukemias

Histological diagnosis	Patient numbers	ADA activity[a]		Reference(s)
		Above normal	Below normal	
CML	9	6	0	93–95
CML/BC	9	6	0	93,95
CLL				
Not classified	33	2	5	96,97
B-cell	85	0	21	93,95,98–100
T-cell	14	2	3	100,101
Prolymphocytic leukemia	7	0	7	99
AML	69	38	6	93,95,97,100
ALL				
Not classified	81	63	9	93,95,97
Non-T-cell	16	12	2	80,100
T-cell	38	38	0	80,94,96,100
Non-T-, non-B-cell	24	21	0	80,100

[a]ADA was detected by different methods. Values were classified as above or below normal by individual authors using a variety of criteria. Patients were excluded unless malignant cells were studied prior to treatment.

(ALL and AML), significantly higher levels of ADA are observed in lymphoblasts than in chronic neoplasias. Approximately 50% of patients diagnosed with acute myelogenous leukemia (AML) have elevated activities. The highest content of ADA is observed in patients with acute lymphocytic leukemia (ALL), particularly those with T-cell ALL, where levels of enzyme may be 20–30 times greater than in normal cells. Because normal tissues contain high levels of ADA, the definition of abnormal ADA levels in leukemia subtypes is complicated and requires analysis of large patient populations to establish normal ranges of ADA. Therefore, determination of ADA levels may not be feasible for routine clinical diagnosis.

PNP IN LEUKEMIA

Studies on PNP deficiency have demonstrated that this enzyme plays an important role in differentiation and immune function of lymphoid cells.[27,102,103] Since expression of PNP varies as hemopoietic cells differentiate, levels of PNP in leukemia may reflect the maturity of the proliferating neoplastic population. Investigators have, therefore, examined PNP activities in lymphoblasts from peripheral blood and bone marrow samples. A summary of these studies is presented in Table 8.3. PNP levels appear to vary dramatically in the myelogenous variants (CML and CML/BC, and AML), whereas 75% of lymphoblasts from lymphocytic leukemias (CLL and ALL) exhibit subnormal PNP activity. CLL and prolymphocytic leukemia (PLL) are closely related disorders which are difficult to distinguish. Although PNP levels are below normal in both leukemias, there is evidence that PNP activities are slightly higher in PLL.[99] Thus, PNP may be a useful marker to delineate PLL from CLL. As is the case with ADA, PNP has only limited utility as a biomarker in the diagnosis of subtypes of leukemias.

CHEMOTHERAPEUTIC TARGETS

TERMINAL DEOXYNUCLEOTIDYL TRANSFERASE

The in vivo function of TdT is not clearly understood, although this enzyme is thought to be involved in the development of T- and B-cells. In leukemic cells, the normal development

Table 8.3 PNP activity in leukemic patients

Histological diagnosis	Patient numbers	PNP activity[a]		Reference(s)
		Above normal	Below normal	
CML	6	3	2	95
CML/BC	6	1	3	95
CLL				
Not classified	32	0	27	97
B-cell	39	0	27	98,99
T-cell	7	0	5	100
Prolymphocytic	4	0	4	99
AML	14	3	7	95
ALL	17	1	14	94,95

[a]PNP was detected by several methods. Values were classified as above or below normal by individual authors using a variety of criteria. Patients were excluded unless malignant cells were studied before treatment of the leukemia.

process is disturbed and TdT may be aberrantly expressed. Several investigators have sought specific inhibitors of TdT to test the hypothesis that inhibition of TdT in leukemic cells might constitute a lethal event for such cells.[104] As yet, potent, specific inhibitors have not been described and will probably not be available until more detailed data concerning the enzyme active site are available.

ADENOSINE DEAMINASE

The profound immunodeficiency associated with ADA deficiency suggested that ADA inhibitors might be effective immunosuppressant and chemotherapeutic agents. In vitro studies of T- and B-lymphocytes cultured with deoxyadenosine along with ADA inhibitors indicated that T-cells were selectively killed.[105] The selection of a single ADA inhibitor appropriate for in vivo studies was based on solubility in aqueous solutions and potency of enzyme inactivation. Of the ADA inhibitors examined, deoxycoformycin (dCF) (Fig. 8.2) was water soluble and had a K_i of 10^{-12} mol/l. The first patients treated with dCF exhibited the type of leukemic cells known to be sensitive to the drug in vitro. As expected, after administration of dCF, ADA levels dropped rapidly in peripheral blood and lymphoblasts were lysed. The dATP levels in blood cells rose rapidly, but, unexpectedly, ATP levels dropped and unacceptable toxicity was observed in patients.[106,107]

The biochemical mechanism responsible for ATP depletion upon administration of high doses of dCF is not understood. The dCF is phosphorylated in cells and these phosphorylated derivatives may precipitate the loss of ATP.[108] Essential to the development of safe dosing regimens of dCF was the biochemical monitoring of dATP and ATP to prevent intracellular depletion of the latter. In a large clinical trial, the authors' laboratory demonstrated that the most important predictor of the onset of clinical toxicity was the ratio of dATP to ATP in erythrocytes. When dATP/ATP was greater than 0.5, toxicity was inevitable.[109] Subsequently, doses of dCF have been established (4 mg/m^2) that can be administered safely while producing responses in refractory lymphoid neoplasms. In the clinical trials of dCF, the inclusion of patients who exhibit relatively low cellular levels of ADA (chronic leukemias) has produced encouraging results. The most promising clinical response to dCF is observed in chronic leukemias and in particular in hairy cell leukemia

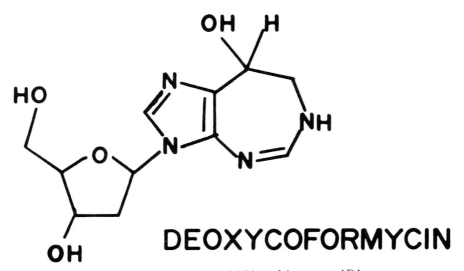

Fig. 8.2 Structure of deoxycoformycin, a potent inhibitor of the enzyme ADA.

(90% responses),[110] in chronic lymphocytic leukemia (30% responses)[111] and in cutaneous T-cell lymphoma (about 40% responses).[112] It appears likely that dCF or other ADA inhibitors will emerge as important chemotherapeutic agents for certain lymphoid neoplasms.

PURINE NUCLEOSIDE PHOSPHORYLASE

Like ADA, this enzyme is an inviting target for chemotherapy because the deficiency state is T-cell specific. Presumably a potent enzyme inhibitor would selectively lyse leukemic cells of T-cell origin. The search for specific PNP inhibitors has thus far been disappointing and no inhibitors suitable for clinical trials have been described. However, the recent elucidation of the three-dimensional structure of PNP should yield information useful for the synthesis of good enzyme inhibitors.[46]

ASSAY METHODS

Detailed procedures for detection of each of the three enzymes are presented in the references cited. In the sections that follow, the salient aspects of these technics are reviewed and, where possible, evaluation offered.

TDT QUANTITATIVE BIOCHEMICAL ASSAY

The in vitro reaction catalyzed by TdT that forms the basis of the biochemical assay is:

$$n\text{dGTP} + d(pY)_m \xrightarrow{Mg^{2+}} d(pY)_m(pG)_n + n\text{PP}_i$$

where $d(pY)_m$ is the DNA substrate, $d(pY_m)(pG)_n$ is the elongated DNA product and PP_i is inorganic pyrophosphate. The DNA substrates most often used are $d(pA)_{50}$ or $d(pA)_{12-18}$. The radioactive nucleotide substrate in this reaction is generally $d[^3H]$ GTP.[60,113,114] At least 2×10^7 nucleated cells from marrow, blood or other lymphoid tissue are necessary to assay TdT reliably. Blood samples should be collected in EDTA which serves as an anticoagulant. The nucleated cells should be separated and quantified.[60] The cells may be frozen in a pellet for enzyme assay at a later date. Enzyme extracts are prepared by sonication of cell pellets suspended in phosphate buffer (0.25 mol/l, pH 7.4) at a concentration of at least 1×10^8 cells/ml. Following the centrifugation of the extract, the supernatant is assayed. The advantage of the enzyme assay is that the interpretation of positive values is relatively unambiguous. Peripheral blood cells have virtually no detectable TdT activity. Normal bone marrow cells have very low levels of TdT activity (the mean is slightly higher in children than in adults). Reagents for use in enzyme activity measurements are commercially available, but these have not been standardized. Therefore, it is essential that each laboratory establish positive and negative control ranges with in-house samples. The principal disadvantages of this technic are lack of commercial test kits, the high number of nucleated cells required and necessity for a radioactive reagent in the assay.

TDT IMMUNOLOGIC METHODS

When specific polyclonal antibodies to TdT became widely available[36,115] immunocytochemical procedures for detection of TdT were developed.[116] These procedures (based on fluorescein or peroxidase labeling) require a film or cytospin preparation of cells on a glass slide. The dried slides are best if prepared just prior to use although slides have a storage life of about 2 weeks in a dessicated chamber. The films should be fixed in absolute methanol (4°C) immediately before the staining but should be constantly hydrated during the entire staining procedure.[116] Indirect immunofluorescence technics have been used successfully in many laboratories to detect TdT antigen in single cells.[116-119] Depending on the quality of the anti-TdT antibody used, this test is sensitive (500-1000 cells on a slide) and specific. Immunoperoxidase procedures have also been developed.[120] Theoretically, immunoperoxidase technics are preferable because of sample examination by light microscopy, absence of autofluorescence or quenching, long storage life of stained smears and improved visibility of cellular morphology.[121,122] Comparisons of the two technics confirm that both give reliable detection of TdT antigen in single cells. It has been observed that immunoperoxidase methods give heightened sensitivity in myelogenous leukemic cells.[120,123] However, the significance of these findings is not yet understood and should be the subject of further investigations.

Double fluorochrome analysis of leukemic cells has been useful in correlating the presence of TdT antigen with the expression of selected cell surface markers. The technics used have combined rhodamine-labeled cell surface monoclonal antibodies and indirect immunofluorescence staining for TdT.[124] Simultaneous labeling of TdT and membrane antigens has likewise been described using an immunoperoxidase method for TdT detection coupled with immunogold for membrane antigens.[125] These studies are useful for determination of the lineage designation of TdT positive leukemic cells.

The reagents for immunofluorescence and immunoperoxidase TdT tests are available from P. L. Biochemicals (Milwaukee, WI, USA), Life Sciences (St Petersburg, FL, USA) and Supertechs (Bethesda, MD, USA).

Monoclonal antibodies have also been developed against TdT[126,127] and utilized for immunoperoxidase staining. Whilst the McAbs give very specific staining of cells containing high levels of TdT,[127] these antibodies are not very sensitive[128] and thus may not be useful for general clinical situations where wide ranges of TdT antigen define lymphoid-type leukemic cells.

The single-cell immunocytochemical tests for TdT antigen are advantageous when only small numbers of leukemic cells are available or when double marker studies might yield additional diagnostic discrimination.[129] However, immunocytochemical procedures are limited by the instability of antigen in unprocessed dried smears and the difficulty in maintaining stable positive control films in a routine clinical setting.[117] It is essential that each laboratory establish positive and negative patient ranges since control slides are not provided in test kits. It has been reported that, using immunocytochemical reagents, positive smears should contain greater than 40% stained cells.[119,121] Since standard positive samples are not readily available, each laboratory should confirm this value with the antibodies obtained for the test.

Quantitative enzyme-linked immunoassays have considerably simplified tests for TdT antigen, but these tests do not allow simultaneous examination of leukemic cell morphology. A solid-phase immunoassay has been extensively compared with immunocytochemical[130] and enzyme activity measurements for TdT.[131,132] The immunoassay uses anti-TdT antibody linked to polystyrene beads. Individual beads are incubated with nucleated cell extracts, washed and incubated with a second anti-TdT antibody conjugated with peroxidase. Following a final washing, the bead complex is incubated with a chromogenic peroxidase substrate. The amount of TdT antigen in the sample is quantified by comparing color development with a standard curve. This quantitative immunoassay is greater than 100 times more sensitive than previously described tests for enzyme activity with a sensitivity of 0.99 and specificity of 0.99 when compared with TdT activity. The solid-phase immunoassay is particularly convenient when large numbers of specimens are being processed. Since the test utilizes and contains frozen positive and negative standards, the laboratory need not maintain TdT-positive cell lines for use as controls. Defined positive samples to generate a standard curve are provided with the assay kit. Recent studies also indicate that the solid-phase immunoassay will reliably detect TdT antigen in whole blood samples, thus obviating the necessity of isolating nucleated cells, a step which is essential in all other quantitative tests for TdT.[132] Reagents for the solid-phase immunoassay for TdT are available in kit form from the author's laboratory (Chapel Hill, NC, USA).

METHODS FOR DETECTION OF ADA

The in vitro reaction catalyzed by ADA and used for measurement of enzyme activity is:

$$[^{14}C]Adenosine \xrightarrow{ADA} [^{14}C]Inosine + NH_3$$

A micromethod for measuring enzyme activity, which monitors the conversion of $[^{14}C]$adenosine to $[^{14}C]$inosine, has been reported.[133] This assay is simple to perform and may be used with small numbers of cells. The radioactive product is separated from the substrate by chromatography on DE-81 paper. Radioactive adenosine is available from commercial sources, but not in a kit form. Positive controls are easy to obtain since virtually all cells contain ADA activity. Nucleated cells are isolated and cell extracts may be prepared in the same manner as described for TdT. Since ADA is present in high amounts in blood cells, small numbers of cells, fewer than 10^6, are required for the assay.

Polyclonal antibody to human ADA has been prepared in several laboratories[41,134] and has been adapted for use in radioimmunoassays,[41] in immunocytochemical methods[134] and in flow cytometric methods.[135] McAbs against human ADA have also been produced.[136] Because none of these antibodies is yet commercially available, routine immunologic assays for ADA are not accessible to clinical laboratories.

METHODS FOR DETECTION OF PNP

PNP is the second enzyme after ADA, in the purine salvage pathway:

$$P_i + Inosine \xrightarrow{PNP} Hypoxanthine$$
$$+ \text{ribose-1-P} \xrightarrow{\text{Xanthine oxidase}} Xanthine \xrightarrow{\text{Xanthine oxidase}} \text{Uric acid}$$

Most PNP assays are based on the conversion of radioactive inosine to uric acid in a coupled reaction employing xanthine oxidase.[45] The $[^{14}C]$inosine and $[^{14}C]$uric acid are separated by paper chromatography. The reagents and enzyme necessary for the reaction are available from commercial suppliers. This assay is sensitive, specific and relatively easy to perform. Nucleated cells must be separated for use in the assay. Extracts may be made in a 0.25 mol/l potassium phosphate buffer pH 7.4. Since the enzyme is present in large quantity, fewer than 10^6 cells are sufficient for the assay. Spectrophotometric assays have also been developed, and these are also rapid and sensitive.[137] Whilst antibodies directed against human PNP have been developed,[45] these have not been used systematically to measure PNP by immunocytochemical methods.

SUMMARY AND PROSPECTUS

Three enzymes, TdT, ADA and PNP, have been used in the differential diagnosis or as targets in treatment of leukemias and lymphomas. Clear patterns for expression of these proteins in neoplasia have emerged and methods of rapid detection of each enzyme have been developed. The level of TdT antigen or activity constitutes an objective and significant marker for the classification of human neoplasms. Inhibitors of ADA have induced selective lysis of lymphoid cells and may be the treatment of choice in certain forms of leukemia. Inhibitors of PNP hold great promise as even more selective lympholytic agents with enhanced specificity. Recent advances in the determination of protein and gene structure of these enzymes will allow detailed comparison of their regulation and mechanisms of action in normal and neoplastic cells.

Acknowledgements

The authors are grateful to Dr J. Lesnaw for her critical reading of the manuscript, to Mr John May for technical assistance and to Ms Sara Thompson for editorial and typing assistance. The authors' work is supported by grants CA26391 and CA19492 from the National Cancer Institute of the National Institutes of Health, USA.

REFERENCES

1. Greaves M F, Delia D, Newman R A, Vodinelich L 1982 Analysis of leukaemic cells with monoclonal antibodies. In: McMichael A J, Fabre J W (eds) Monoclonal antibodies in clinical medicine. Academic Press, London, pp. 129–165
2. Foon K A, Todd R F 1986 Immunologic classification of leukemia and lymphoma. Blood 68: 1–31
3. Coleman M S, Greenwood M F, Hutton J J et al 1978 Adenosine deaminase, terminal deoxynucleotidyl transferase (TdT) and cell surface markers in childhood acute leukemia. Blood 52: 1125–1131
4. McCaffrey R, Lillquist A, Sallan S, Cohen E, Osband M 1981 Clinical utility of leukemia cell terminal transferase measurements. Cancer Research 41: 4814–4820
5. Alt F W, Yancopoulos G D, Blackwell T K et al 1984 Ordered rearrangements of immunoglobulin heavy chain variable region segments. EMBO Journal 3: 1209–1219
6. Reth M G, Ammirati P, Jackson S, Alt F W 1985 Regulated progression of a cultured pre-B-cell line to the B-cell stage. Nature 317: 353–355
7. Furley A J, Mitzutani S, Weilbaecher K et al 1986 Developmentally regulated rearrangement and expression of genes encoding the T-cell receptor–T3 complex. Cell 46: 75–87
8. Knowles D M II, Pelicci P-G, Dalla-Favera R 1986 T-cell receptor beta chain gene rearrangements: genetic markers of T-cell lineage and clonality. Human Pathology 17: 546–551
9. Greenberg J M, Kersey J H 1987 Terminal deoxynucleotidyl transferase expression can precede T-cell receptor β-chain and λ-chain rearrangement in T-cell acute lymphoblastic leukemia. Blood 69: 356–360
10. Tawa A, Hozumi N, Minden M, Mak T W, Gelfand E W 1985 Rearrangement of the T-cell receptor B-chain gene in non-T-cell, non-B-cell acute lymphoblastic leukemia of childhood. New England Journal of Medicine 313: 1033–1037
11. Greaves M F, Paxton A, Janossy G, Pain C, Johnson S, Lister T A 1980 Acute lymphoblastic leukaemia associated antigen. III Alterations in expression during treatment and in relapse. Leukemia Research 4: 1–14
12. Bradstock K F, Hoffbrand A V, Ganeshaguru K et al 1981 Terminal deoxynucleotidyl transferase expression in acute non-lymphoid leukaemia: an analysis by immunofluorescence. British Journal of Haematology 47: 133–143
13. Donlon J A, Jaffe E S, Braylan R C 1977 Terminal deoxynucleotidyl transferase activity in malignant lymphomas. New England Journal of Medicine 297: 461–464
14. Greaves M F, Verbi W, Reeves B R et al 1979 'Pre-B' phenotypes in blast crisis of Ph[1] positive CML: evidence for a pluripotential stem cell 'target'. Leukemia Research 3: 181–191
15. Janossy G, Hoffbrand A V, Greaves M F et al 1980 Terminal transferase enzyme assay and immunological membrane markers in the diagnosis of leukaemia: a multiparameter analysis of 300 cases. British Journal of Haematology 44: 221–234
16. San Miguel J F, Gonzalez M, Cañizo M C, Anta J P, Portero J A, Lopez Borrasca A 1986 TdT activity in acute myeloid leukemias defined by monoclonal antibodies. American Journal of Hematology 23: 9–17
17. Peterson L C, Bloomfield C D, Brunning R D 1976 Blast crisis as an initial or terminal manifestation of chronic myeloid leukemia. A study of 28 patients. American Journal of Medicine 60: 209–220
18. Grever M R, Coleman M S, Balcerzak S P 1983 Adenosine deaminase and terminal deoxynucleotidyl transferase: biochemical markers in the management of chronic myelogenous leukemia. Cancer Research 43: 1442–1445

19 Bollum F J 1960 Oligodeoxynucleotide primers for calf thymus polymerase. Journal of Biological Chemistry 235: PC18–PC20
20 Chang L M S 1971 Development of terminal deoxynucleotidyl transferase activity in embryonic calf thymus gland. Biochemical and Biophysical Research Communications 44: 124–131
21 Coleman M S, Hutton J J, De Simone P, Bollum F J 1974 Terminal deoxynucleotidyl transferase in human leukemia. Proceedings of the National Academy of Sciences of the USA 71: 4404–4408
22 McCaffrey R, Smoler D F, Baltimore D 1973 Terminal deoxynucleotidyl transferase in a case of childhood acute lymphoblastic leukemia. Proceedings of the National Academy of Sciences of the USA 70: 521–525
23 Baltimore D 1974 Is terminal deoxynucletotidyl transferase a somatic cell mutagen in lymphocytes? Nature 248: 409–411
24 Bollum F J 1975 Terminal deoxynucleotidyl transferase: source of immunological diversity? In: Zahn R K (ed) Karl-August-Forster Lectures, vol. 14, Franz Steiner Verlag GmbH, Wiesbaden, pp. 1–41
25 Desiderio S V, Yancopolous G D, Paskind M et al 1984 Insertion of N regions into heavy-chain genes is correlated with expression of terminal deoxy-transferase in B-cells. Nature 311: 752–755
26 Kronenberg M, Siu G, Hood L E, Shastri N A 1986 The molecular genetics of the T-cell antigen receptor and T-cell antigen recognition. Annual Review of Immunology 4: 529–591
27 Barton R, Martiniuk F, Hirschhorn R, Goldschneider I 1980 Inverse relationship between adenosine deaminase and purine nucleoside phosphorylase in rat lymphocyte populations. Cellular Immununology 49: 208–214
28 Giblett E R, Anderson J E, Cohen F, Pollara B, Meuwissen H J 1972 Adenosine-deaminase deficiency in two patients with severely impaired cellular immunity. Lancet ii: 1067–1069
29 Giblett E R, Ammann A J, Wara D W, Sandman R, Diamond L K 1975 Nucleoside-phosphorylase deficiency in a child with severely defective T-cell immunity and normal B-cell immunity. Lancet 1: 1010–1013
30 Coleman M S, Donofrio J, Hutton J J et al 1978 Identification and quantitation of adenine deoxynucleotides in erythrocytes of a patient with adenosine deaminase deficiency and severe combined immunodeficiency. Journal of Biological Chemistry 253: 1619–1626
31 Donofrio J, Coleman M S, Hutton J J, Daoud A, Lampkin B, Dyminski J 1978 Overproduction of adenine deoxynucleosides and deoxynucleotides in adenosine deaminase deficiency with severe combined immunodeficiency disease. Journal of Clinical Investigation 62: 884–887
32 Cohen A, Hirschhorn R, Horowitz S D et al 1978 Deoxyadenosine triphosphate as a potentially toxic metabolite in adenosine deaminase deficiency. Proceedings of the National Academy of Sciences of the USA 75: 472–476
33 Cohen A, Gudas L J, Ammann A J, Staal G E J, Martin D W, Jr 1978 Deoxyguanosine triphosphate as a possible toxic metabolite in the immunodeficiency associated with purine nucleoside phosphorylase deficiency. Journal of Clinical Investigation 61: 1405–1409
34 Ullman B, Gudas L J, Cohen A, Martin D W, Jr 1978 Deoxyadenosine metabolism and cytotoxicity in cultured mouse T lymphoma cells: a model for immunodeficiency disease. Cell 14: 365–375
35 Kredich N M, Hershfield M S 1979 S-Adenosylhomocysteine toxicity in normal and adenosine kinase-deficient lymphoblasts of human origin. Proceedings of the National Academy of the Sciences of the USA 76: 2450–2454
36 Deibel M R, Jr, Coleman M S, Acree K, Hutton J J 1981 Biochemical and immunological properties of human terminal deoxynucleotidyltransferase purified from blasts of acute lymphoblastic and chronic myelogenous leukemia. Journal of Clinical Investigation 67: 725–734
37 Peterson R C, Cheung L C, Mattaliano R J, Chang L M S, Bollum F J 1984 Molecular cloning of human terminal deoxynucleotidyltransferase. Proceedings of the National Academy of the Sciences of the USA 81: 4363–4367
38 Koiwai O, Yokota, T, Kageyama T, Hirose T, Yoshida S, Arai K 1986 Isolation and characterization of bovine and mouse terminal deoxynucleotidyltransferase cDNAs expressible in mammalian cells. Nucleic Acids Research 14: 5777–5792
39 Beach C M, Chan S K, Vanaman T C, Coleman M S 1985 Terminal deoxynucleotidyltransferase: alignment of α- and β-subunits of the core enzyme along the primary translation product. Biochemical Journal 227: 1003–1007
40 Van der Weyden M B, Kelley W N 1976 Human adenosine deaminase: distribution and properties. Journal of Biological Chemistry 251: 5448–5456
41 Wiginton D A, Coleman M S, Hutton J J 1981 Purification, characterization and radioimmunoassay of adenosine deaminase from human leukaemic granulocytes. Biochemical Journal 195: 389–397

42 Wiginton D A, Adrian G S, Friedman R L, Suttle D P, Hutton J J 1983 Cloning of cDNA sequences of human adenosine deaminase. Proceedings of the National Academy of Sciences of the USA 80: 7481–7485
43 Daddona P E, Shewach D S, Kelley W N, Argos P, Markham A F, Orkin S H 1984 Human adenosine deaminase: cDNA and complete primary amino acid sequence. Journal of Biological Chemistry. 259: 12101–12106
44 Wiginton D A, Kaplan D J, States J C et al 1986 Complete sequence and structure of the gene for human adenosine deaminase. Biochemistry 25: 8234–8244
45 Wiginton D A, Coleman M S, Hutton J J 1980 Characterization of purine nucleoside phosphorylase from human granulocytes and its metabolism of deoxyribonucleosides. Journal of Biological Chemistry 255: 6663–6669
46 Stoeckler J D, Ealick S E, Bugg C E, Parks R E, Jr 1986 Design of purine nucleoside phosphorylase inhibitors. Federation Proceedings 45: 2773–2778
47 Williams S R, Goddard J M, Martin D W, Jr 1984 Human purine nucleoside phosphorylase cDNA sequence and genomic clone characterization. Nucleic Acids Research 12: 5779–5787
48 Carson D A, Kaye J, Seegmiller J E 1977 Lymphospecific toxicity in adenosine deaminase deficiency and purine nucleoside phosphorylase deficiency: possible role of nucleoside kinase(s). Proceedings of the National Academy of Sciences of the USA 74: 5677–5681
49 Jani P, Verbi W, Greaves M F, Bevan D, Bollum F 1983 Terminal deoxynucleotidyl transferase in acute myeloid leukaemia. Leukemia Research 7: 17–29
50 Janossy G, Woodruff R K, Pippard M J et al 1979 Relation of 'lymphoid' phenotype and response to chemotherapy incorporating vincristine-prednisolone in the acute phase of Ph' positive leukemia. Cancer 43: 426–434
51 Hoffbrand A V, Ganeshaguru K, Janossy G, Greaves M F, Catovsky D, Woodruff R K 1977 Terminal deoxynucleotidyl-transferase levels and membrane phenotypes in diagnosis of acute leukemia. Lancet ii: 520–523
52 Kung P C, Long J C, McCaffrey R P, Ratliff R, Harrison T A, Baltimore D 1978 Terminal deoxynucleotidyl transferase in the diagnosis of leukemia and malignant lymphoma. American Journal of Medicine 64: 788–794
53 Mertelsmann R, Koziner B, Filippa D A et al 1979 Clinical significance of TdT, cell surface markers and CFU-C in 297 patients with hematopoietic neoplasias. In: Neth R, Gallo R C, Hofschneider P-H, Mannweiler K (eds) Haematology and Blood Transfusion, vol. 23, Modern trends in human leukemia III. Springer-Verlag, Berlin, pp. 131–138
54 Modak M J, Mertelsmann R, Koziner B et al 1980 A micromethod for determination of terminal deoxynucleotidyl transferase (TdT) in the diagnostic evaluation of acute leukemias. Journal of Cancer Research and Clinical Oncology 98: 91–104
55 Mertelsmann R, Gillis S, Steinmann G et al 1981 T-cell growth factor (Interleukin 2) and terminal transferase activity in human leukemias and lymphoblastic cell lines. Blut 43: 99–103
56 Benedetto P, Mertelsmann R, Szatrowski T H et al 1986 Prognostic significance of terminal deoxynucleotidyl transferase activity in acute nonlymphoblastic leukemia. Journal of Clinical Oncology 4: 489–495
57 Greenwood M F, Coleman M S, Hutton J J et al 1977 Terminal deoxynucleotidyl transferase distribution in neoplastic and hematopoietic cells. Journal of Clinical Investigation 59: 889–899
58 Gordon D S, Hutton J J, Smalley R V, Meyer L M, Vogler W R 1978 Terminal deoxynucleotidyl transferase (TdT), cytochemistry, and membrane receptors in adult acute leukemia. Blood 52: 1079–1088
59 Hutton J J, Coleman M S, Keneklis T P, Bollum F J 1979 Terminal deoxynucleotidyl transferase as a tumor cell marker in leukemia and lymphoma: results from 1000 patients. In: Fox M (ed) Advances in medical oncology research and education, vol. 4, Biological basis for cancer diagnosis. Pergamon Press, Oxford, pp. 165–175
60 Coleman M S, Hutton J J 1981 Terminal transferase. In: Catovsky D (ed) Methods in hematology, vol. 2, The leukemic cell. Churchill Livingstone, Edinburgh, pp. 203–219
61 McCaffrey R, Lillquist A, Sallan S, Cohen E, Osband M 1981 Clinical utility of leukemia cell terminal transferase measurements. Cancer Research 41: 4814–4820
62 Bell R, Lillquist A, Abelson H, McCaffrey R 1982 Chromatographic forms of terminal deoxynucleotidyl transferase in normal lymphoid cells and in leukemia cells at presentation and relapse. Leukemia Research 6: 775–780
63 Drexler H G, Menon M, Minowada J 1986 Incidence of TdT positivity in cases of leukemia and lymphoma. Acta Haematologica 75: 12–17
64 Sakamoto S, Kano Y, Hida K et al 1981 Terminal transferase in various kinds of leukemia cells and its usefulness as a marker enzyme for vincristine and prednisolone treatment. Acta Haematologica 44: 43–52

65 Sawada H, Tashima M, Kanishi H et al 1981 Characteristics of the blastic crisis with terminal deoxynucleotidyl transferase positive blasts in chronic granulocytic leukemia. Acta Haematologica 44: 872–880
66 Watanabe Y, Tsutsumi Y, Shimosato Y, Shimoyama M, Minato K, Nasao S 1980 Terminal deoxynucleotidyl transferase activity in leukemia and lymphoma, with special reference to adult T-cell related neoplasms. Acta Haematologica 43: 15–25
67 Sasaki R, Takaku F, Aoki T, Bollum F J, Saito T, Dan S 1981 Terminal deoxynucleotidyl transferase activities and glucocorticoid receptors in leukemia. British Journal of Cancer 48: 63–67
68 Bertazzoni U, Brusamolino E, Isernia P et al 1982 Prognostic significance of terminal transferase and adenosine deaminase in acute and chronic myeloid leukemia. Blood 60: 685–692
69 Brusamolino E, Isernia P, Lazzarino M, Scovassi I, Bertazzoni U, Bernasconi C 1984 Clinical utility of terminal deoxynucleotidyl transferase and adenosine deaminase determinations in adult leukemia with a lymphoid phenotype. Journal of Clinical Oncology 2: 871–880
70 Sarin P S 1977 Terminal transferase as a biological marker for human leukemia. Recent Advances in Cancer Research 1: 131–138
71 Wiernik P H, Edwards L S, Sarin P S 1979 Marrow terminal deoxynucleotidyl transferase activity in adult acute leukemia. In: Neth R, Gallo R C, Hofschneider P-H, Mannweiler K (eds) Haematology and Blood Transfusion, vol. 23, Modern trends in human leukemia III. Springer-Verlag, Berlin, pp. 125–130
72 Krause J R, Brody J P, Kaplan S S, Penchansky L 1986 Terminal deoxynucleotidyl transferase activity in acute leukemia: a study of 100 cases comparing an immunoperoxidase (PAP) vs immunofluorescent method. American Journal of Hematology 22: 179–184
73 Srivastava B I S, Khan S A, Henderson E S 1976 High terminal deoxynucleotidyl transferase activity in acute myelogenous leukemia. Cancer Research 36: 3847–3850
74 Srivastava B I S, Khan S A, Minowada J, Henderson E S, Rakowski I 1980 Terminal deoxynucleotidyl transferase activity and blast cell characteristics in adult acute leukemias. Leukemia Research 4: 209–215
75 Ho A D, Helmstädter V, Hunstein W 1982 Immunocytochemical method for the detection of terminal deoxynucleotidyl transferase in acute leukemia. Klinische Wochenschrift 60: 451–455
76 Ho A D, Hunstein W, Ganeshaguru K, Hoffbrand A V, Brandeis W E, Denk B 1982 Therapeutic and prognostic implications of glucocorticoid receptors and terminal deoxynucleotidyl transferase in acute leukemia. Leukemia Research 6: 1–8
77 San Miguel J F, Gonzalez M, Canizo M C, Anta J P, Portero J A, Lopez-Borrasca A 1986 TdT activity in acute myeloid leukemias defined by monoclonal antibodies. American Journal of Hematology 23: 9–17
78 Skoog L, Öst A, Biberfeld P et al 1984 Prognostic significance of terminal transferase activity and glucocorticoid receptor levels in acute myeloid leukemia. British Journal of Cancer 50: 443–449
79 Bearman R M, Winberg C D, Maslow W C et al 1981 Terminal deoxynucleotidyl transferase activity in neoplastic and nonneoplastic hematopoietic cells. American Journal of Clinical Pathology 75: 794–802
80 Bodner S M, Casavant C H, McHugh T M, Stites D P 1985 Comparison of the expression of terminal deoxynucleotidyl transferase and common acute lymphoblastic leukemia antigen in selected hematologic malignancies. Diagnostic Immunology 3: 139–144
81 Castella A, Davey F R, Kurec A S, Thompson N A 1982 Terminal deoxynucleotidyl transferase activity in non-hematologic and hematologic neoplasms. Annals of Clinical and Laboratory Science 12: 403–407
82 Yasmineh W G, Smith B M, Bloomfield C D 1980 DNA nucleotidyldeoxytransferase of normal persons and leukemia patients. Clinical Chemistry 26: 891–895
83 Vogler L B, Christ W M, Bockman D E, Pearl E R, Lawton A R, Cooper M D 1978 Pre-B-cell leukemia. A new phenotype of childhood lymphoblastic leukemia. New England Journal of Medicine 298: 872–878
84 Furukawa K, Tanaka M, Kaneda T et al 1980 Terminal deoxynucleotidyl transferase activity in the blastic cells of acute lymphoblastic leukemia of childhood and adolescents — a predictor of responsiveness to vincristine-prednisolone therapy. Acta Haematologica Japanica 43: 26–32
85 Shurin S, Scillian J J 1983 Absence of terminal transferase may predict failure of remission induction in childhood ALL. Blood 62: 81–84
86 Hutton J J, Coleman M S, Moffitt S et al 1982 Prognostic significance of terminal transferase activity in childhood acute lymphoblastic leukemia: a prospective analysis of 164 patients. Blood 60: 1267–1276
87 Lauer S J, Lyman S, Kirchner P A, Gottschall J L, Camitta B M, Casper J T 1985 Terminal transferase surveillance of remission bone marrows in childhood acute lymphoblastic leukemia:

improved sensitivity with countercurrent centrifugal elutriation. Journal of Clinical Laboratory Immunology 16: 17–22
88 Froehlich T W, Buchanan G R, Cornet J A, Sartain P A, Smith R G 1981 Terminal deoxynucleotidyl transferase-containing cells in peripheral blood: implications for the surveillance of patients with lymphoblastic leukemia or lymphoma in remission. Blood 58: 214–220
89 Barr R D, Koekebakker M, Sarin P S 1984 Early relapse of acute lymphoblastic leukemia is not predictable by serial biochemical assays of terminal transferase activity in cells from peripheral blood. Leukemia Research 8: 351–354
90 Barr R D, Koekebakker M 1984 Detection of circulating 'terminal transferase-positive' cells does not predict relapse in acute lymphoblastic leukemia. Leukemia Research 8: 1051–1055
91 Stass S A, McGraw T P, Folds J D, Odle B, Bollum F J 1981 Terminal transferase in acute lymphoblastic leukemia in remission. American Journal of Clinical Pathology 75: 838–840
92 Mertelsmann R, Moore M A S, Clarkson B 1982 Leukemia cell phenotype and prognosis: an analysis of 519 adults with acute leukemia. Blood Cells 8: 561–583
93 Morisaki T, Fujii H, Miwa S 1985 Adenosine deaminase (ADA) in leukemia: clinical value of plasma ADA activity and characterization of leukemic cell ADA. American Journal of Hematology 19: 37–45
94 Smith S D, Shatsky M, Cohen P S, Warnke R, Link M P, Glader B E 1984 Monoclonal antibody and enzymatic profiles of human malignant T-lymphoid cells and derived cell lines. Cancer Research 44: 5657–5660
95 Morisaki T, Horiuchi N, Fujii H, Miwa S 1986 Characterization of purine nucleoside phosphorylase in leukemia. American Journal of Hematology 23: 263–269
96 Ma D A F, Sylwestrowicz T A, Granger S et al 1982 Distribution of terminal deoxynucleotidyl transferase and purine degradative and synthetic enzymes in subpopulations of human thymocytes. Journal of Immunology 129: 1430–1435
97 Babusikova O, Hrivnakova A, Pechan I, Ujhazy P 1984 Enzymes of purine metabolism and membrane phenotype in malignant cells of some leukemia patients. Neoplasma 31: 661–666
98 Ho A D, Dorken B, Ma D D F, Pezzuto A, Hunstein W, Hoffbrand A V 1986 Purine degradative enzymes and immunological phenotypes in chronic B-lymphocytic leukemia: indications that leukaemic immunocytoma is a separate entity. British Journal of Haematology 62: 545–555
99 Ratech H, Borer W Z, Winberg C D, Rappaport H 1985 Enzymatic differences between chronic lymphocytic leukemia and prolymphocytic leukemia. Leukemia Research 9: 1271–1275
100 Ganeshaguru K, Lee N, Llewellin P et al 1981 Adenosine deaminase concentrations in leukaemia and lymphoma: relation to cell phenotypes. Leukemia Research 5: 215–222
101 Ma D D F, Massaia M, Sylwestrowicz T A, Price G, Hoffbrand A V 1983 Comparison of purine degradative enzymes and terminal deoxynucleotidyl transferase in T-cell leukaemias and in normal thymic and post-thymic T-cells. British Journal of Haematology 54: 451–457
102 Carson D A, Kaye J, Seegmiller J E 1977 Lymphospecific toxicity in adenosine deaminase deficiency and purine nucleoside phosphorylase deficiency: possible role of nucleoside kinase(s). Proceedings of the National Academy of Sciences of the USA 74: 5677–5681
103 Carson D A, Wasson D B, Lakow E, Kamatani N 1984 Biochemical basis for lymphocyte dysfunction in adenosine deaminase and purine nucleoside phosphorylase deficiencies. In: DeBruyn C H M M, Simmonds H A, Muller M M (eds) Advances in experimental medicine and biology, vol. 165B, Purine metabolism in man IV, Part B, Plenum Press, New York, pp. 133–139
104 McCaffrey R, Bell R, Lillquist A, Wright G, Baril E, Minowada J 1983 Selective killing of leukemia cells by inhibition of TdT. In: Neth R, Gallo R C, Greaves M F, Moore M A S, Winkler K (eds) Haematology and blood transfusion, vol. 28, Modern trends in human leukemia. Springer-Verlag, Berlin, pp. 24–27
105 Mitchell B S, Mejias E, Daddona P E, Kelley W N 1978 Purigenic immunodeficiency diseases: selective toxicity of deoxyribonucleosides for T-cells. Proceedings of the National Academy of Sciences of the USA 75: 5011–5014
106 Siaw M F E, Mitchell B S, Koller C A, Coleman M S, Hutton J J 1980 ATP depletion as a consequence of adenosine deaminase inhibition in man. Proceedings of the National Academy of Sciences of the USA 77: 6157–6161
107 Grever M R, Siaw M F E, Jacob W F et al 1981 The biochemical and clinical consequences of 2'-deoxycoformycin in refractory lymphoproliferative malignancy. Blood 57: 406–417
108 Siaw M F E, Coleman M S 1984 In vitro metabolism of deoxycoformycin in human T lymphoblastoid cells: phosphorylation of deoxycoformycin and incorporation into cellular DNA. Journal of Biological Chemistry 259: 9426–9433

109 Grever M R, Coleman M S, Gray D P, Malspeis L, Balcerzak S P, Neidhart J A 1984 Definition of a safe, effective dosing regimen of 2'-deoxycoformycin with biochemical investigation. Cancer Treatment Symposium 2: 43–49
110 Kraut E H, Bouroncle B A, Grever M R 1985 Treatment of hairy-cell leukemia with low dose 2'-deoxycoformycin. Blood 66: 203a
111 Grever M R, Leiby J M, Kraut E H et al 1985 Low dose deoxycoformycin and lymphoid malignancy. Journal of Clinical Oncology 3: 1196–1201
112 Grever M R, Chapman R A, Ratanandotharathorn V, Siease R B 1985 An investigation of deoxycoformycin in advanced cutaneous T-cell lymphoma (CTCL). Clinical Research 33: 853A
113 Coleman M S 1977 Terminal deoxynucleotidyl transferase: characterization of extraction and assay conditions from human and calf tissue. Archives of Biochemistry and Biophysics 182: 525–532
114 Coleman M S 1977 A critical comparison of commonly used procedures for the assay of terminal deoxynucleotidyl transferase in crude tissue extracts. Nucleic Acids Research 4: 4305–5312
115 Bollum F J 1975 Antibody to terminal deoxynucleotidyl transferase. Proceedings of the National Academy of Sciences of the USA 72: 4119–4122
116 Bollum F J 1979 Terminal deoxynucleotidyl transferase as a hematopoietic cell marker. Blood 54: 1203–1215
117 Cibull M L, Coleman M S, Nelson O, Hutton J J, Gordon D, Bollum F J 1982 Evaluation of methods of detecting terminal deoxynucleotidyl transferase for human hematologic malignancies. Comparison of immunofluorescence and enzymatic assays. American Journal of Clinical Pathology 77: 420–423
118 Okamura S, Crane F, Jamal N, Messner H A, Mak T W 1980 Single-cell immunofluorescence assay for terminal transferase: human leukemic and non-leukemic cells. British Journal of Cancer 41: 159–167
119 Bradstock K F, Papageorgiou E S, Janossy G 1981 Diagnosis of meningeal involvement in patients with acute lymphoblastic leukemia: immunofluorescence in terminal transferase. Cancer 47: 2478–2481
120 Lanham G R, Melvin S L, Stass S A 1985 Immunoperoxidase determination of terminal deoxynucleotidyl transferase in acute leukemia using PAP and ABC methods: experience in 102 cases. American Journal of Clinical Pathology 83: 366–370
121 Stass S A, Dean L, Peiper S C, Bollum F J 1982 Determination of terminal deoxynucleotidyl transferase on bone marrow smears by immunoperoxidase. American Journal of Clinical Pathology 77: 174–176
122 Taylor C R 1978 Immunoperoxidase techniques. Archives of Pathology and Laboratory Medicine 102: 113–121
123 Krause J R, Brody J P, Kaplan S S, Penchansky L 1986 Terminal deoxynucleotidyl transferase activity in acute leukemia: a study of 100 cases comparing an immunoperoxidase (PAP) vs immunofluorescent method. American Journal of Hematology 22: 179–184
124 Bettelheim P, Paietta E, Majdic O, Gadner H, Schwarzmeier J, Knapp W 1982 Expression of a myeloid marker on TdT-positive acute lymphocytic leukemic cells: evidence by double-fluorescence staining. Blood 60: 1392–1396
125 Tavares de Castro J, San Miguel J F, Soler J, Catovsky D 1984 Method for the simultaneous labelling of terminal deoxynucleotidyl transferase (TdT) and membrane antigens. Journal of Clinical Pathology 37: 628–632
126 Bollum F J, Augl C, Chang L M S 1984 Monoclonal antibodies to human terminal transferase. Journal of Biological Chemistry 259: 5848–5850
127 Fuller S A, Philips A, Coleman M S 1985 Affinity purification and refined structural characterization of terminal deoxynucleotidyl transferase. Biochemical Journal 231: 105–113
128 Lanham G R, Bollum F J, Stass S A 1986 Detection of terminal deoxynucleotidyl transferase in acute leukemias using monoclonal antibodies directed against native and denatured sites. American Journal of Clinical Pathology 86: 88–91
129 Paietta E, Dutcher J P, Wiernik P H 1985 Terminal transferase positive acute promyelocytic leukemia: in vitro differentiation of a T-lymphocytic/promyelocytic hybrid phenotype. Blood 65: 107–114
130 Coleman M S, Cibull M L, Manderino G L 1985 A new solid-phase immunoassay for terminal deoxynucleotidyl transferase: analysis of TdT antigen in cells, plasma, and serum. Blood 65: 41–45
131 Coleman M S, Ahn Y H, Fairbanks T, Manderino G, Cibull M 1986 Evaluation of a new enzyme-linked immunoassay for terminal deoxynucleotidyl transferase in haematologic malignancies. British Journal of Haematology 62: 311–316
132 Fairbanks T R, King W J, Coleman M S et al 1987 Solid-phase enzyme immunoassay for terminal deoxynucleotidyl transferase (Abbott TdT-EIA) in extracts of whole blood and

mononuclear cells isolated from bone marrow and blood. Journal of Clinical Laboratory Analysis 1: 175–183

133 Coleman M S, Hutton J J 1975 Micromethod for quantitation of adenosine deaminase activity in cells from human peripheral blood. Biochemical Medicine 13: 46–55

134 Chechik B E, Sen Gupta S 1981 Detection of human, rat and mouse adenosine deaminase by immunochemical and immunomorphologic methods using antiserum to calf enzyme. Journal of Immunological Methods 45: 165–176

135 Sen Gupta S, Petsche D, Gelfand E W, Chechick B E 1985 A flow cytometric method for the detection of adenosine deaminase in mononuclear cells. Journal of Immunological Methods 80: 155–162

136 Philips A V, Robbins D R, Barkley M D, Coleman M S 1987 Immunoaffinity purification and fluorescence studies of human adenosine deaminase. Biochemistry 26: 2893–2903

137 Renouf J A, Thong Y H, Chalmers A H 1985 A rapid, simple method for the micro-estimation of purine nucleoside phosphorylase activity in peripheral blood lymphocytes. Clinica Chimica Acta 151: 311–316

9
Lymphocyte Functional Assays

F. Miedema

INTRODUCTION

The development of monoclonal antibodies (McAbs) recognizing leukocyte differentiation antigens has allowed precise definition of lymphocyte and granulocyte/monocyte differentiation stages in humans. Moreover, genomic probes that identify rearranging genes of the immunoglobulin (Ig) and the T-cell receptor have become available in the last years. Together with the classic technics of characterizing B-cells by surface or cytoplasmic Ig and myeloid and lymphoid cells by histocytochemical (enzyme) staining, these new methods have resulted in a significant progress in the classification of leukemia and lymphoma (reviewed by Foon and Todd[1]). Concomitantly, the identification of B-and T-cell differentiation stages, subpopulations and lineages has led to detailed functional studies of these McAb-defined lymphoid subpopulations.

In this chapter, the variety of functional properties exhibited by mature T-cell subpopulations and B-cells will be dealt with. First, how these functional activities can be measured in the laboratory will be outlined. Secondly, results of functional studies on human B- and T-cell malignancies will be reviewed, and their contribution to classification and possible clinical relevance briefly discussed.

LYMPHOCYTE FUNCTIONAL ASSAYS

T-CELL PROLIFERATION TESTS

In the normal immune response, T-cells are activated through binding of antigen in the context of major histocompatibility complex (MHC) to the T-cell receptor (TCR) for antigen. T-cells can be stimulated in vitro by soluble antigen, but this induces only weak responses because only a minority of peripheral blood cells have specificity for a particular antigen. A larger portion of T-cells can be stimulated in a mixed leukocyte reaction (MLR), where the stimulating antigen is an alloantigen on stimulator cells, i.e. monocytes and B-cells. Traditionally, T-cell activation was studied with lectins such as phytohemagglutinin (PHA), concanavalin A (ConA) and pokeweed mitogen (PWM). These lectins are polyclonal stimulators and induce proliferation in almost all T-cells. Recently, it has become clear that membrane molecules expressed on T-cells may act as signal transducers in T-cell activation. These structures, which are defined by McAbs, include the TCR in complex with CD3,[2] CD2 (the E-rosette receptor)[3] and Tp44/CD28.[4,5] McAbs against these molecules induce T-cell proliferation when combined with each other.[5,6] It has been shown that the lectins PHA and ConA trigger T-cells by binding to TCR/TCD3 and CD2 antigens.[7,8]

T-cell proliferation induced either by lectins, MLR or McAbs involves production of the T-cell-derived lymphokine interleukin-2 (IL-2)[9,10] and the induction of IL-2 receptors (IL-2R) detected by the McAb anti-Tac.[11,12] Anti-IL-2R McAbs inhibit these IL-2-induced T-cell functions.[12] The dependence of T-cell proliferation on monocytes has been shown to be due most probably to monocyte-derived IL-1.[12] Recently, it has been shown that triggering by CD3, antigen or lectins induces a rise in intracellular Ca^{2+} and that the phorbol ester PMA (phorbol myristate acetate) can replace the IL-1/monocyte signal. Together, PMA and calcium ionophore, which aspecifically give(s) rise to intracellular Ca^{2+}, can mimic the monocyte-dependent induction of T-cell proliferation by lectins or McAbs.[13] PMA is structurally related to diacylglycerol which, upon activation of cells, activates protein kinase C.[13] Both the rise in Ca^{2+} and activation of protein kinase C are believed to be important events leading to IL-2 production and IL-2R expression, and to cell proliferation.

METHODS

Isolation of peripheral blood mononuclear cells (MNC) from anti-coagulated blood by Ficoll–Isopaque density gradient centrifugation is a routine procedure.[14] For lectin-, McAb- or IL-2-induced T-cell proliferation, 40 000 cells are cultured in flat-bottomed wells of microtiter plates (Nunc, 96F, Roskilde, Denmark), in 200 µl Iscove's Modified Dulbecco's medium (IMDM: Gibco, Grand Island, NY, USA) supplemented with 5% human pooled serum, penicillin (100 IU/ml) and streptomycin (100 µg/ml). The following stimuli can be used: PHA, 1 µg/ml (Wellcome, Beckenham, UK); ConA, 10 µg/ml (Sigma, St Louis, MO, USA); PWM, 50 µg/ml (Gibco); rIL-2, 10 U/ml (Biogen or Sandoz); CD2, CD3 and CD28 McAbs are used as diluted ascites; PMA is used at 1–10 ng/ml. In the MLR, T-cells are stimulated in a 1:1 ratio with 30 gy irradiated allogeneic MNC. Proliferation induced by PMA, ConA, CD3 and CD2 is measured by a 4-h [^{3}H]thymidine pulse (0.2 µCi/well = 7.4 kBq/well, specific activity 2 Ci/mol) on day 3, whereas proliferation induced by PWM, IL-2 or MLR is measured on day 7. When highly purified T-cells or monocyte-poor patient cells are tested in proliferation assays, 10 000–20 000 irradiated normal donor monocytes should be added.[15]

HELPER T-CELL ACTIVITY

For the evaluation of T-cell regulatory functions, a culture system is used in which B-cells are polyclonally stimulated by PWM in the presence of T-cells and accessory cells (monocytes) (reviewed by Waldmann and Broder[16]). PWM does not directly bind to and stimulate purified B-cells,[17-18] but is thought to bind monocytes (accessory cells) and is presented by monocytes to T-cells.[19] T-cells with helper activity reside in the T-cell subpopulation that has the CD3+, CD4+ CD8- phenotype.[20,21] Evidence has accumulated that distinct functional subpopulations within the CD4+ T-cell population can be defined, which harbor the actual helper-cell activity.[22-24]

It has been shown that, regarding the mechanism of T-helper activity, rIL-2, like PWM can induce Ig synthesis in a fashion that is dependent on T-helper cell.[25,26] Since anti-IL-2R McAb inhibits PWM-induced B-cell differentiation, PWM induces IL-2 production[25] and IL-2 induces release of helper factors by T-helper cells,[27] it was concluded that PWM acts via the induction of IL-2 production as a first important step[28] (Fig. 9.1).

Recently it has been found that anti-CD3 McAbs induce T-cell-dependent Ig synthesis.[29] The triggering of T-cells via the TCR/CD3+ complex to release helper factors for B-cell differentiation was not dependent on the production of IL-2.[29] These results indicate that T-cells triggered by antigen/MHC via the TCR/CD3 complex may respond by independently releasing IL-2 and helper factors, whereas the PWM-induced helper factor release seems to be dependent on IL-2 production. Over the last 5 years, antigen-specific T-helper activity has been described in systems driven by influenza, tetanus toxoid and keyhole limpet hemocyanin (KLH).[30-32] Antigen-specific culture systems, however, cannot be used to analyse functional properties of clonal neoplastic T- or B-cells and will not, therefore, be further discussed.

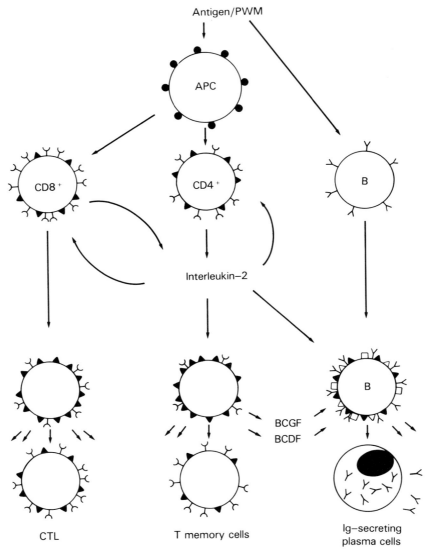

Fig. 9.1 Pivotal role for IL-2 in both the humoral and cellular immune response. ▲, IL-2 receptor; △, BCGF receptor; □, BCDF receptor.

METHODS

In the authors' laboratory, a microculture system has been developed that allows the study of a large number of culture conditions with only a small number of B-cells or T-helper cells per culture.[33–36]

Lymphocyte preparation

Mononuclear cells from healthy donors and patients are isolated from defibrinated or heparinized blood by Percoll (Pharmacia, Uppsala, Sweden) density gradient centrifugation.[14] To remove residual serum Ig, the cells are washed six times in Earle's balanced salt solution supplemented with 5% fetal calf serum (FCS).

T- and non-T-cells are separated by E-rosette sedimentation, using sheep red blood cells treated with neuraminidase[33] or 2-amino-ethyl-isothiouronium bromide hydrobromide (Sigma).[37] For the separation of human T-cell subpopulations, based on their reactivity with anti-T-cell McAbs, a panning technic is used.[38] Briefly, plastic dishes (Falcon 3002F) are coated overnight with 300 µg affinity-purified sheep anti-mouse IgG in phosphate-buffered saline (PBS). Pelleted cells (5×10^6) are incubated with 1:500 diluted McAb-containing ascites or purified McAb, for 30 min at 4°C. The cells are washed and applied to the dishes (15×10^6/dish). After 60–120 min incubation on ice, the non-adherent cells are harvested.

Lymphocytes from normal donors, either separated in non-T- and T-cells or unseparated, and patients' cells can be cryopreserved without loss of functional capacity.

Assessment of helper activity on IgM and IgG production by B-cells

To measure T-helper activity, graded numbers ($0-160 \times 10^3$) of T-cells are added to a constant number of B-cells, or non-T-cells containing 10–30% B-cells ($20-40 \times 10^3$), in wells of round-bottomed microtiter plates (Greiner, Nürtingen, FRG), in a final volume of 170 µl IMDM (Iscore's Modified Dulbecco's Medium), supplemented with 10% FCS and antibiotics. Careful selection of FCS batches, to avoid toxic effects and high background Ig production is recommended in the absence of PWM. The cultures are stimulated either with: PWM (50 µg/ml), rIL-2 (10 U/ml) or insolubilized (coated) anti-CD3 McAbs (1:8000 ascites dilution; 0.5 µg/ml) (Van Lier and Aarden, unpublished data). Supernatants are harvested after 7 days of culture and stored at −20°C.

Enzyme-linked immunoassay (ELISA) for quantitation of Ig production in supernatants

IgM and IgG concentrations in culture supernatants are measured by an enzyme-linked immunosorbent assay (ELISA). The ELISA is performed in flat-bottomed wells of polystyrene 96-well microtiter plates (Dynatech M129A), coated with rabbit anti-IgM or anti-IgG antibodies that have been affinity purified (obtained from the authors' institute). Wells are coated with 0.1 ml antibody (2 µg/ml) in 0.02 mol/l phosphate buffer pH 7.5 overnight at 4°C. The plates are washed four times with tap water; then 0.1 ml of sample is added and incubated for 2 h at 37°C. After washing, 0.1 ml peroxidase-conjugated rabbit antibodies against human IgM or IgG (Dakopatts, Copenhagen, Denmark) are added in Tris-HCl buffer (0.2 mol/l, pH 7.5), supplemented with 20% normal rabbit serum and 0.1% Tween 20. After incubation (2 h, 37°C) and washing, 0.1 ml substrate (3,5,3′,5′-Tetramethylbenzidin (Merck), 0.1 mg/ml and H_2O_2 (0.015%) in citrate buffer are added. The enzymatic reaction is stopped by adding 100 µl 4 N sulfuric acid per well. The absorbance at 450 nm of individual wells is determined with a Titertek Multiscan. Ig contents are quantified using a reference sample with known IgM and IgG content.[34]

Results of a typical experiment, comparing the helper activity of normal CD4+ and CD8+ T-cells in the system driven by PWM and IL-2, are shown in Fig. 9.2.[25] Note that non-T-cells alone do not produce any IgM, and helper activity is delivered by T4+ (CD4+) but not T8+ (CD8+) cells.

SUPPRESSOR T-CELL ACTIVITY

The regulatory activity of T-cells with suppressor activity is measured in the same microculture system described on the previous pages. Suppressor activity, defined as abrogation of B-cell differentiation by relatively low suppressor effector cell numbers, resides in the CD8+ T-cell subpopulation.[20,21] CD8+ cells can be divided into two populations defined by reactivity with the McAb Leu8;[39] the two populations themselves have no suppressor activity but mixtures of the two act as suppressor cells.[39] In addition, suppressor activity has been demonstrated in CD4+ cells that had been pre-activated.[40,41]

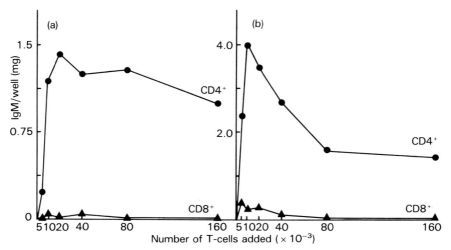

Fig. 9.2 Kinetics of helper activity in PWM- and IL-2-driven culture systems. Graded numbers of either CD4+ cells or CD8+ cells were added to 40 000 non-T-cells and cultured 7 days in the presence of 50 µg/ml PWM (A) or 30 U/ml IL-2 (B). (Reproduced from Miedema et al[25] with permission of the publishers.)

Once it had been established that IL-2 is an important intermediary lymphokine in PWM-driven Ig synthesis by B-cells, investigations were carried out as to whether depletion of IL-2 by suppressor cells caused suppression. The data suggest that the suppressive effect is not at the IL-2 level but probably at the level of helper-factor production by CD4 + helper cells.[25,28,42]

SUPPRESSOR-INDUCER ACTIVITY

It has been shown that collaborative interactions between T-cells are required for the induction of T-suppressor effector cells.[39,43,44] Recently, a McAb 2H4 was described that binds to the suppressor-inducer cells in the CD4 + compartment.[45]

METHODS

Suppressor activity of T-cell populations is tested by adding graded numbers of the cells to a mixture of 20–40 × 10^3 non-T-cells and 10–20 × 10^3 CD4 + cells of a normal donor in the presence of PWM or rIL-2. Culture conditions and Ig measurement are the same as for helper assays. The numbers of CD4 + helper cells are chosen such that the amount of help is suboptimal, allowing an optimal differentiation between help and suppression when effector cells are added.[33,39] Figure 9.3 shows suppressor activity by CD8 + cells and activated CD4 + (T4 +) cells, and the abrogating effect of irradiation on suppressor activity.

CYTOTOXIC ACTIVITIES: ANTIBODY-DEPENDENT CELLULAR CYTOTOXICITY (ADCC) OR KILLER (K) CELL ACTIVITY AND NATURAL KILLER (NK) ACTIVITY

Cytotoxic CD8 + T-cells recognize antigens, such as viral proteins expressed on the cell membrane of infected cells, in the context of predominantly class I major histocompatibility complex (MHC) antigens.[20] For functional analysis of neoplastic T-cell populations,

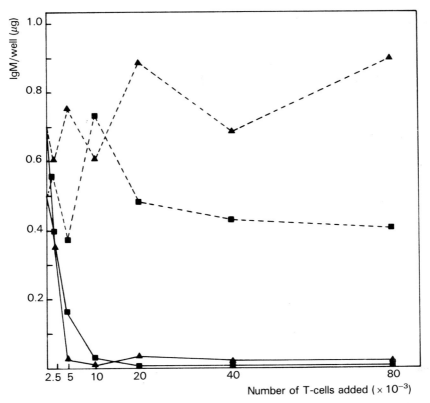

Fig. 9.3 Suppression of PWM-induced IgM synthesis by normal CD8 + and PWM-activated CD4 + cells. Graded numbers of either CD8 + cells (■——■), 40 Gy irradiated CD8 + cells (■---■), PWM-activated CD4 + cells (▲——▲) or 40 Gy irradiated activated CD4 + cells (▲---▲) were added to a mixture of 20 000 non-T-cells and 5000 CD4 + cells. IgM was measured on day 7.

antigen-specific cytotoxicity cannot be evaluated and, therefore, only non-specific cytotoxicity will be discussed here.

Next to specific cytotoxicity, exhibited by CD3 + T-cells restricted by MHC molecules, cytotoxicity, which is non-MHC restricted by human lymphocytes, has been described. In the case of ADCC, target cells sensitized by antibodies are lysed by lymphocytes that express receptors for the Fc portion of IgG (FCR), detected by McAbs of the CD16 group (CLB-FCR1, B73.1/Leu11).[46–48] NK cell activity is the non-specific lysis of tumor cells by lymphoid cells in the MNC fraction. Phenotypically, cells with ADCC and NK cell activity are: CD3 +, CD16 +, CD11b +, CD11b – or CD3 –, CD11b +, CD16 +.[49–51] Proportionally the largest population mediating ADCC and NK cell activity is the CD3 –, CD11b +, CD16 + population.[51]

METHODS

K cell activity is measured with P815 mouse mastocytoma cells, sensitized with rabbit IgG antibodies, as target cells.[46] NK cell activity is measured using myeloid/erythroblastoid K562 cells as target cells. The K562 cell line is cultured continuously in IMDM/20% FCS. Lymphocytes to be tested as effector cells are routinely precultured overnight in IMDM-/FCS, after being thawed out or isolated from the blood. Target cells are labeled with

100 μCi (3.7 MBq) Na$_2^{51}$CrO$_4$ by incubation at 37°C for 1 h. In the case of P815 cells, rabbit antibodies are added during the last half hour of the incubation. Then, the cells are washed extensively to remove free ^{51}Cr and excess rabbit antibody. In the K cell assay, 40 000 target cells are used per well of a round-bottomed microtiter plate, in the NK cell assay 10 000 target cells are used. Effector cells in a E:T ratio of maximally 2.5 and 20, respectively, in the K and the NK cell assay are used. The final volume per well is adjusted to 200 μl. The plates are incubated for 4 h at 37°C after centrifugation (10 min, 400 × g). After incubation, ^{51}Cr release in the supernatant is counted in a gamma counter. Supernatants are harvested by harvesting devices of the Titertek Supernatant Collection System (Flow Laboratories). Controls should include determination of ^{51}Cr release from target cells in the absence of effector cells (spontaneous release: S), and in the presence of 5% saponin (maximal release: M). The percentage of specific release (R) can be calculated as follows:

$$R = \frac{E - S}{M - S} \times 100\%$$

in which E represents the experimental release.

Figure 9.4 shows the results of NK and K cell assay for two controls and a patient. Lymphocytes of all three individuals, including the patient, showed good cytotoxic activities.

B-CELL ACTIVATION AND PROLIFERATION

B-cells are activated by binding of antigen to its receptor, the membrane Ig molecule and by a subsequent interaction with T-helper cells. T-cells become activated by antigen presented by the antigen-specific B-cells or by antigen-presenting cells,[53] both cell–cell interactions being MHC restricted. The activation of T-helper cells induces them to release soluble factors that act on B-cells.[54] The activation of resting B-cells by antigen can be mimicked by

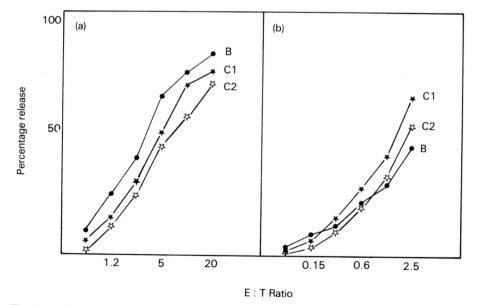

Fig. 9.4 NK (A) and K (B) cell activity of mononuclear cells of two normal controls (C1 and C2) and of a patient (B). Abscissa: effector:target ratio; ordinate; percentage ^{51}Cr release from target cells. (Reproduced from Miedema et al[52] with permission of the publishers.)

anti-μ, anti-δ and *Staphylococcus* Cowan I (SAC), which directly bind membrane Ig.[55,56] T-cell-derived factors, which co-stimulate in anti-μ and SAC-induced B-cell proliferation, have been described.[54,58,59] A small number have been fully characterized and cloned, including IL-2,[59] BSF-1(IL-4)[60] and interferon-γ.[57,61] In addition, a high-molecular-weight B-cell growth factor (HMW-BCGF) has been described.[62] B-cells which respond to anti-μ have been shown to be CD20+, CD21+, whereas the more differentiated CD20+, CD21− cells do not proliferate to anti-μ.[63]

Recent work, analogous to functional studies on T-cell antigens,[3-8] has identified some of the B-cell differentiation antigens to be involved in B-cell proliferation: CD20,[64-68] CD21,[69,70] CD19,[68] CD22,[71] CDW40 (BP50)[66,72] and CD23 (P45).[73] What the natural, physiological ligands for these receptors are and what signals are transduced through the membrane has not been disclosed as yet. The intracellular signals induced by anti-μ are composed of both a rise in free Ca^{2+} concentration and protein kinase C activation, and can be mimicked by PMA in combination with calcium ionophore.[74-77]

B-CELL DIFFERENTIATION

Terminal differentiation of B-cells following the induction to proliferation is also dependent on T-cells or T-cell-derived factors. B-cell differentiation can be studied in the PWM- and SAC-driven systems.[15-17,25,56,78] The major B-cell population in peripheral blood tonsil or spleen populations, which is responsive to PWM, SAC and supplemental T-helper cells, has been described as belonging to an sIgD−, large-size and low-density B-cell population which expresses the B-cell activation antigen 4F2.[78-80] These in vivo activated memory B-cells produce IgG, with IgA and IgM as well.[80] Only a little IgM, but no IgG or IgA, is produced by virgin IgD+ B-cells.[80] A small population of resting memory B-cells which are IgD− and 4F2− produce IgM, IgG and IgA.[80] Because it is difficult to prepare B-cell populations free from residual T-cells or monocytes, some work has been carried out with Epstein–Barr virus-transformed B-cell lines[81] that are mature and respond to BCDF-like factors (BCDF = B-cell differentiation factor, or interleukin-6). Recently, a factor IL-6 has been cloned with BCDF activity[81] that appeared to be identical to a previously cloned gene product designated interferon β2,[82] and a monocyte-derived factor with BCGF-like (B-cell growth factor) activity cloned in the authors' institute by Aarden and co-workers.[83]

METHODS

B-cells are isolated from MNC or tonsillar lymphocytes by depletion of T-cells through E-rosette sedimentation and subsequent treatment of the non-T-cell fraction with anti-pan-T-cell McAb, anti-monocyte/myeloid McAb and complement.[26] Suspensions obtained are up to 85% CD19+ and less than 2% CD3/CD2+.[26] For B-cell proliferation a variety of culture conditions is used. In general, relatively large numbers ($5-10 \times 10^4$) of B-cells are cultured in flat-bottomed wells of microtiter plates (Nunc) in RPMI or IMDM, 10% FCS or human pooled serum, 5×10^{-5} mol/l 2-mercaptoethanol.[57,59,61] PWM (50 μg/ml) plus irradiated T-cells, and SAC plus irradiated T-cells, may be used as classic stimulators. SAC and anti-μ antibodies, in combination with T-cell-conditioned medium or well-defined factors such as interleukin-4 (IL-4), γ-interferon and IL-2, may be used.[57,60,61,78] As stimulus, a combination of PMA (1–3 ng/ml) and calcium ionophore A23187 can also be used.[77] [^{3}H]Thymidine incorporation after an 18-h pulse on day 3 or day 4 is measured.

For B-cell differentiation measured by Ig synthesis in the culture supernatant, cultures are performed in round-bottomed wells of microtiter plates (Greiner) in 200 μl of RPMI-1640 or IMDM as described above. Cells can be stimulated by SAC and PWM (50 μg/ml) in the presence of T-cells[25-27,33-36] or soluble T-cell-derived factors.[84-86] Cumulative Ig production is measured from day 7 to day 12 of culture, depending on the system used. High numbers of B-cells are cultured when soluble factors are used combined with SAC or anti-μ;[85,86] relatively low numbers (20 000–40 000) are cultured when T-cells are present.[25-27,33-36]

FUNCTIONAL STUDIES WITH NEOPLASTIC T-AND B-LYMPHOCYTES

INTRODUCTION

Functional studies employing cloned T-cells or clonal neoplastic T-cells have contributed to the understanding of the relationship between T-cell phenotype and function. These investigations have contributed to a better insight into the maturation arrest of the malignant cells, and to a better classification of the various lymphoproliferative disorders. Below, the contribution of these studies to solving controversies regarding classification of CD4+ T-cell neoplasia and to the recognition of Tγ lymphocytosis as a more benign T-cell expansion within the spectrum of T-cell malignancies will be discussed.

Recent advances in functional studies of B-cell neoplasia will be reviewed in the light of newly identified growth and differentiation signals for B-cells.

FUNCTIONAL ANALYSES OF CD4+ T-CELL MALIGNANCIES

Sézary syndrome

The best known example of a T-cell malignancy with helper activity on polyclonal B-cell differentiation is Sézary syndrome.[87-89] The original reports on helper activity provided by Sézary T-cells appeared before T-cell differentiation antigens CD4 and CD8 were described. Later it was demonstrated that the neoplastic T-cells were CD2+, CD3+, CD4+, CD7−, CD8−.[89,90] Generally, CD7 is expressed on all T-cell neoplasias except Sézary syndrome and adult T-cell leukemia/lymphoma (ATLL).[91,92] Helper activity in vitro is not always reflected in in vivo hypergammaglobulinemia.[87-89,91] In one Sézary patient with a marked IgE hypergammaglobulinemia, the malignant T-cells provided strong subclass-specific helper activity for IgE synthesis in vitro by normal B-cells.[93] The neoplastic T-cells of a non-allergic, non-Hodgkin's lymphoma patient with elevated serum IgE, released factors that induced IgE synthesis in B-cells of patients with allergic rhinitis.[94] The leukemic helper cells expressed Fc_E receptors.[80] Recently a Sézary T-cell ('switch T-cell') was described that, in contrast to normal T-cells, could induce IgG and IgA synthesis in B-cells of patients with hyper-IgM syndrome and IgA deficiencies.[95,96]

Contrary to previously published reports,[73,74,76] in a series of six Sézary syndrome patients studied in the authors' laboratory, leukemic CD4+ cells with helper activity in the PWM-driven system were not present.[96,97] However, when tested on IL-2-driven B-cell differentiation, which is also CD4+ T-helper cell dependent,[25] T-cells of one Sézary patient showed good helper activity.[97] The tumor cells lacked helper activity in the PWM-driven system due to the inability to produce IL-2 upon stimulation with PWM and other lectins.[27,97] In these neoplastic T-cells the capacity to produce IL-2 and the capacity to release helper factors for B-cell differentiation are dissociated.[27,97,98] In these studies, the clonal CD4+ T-cells were used to prove that, in the PWM-driven system, two distinct events are required, which are separated in the neoplastic T-cells but inseparable in normal CD4+ T-cell population.[97,98] Lack of helper activity in the PWM-driven system, observed with neoplastic T-cells of many patients with T-ALL, T-PLL, ATL and T-CLL, may well be due to lack of IL-2 production capacity.[97-99] Since anti-CD3 induces Ig synthesis by normal B-cells in a T-cell-dependent manner, the non IL-2-producing, T-CLL cells were also tested in that system. It was found that the neoplastic CD4 + cells that were able to help in the IL-2-driven system also provided helper activity in the anti-CD3-driven system.[29] In a restricted number of patients with mature T-cell leukemia, with CD4 +, CD8 - helper phenotype, helper activity in the PWM-driven system has been reported (reviewed by Miedema and Melief[98]).

T-PLL

A number (eight) of these patients suffered from T-prolymphocytic leukemia (T-PLL) with the characteristic morphology of large non-granular lymphocytes with nucleoli.[97,100-104] Although a substantial portion of T-PLL cases lack functional activity,[97,99,100,103,104] these results indicate that T-PLL cells are derived from phenotypically and functionally mature T-cells that have sometimes retained helper functions, and the capacity to proliferate and produce IL-2.[97] This is an example where functional studies may contribute to the classification of T-cell leukemias, showing that the term 'prolymphocytic' may be at least misleading.[99,101,102]

T-CLL

T-helper activity has been reported for a few cases of CD4 + T-CLL;[101,102-107] however, most cases of T-CLL with helper phenotype tested in the authors' laboratory lacked functional activity.[36,97,98,104]

ATLL

Within the CD4 + T-cell malignancies of the mature type, ATLL is a distinct clinicopathological entity. There is controversy as to whether ATLL can be morphologically and clinically discriminated from T-PLL[100-102] or from Sézary syndrome and T-CLL by the expression of IL-2R.[89,99] The major distinction is the etiological involvement in ATLL of human T-cell leukemia virus (HTLV-I).[108,109] Functionally, the leukemic CD4 + ATLL cells have suppressor activity in the majority of cases tested.[89,92,110-113] Helper function by neoplastic CD4 + T-cells of patients with HTLV-I-associated T-cell lymphoma, clinically distinct from ATLL, has been reported.[114] The classification of CD4 + T-cell neoplasia, however, is complex, since HTLV-I -, IL-2R + or IL-2R - Sézary cells have been described that have suppressor activity like ATLL cells.[39,90,115]

Despite the expression of IL-2R on ATLL cells, the neoplastic T-cells do not proliferate in response to IL-2.[116] It appears that IL-2R expression is abnormally regulated and non-functional, since the receptor is not down-regulated by anti-IL-2R McAbs.[116,117]

DISCRIMINATION OF Tγ LYMPHOCYTOSIS BY IMMUNOLOGICAL AND FUNCTIONAL STUDIES FROM T-CLL

Detailed immunological studies with the expanded T-cells in a large series of patients revealed that, within the spectrum of T-CLL, a distinct subgroup of patients suffering from a benign form of T-cell leukemia could be distinguished.[104,118-126] The leukemic cells have the morphological characteristics of granular lymphocytes that are also designated NK cells in normal blood.[126,127] Generally, the proliferating T-cells have the CD2 +, CD3 +, CD8 + phenotype, bear receptors for Fcγ (CD16) and sometimes express the myeloid marker OKM1/Mol (CD11b) (reviewed by Miedema and Melief[98] and Miedema et al[121]). In some rare cases the Tγ-cells co-express CD4 and CD11b markers.[124] Both normal Tγ-cells and expanded Tγ-cells in patients express large amounts of CD11a (LFA-1α) and CD18 (LFA-1β) leukocyte-adhesion molecules compared to CD16 - T-cells.[128,129] The clonality and hence malignant character of Tγ lymphocytosis has been amply documented over the last 5 years. Clonal rearrangements of genes encoding the T-cell receptor for antigen have been shown in at least the CD3-expressing neoplastic Tγ-cells.[130-132]

Functional studies have made a major contribution to the recognition of Tγ lymphocytosis within the T-CLL group.[104,118,133] Unlike malignant T-cells in other leukemias, the Tγ-cells exerted K cell (ADCC) activity in most of the patients tested.[121,134] In a minority of cases the Tγ-cells had both K and NK activity.[104,123] In one patient studied in the authors' laboratory, the expanded Tγ-cells were active as suppressor cells in PWM-driven Ig synthesis.[104]

Recognition of a T-CLL being Tγ lymphocytosis is of clinical importance since it is now clear that generally these patients have a favorable prognosis and do not require cytotoxic chemotherapy, unlike the outright T-CLL or T-PLL patients.[104,110,118,121,125,126,134] Moreover, spontaneous regression in a Tγ-lymphocytosis patient, which is associated with reversal of the anemia and neutropenia often found with Tγ lymphocytosis,[120,121,125,126] has been described.[135]

FUNCTIONAL STUDIES WITH NEOPLASTIC B-CELLS

Investigations aimed at the elucidation of the maturation arrest in B-cell neoplasias, in relationship to normal B-cell ontogeny, have used phenotypic, molecular biological and functional methods. On the basis of the newly developed B-cell differentiation markers, B-cell tumors may be ranked in maturation order from B-ALL, B-NHL, B-CLL, B-PLL, HCL to plasmacytomas and myelomas.[1]

B-CLL

Functional studies with malignant B-cells have demonstrated that it is possible to induce some B-CLL cells to proliferate and differentiate with SAC, PWM, and PWM together with SAC and allogeneic helper cells or soluble factors.[136-142] B-CLL cells never responded to anti-μ alone,[142,143] nor to a combination of anti-μ and BCGF.[143] In almost all cases tested, B-CLL cells could be induced to differentiate to Ig-secreting plasma cells by PMA.[144-147] PMA induces IL-2 receptors on B-CLL cells, and some B-CLL cells have been shown to proliferate and differentiate to recombinant IL-2.[148-150] The latter findings and the observation that B-CLL cells absorb IL-2,[150] strongly suggest a role in vivo for IL-2 in the growth of malignant B-cells.

In the authors' laboratory a series of seven B-PLLs, were studied for functional properties in PWM, SAC, IL-2 and PMA inducibility. The neoplastic B-cells of one B-PLL showed a good proliferative response to interferon-γ and were induced to Ig synthesis by as few as 300 T-helper cells in the presence of PWM, IL-2 or the McAb anti-CD3.[151,152] Interestingly, the neoplastic cells proliferated in response to anti-class II McAbs in combination with PMA, whereas normal B-cell functions were not directly affected by this class II McAb.[153,154]

Hairy cell leukemia

The neoplastic B-cells in hairy cell leukemia (HCL) are believed to be mature B-cells. Phenotypically, the HCL cells are characterized by the expression of IL-2 receptors on fresh tumor cells[155] and of the myeloid monocytic marker CD11c (gp 150, 95), a member of the family of cellular adhesion molecules.[156] Although HCL cells were found to be unable to proliferate and differentiate when stimulated with standard B-cell mitogens (anti-μ, SAC, PWM), proliferation could be induced by BCGF preparations.[157,158] This BCGF-induced proliferation was somewhat enhanced by anti-μ antibodies, and was inhibited by $α_2$-interferon but not γ-interferon.[158] Since the mechanism of $α_2$-interferon therapy of HCL is not precisely known, these studies implicate a direct growth-inhibiting effect to be one mechanism.

B-cell-derived B-cell growth factors
Of interest is the finding that malignant B-cells or EBV-transformed B-cells produce B-cell growth factors.[157,159-161] This opens up the possibility of an autocrine model of B-cell growth which may be important in B-cell neoplasia. It could be envisaged that dysregulation of B-cell growth factors can, via an autocrine pathway, lead directly to uncontrolled B-cell proliferation in B-cell malignancy.

Anti-idiotype antibodies and B-cell growth
Since immunotherapy with anti-idiotype McAbs has been tried on patients,[162,163] although with little success, effects of these McAbs on the function of the neoplastic B-cells has been studied in the authors' laboratory. Interestingly, with a panel of anti-idiotypic McAbs, differential effects were observed on B-PLL cell functions in vitro.[164] These results suggest that functional studies in vitro may provide immunobiological criteria for selection of the McAbs to be used for immunotherapeutic protocols.

ACKNOWLEDGEMENTS

The author is indebted to Drs M A de Rie, R A W Van Lier, W P Zeijlemaker and A E G Kr von dem Borne for critical reviewing of the manuscript.

The work was supported by grant CLB-80-2 and IKA 87-20 of the Koningin Wilhelmina Fonds, The Netherlands Cancer Organization.

Since the submission of this chapter, ample evidence has been reported on the role of IL-6 in B-cell malignancies, in particular myelomas.

REFERENCES

1. Foon K A, Todd R F 1986 Immunological classification of leukemia and lymphoma. Blood 68: 1-31
2. Wauwe J P V van, de Mey J R, Goossens J G 1980 OKT3: a monoclonal anti-human T lymphocyte antibody with potent mitogenic properties. Journal of Immunology 124: 2708-2713
3. Meuer S C, Hussey R E, Fabbi M et al 1984 An alternative pathway of T-cell activation. A functional role for the 50 kd T11 sheep erythrocyte receptor. Cell 36: 897-906
4. Hara T, Fu S M, Hansen J A 1985 Human T cell activation. II. A new activation pathway used by a major T cell population via a disulfide-bonded dimer of a 44 kD polypeptide (9.3). Journal of Experimental Medicine 161: 1513-1524
5. Van Lier R A W, Brouwer M, Zeijlemaker W P, Aarden L A 1987 Induction of T cell proliferation by monoclonal antibodies. Anti-Tp44 monoclonal antibodies link the CD3 and CD2 pathways of T-cell activation. In: McMichael A J (ed) Leucocyte typing III. Oxford, Oxford University Press, pp 170-172
6. Clark E A, Ledbetter J A 1986 Amplification of the immune response by agonistic antibodies. Immunology Today 7: 267-270
7. Valentine M A, Tsoukas C D, Rhodes G, Vaughan J H, Carson D A 1985 Phytohemagglutinin binds to the 20 kDa molecule of the T3 complex. European Journal of Immunology 15: 851-854
8. Roosnek E E, van Lier R A W, Aarden L A 1987 Personal communication
9. Robb R J 1984 Interleukin 2: the molecule and its function. Immunology Today 5: 203-209
10. Roosnek E E, Brouwer M C, Kipp J B, Aarden L A 1986 Monocyte-dependent induction of proliferation of human peripheral T cells by recombinant IL-2. European Journal of Immunology 16: 35-40
11. Meuer S C, Hussey R E, Cantrell D A, Hogdon J C, Schlossman S F 1984 Triggering of the T3-Ti antigen-receptor complex results in clonal T-cell proliferation through an interleukin 2-dependent autocrine pathway. Proceedings of the National Academy of Sciences of the USA 81: 1509-1513
12. Depper J M, Leonard W J, Robb R J, Waldmann T A, Greene W C 1983 Blockade of the interleukin-2 receptor by anti-Tac antibody: inhibition of human lymphocyte activation. Journal of Immunology 131: 690-696

13 Imboden J B, Weiss A, Stobo J D 1985 Transmembrane signalling by the T3-antigen receptor complex. Immunology Today 6: 328-331
14 Boyum A 1976 Isolation of lymphocytes from peripheral blood. Scandinavian Journal of Immunology 5 (supplement)
15 Rümke H C, Terpstra F G, Huis B, Out Th A, Zeijlemaker W P 1982 Immunoglobulin production in human mixed lymphocyte cultures: implications for co-cultures of cells from patients and healthy donors. Journal of Immunology 128: 696-701
16 Waldmann T A, Broder S 1982 Polyclonal B-cell activators in the study of the regulation of immunoglobulin synthesis in the human system. Advances in Immunology 32: 1-63
17 Keightley R G, Cooper M D, Lawton A R 1976 The T-cell dependence of B cell differentiation induced by pokeweed mitogen. Journal of Immunology 117: 1538-1544
18 Janossy G, Greaves M 1975 Functional analysis of murine and human B lymphocyte subsets. Transplantation Reviews 24: 177-236
19 Stevenson H C, Miller P J, Waxdal M J, Haynes B F, Thomas C A, Fauci A S 1983 Interaction of pokeweed mitogen with monocytes in the activation of human lymphocytes. Immunology 49: 633-640
20 Reinherz E L, Meur S C, Schlossman S F 1983 The human T-cell receptor: analysis with cytotoxic T cell clones. Immunological Reviews 74: 83-112
21 Thomas Y, Rogozinski L, Chess L 1983 Relationship between human T cell functional heterogeneity and human T cell surface molecules. Immunological Reviews 74: 113-128
22 Morimoto C, Letvin N L, Boyd A W et al 1985 The isolation and characterization of the human helper inducer T-cell subset. Journal of Immunology 134: 3762-3769
23 Van Lier R A W, Borst J, Vroom T M et al 1987 Tissue distribution, biochemical and functional properties of Tp55 (CD27), a novel T-cell differentiation antigen. Journal of Immunology 139: 1589-1596
24 Van Lier R A W, Oudkerk-Pool M, Mous S et al 1988 Anti-CD27 monoclonal antibodies identify CD27 two functionally distinct T cells within the CD4 T-cell subset. European Journal of Immunology 18: 811-816
25 Miedema F, van Oostveen J W, Sauerwein R, Terpstra F G, Aarden L A, Melief C J M 1985 Induction of immunoglobulin synthesis by interleukin-2 is T4 + 8 - cell dependent. A role for interleukin 2 in the pokeweed mitogen-driven system. European Journal of Immunology 15: 107-112
26 Sauerwein R W, van der Meer W G J, Dräger A, Aarden L A 1985 Interleukin 2 induces T cell dependent IgM production in human B cells. European Journal of Immunology 15: 611-616
27 Miedema F, Sauerwein R W, Terpstra F G, van Oostveen J W, Melief C J M 1986 Dual role of T4 + helper cells in in-vitro immunoglobulin synthesis by human B cells: IL-2 production and IL-2-induced release of helper factors. In: Sauerwein R W, Thesis, University of Amsterdam, Amsterdam
28 Miedema F, Melief C J M 1985 T-cell regulation of human B-cell activation. A reappraisal of the role of IL-2. Immunology Today 6: 258-259
29 Sauerwein R W, van der Meer W G J, van Oostveen J W, Miedema F, Aarden L A 1988 Anti-CD3 antibodies induce T-helper function for human B-cell differentiation in vitro by an interleukin 2-independent pathway. European Journal of Immunology 18: 133-137
30 Yarchoan R, Murphy B R, Strober W, Schneider H S, Nelson D L 1981 Specific anti-influenza virus antibody production in vitro by human peripheral blood mononuclear cells. Journal of Immunology 127: 2588-2598
31 Volkman D, Lane H C, Fauci A S 1981 Antigen-induced in vitro antibody production in humans. A model for B cell activation and immunoregulation. Proceedings of the National Academy of Sciences of the USA 78: 2528-2531
32 Lane H C, Whalen G, Fauci A S 1983 Antigen induced human T cell help. Journal of Clinical Investigation 72: 636-647
33 Rümke H C, Terpstra F G, Out T A, Vossen J M, Zeijlemaker W P 1981 Immunoglobulin production by human lymphocytes in a microculture system: culture conditions and cellular interactions. Clinical Immunology and Immunopathology 19: 338-350
34 Rümke H C, Terpstra F G, Roos M Th L et al 1984 Bone marrow transplantation in man. Analysis of T and B cell functions in PWM driven Ig production. Clinical and Experimental Immunology 57: 467-478
35 Rümke H C 1986 Pokeweed mitogen driven immunoglobulin synthesis. A study of B and T cell functions in health and disease. Thesis, University of Leiden, Leiden
36 Miedema F 1985 Immunobiology of normal and neoplastic human T cells. Thesis, University of Amsterdam, Amsterdam

37 Pellegrino M A, Ferrone S, Dierich M P, Reisfeld R A 1975 Enhancement of sheep red blood-cell human lymphocyte rosette formation by the sulfhydryl compound 2-amino-ethyl isothiouronium bromide. Clinical Immunology and Immunopathology 3: 324–333
38 Reinherz E L, Penta A C, Hussey R E, Schlossman S F 1981 A rapid method for separating functionally intact human T lymphocytes with monoclonal antibodies. Clinical Immunology and Immunopathology 21: 257–266
39 Gatenby P A, Kansas G S, Zian C Y, Evans R L, Engleman E G 1982 Dissection of immunoregulatory subpopulations of T lymphocytes within the helper and suppressor sublineages in man. Journal of Immunology 129: 1997–2000
40 Miedema F, Willemze R, Terpstra F G, van Vloten W A, Meijer C J L M, Melief C J M 1984 Regulatory activity of neoplastic T cells in Sézary syndrome on in-vitro immunoglobulin production. Leukemia Research 8: 873–884
41 Thomas Y, Rogozinski L, Irigoyen O et al 1982 Functional analysis of human T-cell subsets defined by monoclonal antibodies. V. Suppressor cells within the OKT4+ population belong to a distinct subset. Journal of Immunology 128: 1386–1390
42 Thomas Y, Sosman Y, Rogozinski L et al 1981 Functional analysis of human T cell subsets defined by monoclonal antibodies. III Regulation of helper factor production by T cell subsets. Journal of Immunology 126: 1948–1951
43 Thomas Y, Sosman J, Irigoyen O et al 1980 Functional analysis of human T-cell subsets defined by monoclonal antibodies. Collaborative T–T interaction in the immunoregulation of B cell differentiation. Journal of Immunology 125: 2402–2408
44 Morimoto C, Reinherz E L, Borel Y, Schlossman S F 1983 Direct demonstration of the human suppressor-inducer subset by anti-T cell antibodies. Journal of Immunology 130: 157–161
45 Morimoto C, Letvin N L, Distaso J A, Aldrich W R, Schlossman S F 1985 The isolation and characterization of the human suppressor inducer T-cell subset. Journal of Immunology 134: 1508–1515
46 Van Oers M H J, Zeijlemaker W P, Schellekens P Th A 1977 Separation and properties of EA-rosette-forming lymphocytes in humans. European Journal of Immunology 7: 143–150
47 Werner G, von dem Borne A E G Kr, Bos M J E et al 1986 Localization of the human NA1 alloantigen on neutrophil Fc-γ-receptors. In: Reinherz E L, Haynes B F, Nadler L M, Bernstein I (eds) Leucocyte typing II (vol. 3) Springer Verlag, New York, pp 109–121
48 Perussia B, Acuto O, Terhorst C et al 1983 Human natural killer cells analysed by B73. A monoclonal antibody blocks Fc receptor functions. Journal of Immunology 130: 2142–2148
49 Griend R J van de, Ten Berge I, Tanke H J et al 1982 Characterization of subsets of human Tγ cells. Journal of Immunology 128: 1979–1985
50 Zarling J M, Clouse K A, Biddison W E, Kung P C 1981 Phenotypes of human natural killer cell populations detected with monoclonal antibodies. Journal of Immunology 127: 2575–2580
51 Lanier L L, Phillips J H 1986 Evidence for three types of human cytotoxic lymphocytes. Immunology Today 7: 132–134
52 Miedema F, Tetteroo P A T, Terpstra F G et al 1985 Immunological studies with LFA-1 and Mo1 deficient lymphocytes from a patient with recurrent bacterial infections. Journal of Immunology 134: 3075–3081
53 Lanzavecchia A 1985 Antigen-specific interaction between T and B cells. Nature 314: 537–539
54 Paul W E 1985 Living with lymphocytes. International Archives of Allergy and Applied Immunology 77: 7–12
55 Sieckmann D G 1980 The use of anti-immunoglobulin to induce a signal for cell division in B lymphocytes via their surface membrane IgM and IgD. Immunological Reviews 52: 181–220
56 Romagnino S, Giudizi M G, Biagotti T et al 1981 Surface immunoglobulins are involved in the interaction of protein A-containing *Staphylococcus aureus*. Journal of Immunology 127: 1307–1313
57 Kehrl J H, Muraguchi A, Butler J L, Falkoff R J M, Fauci A S 1984 Human B cell activation, proliferation and differentiation. Immunological Reviews 78: 75–96
58 Saiki O, Ralph P 1982 Induction of human immunoglobulin secretion. T lymphocyte dependency and radiosensitivity of T-cell help for induction of B-cell differentiation by *S. aureus* Cowan I. Cellular Immunology 70: 301–310
59 Mingari M C, Gerosa F, Carra G et al 1984 Human interleukin-2 promotes proliferation of activated B cells via surface receptors similar to those of activated T cells. Nature 312: 641–643
60 Lee F, Yokota T, Otsuka T et al 1986 Isolation and characterization of a mouse interleukin cDNA clone that expresses B cell stimulating factor 1 activities and T-cell and mast-cell stimulating activities. Proceedings of the National Academy of Sciences of the USA 83: 2061–2065

61 Romagnino S, Giudizi G M, Maggi E et al 1985 Synergy of B cell growth factor and interleukin 2 in the proliferation of activated human B cells. European Journal of Immunology 15: 1158–1164
62 Ambrus J L, Jurgensen C H, Brown E J, Fauci A S 1985 Purification for homogeneity of a high molecular weight human B cell growth factor: demonstration of specific binding to activated B cells, and development of a monoclonal antibody to the factor. Journal of Experimental Medicine 162: 1319
63 Anderson K C, Boyd A W, Fisher D C et al 1985 Isolation and functional analysis of human B cell populations. I. Characterization of the B1 + B2 + and B1 + B2 − subsets. Journal of Immunology 134: 820–827
64 Golay J T, Clark E A, Beverley P C L 1985 The CD20 (Bp35) antigen is involved in activation of B cells from the G0 to the G1 phase of the cell cycle. Journal of Immunology 135: 3795–3801
65 Tedder T F, Boyd A W, Freedman A S, Nadler L M, Schlossman S F 1985 The B cell surface molecule B1 is functionally linked with B cell activation and differentiation. Journal of Immunology 135: 973–979
66 Clark E A, Ledbetter J A 1986 Activation of human B cells mediated through two distinct cell surface differentiation antigens, Bp35 and Bp50. Proceedings of the National Academy of Sciences of the USA 83: 4494–4498
67 Clark E A, Shu G 1987 Activation of human B-cell proliferation through surface Bp35 (CD20) polypeptides or immunoglobulin receptors. Journal of Immunology 138: 720–725
68 de Rie M A, Terpstra F G, van Lier R A W, von dem Borne A E G Kr, Miedema F 1987 Identification of functional epitopes on Workshop-defined B-cell membrane molecules. In: McMichael et al (eds) Leucocyte typing III, Oxford University Press, Oxford, p 402
69 Wilson B S, Platt J L, Kay N E 1985 Monoclonal antibodies to the 140 000 mol wt glycoprotein of B lymphocyte membranes (CR2 receptor) initiates proliferation of B cells in vitro. Blood 66: 824–829
70 Nemerow G R, McNaughton M E, Cooper N R 1985 Binding of monoclonal antibody to the Epstein Barr virus/CR2 receptor induces activation and differentiation of human B lymphocytes. Journal of Immunology 135: 3068–3073
71 Pezzuto A, Dörken B, Moldenhauer G, Clark E A 1987 Amplification of human B cell activation by a monoclonal antibody to the B cell-specific antigen CD22, Bp130/140. Journal of Immunology 138: 98–103
72 Ledbetter J A, Shu G, Gallagher M, Clark E A 1987 Augmentation of normal and malignant B cell proliferation by monoclonal antibody to the B cell specific antigen Bp50 (CDW 40). Journal of Immunology 138: 788–794
73 Gordon J, Rowe M, Walker L, Guy G 1986 Ligation of the CD23, p45 (Blast-2, EBVCS) antigen triggers the cell-cycle progression of activated B lymphocytes. European Journal of Immunology 16: 1075–1080
74 Pozzan T, Arslan P, Tsien R Y, Rink T J 1982 Anti-immunoglobulin, cytoplasmic free calcium and capping in B lymphocytes. Journal of Cell Biology 94: 335–340
75 Bijsterbosch M K, Meade C J, Turner G A, Klaus G G B 1985 B lymphocyte receptors and phosphoinositide degradation. Cell 41: 999–1006
76 Paul W E, Mizuguchi J, Brown M et al 1986 Regulation of B-lymphocyte activation, proliferation and immunoglobulin secretion. Cell Immunology 99: 7–13
77 Clevers M C, Verstegen J M T, Logtenberg T, Gmelig-Meyling F H J, Ballieux R E 1985 Synergistic action of A23187 and phorbol ester on human B cell activation. Journal of Immunology 135: 3827–3830
78 Saiki O, Ralph P 1981 Induction of immunoglobulin secretion. Synergistic effect of B cell mitogen Cowan I plus T cell mitogens or factors on induction of immunoglobulin synthesis. Journal of Immunology 127: 1044–1047
79 Kuritani T, Cooper M D 1982 Human B cell differentiation. II Pokeweed mitogen responsive B cells belong to a surface immunoglobulin-D negative subpopulation. Journal of Experimental Medicine 155: 1561–1566
80 Jelinek D F, Splawski J B, Lipsky P E 1986 Human peripheral blood B lymphocyte subpopulations: function and phenotypic analysis of surface IgD positive and negative subsets. Journal of Immunology 136: 83–92
81 Hirano T, Yasukawa, Harada H et al 1986 Complementary DNA for a novel human interleukin (BSF-2) that induces B lymphocytes to produce immunoglobulin. Nature 324: 73–76
82 Billiau A 1986 BSF-2 is not just a differentiation factor: Letter. Nature 324: 415

83 Brakenhoff J P J, De Groot E R, Evers R F, Pannekoek H, Aarden L A 1987 Molecular cloning and expression of hybridoma growth factor in *E. coli*. Journal of Immunology 139: 4116–4121
84 Muraguchi A, Fauci A S 1982 Proliferative responses of normal human B lymphocytes. Development of an assay system for human B cell growth factor. Journal of Immunology 129: 1104–1108
85 Nakagawa T, Hirano T, Nakagawa N, Yoshizaki K, Kishimoto T 1985 Effect of recombinant IL-2 and γIFN on proliferation and differentiation of human B cells. Journal of Immunology 134: 959–966
86 Kehrl J H, Muraguchi A, Goldsmith P K, Fauci A S 1985 The direct effects of interleukin 1, interleukin 2, interferon-α, interferon-γ, B cell growth factor, and a B-cell differentiation factor on resting and activated human B cells. Cell Immunology 96: 38–48
87 Broder S, Edelson R L, Lutzner M A et al 1976 The Sézary syndrome. A malignant proliferation of helper T cells. Journal of Clinical Investigation 58: 1297–1306
88 Siegal F P, Siegal M 1977 Enhancement by irradiated T cells of human plasma cell production: dissection of helper and suppressor functions in vitro. Journal of Immunology 118: 642–647
89 Waldman T A, Greene W C, Sarin P S et al 1984 Functional and phenotypic comparison of human T cell leukemia/lymphoma virus positive adult T cell leukemia with HTLV negative Sézary leukemia, and their distinction using anti-Tac. Journal of Clinical Investigation 73: 1711–1718
90 Greaves M F, Rao J, Hariri G et al 1981 Phenotypic heterogeneity and cellular origins of T-cell malignancies. Leukemia Research 5: 281–299
91 Haynes B F, Bunn P, Mann D L et al 1981 Cell surface differentiation antigens of the malignant T cells in Sézary syndrome and mycosis fungoides. Journal of Clinical Investigation 67: 523–530
92 Miedema F, Terpstra F G, Smit J W et al 1984 Functional properties of neoplastic T cells in adult T cell lymphoma/leukemia patients from the Caribbean. Blood 63: 477–481
93 Mitsuya H, Sato M, Hirano T, Fujimoto K, Kawano F, Kishimoto S 1983 Evidence for a malignant proliferation of IgE-class specific helper T cells in a patient with Sézary syndrome exhibiting massive hyperimmunoglobulinemia E. Clinical Immunology and Immunopathology 26: 171–183
94 Young M C, Harfi H, Sabbah R, Leung D Y, Geha R S 1985 A human T cell lymphoma secreting an immunoglobulin E specific helper factor. Journal of Clinical Investigation 75: 1977–1982
95 Mayer L, Posnett D N, Kunkel H G 1985 Human malignant T cells capable of inducing an immunoglobulin class switch. Journal of Experimental Medicine 161: 134–144.
96 Mayer L, Kwan S P, Thompson C et al 1986 Evidence for a defect in switch T cells in patients with immunodeficiency and hyperimmunoglobulinemia. New England Journal of Medicine 314: 409–413
97 Miedema F, van Oostveen J W, Terpstra F G et al 1985 Analysis of helper activity on PWM- and IL-2-driven immunoglobulin synthesis by neoplastic T4+ cells. Journal of Clinical Investigation 76: 2139–2143
98 Miedema F, Melief C J M 1986 Immunobiology of the expanded T cells in T cell leukemia and Tγ lymphocytosis. Leukemia Research 10: 469–474
99 Pandolfi F, de Rossi G, Ranucci A et al 1985 Tac-positive, HTLV-negative T helper phenotypic chronic lymphocytic leukemia cells. Blood 65: 1531–1537
100 Pandolfi F, de Rossi G, Lauria F et al 1985 T helper phenotype chronic lymphocytic leukaemia and adult T-cell leukaemia in Italy. Lancet II: 633–636
101 Catovsky D, Matutes E, Moss V, Brito-Babapulle V 1985 T-cell leukaemias with helper phenotype in adults. Lancet ii: 945–946
102 Pandolfi F, de Rossi G, Semenzato G 1985 T-helper-phenotype leukaemias: role of HTLV-I. Lancet ii: 1367–1368
103 Lauria F, Foa R, Raspadori D et al 1985 T-cell prolymphocytic leukemia: a clinical and immunological study. Scandinavian Journal of Haematology 35: 319–324
104 Rümke H C, Miedema F, ten Berge I J M et al 1982 Functional properties of T cells in patients with chronic Tγ lymphocytosis and chronic T-cell neoplasia. Journal of Immunology 129: 419–426
105 Foon F A, Naiem F, Saxon A, Stevens R, Gale R P 1981 Leukemia of T-helper lymphocytes: clinical and functional features. Leukemia Research 5: 1–10.
106 Gramatzki M, Dolan M F, Fauci A S, Maples J A, Bonnard G D, Strong D M 1982 Immunological characterization of a helper T-cell lymphoma. Blood 59: 702–708

107 Simpkins H, Kiprov D D, Davis J L, Morand P, Puri S, Grahn E P 1985 T cell chronic lymphocytic leukemia with lymphocytes of unusual immunological phenotype and function. Blood 65: 127–133
108 Hinuma Y, Komoda H, Chose T et al 1982 Antibodies to adult T-cell leukemia virus-associated antigen (ATLA) in sera from patients with ATL and controls in Japan. A nation-wide sero-epidemiologic study. International Journal of Cancer 29: 631–635
109 Blattner W A, Kalyanaraman V S, Robert-Guroff M et al 1982 The human type-C retrovirus, HTLV, in blacks from the Caribbean region and relationship to adult T-cell leukemia/lymphoma. International Journal of Cancer 30: 257–264
110 Uchiyama T, Yodoi J, Sagawa K, Takatsuki K, Uchino H 1977 Adult T-cell leukemia: clinical and hematological features in 16 cases. Blood 50: 481–492
111 Hattori T, Uchiyama T, Toibana T, Takatsuki K, Uchino H 1981 Surface phenotype of Japanese adult T-cell leukemia cells characterized by monoclonal antibodies. Blood 58: 645–647
112 Yamada Y 1983 Phenotypic and functional analysis of leukemic cells from 16 patients with adult T-cell leukemia/lymphoma. Blood 61: 192–199
113 Morimoto C, Matsuyama T, Oshige C et al 1985 Functional and phenotypic studies of Japanese adult T-cell leukemia cells. Journal of Clinical Investigation 75: 836–843
114 Yamada Y, Amagasaki T, Kamihira S et al 1985 T lymphomas associated with human T-cell leukemia-lymphoma virus may show phenotypic and functional differences from adult-T cell leukemias. Clinical Immunology and Immunopathology 36: 306–319
115 Golstein M M, Farnarier-Seidel C, Daubrey P, Kaplanski S 1986 An OKT4+ T-cell population in Sézary syndrome: attempts to elucidate its lack of proliferative capacity and its suppressive effect. Scandinavian Journal of Immunology 23: 53–64
116 Uchiyama T, Hori T, Tsudo M et al 1985 Interleukin-2 receptor (Tac antigen) expressed on adult T cell leukemia cells. Journal of Clinical Investigation 76: 446–453
117 Tsudo M, Uchiyama T, Uchino H, Yodoi J 1983 Failure of regulation of Tac antigen/TCGF receptor on adult T-cell leukemia cells by anti-Tac monoclonal antibody. Blood 61: 1014–1016
118 Bom-van Noorloos A A, Pegels H G, van Oers R J et al 1980 Proliferation of Tγ cells with killer-cell activity in two patients with neutropenia and recurrent infections. New England Journal of Medicine 302: 933–937
119 Aisenberg A C, Wilkes B H, Harris N L, Ault K A, Carey R W 1981 Chronic T-cell lymphocytosis with neutropenia: report of a case studied with monoclonal antibodies. Blood 58: 818–822
120 Reynolds C W, Foon K A 1985 Tγ lymphoproliferative disease and related disorders in humans and experimental animals: a review of the clinical, cellular and functional characteristics. Blood 64: 1146–1158
121 Miedema F, Terpstra F G, Smit J W, van der Veen J P W, Melief C J M 1985 Tγ lymphocytosis is clinically non-progressive but immunologically heterogeneous. Clinical and Experimental Immunology 61: 440–449
122 Itoh K, Tsuchikawa K, Awataguchi T, Scriba K, Kumagai K 1983 A case of chronic lymphocytic leukemia with properties characteristic of natural killer cells. Blood 61: 940–948
123 Schlimok G, Thiel E, Rieber E R et al 1982 Chronic leukemia with a hybrid surface phenotype (T lymphocytic/myelomonocytic): leukemia cells displaying natural killer activity and antibody-dependent cellular cytotoxicity. Blood 59: 1157–1162
124 Moss V, Miedema, F, Matutes E et al 1986 An unusual variant of T-CLL: evidence for the existence of a hitherto unrecognised T-cell subset. Clinical and Experimental Immunology 63: 303–311
125 Newland A C, Catovsky D, Linch D et al 1984 Chronic T cell lymphocytosis: a review of 21 cases. British Journal of Haematology 58: 433–446
126 Pandolfi F, Mandelli F, Semenzato G, Ranucci A, Aiuti F 1984 Classification of patients with T cell chronic lymphocytic leukemia and expansions of granular lymphocytes: heterogeneity of Italian cases by a multi-parameter analysis. Journal of Clinical Immunology 4: 174–184
127 Smit J W, Blom N R, van Luyn H J A, Miedema F, Melief C J M, Halie M R 1985 T cells in patients with chronic Tγ lymphocytosis: morphology, cytochemistry, ultrastructure and immunological characteristics. Blut 51: 83–95
128 Miedema F, Tetteroo P A T, Hesselink W G, Werner G, Spits H, Melief C J M 1984 Both Fc receptors and lymphocyte function-associated antigen 1 on human Tγ lymphocytes are required for antibody-dependent cellular cytotoxicity. European Journal of Immunology 14: 518–522
129 Miedema F, Tromp H, van 't Veer M B, Poppema S, Melief C J M 1985 LFA-1 is a marker of mature immunocompetent cells. A survey of lymphoproliferative diseases in man. Leukemia Research 9: 1099–1104

130 Knowles D M, Dalla-Favera R, Pelicci P-G 1985 T-cell-receptor β-chain gene rearrangements. Lancet ii: 159–160
131 Rambaldi A, Pelicci P-G, Allavena P et al 1985 T cell receptor β chain rearrangements in lymphoproliferative disorders of large granular lymphocytes/mature killer cells. Journal of Experimental Medicine 162: 2156–2162
132 Waldmann T A, Davis M M, Bongiovanni K F, Korsmeyer S J 1985 Rearrangements of genes for the antigen receptor on T cells as markers of lineage and clonality in human lymphoid neoplasms. New England Journal of Medicine 313: 776–783
133 Pandolfi F, Strong D M, Slease R B, Smith M L, Ortaldo J R, Herberman R B 1980 Characterization of a suppressor T-cell chronic lymphocytic leukemia with ADCC but not NK activity. Blood 56: 653–660
134 Gastl G, Rumpold H, Kraft D et al 1986 Abnormal expansions of granular lymphocytes: reactive lymphocytosis or chronic leukemia. Case report and literature review. Blut 52: 73–89
135 Winton E F, Chan W C, Check I, Colenda K W, Bongiovanni K F, Waldmann T A 1986 Spontaneous regression of a monoclonal proliferation of large granular lymphocytes associated with reversal of anemia and neutropenia. Blood 67: 1427–1432
136 Fu S M, Chiorazzi N, Kunkel H G, Halper J P, Harris S R 1978 Induction of in vitro differentiation and immunoglobulin synthesis of human leukemic B lymphocytes. Journal of Experimental Medicine 148: 1570–1578
137 Nowell P, Shankey T V, Finan J, Guerry D, Besa E 1981 Proliferation, differentiation and cytogenetics of chronic leukemic B lymphocytes cultured with mitomycin-treated normal cells. Blood 57: 444–451
138 Robert K-H 1979 Induction of monoclonal antibody synthesis in malignant human B cells by polyclonal B-cell activators. Immunological Reviews 48: 123–143
139 Rubartelli A, Sitia R, Grossi C E, Ferrarini M 1985 Maturation of chronic lymphocytic leukemia B cells: correlation between the capacity of responding to T-cell factors in vitro and the stage of maturation reached in vivo. Clinical Immunology and Immunopathology 34: 296–303
140 Bloem A C, Bast E J E G, Gmelig Meyling F H J, de Gast G C, Ballieux R E 1982 Mitogenic stimulation of malignant B cells. Chronic lymphocytic leukaemia: relationship between stimulation and surface phenotype. Clinical and Experimental Immunology 50: 355–359
141 Johnstone A P, Jensenius J C, Millard R E, Hudson L 1982 Mitogen-stimulated immunoglobulin production by chronic lymphocytic leukaemic lymphocytes. Clinical and Experimental Immunology 47: 697–705
142 Tamaki T, Yonezawa T, Kanakura Y et al 1986 Mitogenic response of neoplastic B cells: comparison of reactivity to *Staphylococcus aureus* Cowan I and anti-immunoglobulins. Clinical and Experimental Immunology 64: 181–187
143 Perri R T 1986 Impaired expression of cell surface receptors for B cell growth factor by chronic lymphocytic leukemia B cells. Blood 67: 943–948
144 Tötterman T H, Nilsson K, Sundström C 1980 Phorbol ester-induced differentiation of chronic lymphocytic leukaemia cells. Nature 288: 176–178
145 Cossman J, Neckers L M, Braziel R M, Trepel J B, Korsmeyer S J, Bakhsh A 1984 In vitro enhancement of immunoglobulin gene expression in chronic lymphocytic leukemia. Journal of Clinical Investigation 73: 587–592
146 Efremidis A P, Haubenstock H, Holland J F, Bekesi J G 1985 TPA-induced maturation in secretory human B-leukemic cells in vitro, DNA synthesis, antigenic changes and immunoglobulin secretion. Blood 66: 953–960
147 Gordon J, Mellstedt H, Aman P, Biberfeld P, Klein G 1984 Phenotypic modulation of chronic lymphocytic leukemia cells by phorbol ester: induction of IgM secretion and changes in the expression of B-cell associated surface antigens. Journal of Immunology 132: 541–547
148 Kabelitz D, Pfeffer K, von Steldern D, Bartmann P, Brudler O, Nerl C, Wagner H 1985 In vitro maturation of B cells in chronic lymphocytic leukemia. Synergistic action of phorbol ester and interleukin 2 in the induction of Tac antigen expression and interleukin 2 responsiveness in leukemic B cells. Journal of Immunology 135: 2876–2881
149 Mayer L, Crow M K, Thompson C 1985 Synergy between B-cell differentiation factors and interleukin 2, using a monoclonal system. Journal of Immunology 135: 3272–3276
150 Foa R, Giovarelli M, Jemma C et al 1985 Interleukin 2 (IL-2) and interferon γ production by T lymphocytes from patients with chronic lymphocytic leukemia: evidence that normally released IL 2 is absorbed by the neoplastic B cell population. Blood 66: 614–619
151 Sauerwein R W 1986 Regulation of human B cell proliferation and differentiation by T cells and T-cell-derived factors. Thesis, University of Amsterdam, Amsterdam

152 Sauerwein R W, van der Meer W G J, Aarden L A 1987 Induction of proliferation of B-prolymphatic leukemia cells by phorbol ester and native or recombinant interferon-γ. Blood 70: 670–675
153 Rie M A de, Kabel P, Sauerwein R W, van Lier R A W, von dem Borne A E G Kr, Melief C J M, Miedema F 1987 Anti-HLA class-II monoclonal antibodies inhibit polyclonal B-cell differentiation in vitro at the accessory-cell level. European Journal of Immunology 17: 881–886
154 Sauerwein R W, de Rie M A, Van der Meer W G J, Miedema F, Aarden L A 1988 Regulation of malignant B-cell proliferation by direct binding of HLA class II antibodies. Cell Immunology 114: 424–431
155 Korsmeyer S J, Greene W C, Cossman J et al 1983 Rearrangement and expression of immunoglobulin genes and expression of Tac antigen in hairy cell leukemia. Proceedings of the National Academy of Sciences of the USA 80: 4522–4526
156 Schwarting R, Stein H, Wang C Y 1985 The monoclonal antibodies αS-HCL 1 (αLeu14) and αS-HCL 3 (αLeuM5) allow the diagnosis of hairy cell leukemia. Blood 65: 974–983
157 Ford R J, Kwok D, Quesada J, Sahasrabuddhe C G 1986 Production of B cell growth factor(s) by neoplastic B cells from hairy cell leukemia patients. Blood 67: 573–577
158 Paganelli K A, Evans S S, Han T, Over H 1986 B cell growth factor-induced proliferation of hairy cell lymphocytes and inhibition by Type I interferon in vitro. Blood 67: 937–942
159 Jurgensen C J, Ambrus J L, Fauci A S 1986 Production of B-cell growth factor by normal human B cells. Journal of Immunology 136: 4542–4547
160 Gordon J, Ley S C, Melamed M D, English L S, Hughes-Jones N C 1984 Immortalized B lymphocytes produce B-cell growth factor. Nature 310: 145–147
161 Ambrus J L, Fauci A S 1985 Human B cell lymphoma cell line producing B cell growth factor. Journal of Clinical Investigation 75: 732–739
162 Miller R A, Maloney D G, Warnke R, Levy R 1982 Treatment of B-cell lymphoma with monoclonal anti-idiotype antibody. New England Journal of Medicine 306: 517–522
163 Meeker T C, Lowder J, Maloney D G, Miller R A, Thielemans K, Warnke R, Levy R 1985 A clinical trial of anti-idiotype therapy for B-cell malignancy. Blood 65: 1349–1363
164 de Rie M A, van Lier R A W, Imholz M J M, Schumacher T N M, Van Schyndel G M W, Miedema F 1989 Requirements for induction of activation and proliferation of human B-cells analysed with anti-idiotype monoclonal antibodies. Scandinavian Journal of Immunology 30: 249–257
165 Kishimoto T 1989 The biology of interleukin-6. Blood 74:1–10

10
The Clonal Culture in vitro of Human Myeloid Leukemic Cells

Donald Metcalf

INTRODUCTION

This chapter will be restricted to a discussion of methods for the primary culture of myeloid leukemic cells in semisolid cultures and discussion of what the in vitro culture of leukemic cells has revealed about the nature and origin of leukemia. A number of continuously propagatable culture lines of human leukemic cells exist but the establishment of such lines often involves major cell selection during initiation of the cultures, and subsequent mutations are common when cell lines proliferate continuously in vitro. Because of this, continuous lines cannot provide reliable information on the nature of primary leukemia, and, of course, cannot provide information on the subsets of leukemic cells in an individual patient or on the interactions between normal and leukemic populations in a given patient. Liquid culture systems for hemopoietic cells have many uses but changes in the number or differentiation of a particular cell type in cultures of complex hemopoietic populations are difficult to interpret. Cell input and output can be monitored well enough but liquid cultures are 'black boxes' that do not permit events such as proliferation of differentiation to be related to individual cells or their progeny.

Progress in recent years in understanding the cellular events in normal or leukemic hemopoiesis has come almost entirely from the application of semisolid culture technics in which the progeny of individual cells can be identified because they remain in a fixed location as a colony or cluster of cells. By means of this technology, most of the various hemopoietic ancestral cells can now be enumerated and characterized (see review by Metcalf[1]), and the same cultures have proved to be very sensitive bioassay systems for the detection and analysis of regulatory factors controlling both normal and leukemic hemopoiesis. Based on this newer information, it is now possible to perform fairly selective liquid cultures for certain cell types. These liquid cultures certainly have some uses, but semisolid cultures remain the most useful method for the characterization of normal and leukemic populations sampled directly from the human subject.

A SHORT HISTORY OF SEMISOLID CLONING

The first semisolid culture technics were introduced in 1966 with the simultaneous demonstration by Bradley and Metcalf[2] and Ichikawa et al[3] that colonies of normal mouse neutrophilic granulocytes and/or macrophages could be grown in semisolid agar cultures of mouse hemopoietic cells. Such colonies were shown to be clones produced by the proliferation and differentiation of the specific precursor cells (progenitor or colony-forming cells) of this double hemopoietic family. Most mouse granulocyte–macrophage colony-forming cells (GM-CFC or CFU-C) were shown to be bi-potential and capable of giving rise to both polymorphs and monocyte–macrophages.[1,4] The proliferation of such colonies was shown to depend absolutely on the presence in the culture medium of an adequate concentration of one or more of a group of specific glycoproteins, known as the colony-stimulating factors (CSFs).[1]

In subsequent studies, it was shown that mouse myeloid or myelomonocytic leukemic cells could be grown in the same type of agar culture, and again colony formation and differentiation of the leukemic colony cells were found to depend on stimulation by CSF.[5-7]

The agar culture system was adapted by Pike and Robinson[8] to permit the clonal growth in vitro of colonies of human granulocytes and monocyte–macrophages. Much of the initial work with this system was performed using underlayers of peripheral blood cells to stimulate colony formation and analysis showed that the cells in the underlayer released the CSF necessary for stimulation of colony formation.[9-11] Media conditioned by peripheral blood cells were also found to be able to stimulate colony formation.[12]

It was pointed out by Chervenick and Boggs[13] that this type of human marrow culture also developed colonies of eosinophils and these have since been analysed by morphological and histological studies.[14-17]

During this work, it was demonstrated that colonies or clusters of granulocyte–macrophage cells could regularly be grown from the marrow or blood of patients with acute or chronic myeloid leukemia and the neoplastic nature of the cells was confirmed by karyotypical examination of the proliferating cells.

Stephenson et al[18] introduced a semisolid culture technic, based on plasma clots and the use of erythropoietin, that permitted the clonal proliferation of relatively mature erythroid precursors (colony-forming units–erythroid; CFU-E). Following improvements in the media and the use of higher concentrations of erythropoietin, these cultures also supported the growth of large, often multicentric, erythroid colonies originating from the most ancestral progenitor cells in the erythropoietic series – the so-called burst colony-forming units–erythroid (BFU-E).[19] Both technics have been modified to permit the growth of corresponding cells from human marrow and peripheral blood.[20]

Further studies developed methods for culturing megakaryocyte colonies from murine hemopoietic cells,[21] and this procedure has also been adapted for the culture of human megakaryocytic colonies.[22] Subsequently, a method was developed for growing multipotential colonies containing differentiating erythroid, granulocytic, macrophage, eosinophilic and megakaryocytic cells[23] and finally a method was described for growing pure colonies of undifferentiated (blast) cells which analysis showed to contain hemopoietic stem and progenitor cells.[24,25] Both of these latter colony types can now also be grown from human hemopoietic populations.[26-28]

These developments have made it possible to clonally analyse all the major hemopoietic stem and progenitor populations in semisolid cultures using cells taken directly from the animal or patient. The cells involved are shown schematically in Figure 10.1.

THE HETEROGENEITY OF GRANULOCYTE–MONOCYTE PROGENITORS

Within the granulocyte–monocyte precursor population, considerable heterogeneity exists of two general types:

1. Heterogeneity between cells of equivalent ancestral stage based on varying differentiation commitment. This is seen more clearly with murine cells where progenitors with equivalent proliferative potential can be pre-committed either to granulocyte or macrophage formation or commonly to be bi-potential.
2. Heterogeneity based on proliferative potential and probably reflecting a parent–progeny relationship. For example, human promyelocytes generate small transient clones of granulocytes and these promyelocytes are the likely progeny of ancestral progenitors forming larger granulocytic or granulocyte–monocyte colonies.[29]

Not only can three types of granulocyte–monocyte colony be grown from normal human hemopoietic populations (granulocytic, granulocyte–monocyte and monocyte–macrophage)

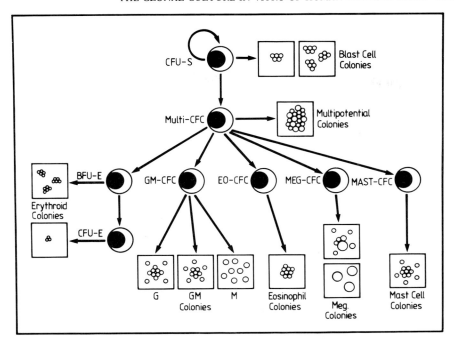

Fig. 10.1 Schematic representation of the various human stem and progenitor cells able to be grown clonally in vitro.

but such colonies develop, mature and disintegrate in cultures asynchronously, requiring cultures to be scored at several timepoints to detect all clones.

It also follows from this complexity that it is not sufficient simply to score total colony or clone numbers but the cultures must be stained and differential colony counts performed to establish the exact frequency of each colony subtype. This staining and typing step is all the more necessary since, with many stimuli, other colony types e.g. eosinophil, develop in the same culture dish and need to be distinguished from granulocyte-monocyte colonies.

Multiple lines of evidence indicate that all myeloid leukemias are monoclonal in nature. In the case of chronic myeloid leukemia it is likely that the initiating clonogenic cell must be a member of the multipotential stem cell compartment. In many cases of acute myeloid leukemia it is possible that the cell initiating the leukemic clone is a member of the committed granulocyte-monocyte progenitor population. However, for some cases of acute myeloid leukemia it may be that the erythroid, eosinophil, megakaryocytic and mast cell populations are also members of the leukemic clone and this question is certainly in need of further investigation. Indeed, a contrary view has been advanced that acute myeloid leukemias are derived from cells properly assignable to the stem cell compartment.[30] The mixed lineage membrane markers exhibited by many acute myeloid leukemic blast cells[31] further confuses the issue, although these may well be anomalous and may merely reflect the derangements in the genome of the leukemic cells concerned.

REGULATORS CONTROLLING HEMOPOIETIC POPULATIONS

Whilst quite adequate clonal cultures of leukemic cells can be achieved without the use of sophisticated reagents, it is necessary to understand some details of the control mechanisms known to operate on hemopoietic cells if cultures are to be used to pose useful questions regarding the nature of leukemia.

For the mouse, current evidence indicates that four distinct glycoprotein colony-stimulating factors interact to control the proliferation and function of granulocyte–monocyte populations.[1,32] These are GM-CSF, G-CSF M-CSF (CSF-1) and multi-CSF (IL-3). Each has been purified, cDNAs cloned for each and the full structure of the polypeptides has been deduced from such clones. The essential data on these CSFs are tabulated in Table 10.1.

The CSFs have multiple actions on responding granulocyte–monocyte populations:

1. They are necessary for, or prolong, cell survival in vitro.
2. They are mandatory continuous stimuli for every cell division, the concentration of the CSF determining the mean cell cycle time and the number of progeny produced.
3. They have the ability to irreversibly commit bi-potential cells to produce either granulocytes or monocytes.
4. They are able to increase the functional activity of mature granulocytes and monocytes.

The control exerted by the CSFs exhibits considerable overlap. Most granulocytic and monocytic cells simultaneously express receptors for all four CSFs and, because of this, more than one CSF can act on an individual cell giving an overlapping and, to some degree, a redundant, control system.

In humans, a comparable situation exists with four human CSFs analogous to the four murine CSFs. There are close parellels in the action of two of these CSFs: GM-CSF in both mouse and humans is also an effective stimulus for eosinophil proliferation[33,34] whilst in both species G-CSF tends to be an exclusive proliferative stimulus for granulocytes.[35,36] Human multi-CSF has only recently been identified[37] and it is not yet certain whether the range of responding target cells is as broad as is the case for murine multi-CSF, which also has proliferative effects on erythoid, multipotential, eosinophil, megakaryocytic and mast cells.[38] Human M-CSF is somewhat anomalous in appearing to have weak or no direct proliferative effects on human cells,[39,40] although it is functionally equivalent to murine M-CSF as a proliferative stimulus when acting on mouse cells.

Thus, currently the culture of normal or human leukemic granulocyte–monocyte cells can be achieved using stimulation either by purified native or recombinant GM-CSF or G-CSF, or by crude preparations, most of which contain both molecules, e.g. placental conditioned medium, phytohemagglutinin-stimulated, leukocyte-conditioned media or media conditioned by several human tumor cell lines. Although a theoretical possibility exists that a clonal leukemic population could be derived from a cell selectively responsive only to GM-CSF or G-CSF, a survey of myeloid leukemic patients has failed to document examples of this.[41]

Table 10.1 The known granulocyte–macrophage colony stimulating factors

Species	Name	Molecular weight	Chromosomal location of gene
Mouse	GM-CSF	23 000	11
	G-CSF	25 000	11
	M-CSF(CSF-1)	70 000 (dimer)	3
	Multi-CSF (IL-3)	23 000–28 000	11
Human	GM-CSF	22 000	5
	G-CSF	18 000	17
	M-CSF(CSF-1)	45 000 (dimer)	5
	Multi-CSF (IL-3)	15 000	5

In CSF-stimulated cultures, a sigmoid dose–response curve exists between CSF concentration and the number of colonies developing. The mid-point on the linear portion of this dose–response curve is assigned the value of 50 units/ml and, to ensure that all available progenitors are stimulated to proliferate, it is necessary to use a CSF concentration at least two to four times that required to stimulate the formation of maximal colony numbers (Fig. 10.2).

TECHNICAL PROCEDURES

GENERAL CONSIDERATIONS

For convenience, semisolid cultures are usually performed in 35 mm plastic Petri dishes although the methods are equally applicable to the growth of cells in larger dishes, tubes, capillary tubes or microtiter trays. In principle, the culture technic involves adding a

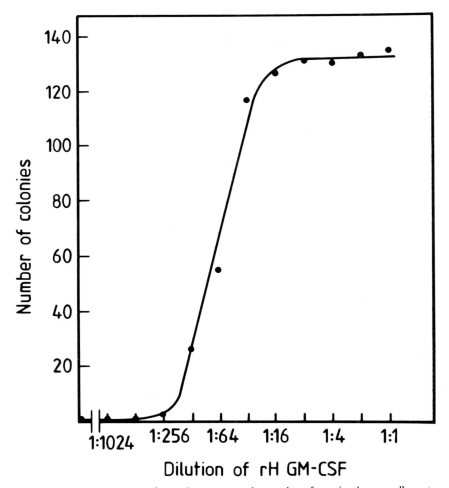

Fig.10.2 Dose–response curve of granulocyte–macrophage colony formation by non-adherent human marrow cells after stimulation by purified recombinant human GM-CSF. The GM-CSF concentration of the preparation was 1 μg/ml.

dispersed suspension of marrow or peripheral blood cells to culture medium containing an agent that will produce either a firm gel or a highly viscous solution. Three agents are used commonly to produce this semisolid state: agar, plasma clot or methylcellulose.

Methylcellulose, which produces merely a highly viscous solution, has the theoretical advantage of allowing colonies to be harvested more readily than from genuine semisolid cultures. However, it is difficult to fix and stain an intact methycellulose culture although this has been achieved. [42]

Furthermore, with some methylcellulose formulations the cells settle continuously during the culture period and the growing colonies and clusters tend to form a carpet over the bottom of the culture dish. Although this need not prevent colony counting, it makes the identification and enumeration of clusters impossible. As shall be discussed later, cluster formation is of critical importance in the analysis of cultures from patients with acute myeloid leukemia (AML). Use of methylcellulose is not ideal, therefore, for cultures of preleukemic or acute leukemic cells and it is strongly recommended that all semisolid cultures be performed using agar (final concentration 0.3%) with which no scoring problems arise and from which colonies or clusters can readily be harvested for further study.

Plasma gel cultures are unsatisfactory because of their rubbery consistency which essentially prevents the harvesting of growing colonies or clusters.

As discussed in more detail elsewhere[1] there are three requirements for successful semisolid cultures of hemopoietic cells: use of a satisfactory batch of serum in the medium, proper incubating conditions, and use of an adequate concentration of the specific stimuli required to stimulate the proliferation of the cells under study.

Serum

Whilst it has been possible to grow granulocyte–macrophage colonies in serum-free, fully characterized culture medium,[43] this requires high levels of technical expertise and the procedure is only of value in special studies. For routine purposes, semisolid cultures are performed using a relatively high concentration of 15–25% serum. As is true for all tissue cultures, the nature of this serum is of critical importance. 'Bad' batches of serum will support neither survival nor proliferation of cells and 'good' batches will support colony formation with varying degress of efficiency. Analysis of this phenomenon has revealed a more serious situation than previously suspected. Progenitor (colony-forming) cells are a heterogeneous population and, where a 'fair' batch of serum supports some colony formation, the situation commonly exists that the colony formation by subsets of progenitors is supported whereas the colony formation by others is not. It is essential, therefore, that the very best serum be used in cultures if all subsets of progenitor cells are to be analysed satisfactorily.

Choice of a 'good' serum batch can only be made by trial and error – i.e. by tests using normal marrow cells. It should be emphasized that the properties of the serum which are good for one type of culture are not necessarily the same as those required for other types of cultures. Thus a serum may support good phytohemagglutinin (PHA)-stimulated proliferation of human lymphocytes in liquid cultures, but be useless for the culture of granulocyte–macrophage colonies. Even a serum supporting relatively good granulocyte–macrophage colony formation may be poor when eosinophil or erythroid colony formation is considered.

In general, fetal calf serum is the most satisfactory serum for human hemopoietic cultures using a final concentration of 20%. Preheating sera to 56°C for 30 min is often used to inactivate complement, but in most cases this has little influence on the performance of the serum. Most suppliers of serum allow pre-testing of batches before a definitive purchase is made. Fetal calf serum retains its activity best when stored at 4°C but, as the activity of serum may fall progressively on storage, it is possibly unwise to purchase in advance more than is sufficient for 6 months' work. It is preferable to avoid excessive millipore filtering of media, sera or stimulatory preparations since the filters can release cytotoxic material and/or inactive proteins in low concentrations. Since sera are supplied prefiltered, such sera can be added without refiltration to filtered batches of serum-free culture medium immediately before use.

Unsatisfactory serum is the most common cause of poor cultures and this cause must always be excluded when difficulties arise with semisolid cultures.

Incubating conditions
Semisolid cultures are usually incubated at 37°C in a fully humidified atmosphere of 10% carbon dioxide in air. It has been shown that incubation in 10% carbon dioxide and only 5% oxygen produces better and more sustained colony growth.[44] Although the latter gas mixture is more expensive, its use for special purposes may be worth while. For the special purpose of growing erythroid colonies, 5% carbon dioxide is better than 10% in supporting the growth of maximal colony numbers and allowing good hemoglobinization of the colonies.

On continued incubation, Petri dish cultures tend to dry out, a process resulting in inhibition of colony formation, because of the large surface area of a 35-mm culture dish in proportion to the standard 1 ml volume of the culture. This is of special importance for human cultures which must be kept for 2 weeks. Drying out can be avoided by a number of procedures: (1) use of a 2 ml volume in the culture dish; (2) reduction of the gas flow rate to less than 2l per min; (3) use of a water bath in the bottom of the incubator through which the gas mixture enters the incubator via a scintered glass filter; and (4) placing two culture dishes in a 90-mm culture dish together with a third 35-mm Petri dish without a lid and filled with distilled water — a procedure enchancing local humidity around the two culture dishes.

A fully humidified incubator should show condensed water on the glass door and the lids of the Petri dishes. If such condensation is not present, the door seal should be checked and possibly filter paper introduced into the water bath and taped to the back wall of the incubator to increase the moist surface area. Water jacketed incubators keep a more uniform temperature than incubators with solid insulation, but the water level in the jacket must be constantly checked. If the water level falls, cultures on the top trays and on the edges of trays will dry out.

A continuous gas flow is not essential for semisolid cultures and a more cumbersome, but quite satisfactory, method is to culture the dishes in a gas-tight plastic box that is regassed every time the box is opened.

As Petri dish lids fit loosely, and are essentially open to liquid droplets in the atmosphere of the incubator, under no conditions should toxic antifungal or antibacterial agents of any type be put in the water bath. Water baths regularly become contaminated and, whilst this does not necessarily cause problems with contamination of cultures, eventually the quality of colony formation diminishes. This can be avoided by thorough washing of the incubator with soap and water every 2-3 months.

For the same general reasons, use of incubators with a fan for circulating the atmosphere within the incubator should be avoided as this causes frequent contamination of the cultures.

The final common problem of incubators is maintenance of a satisfactory pH as indicated by the yellow-salmon pink color of the phenol red indicator in the culture medium. Where incubator doors are opened at regular intervals throughout the working day, the pH of the incubator is usually alkaline (red color in the medium). This requires the use of an incubator, e.g. a National incubator, possessing a valve which is used to pulse pure carbon dioxide through the incubator for 45-60 seconds each time the door is opened. Ideally, the percentage carbon dioxide in an incubator should be checked at regular intervals using a Fyrite carbon dioxide indicator (Bacharach Instrument Co., Pittsburgh, Pa.) with adjustment of the relative gas flows of carbon dioxide and air to maintain the correct percentage.

GENERAL CULTURE TECHNICS

COLLECTION OF CELLS

Marrow aspirates, preferably less than 2 ml in volume to avoid excessive hemodilution, are collected in 200 units of preservative-free herapin. To these aspirates are added 3 ml of Eisen's balanced salt solution or single strength culture medium, and a dispersed cell suspension prepared by pipetting. It is important that no cell clumps are allowed to remain in the cultured cell suspension, and visible bone fragments or undispersed cell clumps should be allowed to settle, the supernatant cell suspension then being transferred to another tube. The cell suspension is centrifuged at 400 × g for 7 min and the buffy coat containing nucleated cells carefully removed and resuspended in fresh medium. Viable cell counts are performed using eosin and, if undispersed cell clumps are seen in the counting chamber, the suspension should be redispersed.

Rib fragments and sternal curettings are a useful source of normal human hemopoietic cells for culture. Rib fragments can be broken open using bone cutters and the marrow flushed out using a syringe and needle. Sternal curettings can be processed by adding 15 ml of balanced salt solution and a cell suspension obtained by pipetting. The subsequent steps are as for marrow aspirates, taking care to exclude fat droplets on the surface of the cell suspension when harvesting the cells.

Peripheral blood cells can be collected for culture in preservative-free heparin and the buffy coat cells removed and washed by centrifugation using methods similar to those described for marrow aspirates.

Contaminating red cells do not interfere with the growth of granulocyte–macrophage colonies and in fact can improve cell growth. If excessive numbers of red cells in the culture dishes impede visibility during colony scoring, these can be lysed by the addition of 0.5 ml of 3% acetic acid immediately prior to counting.

PRECULTURE FRACTIONATION PROCEDURES

Marrow cell suspensions should be washed by centrifugation through culture medium or buffered saline to remove inhibitory substances and/or damaged cells as this process has been shown to increase colony numbers.[45]

Density separation

It has been shown that high concentrations of polymorphs are inhibitory for granulocyte–macrophage colony formation, particularly in culture systems depending on endogenous production of CSF (e.g. by feeder layers).[46] Such cells can be removed by prefractionation of the marrow cell suspension by density separation. Most progenitor cells are of lower density than 1.077 g/cm^3 and, to obtain such a preparation, 10 ml of the cell suspension in Eisen's balanced salt solution is layered onto 10 ml of Ficoll-Paque (Pharmacia, Uppsala). The tube is centrifuged at $400 \times g$ for 20 min at room temperature, then the interface cells removed and washed twice in balanced salt solution before culture.

Adherent cell removal

For some purposes the preliminary removal of adherent cells is desirable prior to culture, either because such cells can produce CSF or factors inhibiting colony formation. Removal of adherent cells leads to an approximate doubling of the observed frequency of progenitor cells.

A simple method for removing adherent cells is to place 1×10^7 cells in 20 ml of culture medium containing 20% fetal calf serum (FCS) in 25 cm^2 tissue culture flasks (Corning, New York) and to incubate the flasks at 37°C for 1 h. The flask is then gently shaken and the non-adherent cells removed. A second cycle of adherence removal is probably desirable,[47] making the procedure somewhat lengthy.

A more efficient and more rapid method for removing adherent cells is to use carbonyl iron.[48] In this procedure, 10 ml of marrow cell suspension in medium containing serum is incubated at 37°C for 1 h with 200-500 mg carbonyl iron. The adherent cells phagocytose and adhere to sufficient iron particles to allow them to be removed using a magnet. The flat-sided culture bottle is placed on a magnet and the supernatant cells gently removed from the adherent cells that are held to the side of the culture bottle by the magnetic field.

Although it is common to read papers in which human hemopoietic populations have been cultured following removal of high density and adherent cells, for many types of experiment these prefractionation procedures are not strictly necessary and their efficiency and wisdom can be debated.

More recent studies on the culture of human cells[49] have revealed a serious problem in that the culture of unfractionated populations may permit the detection of only a fraction (possibly one-sixth) of the progenitor cells actually present, due to the suppressive effects of other cells in the culture. Neither density separation, nor adherent cell separation, efficiently removes such inhibitory cells whose elimination can be achieved using immunomagnetic beads and a battery of monoclonal antisera. This is a worrying situation since it suggests that existing data on progenitor cell numbers may be underestimates and that future survey work needs to be performed on cells pre-treated with monoclonal antisera to remove inhibitory cells. Although the procedure is relatively fast and simple, it becomes more difficult to survey the large numbers of samples that might be desirable in a clinical study.

It needs to be accepted therefore that present data from the culture of normal and leukemic cells may have seriously underestimated actual progenitor cell levels and will ultimately need revision.

However it can be argued that any routine of prefractionation is potentially dangerous when an unknown, potentially abnormal, cell population is to be cultured and analysed. The prefractionation steps are based on the properties of normal cells and, in an abnormal population, these properties may differ. Thus, prefractionation may result in a major loss of the cells under study and could generate quite misleading information. At the very minimum, the use of prefractionation steps must be accompanied by the culture of all starting and rejected populations so that an assessment can be made of the distribution of the cells under study following the fractionation steps.

PREPARATION OF CULTURES

Semisolid cultures are prepared by mixing volumes of double strength, serum-free medium, fetal calf serum and 0.6% Bacto-agar (Difco) (boiled for 2 min, then held at 37°C) in the ratios 2:1:3 respectively to produce a final medium containing 20% serum in 0.3% agar. The required number of cells for culture are then added to the medium. Volumes of 1 or 2 ml of this cell suspension in agar medium are then pipetted into 35-mm Petri dishes containing the CSF source, either in the form of 0.1-0.2 ml of conditioned medium or a preparation of purified CSF. The cell suspension is mixed thoroughly by circular movement of the culture dish and the cultures allowed to gel. These are then incubated without further delay in a fully humidified atmosphere of 10% carbon dioxide in air.

A satisfactory formula for the double strength medium is: Dulbecco's Modified Eagle's HG-Instant Tissue Culture Powder (Grand Island Biological Company, New York) 10 g; 390 ml double glass distilled water; 3 ml L-asparagine (6.7 mg/ml – final concentration in medium 20 µg/ml); 1.5 ml DEAE-dextran (50 mg/ml – final concentration in medium 75 µg/ml) (Pharmacia, Sweden, molecular weight = 500 000); 0.575 ml penicillin (2×10^5 IU/ml; 0.375 ml streptomycin (200 mg/ml); 4.9 g $NaHCO_3$.

The double-strength, serum-free medium is millipore filtered and can be gassed by bubbling carbon dioxide through the medium to adjust the pH. This medium can be stored at 4°C for up to 14 days. It is preferable not to add the fetal calf serum to stored medium, but to add the appropriate volume of serum at the time of preparation of cultures.

Human marrow and peripheral blood contain cells (probably including monocytes) that can produce CSF in vitro. If high cell concentrations are cultured, apparently CSF-independent colony formation can occur. This can be a problem if experiments are designed to investigate, for example, the dependency or autonomy of leukemic cells with respect to stimulation by CSF. Analysis of this phenomenon has shown that most 'spontaneous' colony formation is in fact due to the elaboration of CSF with the culture dish by adherent cells in the cultured marrow or peripheral blood population.[9] Methods for removal of adherent cells were described above and the resulting non-adherent (NA) marrow or peripheral blood cells exhibit minimal spontaneous cell proliferation.

Spontaneous colony formation is markedly dependent on cell concentration and usually only becomes evident if more than 50 000 per ml are cultured.[9] A useful procedure for minimizing this phenomenon is therefore simply to culture 25 000–50 000 cells per ml. A more important reason for choosing to culture only 25 000–50 000 marrow cells per dish is that this cell number produces 'comfortable' numbers of discrete colonies to count in a single dish (20–150). Use of higher cell concentrations can lead to colony confluence and serious errors in determining colony numbers and composition. For peripheral blood cells, the frequency of colony-forming cells is so low that higher numbers of cells can be cultured, e.g. 200 000/ml.

It is important not to adhere inflexibly to the above cell concentrations. If it is suspected that either a high frequency of colony - or cluster-forming cells might be present, e.g. in chronic myeloid leukemia (CML), or a regenerating marrow, much lower cell numbers can, and should, be cultured, e.g. 10 000/ml. In cultures of AML cells where it is important to perform cluster counts, it may be necessary to culture even lower cell concentrations, e.g. 1000/ml, otherwise cluster crowding may make accurate counting impossible, obscure the assessment of cluster size or may even lead to the formation of pseudocolonies. Many published studies have used routinely 2×10^5 cells or more per ml regardless of the type of marrow being cultured and the data produced from cultures of AML cells are quite meaningless because of overcrowding.

PROVISION OF COLONY-STIMULATING FACTORS

For growing myeloid leukemia cells, the ideal requirement is to add to the cultures an adequate concentration of both GM-CSF and G-CSF. This can be achieved in one of two ways: (1) use of crude conditioned media containing both CSF's or (2) use of a mixture of purified native or recombinant GM-CSF and G-CSF. In both cases, the preparations used need to be preassayed on normal marrow cells to establish the correct concentration to use, so that addition of 0.1 ml of the stimulus achieves CSF concentrations two- to four-fold in excess of those stimulating maximal colony numbers to develop. Where crude conditioned media are being used it is important to establish that preparations do not exhibit high-dose inhibition which can effect certain marrow suspensions and not others. Since the CSFs are stable at 4°C or – 15°C, once preparations have been preassayed, a batch of CSF can be used repeatedly without further retitrations, although occasional reassays are a useful precaution.

The original method described for stimulating the growth of human granulocyte–monocyte colonies was the use of a 1 ml underlayer of 0.5% agar containing $1-2 \times 10^6$ peripheral blood white cells. The cells actively produced both GM-CSF and G-CSF that then diffuse up into the layer containing the target marrow cells. Whilst this method can result in stimulation of excellent colonies, the method has been superseded by the use of liquid CSF-containing stimuli for several reasons: (1) convenience; (2) the quite variable activity of different batches of underlayer cells and the consequent uncertainty that a particular underlayer had in fact produced adequate concentrations of CSF; and (3) the difficult optics involved in trying to count colonies and distinguishing these against a background of surviving underlayer cells some of which may even have exhibited abortive proliferation.

CRUDE CONDITIONED MEDIA

Human placental conditioned medium (HPCM)

To prepare HPCM, placentas delivered up to 12 hours previously are cut into 1 cm cubes and, after rinsing three times in saline, six cubes are placed in flat-bottomed plastic bottles (Falcon 25 cm^2 growth area) containing 20 ml of RPMI-1640 with 5% FCS. Bottles are incubated flat for 7 days at 37°C in 10% carbon dioxide in air and the media harvested, freed of placental fragments by filtering through a double layer of cotton gauze, then freed of cellular material by centrifugation at 12 000 × g for 20 min. This HPCM contains high levels of human-active CSF but also contains inhibitory material. To obtain material with satisfactory stimulating activity, it is preferable to adsorb the CSFs on calcium phosphate gel and then, after elution and concentration, to further purify the material by gel filtration using Sephadex G-100.[50] The active fractions are pooled and analysis has shown such material to exhibit no high-dose inhibition. The material can then be titrated to establish the dilution capable of delivering a stimulus two to four times that eliciting maximal colony numbers.

HPCM in impure or semipurified form is stable for years on storage. Although this material stimulates the formation of the same number of colonies as does an active underlayer, the colonies tend to be slightly smaller in size.

Phytohemagglutinin-stimulated leukocyte-conditioned media (PHA-LCM)

PHA-LCM can be prepared using buffy coat peripheral blood cells freed of polymorphs by centrifuging over Ficoll-Hypaque. Cells are cultured in RPMI-1640 medium containing 2% FCS using 10^6 cells per ml. Mitogenic stimulation is provided by inclusion of 9 mg per 100 ml of reagent grade phytohemagglutinin (Wellcome, Beckenham, England). Media are harvested after 7 days of incubation at 37°C in an atmosphere of 10% carbon dioxide in air. An alternative method is to achieve mitogenic stimulation by a mixed leukocyte reaction. Here equal numbers of the above cells from three donors are mixed and cultured for 7 days at a total cell concentration of 10^6/ml.

GCT conditioned medium

This is commercially available from Gibco (Grand Island, New York, USA) and is a medium derived from cultures of a human cell line in turn derived from a lung metastasis of a fibrous histiocytoma. The material is a good stimulus for granulocyte–macrophage and eosinophil colony formation but commercially purchased CSF preparations tend to be expensive and, where a lot of culture work is planned, it may prove preferable and cheaper to produce HPCM or PHA-LCM in the laboratory. Similarly there are a number of other human cells, e.g. Mo, T3M-1, which produce conditioned medium with similar biological activity.

PURIFIED COLONY-STIMULATING FACTORS

Following the cloning of cDNAs for human GM-CSF and G-CSF and the demonstration that biologically active recombinant CSF can be synthesized using mammalian, yeast or bacterial expression systems, it can be anticipated that highly purified recombinant human CSFs will shortly become generally available.

The investigator will then have two choices: (1) to run parallel cultures containing GM-CSF and G-CSF to obtain specific information regarding reactivity to either specific stimulus or (2) to use a mixture of both to ensure that all progenitors will be stimulated.

Either way, the same general rules apply as for crude materials.

1. The material must be preassayed to establish the concentration required for delivering a two- to four-fold supramaximal stimulus (*not* in the manufacturer's laboratory but in the investigator's own laboratory using the medium chosen).
2. Avoidance of crowded cultures and the generation of significant levels of CSF by the cultured cells themselves (an occurrence that would confuse any interpretation of apparent responses to single purified CSFs).
3. Periodic rechecking of material to ensure retention of expected levels of biological activity.

STIMULATION OF COLONY FORMATION BY THE OTHER CELL TYPES

Eosinophil colonies

These are adequately stimulated by use of GM-CSF-containing materials and, if specific progenitor cells are present, eosinophil colonies will develop. A novel method for obtaining cultures of human cells that contain only eosinophil colonies is the use of pokeweed mitogen-stimulated, mouse spleen cell-conditioned medium.[51] Of the various CSFs in this preparation (GM-CSF, multi-CSF and EO-CSF), only the EO-CSF is cross-reactive with human cells. An alternative source of this EO-CSF (also called eosinophil differentiation factor, or IL-5) is medium conditioned by the T-lymphocyte hybrid cell line (NIMP-TH1).[52] A cDNA for this CSF has also been cloned and EO-CSF has been shown to be, in addition, a B-lymphocyte mitogen.[53] However, if 2-mercaptoethanol is omitted from the cultures, no B-lymphocyte proliferation will occur and only eosinophil colonies should develop.

Megakaryocyte colonies

This remains a difficult technic but the procedures used by laboratories successful in obtaining megakaryocyte colony formation should be followed.[22,54]

Erythroid colonies

Addition of human urinary erythropoietin (1 unit/ml) will allow erythroid colony formation by CFU-E (day 5 or day 7 erythroid colonies). For burst-erythroid colonies, combination of erythropoietin (1 unit/ml) with an adequate source of GM-CSF probably will allow most burst-erythroid colonies to develop. Fractionation studies have shown that a subset of BFU-E requires only stimulation by erythropoietin whilst another requires GM-CSF as a second stimulus.[55] Some BFU-E may possibly require an additional enchancing factor (BPA) present in various crude source materials, e.g. HPCM, PHA-LCM or medium conditioned by the Mo leukemic cell line (Mo CM). Fractionation studies have also documented the presence of inhibitory cells in most human marrow suspensions that prevent colony formation by some BFU-E, and this is one clear example where the use of unfractionated cells will result in an underestimate of the true clonogenic cell frequency.[49]

Mixed-erythroid (multipotential) colonies

These are stimulated as for BFU-E.

Stem cell colonies

These are stimulated as for BFU-E.

SCORING OF CULTURES

An Olympus dissection microscope is used to score cultures at magnifications of × 35 for colonies and × 40 for clusters. The mirror is tilted to give semi-indirect lighting, counting white colonies against a brown or black background.

Most workers have adopted the convention that human colonies are discrete aggregates of 40 or more cells and clusters are aggregates of 3–39 cells. The reader is cautioned to note carefully the criteria used by individual authors, because some use quite different (less satisfactory) criteria and their results cannot be compared directly with those of most workers.

Scoring of agar cultures, particularly of abnormal marrows, is *not* a task to be delegated to a technician. Technicians often lack sufficient awareness of the potential information present in the culture dish to be sufficiently observant and maintain their concentration. Moreover, no two human cultures are exactly alike and important new information or abnormalities in cultures from a particular patient are easily missed if scoring is treated as a low level routine procedure.

Underlayer- and conditioned medium-stimulated human cultures also develop eosinophil as well as neutrophil–monocyte (GM) colonies. At 10 days of incubation, 20–30% of colonies are composed of eosinophils.[13,16,17] As discussed above, other colony types also develop in cultures stimulated by CSFs and it is not sufficient in scoring a human culture simply to enumerate colonies or clusters. The cellular composition of the colonies needs to be established and thus the relative frequencies of the different colony types. This is most satisfactorily accomplished by fixing and staining the entire culture.

After colony counting, the cultures are *promptly* fixed by gently adding to the surface 1 ml of 2.5% glutaraldehyde. It is important to realize that colony cells disintegrate rapidly at room temperature and alkaline pH, particularly if the room is warm. Unless cultures are fixed within 30 min of removal from the incubator many colony cells, particularly granulocytic cells, will disintegrate and not be scorable in the stained cultures. After fixation for 1–24 hours, the cultures are rimmed using a spatula and the culture dish inverted over a dish filled with water. The intact culture is picked up on a 7.5 × 5 cm microscope slide and allowed to dry completely at room temperature. If the cultures are overlayed with a 50 mm Whatman filter paper, the edges of the culture dry evenly without a meniscus rim that otherwise would result in subsequent uneven staining. The cultures are then stained in a staining dish with Luxol Fast Blue MBS (0.1% w/v) (G.T. Gurr, High Wycombe, Bucks) dissolved in 70% ethanol saturated with urea. Slides are washed gently under running tap water for 2 hours then counterstained with Harris' hematoxylin (3 min). If desired, the cultures can also be stained for benzidine prior to hematoxylin counterstaining.

After staining, preparations can be mounted permanently under coverslips using DPX mounting medium. Colonies are normally typed at × 100 or × 400 magnifications. Provided the cultures are not too crowded and colonies become superimposed during drying, the stained cultures allow accurate estimates of the relative frequency of various colonies and of cluster/colony ratios and cluster cell numbers.

This staining procedure allows ready identification of eosinophil colonies because of the bright apple-green color of the eosinophil granules. Some dead monocytes can also stain green, but this is a duller color and the cytoplasm stains uniformly and is not granular. Monocyte–macrophage colonies are also readily identified from their loose morphology and the bulky cytoplasm of the cells, as are erythroid cells from their distinct, compact, dark, round nuclei. Maturing granulocytic colonies also present little difficulty in identification based on nuclear morphology. However, some immature granulocyte colonies can be difficult to distinguish from granulocyte–monocyte colonies and this problem is compounded in AML-derived clones where cellular differentiation is often highly abnormal. For most purposes, it may be sufficient to group together all granulocytic and/or monocytic-containing colonies. However, where greater precision is required, it may be necessary to use differential esterase staining.[56]

It should be emphasized that colony counts from bone marrow cultures give an estimate of the frequency, *not* the total number of progenitor cells. Where peripheral blood is cultured, the data can be converted to absolute numbers per millilitre. Colony- and cluster-forming cell levels in peripheral blood are extremely low in comparison with those in the marrow, and all marrow samples are potentially diluted by an unknown volume of peripheral blood. This will always raise difficulties in interpretation of data on the frequency of normal or leukemic colony- or cluster-forming cells in cultured specimens. If aspirate volumes are restricted to 1–2 ml and aspirates are obtained without difficulty, colony counts from normal marrow vary from 20 to 150 colony-forming cells (CSFs) per 10^5 cells and this degree of variability is tolerable where major disturbances in CFC levels are being sought, e.g. in AML or CML, etc.

THE INTERPRETATION OF AGAR CULTURES

VARIABILITY IN CULTURE EFFICIENCY

Because there is considerable intrinsic variability in the responsiveness of progenitor cells to stimulation by CSF, it is essential to use supraplateal concentrations of CSF to ensure that all progenitors are stimulated to proliferate and thereby be detected. Use of suboptimal stimuli can give rise to quite misleading information regarding the properties of progenitors, if only the most readily stimulated cells are detected.

This problem is of special importance in cultures of AML or preleukemic cells. The implications of cultures containing only clusters is of great importance, both diagnostically and prognostically. Further, the exact size of clusters is also of importance. Extremely misleading data will be obtained if poor culture conditions lead to the formation only of clusters instead of colonies, or the formation of small clusters instead of medium-sized or large clusters.

To minimize this problem of variability it is essential always to culture control marrow suspensions in which normal colony-forming cells are present. Ideally, such control cultures can also be used to standardize colony numbers grown from an unknown marrow specimen so that the results obtained in one experiment can validly be added to, or compared with, results obtained on the other occasions. Where laboratories have facilities for, and experience with, liquid nitrogen storage of cells, replicate ampoules of a single specimen or normal marrow, or even a CML marrow, can be used as a standard.

TIME OF SCORING OF CULTURES

It is routine with cultures of animal marrow cells to use 7 days as the incubation interval before scoring and a number of workers have also used this convenient end-point for scoring human cultures. However, human colonies grow more slowly than animal colonies and many investigators delay scoring cultures until 14–21 days. Major discrepancies exist in the literature because of the use of these differing timepoints. For example, in cultures of some AML cells, large clusters present at 7 days and scored as such by one investigator may continue slow growth and be scored as colonies by another investigator scoring at 14 days. It is very important in recording data to indicate clearly the timepoints used.

The events occurring in a human culture are extremely complex and, since no one timepoint is entirely satisfactory, it is preferable to use multiple timepoints according to the needs of the experiment.

1. Cluster numbers are maximal early in the culture period (4–5 days) and then decrease due to dispersion and/ or disintegration. Scoring at 5 days is a suitable time to detect promyelocyte-derived clones.
2. With high concentrations of CSF, higher cluster numbers will develop, but their premature dispersion leads to lower cluster counts when such cultures are scored at 10–14 days than in cultures containing low CSF concentrations.
3. Eosinophil colonies exhibit an initial growth lag. No eosinophil colonies are present at day 7 and colony numbers are maximal at 2–3 weeks.
4. Subpopulations of GM-CFC exist that form colonies characteristically dispersing and/or dying between day 7 and 14 of incubation. For this reason cultures at day 7 and 14 do not detect the same progenitor cells.
5. Multipotential colonies containing, for example, erythroid and other cells are best scored at 14 days.
6. Blast cell colonies may need to be scored at day 14 or 21.

In the authors' laboratory, a commonly used procedure is to score duplicate sets of cultures at 7 and 14 days, eosinophil colony counts being derived from day 14 cultures. However, when it is also necessary to monitor the proliferation of promyelocytes, scoring at 3–5 days is performed since many of these clones disintegrate by day 7. Each investigator needs to consider carefully his own requirements. For example, with AML cultures, if it is desired to follow the classification of Moore et al[57] or Spitzer et al,[58] cultures must be scored at 7 days. If other classifications are being followed, the incubation period should be matched to that used by the original investigator.

SPECIALIZED PRECULTURE PROCEDURES

To characterize the nature of cells proliferating in agar cultures, it is often necessary to use a variety of separation or experimental procedures on the marrow or peripheral blood cells prior to culture.

Leukemic colony- and cluster-forming cells are characterized by their abnormally light, buoyant density. An estimate of the proportion of cells of abnormally light, buoyant density can be obtained by centrifuging the cells through bovine serum albumin of density 1.062 g/cm^3, a higher than normal proportion of leukemic cells remaining in suspension. To fully characterize the density profile of proliferating cells, it is necessary to fractionate the cells in a continuous density gradient, culturing and analysing each fraction. It is important *not* to use a discontinuous gradient for this purpose because artefacts occur at the interfaces of the density regions.

For a number of purposes it has proved to be of value to be able to estimate, by selective killing, the fraction of normal or leukemic cells in the S-phase of the cell cycle. Two methods are available for pre-treating human cells in S-phase by preincubation of the cells in vitro either with high concentrations of [^{3}H]TdR[59] or, simply, with hydroxyurea.[60] After washing, the cells are cultured and the proportion of cells in S-phase calculated from the percentage reduction in colony or cluster numbers compared with control cultures.

The most powerful preculture fractionation procedure is fluorescence-activated cell sorting (FACS). To reduce sorting time it is usual to reduce the number of irrelevant cells by a preliminary density fractionation and/or separation of adherent cells. Another very useful initial step involves removing mature cells, e.g. polymorphs, monocytes, nucleated erythroid cells, by relevant specific antibodies bound to Petri dishes (panning) or conjugated to magnetic beads. Even without the use of specific probes, simple sorting based on size and cytoplasmic granularity and/or nuclear convolution can be used to enrich for normal and leukemic progenitor cells. The large size (low angle light scatter) and lack of cytoplasmic granularity of progenitor cells (low, high angle light scatter) results in most of the progenitor cells fractioning into one box on the scatter profile.

Coupling these sorting parameters with specific fluorescein-labeled McAbs greatly enhances the enrichment of progenitor (clonogenic) cells. A useful antibody in this context is My10 (CD34) which positively labels a variety of progenitor cells.[61,62]

Combination of pre-sorting fractionation with three parameter sorting can result in highly enriched progenitor and stem cell populations where more than 60% of the cells are clonogenic. With such preparations, a variety of a single cell cultures becomes feasible and these are of great value in establishing the nature of direct actions of regulators such as the CSFs on normal or leukemic cells.

One initial hope was that the use of McAbs and FACS sorting might allow separation of pure populations of the progenitor cells of individual lineages. However, most McAbs so far tested have been unable to distinguish between progenitor cell subsets, and this expectation from FACS sorting has yet to be fulfilled. Partial segregation of erythroid and megakaryocytic progenitors has been achieved,[63,64] which has been of some value if only in establishing that lineage-committed specific progenitors do exist and that not all progenitor cells are a single population available for commitment into different lineages following exposure to specific regulatory molecules.

A striking feature of hemopoietic precursor cells of any one type in their heterogeneity in cell volume. A very useful procedure for analyzing subpopulations of normal or leukemic progenitor cells is to separate them on the basis of cell volume using a simple sedimentation chamber (velocity sedimentation separation). Details of this procedure have been published elsewhere.[65]

SPECIAL CULTURE TECHNICS FOR LEUKEMIC BLAST CELLS

As will be discussed below, in conventional CSF-stimulated cultures most clonogenic cells from patients with AML form small clusters rather than colonies. Furthermore, resuspension and reculture of such clusters fails to detect clonogenic cells in them. These observations have led to a general view that cultures of this type are not detecting the true clonogenic (stem) cells in the leukemic population that might be expected to be capable, not only of extensive proliferation, but also of a high level of self-generation.

A variety of technical modifications of agar or methylcellulose cultures has been introduced with the claim that these permit the formation of colonies of blast cells by cells that show at least some capacity for self-generation. These blast cell colonies are therefore viewed as identifying more ancestral cells in the leukemic population and possibly even the true stem cells of the population.

The technics used include direct addition of phytohemagglutinin (PHA) to cultures already containing CSF,[66] the use of certain PHA-stimulated, leukocyte-conditioned media[67] and more recently inclusion of membrane preparations from leukemic cells.[68] All of the technics present some technical problems, and only a limited number of laboratories seem to have achieved consistent colony formation. Clearly, a need remains for improving and/or simplifying the technics so that consistent results can be obtained routinely.

Doubt remains as to whether these blast colonies really differ significantly from the familiar clusters that can be grown in most laboratories. There is no clear evidence that the two types of clonogenic cell are separable and, with good general culture conditions, many clusters in CSF-stimulated cultures will achieve colony size on continued incubation. In some laboratories, the size criterion used for blast cell colonies is only 20 cells (classifiable as clusters in most other laboratories) and the capacity for recloning of such leukemic colonies is usually quite restricted. It also seems that combined use of purified GM-CSF with G-CSF is an effective stimulus for such colonies.[69]

It is quite conceivable that none of the existing technics satisfactorily allows the true stem cells of the AML population to be identified and distinguished from the more numerous clonogenic cells that are presumably their progeny.

The use of blast cell culture technics for the culture of cells from patients with CML presents fewer problems in interpretation since most CSF-stimulated colonies grown from CML cells exhibit obvious cellular differentiation, but again there is no available technic for growing only blast cell colonies, no method for fractionating blast progenitors from other progenitors, and there is thus a formidable difficulty in identifying such blast colonies in crowded cultures of other colony types.

CULTURE OF CELLS FROM PATIENTS WITH CML

In stimulated cultures of bone marrow or peripheral blood cells from a patient with untreated CML, a very constant culture pattern is observed. The general size and shape of the clusters and colonies developing are normal but the frequency of colony-forming cells in cultures of marrow cells is markedly elevated above normal (230 per 10^5 cells for 27 such patients versus 28 per 10^5 for normal subjects in one study in the authors' laboratory[70]). The differences are even more striking in the case of peripheral blood – 510 per 10^5 cells in CML blood versus 0.2 per 10^5 cells in normal blood, in the same study. It should be noted from these figures that the frequency of granulocytic precursors in the blood actually exceeds the elevated levels in the marrow, a combination unique to CML. Cells from different patients with CML grow uniformly well in culture and there is remarkably good agreement between the findings of various groups on the elevated frequency of colony-forming cells in CML.[71-77]

In many studies, no effort was made to record separately the frequency of neutrophil and/or monocyte colonies (GM) versus the frequency of eosinophil colonies. In studies performed on cultures after only 1 week of incubation, the data do in fact refer only to GM colonies since, as in cultures of normal cells, eosinophil colonies only become apparent in the second week of incubation. Examination of CML cultures after 2 weeks of incubation indicated a near-normal ratio of eosinophil to GM colonies.[17] Furthermore, metaphases from eosinophil colony cells exhibit the Philadelphia (Ph) chromosome.[78] It can thus be concluded that, in CML, there is a corresponding massive increase also in the total number of eosinophil progenitor cells and that eosinophils are part of the leukemic clone.

GM colonies grown from CML patients increase in size at a normal rate and exhibit the heterogeneity of size and general shape characteristic of normal GM colonies. The apparent normality of CML colonies is further emphasized when the colony populations are examined morphologically. Maturation of colony cells results in the production of what appear to be normal polymorphs, monocytes, macrophages and eosinophils.

Further evidence of the normality of CML colonies was obtained from an analysis of their dependency on CSF-containing material for continued proliferation. As is true for cultures of normal marrow cells, if sufficiently high concentrations of CML cells are cultured, spontaneous colony formation occurs.[79] However, if endogenous CSF-producing cells are removed by preliminary density fractionation or adherence separation, the colony-forming cells are quite unable to proliferate in the absence of an exogenous source of CSF.[79] Furthermore, on exposure in vitro to CSF, non-cycling CML colony-forming cells enter S-phase within 3 hours as is the case for normal cells.[80] Whilst an analysis of the dose–response curve of CML cells after stimulation by CSF suggested that they may be slightly hyporesponsive to stimulation compared with normal cells,[81] this study re-emphasized the absolute dependency of CML cells on CSF for cell division.

Although the growth of CML cells has many resemblances to that of normal marrow cells, analysis has revealed that a number of differences do exist:

1. Karyotypic analysis of dividing CML colony cells has revealed the presence of the Ph chromosome in most colonies.[73,82-84]
2. When CML cells are fractionated in continuous gradients of bovine serum albumin, an abnormally high proportion of the colony-forming cells is found to be of lighter buoyant density than 1.062 g/cm^3.[72,77] This proportion (up to 70-90% in individual patients, versus 5% for normal marrow) is higher in the blood than in the marrow.[77]
3. A lower proportion of CML colony-forming cells is in the S-phase of the cell cycle than normal (less than 10% versus 30% for normal cells).[72] Fluctuations have been reported in the proportion of CML colony-forming cells in cycle, according to whether or not a leukocytosis was developing in the patient[85] and whether the patient was responding to therapy or in relapse.[77]
4. The ratio of clusters to colonies is slightly lower than normal and there is some tendency for the early appearance of monocytes in mixed colonies grown from CML cells.[72]
5. CML colony-forming cells sediment as a single peak with a modal sedimentation velocity of 7-9 mm/h in contrast to the double peak of colony-forming cells observed with normal marrow.[65]
6. CML colony-forming cells are relatively resistant to suppression by prostaglandin E compared with normal colony-forming cells.[86,87]

The abnormally light buoyant density characteristic of most CML colony-forming cells has permitted the morphological identification of these cells. In at least some patients, light density fractions of CML blood or marrow were found to contain up to 100% of cells identifiable on morphological grounds as 'myeloblasts'.[70,72,88] When such fractions were cultured in vitro, up to 100% of the cells formed colonies or clusters. This indicates that at least some of the colony-forming cells in CML must have the morphology of myeloblasts. The findings do not exclude the possibility that some CML colony-forming cells may have a different morphology, although this must be considered unlikely. A similar observation was made using progenitor cells purified by rosetting using a panel of McAbs.[89] With cells purified by both procedures, the colony-forming cells in culture exhibited absolute dependency for growth on exogenous CSF.

Following initiation of myleran therapy, there is a dramatic fall in progenitor cell levels in the blood, preceding and of relatively greater magnitude than the fall in peripheral blood white cell levels.[70] Whilst a similar fall also occurs in marrow levels, in most patients these levels remain somewhat higher than normal in the stable phase of the disease.

Less extensive studies have been performed on erythroid, multipotential and blast cell progenitor levels in CML but the evidence indicates that these populations are also present in greatly increased numbers in CML.[90-93]

Thus the clonal culture data support other lines of evidence indicating that the leukemic clone in CML is multipotential, and indicate that within the leukemic clone there is a disproportionate expansion of the progenitor cell compartment coupled with the presence of grossly elevated levels of progenitor cells in the peripheral blood.

Whilst the hemopoietic populations are dominated by members of the CML clone, more recent studies have shown that the pre-existing normal progenitor cells are not suppressed in this disease. The absolute numbers of these cells is near normal; they are simply diluted to a low frequency by the massive numbers of progenitors from the leukemic clone.[94]

Studies of the behavior on recloning of resuspended CML granulocyte-macrophage colonies have shown that, as for normal colonies of this type, they lack colony-forming cells. This indicates that the CML myeloblasts do not possess any abnormal capacity for self-generation.

When CML terminates in acute transformation, the abnormal populations displacing the original CML clone are usually derived from mutant cells arising in the CML population.

Whereas in some patients the acutely transformed population is lymphoid in nature, in the majority of transformed patients the abnormal cells appear to be members of the neutrophil–monocyte series. The results from agar cloning of such transformed populations have been a little unsatisfactory since, in some cases, the cells fail to proliferate in vitro and cannot therefore be characterized either as being GM in nature or as being responsive to CSF.

In most patients progressing to acute transformation, a progressive fall occurs in the frequency of colony-forming cells with a progressive rise in the ratio of clusters to colonies.[70,72,77,95] In one-third of patients, the transformed population is capable only of forming clusters with an upper size limit of either 20 or 40 cells, a growth pattern characteristic of AML cells (see below).[95] In contrast to the behavior of chronic phase CML cells in vitro, there are evident abnormalities in differentiation in the colony and cluster cells grown from most transformed patients.[70,72] The cluster- and colony-forming cells in acutely transformed patients exhibit the abnormally light buoyant density of corresponding CML cells and their cell cycle status is usually abnormal.[70,72,77] As with CML cells, the proliferation of transformed cells in vitro appears to remain wholly dependent on CSF.

Growth pattern changes characteristic of acute transformation are observable 2–6 months before transformation is demonstrable using conventional clinical parameters.[70,72,95] Agar cultures of this type therefore appear to have a useful role in monitoring the progress of patients with CML.

The resemblance between the growth patterns in vitro of cells from most patients with acute transformation and those of cells from patients with AML supports the conclusion that transformed populations are usually GM in nature, not lymphoid. A similar conclusion has been reached from in vitro culture studies using PHA stimulation of the cultures. As will be described below, it is possible, using PHA, to stimulate some cells in AML populations to form colonies of leukemic blast cells in vitro.[66,96] This same phenomenon has been observed with acutely transformed populations but not with CML populations.[97,98] Indeed, using these special cultures, it seems possible to detect the emergence of transformed clones by their ability to form colonies in PHA-stimulated cultures with no added CSF. Such colony-forming cells are detectable 2–6 months before transformation is demonstrable by conventional morphological examination.

CULTURE OF CELLS FROM PATIENTS WITH AML

The culture patterns exhibited in agar by marrow or peripheral blood cells from an untreated patient with AML are very characteristic. Such cultures either completely lack colonies or exhibit greatly reduced numbers of colonies; the cultured cells either proliferate to form clusters of various sizes or, less commonly, fail to proliferate.

In a study of 127 patients with untreated AML (non-lymphoid leukemia),[57] one of four culture patterns was exhibited by marrow or peripheral blood cells:

1. The cultures showed no colony or cluster formation and contained no living cells; where cells were from patients with monocytic leukemia such cultures often contained numerous single surviving monocytic cells (12% of patients).
2. The cultures exhibited no colonies but varying numbers of clusters 3–20 cells in size (47% of patients).
3. The cultures exhibited no colonies but varying numbers of clusters of up to 40 cells in size (24% of patients).
4. Some colonies or clusters developed but often an abnormally high ratio of clusters to colonies was present (17% of patients).

Comparable results have been reported by Greenberg et al,[99] Spitzer et al[58] and Vincent et al.[100]

Some laboratories (e.g. Senn et al,[101] Iscove et al,[12] Hornsten et al[102]) have reported culture data in which 20 cells were used as the minimum size for classification of a clone as a colony. From the above description, it will be realized that this method of classification raises unnecessary problems in interpretation of the culture data and seems unwise.

The presence of large numbers of cluster-forming cells in the blood is almost diagnostic of AML. In some patients with myeloproliferative disorders in a preleukemic phase, cultures of bone marrow may also exhibit large numbers of clusters. However, cultures of the blood from such patients usually do not exhibit large numbers of clusters and, in fact, may have elevated numbers of colony-forming cells.[70,103]

It is important to emphasize that the data on which the above descriptions are based were collected after 7 days of incubation. In cultures maintained for longer intervals, clusters formed by leukemic cells from some patients can continue to increase in size and exceed the minimum size limit for colonies. Thus, in some publications where cultures are scored at 14 or 21 days, colony formation by AML cells is described. Furthermore, if cultures are re-fed, leukemic clusters can often increase in size to become colonies [104] and the ability to grow colonies from leukemic cells can be of importance for special purposes. However, in routine cultures it seems counterproductive to extend the culture period until some leukemic cells form colonies, since a simple parameter for distinguishing normal from leukemic cells (i.e. colony versus cluster) is thereby lost. Late scoring of cultures becomes particularly confusing if the patient is in partial remission, when it can become impossible to decide without extensive examination which colonies are normal and which leukemic. The observation of colony formation in vitro by AML cells is a useful property to have documented, because it indicates that AML cells really have a more sustained capacity for proliferation in vitro than might be assumed from the cluster formation seen after 7 days of incubation. However, having established this proposition, it appears far simpler in practice to work with 7-day cultures where the differences between leukemic and normal are most clearly evident.

Comparison of culture patterns in vitro with the morphological subtype of AML has indicated that there is no correlation between these parameters and, for example, myeloblastic, promyelocytic or monocytic cells can proliferate in any one of the above four patterns.[57]

It has also been observed that there can be extreme variation from 10 to 40 000 in the absolute number of clusters developing per 10^5 cultured cells, even between patients with similar percentages of blast cells in the marrow or blood.[72,105] The significance of the extreme variability in the apparent frequency of cluster-forming cells per 10^5 cells or per 10^5 blast cells is difficult to assess. Whilst cluster-forming cells in AML are clearly some type of ancestral cell within the leukemic population, it is a little improbable that they are leukemic stem cells in the generally accepted meaning of this word, i.e. a cell capable of self-generation and generating the entire leukemic population. At the present time it seems more reasonable to assume that the variability may be merely an in vitro artefact based on differing metabolic requirements of different leukemic populations in vitro than to postulate extreme differences in kinetics or population hierarchy between different leukemic populations.

The leukemic nature of the clusters and colonies developing in cultures of AML cells has been confirmed by comparison of the karyotype of the dividing cells in such aggregates with karyotypes performed directly on the leukemic tissues. Where marker chromosomes were present in the patient these were also present in the cells dividing in agar culture.[82,83,106]

Fractionation of leukemic populations using buoyant density separation indicated that the proliferating cells were of abnormally light buoyant density (50–60% of the cells were less than 1.062 g/m^3) and abnormally low proportions were cycling as assessed by in vitro exposure of the cells to high concentrations of tritiated thymidine.[72]

In favorable specimens where the majority of cells were myeloblasts and a very high proportion of cultured cells proliferated in vitro, analysis of density-separated fractions indicated that the cluster-forming cells had the morphology of myeloblasts.[70,72] This conclusion may be equally true for other AML patients but the data need to be interpreted with caution since not all 'myeloblasts' may be cluster- or colony-forming cells, and certainly there is no numerical correlation between the frequency of cells proliferating in vitro and the percentage of cells identified on morphological criteria as 'myeloblasts'.[72,107]

Clonogenic cells from the majority of patients with AML exhibit complete dependency on extrinsic CSF for all cell proliferation in vitro and the dose–response curves indicate a similar responsiveness to that of normal clonogenic cells. In this context, it should be remembered that normal clonogenic cells vary in responsiveness and, since AML populations are clones derived from single cells, different AML populations will exhibit a greater or lower degree of responsiveness. A comparative study using purified GM-CSF and G-CSF indicated that most AML populations responded equally to stimulation by either CSF.[41]

There are some patients with AML whose leukemic cells exhibit genuine autonomy in vitro and can proliferate in the absence of exogenous CSF. Such cells have been shown to transcribe and synthesize CSF as the likely basis for this autonomous proliferation.[108,109]

Whilst CSF-stimulated agar cultures have proved to have a number of useful applications in the analysis of AML leukemic cells, several deficiencies prevent the more extensive application of this type of culture:

1. The cultures do not support the *selective* culture of leukemic cells since both leukemic and normal cells are CSF-dependent and will grow in the cultures.
2. AML cells usually grow as clusters similar in size and shape to normal GM clusters. This makes it extremely difficult to detect whether a few residual AML cluster-forming cells are persisting in a regenerating remission marrow.
3. The cultures probably do not detect the genuine stem cells in the leukemic populations, and certainly do not detect the multipotential leukemic stem cells which presumably are present.

Several reports suggest that it may be possible to modify semisolid cultures to overcome some of these problems. If AML cells are preincubated with PHA, and then cultured in agar containing PHA but with no added CSF, colonies can develop that appear to be composed of AML cells.[66,96] It remains to be determined whether this proliferation is genuinely CSF-independent or whether CSF is generated endogenously in the cultures. The latter possibility is almost certain to occur because of the known capacity of lectins to stimulate CSF production by lymphocytes, but the level of resulting CSF production in a PHA-stimulated AML culture has yet to be determined. This PHA culture system appears to be useful in demonstrating the presence of residual leukemic cells in treated AML patients[66] and in detecting the early stages of transformation in CML patients.[97]

The technic often has two technical problems. PHA can induce a marked agglutination of the cultured cells in the preliminary liquid culture step. Unless great care is exercised to ensure adequate redispersion of these aggregates during the subsequent preparation of the semisolid cultures, pseudo-colonies will be present in the cultures. Even if these contain proliferating cells, the significance of such 'colonies' is of course quite different from that of true colonies. The second problem arises from the fact that PHA stimulation procedures are essentially the same as those used to obtain colony formation in agar by normal T-lymphocytes.[110,111] The general morphological appearance of leukemic AML and normal T-lymphocyte colonies is similar and the two types of colony cannot be readily discriminated from one another by simple inspection. Careful morphological examination of the cells in individual colonies may permit the identification of some of the leukemic colonies because of their content of immature granulocytes,[96] and T-lymphocyte colony cells can be identified because of their capacity to form rosettes with sheep red cells.[110,111] Neither procedure lends itself to the simple enumeration of leukemic or normal colonies in a culture dish, and for this reason it is preferable prior to culture to remove all T-lymphocytes by rosetting with sheep red cells or by FACS fractionation, thus eliminating or minimizing subsequent T-lymphocyte colony formation.

The second procedure for growing colonies from AML populations has been described by Minden et al.[67] This involves stimulation of AML peripheral blood cultures by PHA-stimulated, leukocyte-conditioned medium. With this system, small numbers of leukemic colonies composed of blast cells have been grown from AML peripheral blood. Use of cell cycle agents has indicated that these colony-forming cells are in active cell cycle (as distinct from the more slowly proliferating general population of leukemic blast cells) and it has been suggested that these colony-forming cells may be the true stem cells of the leukemic population.[67] The blast cells in such colonies exhibit a limited degree of recloning capacity, suggesting some self-renewal capacity of the original clonogenic cells and blast colony formation remains dependent on CSF stimulation, a combination of GM-CSF plus G-CSF giving best colony formation.

Although it appears that both these newer methods for obtaining colony formation by AML cells offer some interesting possibilities for exploring the biology of AML and detecting residual AML cells, both appear in need of standardization and improvement, and neither may yet be able to provide the badly needed technic for detection of multipotential leukemic stem cells.

Some discrepancies exist in the literature on the question of whether the cells in clusters and colonies generated in vitro by AML cells exhibit normal differentiation. There are some reports of normal differentiation, usually in colonies grown from leukemic patients.[71] As discussed above, there must always be some reservation concerning the nature of 'colonies' grown from AML patients, particularly if the patient had undergone therapy, since an unknown proportion of such colonies may in fact be derived from regenerating normal cells. Where the morphology of cluster cells has been examined in 7-day cultures of AML cells, most workers have noted that the cells exhibit abnormalities in differentiation.[58,70,72] The most common of these are maturation arrest at the myelocyte or promyelocyte stage but, in about one-quarter of cases, cluster cells exhibited qualitative abnormalities in nuclear morphology, nuclear versus cytoplasmic differentiation or degenerative changes.[57] Where Auer rods were present in the leukemic cells in vivo, these were also present in cluster cells grown in vitro.

One of the most striking features of AML marrow is the usual complete absence of normal progenitors. In patients with karyotypic markers in the leukemic population, studies have indicated that, during remission, the proliferating marrow cells exhibit a normal karyotype.[112] This strongly suggests that remission is indeed associated with re-emergence of suppressed normal populations.

A number of groups have investigated what happens when mixtures of normal and leukemic cells are co-cultured. The initial results failed to document convincing suppression of normal GM colony formation.[72,99,113] It was noted, however, that where the percentage of blasts in an AML marrow exceeded 20%, only subnormal numbers of GM colonies could be grown.[114] A number of studies followed in which significant suppression of proliferation by normal colony cells was observed in mixed cultures of normal and leukemic cells.[115,116] Suppression of normal populations in vivo is no doubt a much more complex process, presumably also involving suppression in the stem cell compartment and probably interference with the production of regulatory factors by local stromal cells within the marrow. In this context it is of interest that the frequency of clonogenic fibroblast precursors is abnormally low in the marrow of patients with AML.[117] Since these fibroblasts are an important component of the regulatory hemopoietic stromal population, their suppression in AML may be partly responsible for the absence of normal progenitors in the marrow of pre-treatment AML patients.

In long-term cultures of AML marrow populations, it has been observed that clonogenic AML cells disappear from the culture and simultaneously normal progenitor cells reappear.[118] Whilst providing further evidence that leukemic cells can suppress the generation of normal progenitors, the observations also indicate that normal stem cells persist in such populations and can again generate normal GM progenitors if released from leukemic cell suppression.

Evidence for the return of normal granulopoiesis during remission has been obtained from an analysis of the in vitro growth patterns of remission bone marrow samples. When remission marrow cells are cultured, a normal pattern of colony and cluster formation is observed often with an increased frequency of both cluster- and colony-forming cells.[72,100,114] Early return of colony-forming cells following chemotherapy has been shown to be correlated with a high probability of successful remission induction.[100,102] Analysis of such colonies has shown that granulocyte–macrophage and eosinophil colonies are present in normal proportions,[17] that colony cells exhibit normal differentiation,[70,72] that the colony cells exhibit a normal karyotype[83] and that the colony-forming cells have a normal buoyant density and cell cycle status.[70,72] Marrow cells also exhibit a normal capacity to produce CSF.[72,119]

By all these criteria, the granulopoietic populations in most marrows in remission are of normal origin. Two qualifications need to be made to this conclusion:

1. In a few patients, the growth pattern in remission cultures continues to exhibit abnormalities similar to those seen in cultures of preleukemic marrow, suggesting that in these patients the re-emergent cells are of preleukemic rather than normal type.[100]
2. It has been reported that reverse transcriptase of the type found in leukemic cells is present in remission marrow but not in normal marrow cells.[120] In these patients it is likely that the population rebounding in remission is a preleukemic clone rather than the usual polyclonal normal population.

The in vitro data strongly support the conclusion that in AML two populations, normal and leukemic, coexist on a competitive basis. In relapse, the leukemic clone is dominant and in remission the reverse is true. This conclusion does not eliminate the possibility that in some patients the leukemic population might also be capable of improved differentiation during remission. However, from the existing data, the latter could not be a quantitatively important source of mature cells and is unlikely in most patients to be the origin of the normal hemopoietic population during remission.

AUTOCRINE CONCEPTS OF CARCINOGENESIS

It has been established from studies on carcinogenesis in target tissues of endocrine hormones that prolonged imbalance in regulatory control resulting in chronic excess stimulation can lead to cancer development in the appropriate target cells.[121] In recent years this general principle has been extended by speculation that in some cases cancer may arise following acquisition by a cell of a constitutive capacity to produce its own specific growth factor(s) – the so-called autocrine hypothesis of cancer. As originally proposed, it was envisaged that a cell could secrete elevated levels of an exact replica of its normal growth factor or an abnormal version of such a factor able to function effectively as a growth factor stimulus.[122] In either case, the secreted molecules were envisaged as binding to membrane growth factor receptors and eliciting a proliferative response.

The general weakness in this hypothesis arises from the fact that most cancers are clones formed by a single initiating cell, and it is difficult to imagine a process by which one cell in a dynamic fluid milieu could secrete sufficient numbers of active molecules to build up a high enough concentration of growth factor around the cell to achieve significant binding to membrane receptors. The concept also encounters difficulties in situations, such as with the CSFs, where many cells in the body already produce the growth factor concerned and where adequate levels of circulating factor exist that are already sufficient to elicit proliferative responses.

The concept that growth factor imbalance alone, whether or not of autocrine origin, is sufficient to lead to cancer or leukemia formation also ignores certain key aspects of carcinogenesis. Cancers are clonal in origin and the initiating cell is unlikely to be a normal cell but rather a preneoplastic cell that has already acquired crucial heritable intrinsic changes. These may or may not involve the acquisition of abnormal quantitative responsiveness to stimulation, but certainly include aquisition of a qualitatively abnormal responsiveness to proliferative stimulation resulting in enchanced self-generation by the clonogenic cells. Acquisition of enchanced self-generation (above the normal 50% level) is mandatory if a clonogenic cell is to form a progressively enlarging neoplastic clone, but this property is not in itself sufficient to lead to neoplastic change. Thus, clonogenic cells of continuous hemopoietic cell lines exhibit high self-renewal and often more than 90% of the progeny can be parental in type, but such cell lines are not leukemogenic.[123,124] The key feature, therefore, of the clonogenic process is not the level of proliferative stimulation or necessarily the source of the growth molecules, but the intrinsic pattern of proliferative response exhibited by the cells following proliferative stimulation.

Returning to possible autocrine mechanisms in leukemia development, there are a number of alternative mechanisms that could result in self-stimulation other than the secretion of a factor with subsequent binding of the molecules to membrane receptors. All of the alternatives fit better the situation where a single cell is achieving clonal dominance by self-stimulation, given the abnormal genetic programming allowing the necessary element of abnormal self-generation in the response elicited.

There are three general alternatives:

1. Synthesis by the cell of abnormal numbers or types of growth factor receptors that, with or without any binding of growth factor, are able to elicit the metabolic cascade normally occurring following binding of growth factor to its receptor.
2. Acquisition by a cell of a constitutive capacity to produce its own growth factor, but with growth factor-receptor binding occurring *within* the cytoplasm of the affected cell. Whether or not the cell actually secretes growth factor molecules would be irrelevant because the key events have already occurred within the affected cell.
3. Production within the cell of abnormal, or abnormal numbers of, molecules that form part of the metabolic cascade initiated normally following growth factor-receptor binding. The intermediate molecules could therefore activate the remaining sequence of the cascade and, in effect, deliver the proliferative signal, bypassing the need for the growth factor-receptor initiating signal. Again as in (2), whether or not the altered cell also secretes growth factor would be largely irrelevant to this self-stimulation.

An example of the first situation is likely to be seen in adult T-cell leukemia (HTLV-I induced) where a striking feature of the acquired independence of the cells from their normal growth factor interleukin-2 (IL-2) is expression by the cells of very high numbers of membrane receptors for IL-2.[125] Later in this discussion it will also be seen that probable examples of the second and third situations have also been documented in studies on the induction of leukemia in continuous murine hemopoietic cell lines.

CSF DEPENDENCY OF HUMAN MYELOID LEUKEMIA

The CSFs are the only agents known to stimulate the proliferation of normal and myeloid leukemic cells in vitro. Recent results from the injection of recombinant CSF into animals has shown these molecules to be effective agents in stimulating hemopoiesis in vivo.

Analysis in vitro of the characteristics of myeloid leukemic cells from patients with AML or CML has indicated that, in the large majority of cases, the survival and proliferation of the leukemic cells remains absolutely dependent on the addition of exogenous CSF, either GM-CSF or G-CSF. This applies both to the clonogenic cells forming granulocyte–macrophage colonies and to the cells generating blast cell colonies. In general, the quantitative responsiveness of the leukemic cells is closely similar to that of normal cells and, where estimates of membrane receptor numbers have been made (so far only for G-CSF), the number and affinity of such receptors also appear to be similar to those on corresponding normal cells.[126]

Unless there is some strange anomaly in the behavior of leukemic cells in vitro, as opposed to their behavior in vivo, these observations would lead to the unambiguous conclusion that myeloid leukemias are examples of dependent tumors where all cell proliferation remains dependent on the continued stimulation by normal growth regulators, specifically the colony-stimulating factors.

The in vitro data allow a minimal conclusion that the CSFs are mandatory co-factors in the emergence and progressive expansion of myeloid leukemias. Without continued stimulation by CSF, the original leukemogenic cell and its progeny could not proliferate and no leukemic clone could emerge. For the two CSFs that can be tested (GM-CSF and G-CSF) there has been no evidence that individual myeloid leukemias are selectively responsive only to one of the two types.

Because no method has been developed for suppressing CSF production in vivo, no formal proof of this conclusion has been possible. Since the synthesis of CSF in adult life is dramatically influenced by exposure to microorganisms, the closest model exhibiting significantly reduced CSF levels is the germ-free animal. It is of interest that such animals exhibit a profound resistance to the induction of myeloid leukemia by whole body irradiation, and only develop leukemia if subsequently conventionalized by microbial infection,[127] a process leading to elevation of circulating CSF levels.[1]

Conversely, no clinical state has so far been documented where chronically elevated CSF levels exist and, as a consequence, no information exists on whether chronic elevation of CSF levels might result in an increased frequency of myeloid leukemia development. Recurrent infections presumably would achieve episodic elevation of CSF levels, but no epidemiological surveys have attempted the difficult task of correlating such a situation with predisposition to myeloid leukemia development.

These considerations indicate the importance of attempting to establish what levels of CSF are present in the tissues and serum of patients at risk of developing myeloid leukemia or already with leukemia. Older observations on this question are now of doubtful value since they were made before the existence of multiple types of CSF was recognized. Furthermore, there are formidable difficulties in establishing the CSF concentration within the marrow – the site of most hemopoietic cells. It is technically possible to determine serum and the urine CSF levels which, for a classic hormone of single organ origin, would provide reasonably complete information. However, the CSFs are characterized by their production by multiple cell types in many locations in the body, and these include cells within the marrow cavity itself. Situations have been documented in experimental animals, e.g. following whole-body irradiation, where alterations in bone shaft production of CSF did not parallel those in other tissues.[1] In the context of leukemia development and progression, it is essential to develop methods to determine the levels of CSF production within the marrow cavity itself. In humans, the only feasible approach to this question is to examine the capacity of aspirated or biopsied marrow samples to produce CSF in vitro. This is an artificial system that may neither provide a valid sample of CSF-producing cells nor necessarily establish the actual functional activity of the same cells in vivo.

Earlier studies using human sera and urine in mouse marrow assays could not have detected GM-CSF since this human molecule is inactive on murine cells. The assays could, however, have detected G-CSF and M-CSF. Fewer studies have been performed using human marrow assays and these would potentially have detected, by direct action, human GM-CSF and G-CSF and, by indirect action, human M-CSF. Human M-CSF has little direct proliferative effect on human cells but can stimulate adherent cells in the cultures to elaborate human-active CSF, possibly mainly G-CSF.

MOUSE MARROW ASSAYS

In one early study, urine CSF levels were found to be low or absent in the majority of AML patients prior to treatment or in relapse, levels returning to normal after remission induction.[128] In other studies, serum and urine CSF levels were found to be elevated for varying periods in most patients with AML and CML often, but not exclusively, during episodes of secondary infection.[129] Serum and urine CSF levels were also often elevated in patients with myeloproliferative disorders, being exceptionally high in the serum of patients with CML or myelofibrosis.[130] No differences were observed in CSF levels in relapse versus remission AML patients, excluding the frequent episodes during which relapse patients were suffering secondary infections.

HUMAN MARROW ASSAYS

Production of CSF by human peripheral blood cells has been reported to be abnormally low in AML patients, who subsequently exhibited poor responses to therapy, or in myeloproliferative patients who subsequently progressed to AML. Marrow stromal production of CSF was subnormal in the same two groups of patients.

Serum capacity to stimulate colony formation was claimed to be higher than normal in patients with CML and CLL but to be normal or subnormal in the serum of patients with AML.[131] This was not confirmed in the other studies. Mangalik and Robinson[132] found that the addition of AML sera to cultures of normal or leukemia marrow did not alter the number of colonies stimulated by underlayers of peripheral blood cells. Serum levels of CSF were found to be highly variable in patients with myeloid leukemia.[133,134]

Initial reports suggested that the peripheral blood cells from patients with AML have a decreased capacity to stimulate granulocyte–macrophage colony formation.[47,99] However, other studies reported that, in some cases, colony-stimulating activity was normal.[79,102,135,136] The basis for this variability appears to depend on the morphological subtype of the leukemia involved and on the level of monocytes in the peripheral blood. Where blood monocyte levels were low, e.g. in acute myeloblastic leukemia, low colony-stimulating activity was found, whereas in acute monocytic leukemia activity was often high.[137,138] However, in another study, no correlation was observed between the capacity of peripheral blood cells to stimulate colony formation and their content of monocytes.[102]

The capacity of peripheral blood cells from leukemic patients to stimulate colony formation was relatively resistant to chemotherapy, and was not significantly depressed in contrast to the sharp fall in colony-forming cell levels.[102] In AML patients with full clinical remission following chemotherapy, the colony-stimulating activity of peripheral blood cells was found to be normal.[72,79,99]

An interesting indirect approach to establishing the possible levels of CSF within the marrow cavity has been the analysis of levels of clonogenic fibroblasts in the marrow. This approach is based on the fact that marrow stromal cells have a regulatory influence on hemopoiesis, part at least of which may well be mediated by CSF production. The fibroblasts able to be grown clonally in vitro represent at least one type of marrow stromal population that is now capable of quantification.

Assays for fibroblast colony-forming (F-CFC) have revealed that, in patients with AML in relapse, there is an obvious reduction in the frequency of these cells whilst levels of clonogenic cells returned to normal following remission induction.[117] This approach needs to be coupled with some assessment of the production of CSF and other regulatory molecules by these same stromal clones. Although again this would provide information only on a selected subset of marrow stromal cells, it does approach more closely an accurate assessment of likely intramedullary CSF levels. It could also be possible to develop assays on the fluid from carefully aspirated marrow samples even though there is an obvious problem of an unmeasurable dilution by peripheral blood that would confuse interpretation of any observed CSF levels.

ROLE OF THE CSFs IN MYELOID LEUKEMIA INDUCTION

In the context of the earlier discussion of autocrine mechanisms for achieving CSF stimulation and the consequences of such stimulation, there are a number of recent observations suggesting that derangements in CSF production or CSF signalling pathways could be involved in the development of myeloid leukemia.

1. Several cases of AML have been documented where the leukemic cells proliferate autonomously in vitro with evidence that cells are actively transcribing mRNA for CSF.[108,109] In these cases, which are not typical of most myeloid leukemias, a strong possibility exits that the cells are self-stimulating either via secreted CSF or more probably by synthesized CSF interacting with CSF receptors intracytoplasmically.
2. In humans, the genes for GM-CSF, multi-CSF, M-CSF and M-CSF receptor (c-fms) are all close together at the breakpoint in the 5q– syndrome[139,140] (Kamen R, personal communication) – a syndrome associated with clonal proliferative disorders involving granulocyte–macrophage populations and commonly found in acute myeloid leukemias arising secondary to cytotoxic therapy.
3. In humans, the gene for G-CSF is on chromosome 17 close to the translocation point in acute promyelocytic leukemia (Vadas, M., personal communication), suggesting that the dysregulation of this gene as a consequence of translocation could be relevant in the pathogenesis of this disease.
4. Insertion of GM-CSF cDNA in a non-regulatable mode into immortalized but non-leukemic murine FDC-P1 cells led to their transformation to leukemic cells.[124] Whilst the cells constitutively secreted GM-CSF, the evidence indicated that intracytoplasmic GM-CSF was more likely to be involved in supplying the crucial proliferative signalling involved in the transformation.

Despite the observations linking autonomous production of CSF with leukemic transformation, other observations have shown that leukemic transformation can be accomplished by mechanisms not involving the production of CSF or CSF-receptors. Thus infection of FDC-P1 cells by Abelson virus led to transformation with no evidence of the occurrence of transcription or synthesis either of GM-CSF or multi-CSF (the two CSFs necessary to stimulate the proliferation of these cells), or the expression of abnormal numbers of CSF receptors.[141] The possibility raised here is that the *abl* product may nevertheless achieve proliferative stimulation by influencing or entering the metabolic cascade normally initiated by CSF signalling.

None of the above experimental leukemias is a close model of the majority of human myeloid leukemias since leukemic cells exhibit clear autonomy when cultured in vitro, unlike the CSF dependency exhibited by most human myeloid leukemias. However, recent studies in the author's laboratory, in which FDC-P1 cells were transformed to leukemic cells by infection with a retrovirus containing the cDNA for the polyoma middle-T antigen, have documented transformed populations which are certainly leukemogenic but yet retain absolute CSF dependency in vitro and thus resemble human myeloid leukemia cells (Dunn A R, Metcalf D, unpublished data). Although once more raising the possibility that polyoma middle-T antigen may enter the CSF-induced proliferative cascade and, in effect, mimic CSF signalling, these cells are intriguing in that they can exhibit the same absolute dependency on extrinsic CSF as the untransformed FDC-P1 cells.

SUPPRESSION OF MYELOID LEUKEMIA BY CSFs

The action of the CSFs on responding normal granulocyte-macrophage populations is complex. Not only are they mandatory proliferative stimuli but they are also capable of inducing differentiation commitment and of enhancing mature cell functional activities.[1] These latter two properties are potentially antagonistic to the proliferative actions of the CSFs and raise the possibility that the CSFs could suppress leukemic populations by suppressing self-generation by the clonogenic cells with or without a parallel induction of differentiation.

The clearest evidence on this question has been obtained from studies on the action of murine CSFs on two model mouse leukemias – the WEHI-3B and M1 leukemias. When WEHI-3B cells are grown in the presence of purified murine CSFs, no evidence of suppression is observed with M-CSF or multi-CSF. GM-CSF exhibits a detectable capacity to induce differentiation of WEHI-3B cells to maturing granulocytes and monocytes, but whilst some suppression of clonogenic self-renewal can be observed, it is not sufficient to achieve complete suppression of the leukemic population.[142]

G-CSF exhibits a much more effective capacity both to induce differentiation and to suppress clonogenic self-renewal and complete suppression of a WEHI-3B population can be achieved.[143] The suppression process is slow, requires two to five cycles of culture with G-CSF and is asymmetrical in nature, not all of the progeny being affected at the same cell division or rate.[144]

Not all leukemic cell lines are suppressed or respond to differentiation induction by G-CSF. In one instance, unresponsiveness was shown to be associated with failure of the leukemic cells to express membrane receptors for G-CSF,[145] but in other cases it may well be that the intrinsic abnormalities in the leukemic cell prevent responsiveness. In this context, it is of interest that pre-exposure of unresponsive cells to a variety of cytotoxic drugs can induce responsiveness, but it has yet to be determined what mechanism is involved.

It needs also to be emphasized that the CSFs are not the only agents of biological origin able to induce differentiation in leukemic cells. Another agent, differentiation inducing factor (DIF), can induce differentiation in M1 leukemic cells.[146,147] DIF has no apparent actions on normal granulocyte-macrophage precursors and its function in the normal body remains unknown. A DIF active in suppressing human myeloid leukemic cells has been shown to be tumor necrosis factor[148] and other biological agents with differentiation-inducing activity are hydrocortisone and the retinoids.[149]

It has been more difficult to obtain comparable data for human myeloid leukemic cell lines because of the lack of suitable continuous cell lines. Studies with HL60 cells suggested that both GM-CSF (CSFα) and G-CSF (CSFß) had some capacity to induce differentiation[150] but a subsequent study documented that G-CSF was more potent in suppressing clonogenic cell self-renewal.[151] The interesting point raised by this latter study was that morphological differentiation was not a necessary facet of suppression of clonogenic self-renewal. This latter observation is of potential importance since it has been the experience of most laboratories working with CSF-stimulated clonal cultures of AML cells that cells in the clusters and colonies fail to exhibit convincing evidence of normal maturation.

The possible ability of the CSFs to suppress human myeloid leukemias and to be of potential therapeutic value in the management of myeloid leukemia is therefore largely unassessable at present. In view of the documentation that failure to express membrane receptors for CSF can be a basis for lack of responsiveness, it is necessary to verify whether primary human myeloid leukemias do express membrane receptors for CSF, particularly for G-CSF. The clear ability of G-CSF to stimulate the proliferation of myeloid leukemic cells in vitro indicates that some cells in the clone must express CSF receptors, but since the cloning efficiency of myeloid leukemic cells in vitro is often low, a possibility remains that many cells may not express receptors and are the counterparts of the unresponsive WEHI-3B D− sublines. In this case, attempted suppression by G-CSF would merely lead to the emergence or refractory sublines of the leukemic population.

Analysis of primary human myeloid leukemias for CSF receptors using ^{125}I-labeled G-CSF has indicated that most populations demonstrate detectable binding although the M5 monocytic leukemias may be an exception. However, autoradiography of leukemic cells from individual myeloid leukemic patients has indicated that not all the blast cells in the population exhibit detectable receptors, again raising the possibility that variant cells may exist in many leukemic populations that would be resistant to the effects of G-CSF.[41] The cells exhibiting highest receptor numbers are leukemic promyelocytes (paralleling the high G-CSF receptor numbers on normal promyelocytes) and these leukemias (AML M3) may be the best candidates for suppression by G-CSF.[41]

In view of the current availability of recombinant GM-CSF and G-CSF for clinical trials, it is a matter of urgency to establish from further survey studies the CSF receptor status of leukemic cells, particularly in patients with AML before and following cytotoxic therapy.

Because of the potentially conflicting actions of the CSFs on leukemic populations, i.e. growth stimulation versus suppression, and the differences exhibited between GM-CSF and G-CSF in this regard, it is of importance to reinvestigate the actual levels of these two CSFs in patients with potentially preleukemic disorders in addition to those with established AML. The older observations on this question are not particularly helpful, because they were made before the existence of the two types of CSF was recognized. The situation of patients with potentially preleukemic myeloid disorders should be of particular interest since the differing behavior of these patients may be based on differing CSF levels.

CONCLUSIONS

The use semisolid cultures permits the detection of clonogenic cells in patients with acute or chronic myeloid leukemia and the characterization of these clonogenic cells. In most patients, the clonogenic cells remain dependent on, and responsive to, stimulation by the normal regulatory hormones controlling granulocyte and monocyte formation, the glycoprotein colony-stimulating factors (CSFs). The CSFs are therefore mandatory co-factors in the initiation and progression of myeloid leukemias, a conclusion confirmed in experimental models by evidence that the CSF genes can function as proto-oncogenes.

The ability of G-CSF to suppress some myeloid leukemias by inhibition of clonogenic cell self-renewal indicates the complexity of actions of these regulatory molecules on leukemic populations but raises the possible value of G-CSF in the treatment of some myeloid leukemias.

REFERENCES

1. Metcalf D 1984 The Hemopoietic Colony Stimulating Factors. Elsevier, Amsterdam
2. Bradley T R, Metcalf D 1966 The growth of mouse bone marrow cells in vitro. Australian Journal of Experimental Biology and Medical Science 44: 287-299
3. Ichikawa Y, Pluznik D H, Sachs L 1966 In vitro control of the development of macrophage and granulocyte colonies. Proceedings of the National Academy of Sciences of the USA 56: 488-489
4. Moore M A S, Williams N, Metcalf D 1972 Purification and characterization of the in vitro colony forming cells in monkey hemopoietic tissue. Journal of Cell Physiology 79: 283-292
5. Metcalf D, Moore M A S, Warner N L 1969 Colony formation in vitro by myelomonocytic leukemic cells. Journal of the National Cancer Institute 43: 983-997
6. Ichikawa Y 1964 Differentiation of a cell line myeloid leukemia. Journal of Cell Physiology 74: 223-234
7. Sachs L 1978 Control of normal cell differentiation and the phenotypic reversion of malignancy in myeloid leukemia. Nature 274: 535-539
8. Pike B, Robinson W A 1970 Human bone marrow colony growth in agar gel. Journal of Cell Physiology 76: 77-84
9. Moore M A S, Williams N 1972 Physical separation of colony stimulating from in vitro colony-forming cells in hemopoietic tissue. Journal of Cell Physiology 80: 195-206
10. Golde D W, Cline M J 1972 Identification of the colony-stimulating cell in human peripheral blood. Journal of Clinical Investigation 51: 2981-2987
11. Chervenick P A, Lo Buglio A F 1972 Human blood monocytes: stimulation of granulocyte and mononuclear formation in vitro. Science 178: 164-169
12. Iscove N N, Senn J S, Till J E, McCulloch E A 1971 Colony formation by normal and leukemic human marrow cells in culture. Effect of conditioned medium from human leukocytes. Blood 37: 1-5
13. Chervenick P A, Boggs D R 1971 In vitro growth of granulocytic and mononuclear colonies from blood of normal individuals. Blood 37: 131-135
14. Shoham D, Ben David E, Rozenszajn L A 1974 Cytochemical and morphological identification of macrophages and eosinophils in tissue cultures of normal human bone marrow. Blood 44: 221-233
15. Parmley R T, Ogawa M, Spicer S G, Wright N J 1976 Ultrastructive and cytochemistry of human bone marrow granulocytes in culture. Experimental Hematology 4: 75-89
16. Dao C, Metcalf D, Bilski-Pasquier G 1977 Eosinophil and neutrophil colony-forming cells in culture. Blood 50: 833-839
17. Dresch C, Johnson G R, Metcalf D 1977 Eosinophil colony formation in semisolid cultures of human bone marrow cells. Blood 49: 835-844
18. Stephenson J R, Axelrad A A, McLeod D L, Shreeve M M 1971 Induction of colonies of hemoglobin-synthesizing cells by erythropoietin in vitro. Proceedings of the National Academy of Sciences of the USA 68: 1542-1546
19. Heath D S, Axelrad A A, McLeod D L, Shreeve M M 1976 Separation of the erythropoietin-responsive progenitors BFU-E and CFU-E in mouse marrow by unit gravity sedimentation. Blood 47: 777-792
20. Tepperman A D, Curtis J E, McCulloch E A 1974 Erythropoietic colonies in cultures of human marrow. Blood 44: 659-669
21. Metcalf D, MacDonald H R, Odartchenko N, Sordat B 1975 Growth of mouse megakaryocyte colonies in vitro. Proceedings of the National Academy of Sciences of the USA 72: 1744-1748
22. Vainchenker W, Bouguet J, Guichard J, Breton-Gorius J 1979 Megakaryocyte colony formation from human bone marrow precursors. Blood 54: 940-945
23. Johnson G R, Metcalf D 1977 Pure and mixed erythroid colony formation in vitro stimulated by spleen conditioned medium with no detectable erythropoietin. Proceedings of the National Academy of Sciences of the USA 74: 3879-3882
24. Keller G M, Phillips R A 1982 Detection in vitro of a unique multipotent hemopoietic progenitor. Journal of Cell Physiology (Supplement) 1: 31-36
25. Nakahata T, Ogawa M 1982 Identification in culture of a class of hemopoietic colony-forming units with extensive capability to self-renew and generate multipotential colonies. Proceedings of the National Academy of Science of the USA 79: 3843-3847
26. Fauser A A, Messner H A 1978 Granuloerythropoietic colonies in human marrow, peripheral blood and cord blood. Blood 52: 1243-1248
27. Messner H A, Lim B, Jamal N, Takahashi T 1983 Lymphoid cells in multilineage colonies. In: Killman S-A, Cronkite E P, Muller-Berat C N (eds) Haemopoietic Stem Cells, Munksgaard, Copenhagen, pp 338

28 Nakahata T, Ogawa M 1982 Hemopoietic colony-forming cells in umbilical cord blood with extensive capability to generate mono- and multipotential hemopoietic progenitors. Journal of Clinical Investigation 70: 1324–1328
29 Begley C G, Lopez A F, Vadas M A, Metcalf D 1985 The clonal proliferation in vitro of enriched populations of human promyelocytes and myelocytes. Blood 65: 951–958
30 McCulloch E A, Izaguirre C A, Chang L J-A, Smith L J 1982 Renewal and determination in leukemic blast populations. Journal of Cell Physiology Supplement 1: 103–111
31 Smith L J, Curtis J E, Messner H A, Senn J S, Furthmayr H, McCulloch E A 1983 Lineage infidelity in acute leukemia. Blood 61: 1138–1145
32 Metcalf D 1986 The molecular biology and functions of the granulocyte-macrophage colony-stimulating factors. Blood 67: 257–267
33 Metcalf D, Burgess A W, Johnson G R et al 1986 In vitro action on hemopoietic cells of recombinant murine GM-CSF purified after production in E.coli: Comparison with purified native GM-CSF. Journal of Cell Physiology 128: 421–431
34 Metcalf D, Begley C G, Johnson G R et al 1986 Biologic properties in vitro of recombinant human granulocyte-macrophage colony-stimulating factor. Blood 67: 37–45
35 Metcalf D, Nicola N A 1983 Proliferative effects of purified granulocyte colony-stimulating factor (G-CSF) on normal mouse hemopoietic cells. Journal of Cell Physiology 116: 198–206
36 Welte K, Platzer E, Lu L et al 1985 Purification and biochemical characterization of human pluripotent colony-stimulating factor. Proceedings of the National Academy of Sciences of the USA 82: 1526–1530
37 Yang Y-C, Ciarletta A B, Temple PA et al 1986 Human interleukin 3 (Multi-CSF):identification by expression cloning of a novel hematopoietic growth factor related to murine IL-3. Cell 47: 3–10
38 Metcalf D 1986 The multipotential colony stimulating factor, Multi-CSF (IL-3). In: Schrader J W (ed) Interleukins: the panspecific hemopoietin. Lymphokines 15. Academic Press, New York
39 Metcalf D 1979 Stimulation by human urine or plasma of granulopoiesis by human marrow cells in agar. Experimental Hematology 2: 157–173
40 Motoyoshi K, Suda T, Kusumoto K, Takaku F, Miura Y 1982 Granulocyte-macrophage colony-stimulating and binding activities of purified human urinary colony-stimulating factor to murine and human bone marrow cells. Blood 60: 1378–1386
41 Begley C G, Metcalf D, Nicola N A 1987 Primary human myeloid leukemia cells: comparative responsiveness to proliferative stimulation by GM-CSF or G-CSF and membrane expression of CSF receptors. Leukemia 1: 1–8
42 Ozawa K, Hashimoto Y, Urabe A et al 1982 A new method for permanent preparations of hemopoietic cells cultured in methylcellulose medium. Experimental Hematology 10: 145–150
43 Drouet X, Charbord P, Neel H et al 1985 Human granulocyte colony growth: differences between serum-free and serum-dependent cultures. Experimental Hematology 13: 1133–1137
44 Bradley T R, Hodgson G S, Rosendaal M 1978 The effect of oxygen tension on hemopoietic and fibroblast cell proliferation in vitro. Journal of Cell Physiology 97: 517–522
45 Entringer M A, Robinson W A, Kurnick J E 1977 Colony growth of normal human bone marrow in agar gel. Experimental Hematology 5: 125–135
46 Heit W, Kern P, Kubanek B, Heimpel H 1974 Some factors influencing granulocyte colony formation in vitro by human white blood cells. Blood 44: 511–515
47 Messner H A, Till J E, McCulloch E A 1973 Interacting cell populations affecting granulopoietic colony formation by normal and leukemic human marrow cells. Blood 42: 701–710
48 Lundgren G, Zukoski Ch F, Moller G 1968 Differential effects of human granulocytes and lymphocytes on human fibroblasts in vitro. Clinical and Experimental Immunology 3: 817–836
49 Kannourakis G, Bol S 1987 Fractionation of normal and β-thalassemic human hemopoietic progenitor cells by immunomagnetic beads. Experimental Hematology 15: 1103–1108
50 Nicola N A, Metcalf D, Johnson G R, Burgess A W 1978 Preparation of colony stimulating factors from human placental conditioned medium. Leukemia Research 2: 313–322
51 Metcalf D, Cutler R L, Nicola N A 1983 Selective stimulation by mouse spleen cell conditioned medium of human eosinophil colony formation. Blood 61: 999–1005
52 Sanderson C J, Warren D J, Strath M 1985 Identification of a lymphokine that stimulates eosinophil differentiation in vitro. Its relationship to interleukin 3 and functional properties of eosinophils produced in culture. Journal of Experimental Medicine 162: 60–74
53 Azuma C, Tanabe T, Konishi M et al 1986 Cloning of cDNA for human T-cell replacing factor (interleukin-5) and comparison with the murine homologue. Nucleic Acids Research 14: 9149–9158
54 Hoffman R, Yang H H, Bruno E, Straneva J E 1985 Purification and partial characterization of a megakaryocyte colony stimulating factor from human plasma. Journal of Clinical Investigation 75: 1174–1182

55 Kannourakis G, Johnson G R 1987 Fractionation of subsets of BFU-E from normal bone marrow: responsiveness to erythropoietin, human placental-conditioned medium, or granulocyte-macrophage colony-stimulating factor. Blood 71: 758–765
56 Kubota K, Mizoguchi H, Miura Y, Suda T, Takaka F 1980 A new technique for the cytochemical examination of hemopoietic cells grown in agar gel. Experimental Hematology 8: 339–344
57 Moore M A S, Spitzer G, Williams N, Metcalf D, Buckley J 1974 Agar culture studies in 127 cases of untreated acute leukemia: The prognostic value of reclassification of leukemia according to in vitro growth characteristics. Blood 44: 1–9
58 Spitzer G, Dicke K A, Gehan E A et al 1976 A simplified in vitro classification for prognosis in adult acute leukemia: the application of in vitro results in remission – predictive models. Blood 48: 795–807
59 Iscove N N, Till J E, McCulloch E A 1970 The proliferative states of mouse granulopoietic progenitor cells. Proceedings of the Society for Experimental Biology and Medicine 134: 33–36
60 Sinclair W K 1967 Hydroxyurea. Effects on Chinese hamster cells grown in culture. Cancer Research 27: 297–308
61 Civin C I, Strauss L C, Brovall C, Fackler M J, Schwartz J F, Shaper J H 1984 Antigenic analysis of hematopoiesis III. A hemopoietic progenitor cell surface antigen defined by a monoclonal antibody raised against kg – 1a cells. Journal of Immunology 133: 157–165
62 Strauss L C, Rowley S D, La Russa V F, Sharkis S J, Stuart R K, Civin C I 1986 Antigenic analysis of hematopoiesis V. Characterization of My-10 antigen expression by normal lymphohematopoietic progenitor cells. Experimental Hematology 14: 878–886
63 Watt S M, Metcalf D, Gilmore D J, Stenning G M, Clark R M, Waldmann H 1983 The selective isolation of erythropoietin-responsive progenitor cells (CFU-E) with monoclonal antibodies. Molecular Biology and Medicine 1: 95–115
64 Harris R A, Hogarth P M, Mckenzie I F C, Penington D 1983 Differential expression of Qa-m^2 alloantigen on murine hematopoietic progenitor cells. Selective enrichment for megakaryocyte progenitors. Experimental Hematology 11: 527–541
65 Johnson G R, Dresch C, Metcalf D 1977 Heterogeneity in human neutrophil, macrophage and eosinophil progenitor cells demontrated by velocity sedimentation separation. Blood 50: 823–831
66 Dicke K A, Spitzer G, Cork A, Ahearn M J 1976 In vitro colony growth of acute myelogenous leukemia. Blood Cells 2: 125–137
67 Minden M D, Till J E, McCulloch E A 1978 Proliferative state of blast cell progenitors in acute myeloblastic leukemia (AML). Blood 52: 592–600
68 Nara N, McCulloch E A 1985 Membranes replace irradiated blast cells as a growth requirement for leukemic blast progenitors in suspension culture. Journal of Experimental Medicine 162: 1435–1443
69 Kelleher C, Miyauchi J, Wong G, Clark S, Minden M D, McCulloch E A 1987 Synergism between recombinant growth factors GM-CSF and G-CSF acting on the blast cells of acute myeloblastic leukemia. Blood 69: 1498–1503
70 Moore M A S 1975 In vitro studies in the myeloid leukemias. In: Cleton F J, Crowther D, Malpas J B (eds) Advances in acute leukemia. North-Holland, Amsterdam, p 161
71 Paran M, Sachs L, Barak Y, Resnitsky P 1970 In vitro induction of granulocyte differentiation in hematopoietic cells from leukemic and non-leukemic patients. Proceedings of the National Academy of Sciences of the USA 67: 1542–1549
72 Moore M A S, Williams N, Metcalf D 1973 In vitro colony formation by normal and leukemic human hematopoietic cells. Characterization of the colony-forming cells. Journal of the National Cancer Institute 50: 603–623
73 Shadduck R K, Nankin H R 1971 Cellular origin of granulocytic colonies in chronic myeloid leukemia. Lancet ii: 1097–1098
74 Brown C H, Carbone P P 1971 In vitro growth of normal and leukemic human bone marrow. Journal of the National Cancer Institute 46: 789–795
75 Goldman J M, Th'ng K H, Lowenthal R M 1974 In vitro colony-forming cells and colony stimulating activity in chronic granulocytic leukemia. British Journal of Cancer 30: 1–12
76 Moberg C, Olofsson T, Olsson I 1974 Granulopoiesis in chronic myeloid leukemia. I. In vitro cloning of blood and bone marrow cells in agar culture. Scandinavian Journal of Haematology 12: 381–388
77 Berthier R, Douady F, Holland D 1977 Cellular factors regulating granulopoiesis in myeloid leukemia. Blood Cells 3: 461–474
78 McCarthy J H, Nicola N, Szelag G, Garson O M 1980 Studies on eosinophil colonies grown from leukemic and non-leukemic patients. Leukemia Research 4: 415–426

79 Moore M A S, Williams N, Metcalf D 1973 In vitro colony formation by normal and leukemic human hemopoietic cells. Interactions between colony-forming and colony-stimulating cells. Journal of the National Cancer Institute 50: 591–602
80 Moore M A S, Williams N 1973 Functional, morphologic and kinetic analysis of the granulocyte-macrophage progenitor cell. In: Robinson W A (ed) Hemopoiesis in culture. DHEW Publication NO 74-205, Washington, p 17
81 Metcalf D, Moore M A S, Sheridan J W, Spitzer G 1974 Responsiveness of human granulocytic leukemic cells to colony stimulating factor. Blood 43: 847–859
82 Duttera M J, Whang-Peng J, Bull J M L, Carbone P P 1972 Cytogenetically abnormal cells in vitro in acute leukemia. Lancet i: 715–718
83 Moore M A S, Metcalf D 1978 Cytogenetic analysis of human acute and chronic myeloid leukemic cells cloned in agar culture. International Journal of Cancer 11: 143–152
84 Aye M T, Till J E, McCulloch E A 1973 Cytological studies of granulopoietic colonies from two patients with chronic myelogenous leukemia. Experimental Hematology 1: 115–118
85 Olofsson T, Olsson I 1976 Granulopoiesis in chronic myeloid leukemia. II. Serial cloning of blood and bone marrow cells in agar culture. Blood 48: 351–360
86 Pelus L M, Broxmeyer H E, Clarkson B D, Moore M A S 1980 Abnormal responsiveness of granulocyte–macrophage committed colony-forming cells from patients with chronic myeloid leukemia to inhibition by prostaglandin E. Cancer Research 40: 2512–2515
87 Aglietta M, Piacibello W, Gavosto F 1980 Insensitivity of chronic myeloid leukemia cells to inhibition of growth by prostaglandin E. Cancer Research 40: 2507–2511
88 Metcalf D, Johnson G R, Kolber S, Dresch C 1978 Clonal analysis of chronic myeloid leukemic cells using agar cultures. In: Bentvelson P (ed) Advances in comparative leukemia research 1977, Elsevier/ North-Holland Biomedical Press, Amsterdam, p 307
89 Griffin J D, Beveridge R P, Schlossman S F 1982 Isolation of myeloid progenitor cells from peripheral blood of chronic myelogenous leukemia patients. Blood 60: 30–37
90 Hibbin J A, McCarthy D M, Goldman J M 1983 Antigenic expression and proliferative status of multilineage progenitor cells (CFU-GEMM) in normal individuals and patients with chronic granulocytic leukaemia. Scandinavian Journal of Haematology 31: 454–460
91 Hara H, Kai S, Fushimi M, Taniwaki S et al 1981 Pluripotent, erythrocyte and granulocytic hemopoietic precursors in chronic granulocytic leukemia. Experimental Hematology 9: 871–877
92 Dowding C R, Gordon M Y, Goldman J M 1986 Primitive progenitor cells in the blood of patients with chronic granulocytic leukemia. International Journal of Cell Cloning 4: 331–340
93 Sugiyama H, Yagita M, Takahashi T et al 1987 Type-specific in vitro growth patterns of multilineage hemopoietic progenitors in myeloproliferative disorders and myelodysplastic syndromes. Acta Haematologica Japanica 50: 46–58
94 Dube I D, Kalousek D K, Coulombel L, Gupta C M, Eaves C J, Eaves A C 1984 Cytogenetic studies of early myeloid progenitor compartments in Ph^1-positive chronic myeloid leukemia. II. Long-term culture reveals the persistence of Ph^1-negative progenitors in treated as well as newly diagnosed patients. Blood 63: 1172–1179
95 Moore M A S 1975 Marrow culture – a new approach to classification of leukemias. In: Bessis M, Brecher G (eds) Unclassifiable Leukemias, Springer-Verlag, Berlin, p 149
96 Dicke K A, Spitzer G, Ahearn M J 1976 Colony formation in vitro by leukemic cells in acute myelogenous leukemia with phytohaemagglutinin as stimulating factor. Nature 259: 129–132
97 Spitzer G, Schwarz M A, Dicke K A, Trujillo J M, McKredie K B 1976 Significance of PHA-induced clonogenic cells in chronic myeloid leukemia and early acute myeloid leukemia. Blood Cells 2: 149–159
98 Lowenberg B, Hagemeijer A, Abels J 1985 Detection of the blastic crisis cell clone in chronic myeloid leukemia. British Journal of Haematology 59: 27–36
99 Greenberg P L, Nichols W, Schrier S L 1971 Granulopoiesis in acute myeloid leukemia and preleukemia. New England Journal of Medicine 284: 1225–1232
100 Vincent P C, Sutherland R, Bradley M, Lind D, Gunz F W 1977 Marrow culture studies in adult acute leukemia at presentation and during remission. Blood 49: 903–912
101 Senn J S, McCulloch E A, Till J E 1967 Comparison of colony-forming ability of normal and leukaemic human marrow in cell culture. Lancet ii: 597–598
102 Hornsten P, Granstrom M, Wahren B, Gharton G 1977 Prognostic value of colony-stimulating and colony-forming cells in peripheral blood in acute non-lymphoblastic leukemia. Acta Medica Scandinavica 201: 405–410
103 Moore M A S, Spitzer G R 1974 In vitro studies in the myeloproliferative disorders. In: Lindahl-Kiessling K, Osoba D (eds) Lymphocyte recognition and effector mechanisms. Academic Press, New York, p 431
104 Park C H, Savin M A, Hoogstraten B, Amare M, Hathaway P 1977 Improved growth of in vitro colonies in human acute leukemia with the feeding culture method. Cancer Research 37: 4595–4599

105 Till J E, Lan S, Buick R N, Sousan P, Curtis J E, McCulloch E A 1978 Approaches to the evaluation of human hemopoietic stem cell function. In: Clarkson B, Marks P A, Till J E (eds) Differentiation of normal and neoplastic hematopoietic cells. Cold Spring Harbor Laboratory, New York, p 81
106 Aye M T, Till J E, McCulloch E A 1974 Cytological studies of colonies in culture derived from peripheral blood of cells of two patients with acute leukemia. Experimental Hematology 2: 362–371
107 McCulloch E A, Buick R N, Minden M D, Izaguirre C A 1978 Differentiation programmes underlying cellular heterogeneity in the myeloblastic leukemias of man. In: Golde D W, Cline M J, Metcalf D, Fox C F (eds) Hematopoietic cell differentiation. Academic Press, New York, p 317
108 Young D C, Griffin J D 1986 Autocrine secretion of GM-CSF in acute myeloblastic leukemia. Blood 68: 1178–1181
109 Cheng G Y M, Kelleher C, Miyauchi J et al 1988 Structure and expression of genes of GM-CSF and G-CSF in blast cells from patients with acute myeloblastic leukemia. Blood 71: 204–208
110 Rozenszajn L A, Shoham D, Kalechman I 1975 Clonal proliferation of PHA-stimulated human lymphocytes in soft agar culture. Immunology 29: 1041–1055
111 Claesson M H, Rodger M B, Johnson G R, Whittingham S, Metcalf D 1977 Colony formation by human T lymphocytes in agar medium. Clinical and Experimental Immunology 28: 526–534
112 Rowley J D 1978 The cytogenetics of acute leukemia. Clinical Haematology 7: 385–406
113 Robinson W A, Kurnick J E, Pike B L 1971 Colony growth of human leukemic peripheral blood cells in vitro. Blood 38: 500–508
114 Bull J M, Duttera M J, Stashick E D, Northrup J, Henderson E, Carbone P P 1973 Serial in vitro marrow culture in acute myelomonocytic leukemia. Blood 42: 679–686
115 Morris T C M, McNeill T A, Bridges J M 1975 Inhibition of normal human in vitro colony forming cells by cells from leukemic patients. British Journal of Cancer 31: 641–648
116 Chiyoda S, Mizoguchi H, Kosaka K, Takaku F, Miura Y 1975 Influence of leukaemic cells on the colony formation of human bone marrow cells in vitro. British Journal of Cancer 31: 355–358
117 Kaneko S, Motomura S, Ibayashi H 1982 Differentiation of human bone marrow-derived fibroblastoid colony forming cells (CFU-F) and their roles in haemopoiesis in vitro. British Journal of Haematology 51: 217–225
118 Coulombel L, Eaves C J, Dube I D, Kalousek D K, Eaves A C 1984 Variable persistence of leukemic progenitor cells in long-term CML and AML marrow cultures. In: Wright D G, Greenberger J S (eds) Long-term bone marrow culture. Alan R. Liss, New York, pp 243–254
119 Greenberg P, Mura B 1978 Microenvironmental influences on granulopoiesis in acute myeloid leukemia. In: Clarkson B, Marks P A, Till J E (eds) Differentiation of normal and neoplastic cells. Cold Spring Harbor Laboratory, New York, p 405
120 Mak T W, Aye M T, Messner H A, Sheinin R, Till J E, McCulloch E A 1974 Reverse transcriptase activity. Increase in marrow cultures from leukemic patients in relapse and remission. British Journal of Cancer 29: 433–437
121 Furth J 1953 Conditioned and autonomous neoplasms. Cancer Research 13: 477–492
122 Sporn M B, Roberts A B 1985 Autocrine growth factors and cancer. Nature 323: 745–747
123 Metcalf D 1985 Multi-CSF-dependent colony formation by cells of a murine hemopoietic cell line: specificity and action of Multi-CSF. Blood 65: 357–362
124 Lang R A, Metcalf D, Gough N M, Dunn A R, Gonda T J 1985 Expression of a hematopoietic growth factor cDNA in a factor-dependent cell line results in autonomous growth and tumorigenicity. Cell 43: 531–542
125 Yodoi J, Uchiyama T, Maeda M 1983 T cell growth factor receptor in adult T cell leukemia. Blood 62: 509–511
126 Nicola N A, Begley C G, Metcalf D 1985 Identification of the human analogue of a regulator that induces differentiation in murine leukaemic cells. Nature 314: 625–628
127 Upton A C, Jenkins V K, Walburg H E, Tyndall R L, Conklin J W, Wald N 1966 Observations on viral-, chemical- and radiation-induced myeloid and lymphoid leukemias in Rf mice. National Cancer Institute Monograph 22: 329–347
128 Robinson W A, Pike B L 1970 Leukopoietic activity in human urine. The granulocytic leukemias. New England Journal of Medicine 282: 1291–1297
129 Metcalf D, Chan S H, Gunz F W, Vincent P, Ravich R B M 1971 Colony stimulating factor and inhibitor levels in acute granulocytic leukemia. Blood 38: 143–152
130 Metcalf D, Moore M A S 1975 Growth and responsiveness of human granulocytic leukemic cells in vitro. In: Ito Y, Dutcher R M (eds) Comparative leukemia research 1973, University of Tokyo Press, Tokyo/ Karger Basel, p 235

131 Mintz U, Sachs L 1973 Differences in inducing activity for human bone marrow colonies in normal serum and serum from patients with leukemia. Blood 42: 331–339
132 Mangalik A, Robinson W A 1972 The effect of serum from patients with acute granulocytic leukemia on granulocyte colony formation in vitro: a search for inhibitors. Proceedings of the Society for Experimental Biology and Medicine 141: 515–518
133 Lind D E, Bradley M L, Gunz F W, Vincent P C 1974 The non-equivalence of mouse and human marrow culture in assay of granulopoietic stimulating factors. Journal of Cell Physiology 83: 35–41
134 Metcalf D 1974 Stimulation by human urine or plasma of granulopoiesis by human marrow cells in agar. Experimental Hematology 2: 157–173
135 Aye M T, Till J E, McCulloch E A 1975 Interacting populations affecting proliferation of leukemic cells in culture. Blood 45: 485–493
136 Granstrom M, Gahrton G 1974 Colony-forming and colony-stimulating cells in relation to prognosis in leukemia. Acta Medica Scandinavica 196: 221–226
137 Golde D W, Rothman B, Cline M J 1974 Production of colony-stimulating factor by malignant leukocytes. Blood 43: 749–756
138 Goldman J M, Th'ng K H, Catovsky D, Galton D A G 1973 Production of colony-stimulating factor by leukemic leukocytes. Blood 47: 381–388
139 Le Beau M M, Westbrook C A, Diaz M O et al 1986 Evidence for the involvement of GM-CSF and FMS in the deletion (5q) in myeloid disorders. Science 231: 984–987
140 Huebner K, Isobe M, Croce C M, Golde D W, Kaufman S F, Gasson J C 1985 The human gene encoding GM-CSF is at 5q21–q32. The chromosome region deleted in the 5q anomaly. Science 230: 1282-1285
141 Cook W D, Metcalf D, Nicola N A, Burgess A W, Walker F 1985 Malignant transformation of a growth factor-dependent myeloid cell line by Abelson virus without evidence of an autocrine mechanism. Cell 41: 677–683
142 Metcalf D 1979 Clonal analysis of the action of GM-CSF on the proliferation and differentiation of myelomonocytic leukemic cells. Internal Journal of Cancer 24: 616–623
143 Metcalf D 1980 Clonal extinction of myeloid leukemic cells by serum from mice injection with endotoxin. International Journal of Cancer 25: 225–233
144 Metcalf D 1982 Regulator-induced suppression of myelomonocytic leukemic cells: Clonal analysis of early cellular events. International Journal of Cancer 30: 203–210
145 Nicola N A, Metcalf D 1984 Binding of the differentiation inducer granulocyte colony-stimulating factor to responsive but not unresponsive leukemic cell lines. Proceedings of the National Academy of Sciences of the USA 81: 3765–3769
146 Tomida M, Yamamoto-Yamiguchi Y, Hozumi M 1984 Purification of a factor inducing differentiation of mouse myeloid leukemic M1 cells from conditioned medium of fibroblast L929 cells. Journal of Biological Chemistry 259: 10978–10980
147 Olsson J, Sarngadharan M G, Breitman T R, Gallo R C 1984 Isolation and characterization of a T lymphocyte-derived differentiation inducing factor for the myeloid leukemic cell line HL-60. Blood 63: 510–517
148 Takeda K, Iwamoto S, Sugimoto H et al 1986 Identity of differentiation inducing factor and tumour necrosis factor. Nature 323: 338–340
149 Abrahm J, Rovera G 1981 Inducers and inhibitors of leukemia cell differentiation in culture. In: Baserga R (ed) Tissue growth factors. Springer-Verlag, New York p 405
150 Metcalf D 1983 Clonal analysis of the response of HL60 human myeloid leukemia cells to biological regulators. Leukemia Research 7: 117–132
151 Begley C G, Metcalf D, Nicola N A 1987 Purified colony stimulating factors (G-CSF and GM-CSF) induce differentiation in human HL60 leukemic cells with suppression of clonogenicity. International Journal of Cancer 39: 99–105

11
Cytogenetics of Acute Leukemia
Dorothy L. Williams

INTRODUCTION

The large volume of new information in leukemia cytogenetics has generated considerable excitement recently. The acute leukemias are associated with numerous non-random chromosomal abnormalities, many of which characterize specific subgroups.[1] The most frequent are the translocation and the deletion. The translocation may possibly lead to oncogene deregulation. The deletion of a chromosomal segment or single band may result in loss of a critical DNA sequence. Multiple chromosome abnormalities and multiple abnormal lines have also been observed which are related to clonal evolution, and possibly to clinical aggressiveness. Chromosome analysis is now essential for more accurate diagnosis and prognosis, and for monitoring the course of the disease. In addition, it may be helpful in:

1. Evaluating an accumulation of cells in extramedullary sites.
2. Characterizing a lineage switch[2] (i.e. acute lymphoid leukemia (ALL) to acute myeloid leukemia (AML)); or acute mixed lineage leukemia[3] (lymphocytic and myelocytic).
3. Providing evidence of a secondary leukemia.[4]
4. Distinguishing between leukemia and a non-malignant condition (i.e. a leukemoid reaction).[5]

A summary of chromosome abnormalities and their clinical correlation in the acute leukemias and lymphoma is presented following the description of technics.

The recent increase in information has been generated by newer cytogenetic technics being applied to the study of acute leukemia and lymphoma. These have included direct methodology especially designed for ALL, high resolution (extended banding) technics, other culture technics with or without synchronization, improved banding, and multiple technics or new methods in cases known to be difficult, such as T-cell ALL. A key factor in this success is teamwork between the clinical cytogeneticist and the attending physician, who recognize both the necessity of obtaining adequate specimen samples, and the proper attention to fine detail in achieving a successful end result. Through such efforts, clonal chromosome changes may be recognized in nearly all patients and can consistently be obtained in more than 90% of cases.[6-8]

The classification and subtyping of the acute leukemias requires close cooperation among specialists in cytomorphology, immunology and cytogenetics. Recent advances in technics have afforded cytogeneticists an opportunity to identify leukemia subgroups characterized by consistent and specific chromosomal change.[7,9,11]

METHODS

The preparation and analysis of chromosomes in acute leukemia is a difficult task, requiring attention to fine detail, and the development of skill. Most of the technics presented here are those in use in our laboratory, which have been consistently successful with large numbers of cases. In addition, the high resolution technic for bone marrow developed by Yunis is also presented. This technic has provided a very high rate of success in identifying the abnormal clone in AML, and allows the identification of subtle abnormalities and specific breakpoints that may not otherwise be detected.[7,8] The author and colleagues have been very specific in their description of sequential steps, so they may be followed without variation or misunderstanding. Those technics have been emphasized that appear to be very reliable in the acute leukemias and lymphomas.[10] Through experience it has been learned that ALL responds best to the direct technic, which should be supplemented in selected cases by short-term culture of bone marrow and/or circulating blasts. ALL has not responded satisfactorily to high resolution technics: first, the mitotic index in ALL is usually relatively low, and is not significantly altered by the high resolution technic. Secondly, the amount of bone marrow required for the high resolution technic is not always obtainable in small children and infants, which would be a factor in both ALL and AML. However, AML responds especially well to high resolution technics. It also responds to the other technics mentioned above. However, in occasional cases the abnormal clone may be missed in the direct method although identified in the high resolution method, or in short-term culture of bone marrow or circulating blasts.

At St Jude's Hospital the current rate of successful preparations in ALL is 95–97% of cases.[6] Identification of the abnormal clone is made in 90–94% of the successful cases.[6] This was established over a period of several years and required continual effort, experience, and the dedication of both clinical cytogeneticists and technologists. In order to *maintain* a high success rate, it is also necessary to collaborate closely with the attending physicians: obtaining second samples where cytogenetically indicated and not clinically contraindicated, and using multiple preparations in difficult cases.

DIRECT PROCEDURE FOR BONE MARROW ASPIRATE* (METHOD OF WILLIAMS)[11]

Preparation of solutions

1. Tubes: use heavy duty 12 ml, conical, graduated centrifuge tubes with Pennyhead stoppers.
2. Medium, per tube: 8 ml RPMI-1640 medium containing 30% fetal calf serum (pre-mixed in 100 ml amounts).
3. Anticoagulant: 0.5 ml heparin 1000 units/ml or 0.05 ml heparin, 10 000 units/ml.
4. Arresting solution: 0.05 ml colcemid (10 µg/ml). The arresting solution should reach a final concentration of 0.06 µg/ml.
5. Solution for washing cells: Hanks' balanced salt solution.
6. Hypotonic solution: 0.075 mol/l KCl. Mix 0.54g KCl and 100 ml deionized water.
7. Fixative: methyl alcohol–glacial acetic acid, 3:1 v/v. Use acetone-free, absolute methyl alcohol. Fixative should be refrigerated. Do *not* put in freezer. If too cold it will cause cells to clump. *All solutions should be freshly made each time, and all are used at room temperature, except the fixative.* Deionized water is recommended.

Arrest of mitosis

From 0.2 to 0.3 ml bone marrow is placed into each *pre-prepared* centrifuge tube. Close with cap or stopper and immediately mix contents gently 4–5 min to prevent clotting. Four tubes

---

* This procedure was originally published in Cancer Genetics and Cytogenetics 13: 239–258. It is reprinted here in different format and with slight modification with permission of the publisher: Elsevier Science Publishing Co. Inc. New York, N Y, USA, and the Editor: Dr Avery Sandberg

are usually adequate. Add arresting solution (0.05 ml) and allow to remain 25 min, mixing contents gently every 5-10 min (see below for method of mixing or resuspending cells). During this part of the procedure, observe for blood clots and remove.

Washing of bone marrow cells, and treatment with hypotonic solution

1. Cells are resuspended where indicated by twirling a 25 gauge stainless steel wire between the fingers. The end of the wire has been bent to fit the bottom of the centrifuge tube. The bent wire is more effective than a pipette in dispersing bone marrow pieces and is less damaging to the cells, especially after hypotonic treatment. In addition, fewer cells are lost, since they do not stick to the wire.
2. Centrifuge the tubes at 900 rev./min for 10 min and pipette off supernatant. (A clinical centrifuge is used.)
3. Add 8 ml balanced salt solution to each tube and resuspend, then centrifuge 10 min at 900 rev./min, and pipette off supernatant.
4. Repeat step (3).
5. Add 5 drops of hypotonic solution (0.075 mol/l KCl) to each tube, and carefully resuspend cells. Add up to 3 ml of KCl solution to each tube. Let tubes stand for a further 22 ± min at room temperature. Mix cells gently every 4-6 min. Centrifuge at 600 rev./min for 6 min. Time of exposure to hypotonic solution should total approximately 30-32 min distributed as follows:

	minutes
Time working with suspension	3-4
Time tubes standing (adjusted)	22
Time tubes centrifuging	6
Total time	32

Fixation of cells

1. Remove (with pipette) all but 0.1 ml of supernatant in each tube and resuspend cells. Add 3-4 drops of fixative to each tube and resuspend cells thus stopping the action of the hypotonic solution. To each tube add 0.5-ml amounts of fixative, with mixing, until 3 ml have been added. Cover each tube with top or parafilm and allow to stand for 15 min at room temperature. Centrifuge covered tubes at 600 rev./min for 6 min.
2. Pipette off nearly all of supernatant, add 8-10 drops of fresh fixative and resuspend cells. Add fixative, as before, up to 3 ml in each tube and let stand for 10 min. Centrifuge at 600 rev./min for 6 min. If button is brownish (hemoglobin) at this point, repeat fixative change only. Cell button should be white.
3. Pipette off fixative and add 2-4 drops of fresh fixative to make final suspension.

Slide making (edging)

1. For method see Fig. 11.1: slides are pre-cleaned and chilled in deionized water. Shake off excess water, and add one drop of cell suspension from a disposable pipette. Hold pipette 3-4 inches (7.5-10 cm) above slide, allowing *one drop* to strike the slide approximately midway between the edge of the slide and the center. *Tilt* the slide 15-20° and flame the appropriate edge by bringing it momentarily in contact with a spirit flame so that the fixative is ignited. The slide should not get hot. Allow it to complete drying. Since one drop usually will not go over the edge, the resistance of the edge causes rapid dispersion of the fluid (and cells) towards either end of the slide. This expansion, together with the heat produced by flaming, apparently creates an environment suitable for spreading of cells and chromosomes. In addition, the tilt of

1. EDGING OF DROP

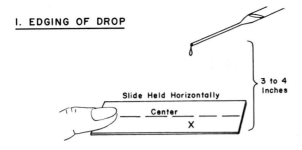

2. FLAMING

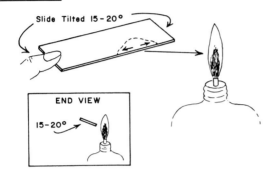

3. FINISHED SLIDE

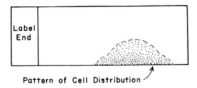

Fig. 11.1 Edging–flaming technic of slide preparation. One drop only of cell suspension delivered from a short Pasteur pipette, 3–4 inches (7.5–10 cm) above the slide, should strike a point approximately midway between the edge of the slide and the center (step 1). The slide is tilted 15–20° to allow the cells to spread toward the edge, and the fixative is ignited by bringing the slide *momentarily* in contact with an alcohol flame (step 2). Care should be taken to avoid overheating. The cold, wet surface causes the cells to spread rapidly. The slight resistance of the edge of the slide causes dispersion of the cells towards either end, with the distribution forming a modified (bell-shaped) half circle. Metaphases with excellent separation of chromosomes appear consistently along the edge. The heat produced by the burning fixative contributes to the rupture of the cell membrane, a better separation of the chromosomes from each other, an increased flattening of the chromosomes, and a very strong adherence of the chromosomes to the glass. A 5.75-inch (14.6-cm) Pasteur pipette is recommended, because it delivers a smaller drop than the long type. (Reprinted from Cancer Genetics and Cytogenetics, 13:239–257, 1984, with permission of the publisher Elsevier Science, New York, USA, and the Editor: Dr Avery Sandberg.)

the slide allows a greater share of the suspension to spread towards the edge. Analyzable spreads will consistently appear along the edge, and these will show excellent separation of chromosomes.

2. Prepare one test slide and examine under the microscope with reduced light (or phase contrast). There should be an even distribution of cells. Chromosomes are observed as dark images. Determine the adjustments needed in the cell suspension, if any, and the number of slides to prepare.

Drying of the slides by natural aging
One of the most important steps in obtaining successful banding in ALL is to achieve optimal drying by *natural* aging. Most quick drying methods, such as the use of a conventional oven or hot plate, are not consistently successful in ALL. One exception which provides acceptable results is the use of a microwave oven (see below). Natural aging requires accurate interpretation of the morphologic pattern which occurs in the G-banded chromosomes at different times in the aging process. The chromosome characteristics of *incomplete* aging are: a blurred image, a rough surface and poor definition of bands. The aging time varies and good G-banding may on rare occasions be obtained immediately after harvest. If

the day of harvest is counted as day 0, the normal time required falls in the range of 1–4 days, with the majority of cases banding well on or before day 3. Banding is attempted at 1-day intervals. At each time interval there will be a range of morphology as follows:

Stage 1: very poor image which appears blurred, bands are hardly perceptible, and the image cannot be brought into 'focus' in the usual manner.

Stage 2: improved image with sharpening of the chromosomes, but the chromosome surface is rough and band definition is poor.

Stage 3: the chromosome surface is smoother, with more bands visible but band detail may remain vague.

Stage 4: bands are sharp with clearly defined gradations of light and dark bands.

The ratio of metaphases representing each morphological stage should shift conspicuously each day towards total improvement. The accurate evaluation of this *shift in ratios* from day to day enables judgment of the proper end point. Occasional cases will appear to be arrested with most metaphases in an intermediate stage and never reaching the desired end point. These, however, may be analyzable, either partially or totally.

Rapid aging (drying) by use of a microwave oven (alternate method)
When the chromosome findings are urgently needed for clinical purposes, rapid drying may be accomplished with consistently adequate results by microwaving the slides. Use of the microwave oven has been previously described for another procedure.[12] For malignant cells the slides are placed in the microwave for 2–5 min on a high setting. Banding is then carried out in the usual manner. *This may not produce the same quality result as natural aging, but it does provide analyzable banded metaphases when the information is urgently needed.* The needs of the patient and attending physician must be met in a timely fashion to be of clinical value. Therefore, some flexibility in the use of reliable procedures is necessary.

G-banding technic (using Wright's stain)

Materials

1. Wright's stain: 0.3 g/100 ml methanol (mix and filter into brown bottle).
2. Trypsin: 0.25%; aliquot 5 ml into each tube.
3. Buffers: stock buffer pH 7.0; working buffer pH 7.0.
4. Working solutions:
    (a) Wright's stain: add 10 ml stain to 40 ml working buffer pH 7.0. Mix well but do not filter;
    (b) Trypsin: to 45 ml physiological saline add 5 ml trypsin. Mix well.

Note: store buffers and stains in refrigerator.

Procedure

1. Treat unstained slide for 5–30 s in trypsin solution. Treatment varies according to age of slide. Increase time for older slides. Run as test slide for the time which produces optimum banding and staining.
2. Rinse in two changes of saline.
3. Stain 3–5 min in buffered Wright's stain.
4. Rinse in distilled water and air dry. *Do not blot slide.* This may cause damage to the DNA content, and transmit dirt or lint to the slides.
5. Coversliping is optional. It is not necessary and may be time consuming where large numbers of slides are stained. However, care must be taken to be sure that slides without coverslips are not damaged.

G-banding technic (using Giemsa stain)
The technic above may be used with Giemsa stain as well as with Wright's, by substituting the appropriate Giemsa stain and buffer. However, in the author's laboratory, the use of Wright's stain has provided more consistent results.

Special comment concerning the direct method of bone marrow preparation
The most important component of the direct method is the slide making procedure: the edging-flaming technic. It is designed for optimum control of the cell suspension and heat distribution, and reduces time spent for microscopic scanning and searching. Bone marrow cells are relatively resistant to heat, and scattering of chromosomes rarely, if ever, occurs. *This technic does not interfere with any type of banding when performed as described.* There are very few 'crossovers' and less 'bunching' of chromosomes. This is of particular importance in the hyperdiploid ALL subgroup with 51–65 chromosomes.

Special problem related to T-cell ALL
Retrospective analysis of results in the author's laboratory in more than 400 banded ALL cases indicates that an abnormal ratio of T-cell cases has been read as normal, as compared to cases of B-cell lineage. The author's recent trials, using interleukin-2 (IL-2), a human T-cell growth factor (TCGF), to stimulate T-cell lymphocytes, has provided promising results in obtaining the abnormal chromosomes of the malignant clone. The method[13] is as follows:

1. Interleukin-2 concentration used: 10%
2. Tissue specimen: bone marrow, lymph node suspension, peripheral blood with circulating blasts.
3. To start a culture, per 8 ml flask:
   (a) 8 ml RPMI-1640 (supplemented with 30% fetal calf serum or FCS), L-glutamine (2%), penicillin streptomycin solution (1%);
   (b) 0.2 ml phytohemagglutinin;
   (c) 0.8 ml IL-2
4. Time in culture: (a) 48 hours, bone marrow and lymph node suspension;
   (b) 72 hours, peripheral blood.
5. Harvest:
   (a) for bone marrow and lymph node suspension, use 25 minutes in colcemid and 25 minutes in KCl
   (b) for peripheral blood, use 55 minutes in colcemid and 6 minutes in KCl.

Special problems related to ALL morphology
Because the malignant cells in acute lymphoblastic leukemia have been historically difficult to work with and slow to respond, several problems related particularly to ALL are presented below in outline form with suggested ways of achieving success.

Fuzzy chromosomes and poor banding quality
There is a marked difference between residual normal cells and leukemic cells.
   The possible causes are:

1. Processing too many cells per tube.
2. Improper drying of slides.
3. Delay in transporting specimens.
4. Poor cellular support during transport.

   The positive results are obtained with:

1. 0.1–0.2 ml sedimented cells per tube.
2. Natural aging of slides with daily monitoring of banding quality, or microwave drying for immediate analysis.
3. Begin direct procedure within 30 min or less of bone marrow aspiration/otherwise use short-term culture of the bone marrow (24–48 hours).

Inadequate number of metaphases
Possible causes are dilute sample, or reduced mitotic index.

Positive results may be obtained with any of the following steps, if not clinically contraindicated:

1. Contact physician to obtain second bone marrow sample.
2. Contact physician to obtain blood specimen for unstimulated culture of circulating blasts (24 hours and/or 48 hours), if circulating blasts are >5%.
3. Recommend that physician routinely obtain some extra cells in an extra syringe at each bone marrow aspiration. Use for direct preparation or culture as needed for each case.
4. If sample is obviously dilute, it should be put in short-term culture (24 and/or 48 hours). If the degree of dilution is in question, a minute portion may be checked under the microscope for cell frequency and type.
5. Routinely culture a portion of all bone marrow samples that are large enough to do so. In most cases the direct bone marrow procedure will provide everything necessary for a complete analysis and identification of the abnormal clone.

Poor spreading or flattening of chromosomes
Possible causes are acute lymphoblastic leukemia cells responding poorly to air drying of slide, blowing on slide or warming of slide.

Positive results are obtained by acute lymphoblastic leukemia cells which respond consistently to flaming by igniting the fixative.

Summary of very important points in achieving consistently good results

1. Careful attention to *detail*.
2. Processing *small amounts* of bone marrow per tube.
3. Use of the *flaming technic* for slide preparation.
4. Routine use of *natural aging* of slides (with monitoring) for appropriate drying. Use of microwave oven for rapid drying when immediate information is needed.
5. *Coordination of effort* among attending physicians, clinical cytogeneticists and technologists (teamwork).
6. Maintaining a technical staff of *qualified and experienced cytogenetic technologists*.
7. Extremely careful analysis requiring adequate time, and based primarily on *direct microscopic analysis*, supplemented by appropriate and adequate karyotyping.
8. Consecutive *reviews* of each finished case by a qualified technologist (i.e. supervisor) and a clinical cytogeneticist.

Photography and processing of film and prints

Chromosome preparations are photographed using Kodak Technical Pan film 2415 with a green filter, preferably 5546 nm Narrow band green filter no. 005 966 4 mm (Vashaw Scientific), or Wratten 58, and processed in Kodak D76 1:1 at 72° for 6 min. Technical Pan requires vigorous agitation in an *up-and-down direction*. This vigorous up-and-down agitation is necessary to allow the developer to work uniformly on the emulsion. This style of agitation should be continued throughout the process, including the stop bath and the fixer. At no time during processing should the tank be rotated in the traditional 180° revolution method of film development.

Exposure with modern automated cameras will vary from one photomicroscope to another. It will be necessary to make test exposures to determine the correct ASA/DIN number to use with your equipment. The ASA/DIN of Technical Pan will also vary with the type of processing and procedures used. Chemistry, time, temperature and technics must be consistent to achieve uniform results from roll to roll.

Photographing with either of the filters listed above, and processing in D76 1:1 for 6 min will generally print on Kodak Polycontrast Rapid II paper without contrast adjustment filtration. In cases where additional separation or emphasis on banding patterns may be needed to separate faintly stained chromosomes from the background, Polycontrast printing filters can be used to adjust the contrast. These filters should be placed in the enlarger light path above the lens. Placing Polycontrast or any other filters between the lens and the paper is not recommended as it can degrade the image.

HIGH RESOLUTION CHROMOSOME TECHNIC OF YUNIS* FOR BONE MARROW ASPIRATE

The use of high resolution chromosomes in clinical medicine has increased recently, especially in the study of AML.[1,7,8] From 400 to 850 bands are identifiable with this technic, in contrast with routine technics which provide 250-320 bands per chromosome spread.

The basic technic involves synchronization of cells with methotrexate, cell block release with thymidine, and brief exposure to colcemid. It is best that no more than two samples be processed each time, unless batches are harvested ½-1 hour apart. Otherwise, the time and temperature related to the processing of colcemid and hypotonic solution will vary. Even minor variations of the hypotonic and fixation treatment, as well as slide preparation, may have a dramatic adverse effect on the result, especially spreading and 'elongation' of mitoses. Technologists who carry out the hypotonic and fixation steps at a moderate speed may obtain nicely elongated and well-spread mitoses. A slow tempo tends to produce more contracted chromosomes and those that are very fast may have good spread but also a high percentage of broken mitoses.

The author compared bone marrow samples from patients with AML using an improved direct method and the methotrexate cell synchronization technic.[13] There was generally a higher mitotic index and a higher percentage of cells with longer chromosomes and chromosome defects observed with the methotrexate cell synchronization method. Several factors may contribute to this: a higher mitotic index is achieved by partial synchronization of marrow cells providing the release of a wave of dividing cells. Secondly, non-leukemic cells may be dividing preferentially in direct cultures whilst the methotrexate synchronization procedure may produce an admixture of dividing normal and leukemic cells, or a selection of dividing leukemic cells. Finally, leukemic cells with abnormal karyotypes may not be observed in direct preparations because chromosomes are sometimes too contracted for certain abnormalities to be detected, especially those with more subtle characteristics. The more elongated chromosomes of the methotrexate synchronization procedure thus facilitate the precise delineation of structural abnormalities.

These superior results with methotrexate cell synchronization suggest that this is the method of choice for the detection and definition of chromosomal abnormalities in patients with AML and other myeloid disorders.

---

* This section was contributed by Dr Jorge J. Yunis, Professor, Department of Laboratory Medicine and Pathology, University of Minnesota Medical School, Box 198, Mayo Memorial Building, 420 Delaware St S.E., Minneapolis, Minnesota 55455, USA.

Collection of bone marrow sample

Draw up a few drops of sodium heparin (1000 units/ml) in a 12 ml syringe. Pull back the plunger and rinse the syringe with the heparin. After rinsing, discard the heparin through the needle, leaving a small amount in the hub of the syringe. Change the needle and draw 3–5 ml of bone marrow.

Once the bone marrow is collected, invert the syringe to mix the marrow with the heparin. Cap the needle and put parafilm around the needle–syringe junction and the plunger end of the syringe. The bone marrow is kept at room temperature and sent to the laboratory for processing. A few hours' delay or local transportation does not affect results.

Concentrating white blood cells from hypocellular bone marrow aspirate

Perform a white blood cell (WBC) count and use marrow at a concentration of $3-5 \times 10^6$ nucleated cells/ml. If the WBC count of the bone marrow aspirate is less than 3×10^6 cells/ml, it is recommended to concentrate the sample. Too many red cells in the culture may detrimentally decrease the amount of nutrients available to the nucleated cells, and they may also cause a dirty cell preparation thus hindering chromosome spreading and banding. Ideally, no more than 0.1 ml bone marrow aspirate should be added to make a 5 ml culture. With hypocellular marrows, do not use more than 1 ml.

Concentrating nucleated cells from marrow

1. Under aseptic conditions, remove the needle from the syringe containing the bone marrow aspirate and slowly transfer the sample into a sterile 15 ml polystyrene (Falcon) centrifuge tube. Cap it and place it vertically in a test tube rack.
2. Let the sample stand for 20–60 min.
3. When the sample has sedimented, the clear plasma layer will be on top of the red blood cells. Aspirate off the plasma and the top of the red blood cell layer, and put it into another sterile 15 ml centrifuge tube containing 5 ml of RPMI-1640–HEPES medium (pH 7.2) warmed to room temperature.
4. Spin in a clinical centrifuge at 1100 rev./min for 8 min.
5. Aspirate off the supernatant and add 1–2 ml of supplemented RPMI-1640–HEPES medium.
6. Do a cell count (of nucleated cells) and dilute the cells in culture medium to a concentration of 3×10^6/ml.

Culture initiation

1. Aseptically add the heparinized bone marrow to 10 ml of room temperature RPMI-1640–HEPES medium in a sterile 15 ml centrifuge tube. Spin at 1100 rev./min for 8 min in a clinical centrifuge.
2. Aspirate off the supernatant leaving approximately 0.5 ml of medium above the cell pellet. Resuspend the pellet and add another 10 ml medium. Spin at 1100 rev./min for 8 min.
3. Aspirate off supernatant and resuspend cell pellet in approximately 5 ml of RPMI-1640–HEPES supplemented medium.
4. Do a cell count, and add $3-5 \times 10^6$ nucleated cells per flask and add supplemented RPMI-1640–HEPES to bring the final volume of each 25 cm^2 polystyrene Falcon flask to 5 ml. Two 5 ml flasks are combined to form one pellet at the time of harvest.
5. Incubate cultures horizontally with the caps loose, at 37°C in a carbon dioxide incubator for 3–7 hours prior to methotrexate block. Less than 3 hours of culture prior to methotrexate exposure is needed to avoid cell toxicity.

6. At the end of this time and under aseptic conditions, gently resuspend the cells and add 0.05 ml of the 10^{-5} mol/l working solution of methotrexate to each 5 ml culture. The final concentration of methotrexate should be 10^{-7} mol/l.
7. Incubate flasks horizontally with the caps loose at 37°C in a carbon dioxide incubator for 17–18 hours. Longer time is toxic to cells.

Releasing the methotrexate block

1. After 17 hours' exposure to methotrexate, aseptically combine the contents of the two 5 ml flasks into a sterile 15 ml round bottomed centrifuge tube and spin at 1100 rev./min for 8 min (higher speed could interfere with subsequent block release—use appropriate tachometer).
2. Remove supernatant and resuspend cells in 10 ml prewarmed unsupplemented RPMI-1640–HEPES medium and spin at 1100 rev./min for 8 min.
3. Repeat step (2).
4. Resuspend cell pellet in 9.4–9.5 ml of freshly prepared RPMI-1640–HEPES supplemented medium pH 7.2. The final volume should be 10 ml. Transfer the cells into a clean flask.
5. Add 0.1 ml of the 10^{-3} mol/l thymidine solution to each 10 ml culture and note exact time. The final concentration of thymidine in the culture should be 10^{-5} mol/l.
6. Exactly 6 hours later proceed to harvest the cells.

Hypotonization and fixation of cells

1. After 6 hours of thymidine cell block release, gently resuspend cells in the flask and add 0.04–0.05 ml of the 10 g/ml colcemid solution to each 10 ml culture. After 8–9 min of colcemid exposure, transfer the contents of the flask into a 15 ml conical centrifuge tube. At 10 min of total colcemid time begin centrifugation.*
2. Centrifuge at 1100 rev./min for 8 min.
3. Aspirate off supernatant leaving approximately 0.5 ml of the medium above the pellet.
4. Resuspend the cells by gently tapping the bottom of the tube with finger.
5. Gently add 8 ml of fresh 0.074 mol/l KCl at 37°C in small amounts with a siliconized Pasteur pipette. Then mix gently but thoroughly either by capping the tube and inverting it or by slowly drawing the cells into the pipette and slowly releasing them.
6. Place cells in an incubator or water bath at 37°C for 10 min.
7. Centrifuge tubes at 1100 rev./min for 5 min.
8. Aspirate off supernatant except for the last 0.1–0.2 ml above the pellet.
9. Fix the cells in fresh 3:1 methanol:acetic acid fixative by resuspending the cell pellet by gently tapping the bottom of the tube and adding fixative drop by drop with a pipette, all the time gently shaking the tube to keep the cells in suspension while fixation is taking place. Add approximately 1–2 ml of fixative in this manner, then thoroughly mix with a pipette, making sure all cell clumps are dispersed. Proper fixation is critical for good spreading and banding.
10. Add an additional 4–5 ml of fixative and mix thoroughly.
11. Tightly seal tubes with parafilm and let cells set at room temperature for 20 min.
12. After 20 min, centrifuge the tubes at 1100 rev./min for 5 min.
13. Aspirate off the fixative, gently resuspend the cell pellet, add 5–7 ml fresh fixative and immediately centrifuge the tubes at 1100 rev./min for 5 min. Do this at least six

---

* To obtain elongated chromosomes, it is critical not to let cells stand in colcemid or hypotonic solution beyond the prescribed time from colcemid exposure to the time of the first cell fixation.

times to ensure that the cell suspension is clean of debris and that the cytoplasmic RNA and proteins are extracted. This then allows the chromosomes to spread and band better. Spread slides the same day or seal the tubes with parafilm and refrigerate overnight. The next day, bring the tubes up to room temperature and wash the cells at least three times with fresh fixative before spreading slides.

Slide making

1. Preclean slides with 70% ethanol.
2. Prepare a thin cell suspension (cell pellet resuspended in 0.5–1.0 ml fresh fixative) and label slides with appropriate identification.
3. Drop 2–3 drops of cell suspension from a distance of 4–5 feet (1.2–1.5 m) onto precleaned slides placed at a 30° angle.
4. Blow air very gently onto slide for a few seconds to allow for rapid evaporation of the fixative. Allow slide to air dry.
5. Check the first slides under the microscope with phase contrast to be sure that the cell suspension is properly diluted and is free of debris, and that the spreading technic is appropriate for the environmental conditions. Both wet cold and dry room temperature slides could be tested since one method may be more successful than the other with a given pellet or time of year. For example, wet cold slides may work in winter and dry slides in the summer. If chromosomes are not spreading well, a few more changes of fixative could be useful. More dilute cell suspensions can also prove helpful. Whatever the season, slides are optimally spread in temperatures at 70–75°F (21–24°C) and at 10–40% humidity.
6. For routine use, slides should be dried 16–24 hours in a 65°C drying oven and then desiccated until they are stained.

Slide staining procedure

1. Place 3 ml of room temperature phosphate buffer in a clean 15 ml polystyrene, round-bottomed tube.
2. Add 1 ml Wright's stain with a 1 ml pipette. Mix quickly by shaking the tube or by pipetting the mixture up and down in the pipette, and pour immediately onto a slide placed on a level staining rack over a sink.
3. After exact timing (see below) with a stop watch, quickly rinse with tepid tap water for 8–15 s and air jet the slide dry.

Important: exact timing

1. To obtain high quality banding exact timing is important, therefore stain one slide at a time.
2. Optimal time is between 2 and 3 min: the authors normally use between 2 and $2\frac{1}{2}$ min. Dilute stock solution with methanol, if necessary, to achieve this range.
3. For each stock solution bottle, make several trials to determine the approximate staining time for that batch of stain. The exact staining time, however, will vary by a few seconds with source of cells, age of slides, type of preparation and temperature.
4. Prometaphase chromosomes require a few seconds longer than metaphase chromosomes.
5. The ideal temperature and humidity for banding appear to be 72–75°F (21–24°C) and less than 40%, respectively.

Comments about the Wright's staining technic

The technic recommended is advantageous in that it requires no special chromosome pre-treatment and yet elicits sharp and well contrasted G-bands with a minimum of time, reagents and equipment. It is, however, important that the details given, such as source of stain, preparation of stock solution and buffer, and the actual staining procedure, are followed closely.

As mentioned above, for staining, the Wright's stock solution is diluted 1:3 with phosphate buffer (4 ml total/slide) in a clean tube, mixed rapidly, and poured immediately onto the slide. After exact timing, the slide is rinsed quickly with tap water and dried with an air jet.

Inadequately stained slides can sometimes be improved by further rinsing and restaining. For example, an additional 5–15 s rinse in running tap water may be employed to improve overstained slides. Understained slides may also be stained for an additional 30–60 s, followed by a brief rinse. Progress of staining is most easily monitored with the use of an Epiplan 80X microscope objective which does not require the application of oil to the slide.

Ideally, slides should not be heated and should age 10–60 days before staining to obtain the best banding possible. For more routine chromosome studies, however, one can forego the aging requirement by heating fresh slide preparations at 65°C for 18–24 hours, followed by heating at 90°C for 10 min. Alternatively, fresh slide preparations could be stained, destained and restained to improve banding quality. To destain, fresh slides which have already been stained are dipped into the following reagents in the given order for the stated time: 70% ethanol–2 min; 80% ethanol–2 min; 95% ethanol with 1% concentrated HCl–2 min; 95% ethanol–2 min; 100% methanol–2 min.

Slides are dried after methanol treatment and solutions are changed daily. Several slides may be destained at the same time. If a slide has previously been checked with the use of an oil immersion objective, the oil must be removed by rinsing in several changes of xylol and dried before destaining. Restaining is carried out in the same manner as the initial staining and for a similar time. For very freshly made preparations, one to two destain/restain series may be best; more than three times usually affects the chromosome morphology. This procedure can also be used to improve slides that were initially over- or understained.

Photography of G-banded preparations

Of critical importance for chromosome analysis and photography is the use of a microscope with high-quality optics (as manufactured by the Zeiss or Leitz Companies). A planapochromat 100 X oil objective (numerical aperture 1.3–1.4) and a planachromat condenser (numerical aperture 1.4) should be used. To achieve optimal photographic detail, it is necessary to use oil (Cargille oil refractive index 1.556) between slide and condenser and a monochromatic light filter such as a Schott filter type PIL, which allows only a narrow wavelength of monochromatic light to pass through the microscope optics.

In photographing elongated and finely banded chromosomes, it is important to use a 4 × 5 inch camera. This attachment when used with a 100× objective and a 10× eyepiece, records the image at 1600× enlargement, thus obtaining maximum resolution. To visualize the very delicate banding pattern of prometaphases through the camera eyepiece, it is also necessary to use a high-intensity xenon lamp instead of one of the more common light systems. The authors have found that 4 × 5 inch Kodak Plus-X professional film 4147 provides appropriate fine grain and tone range and gives excellent results, provided that development of the negatives with Kodak D-76 is carried out for 15 min at room temperature (22°C) instead of the manufacturer's recommended 6 minutes. Overdevelopment with this film results in a darker gray background with greatly improved contrast. Important details in printing include the use of a good dark room enlarger (such as the Omega enlarger with variable condenser and Componon objectives) and Kodabromide F-5 photographic paper to achieve the highest degree of dark and light contrast without significant loss of detail.

Materials and solutions

Glassware
Use 15 ml polystyrene, round-bottomed centrifuge tubes (Falcon) for washing cells; 25 cm^2 growth area polystyrene flasks (Falcon) for culturing the cells; and sterile disposable pipettes for handling cells.

Heparin
Obtained from Upjohn Co., NDC 0009-0268-01, 1000 units per ml, from beef lung. Store at 4°C. Product is stable for 2–3 years.

Washing solution
RPMI-1640–HEPES medium (Gibco) warmed to room temperature.

Media
Make RPMI-1640–HEPES medium (Gibco) supplemented with 15% fetal calf serum (Gibco); 2.0% penicillin–streptomycin, 5000 units/ml penicillin and 5000 g/ml streptomycin (Microbiological Associates); and 2.0% L-glutamine, 29.23 mg/ml (Microbiological Associates). The supplemented medium has a pH of about 7.2. The color of the medium should be a light orange, not yellow or red. If the medium starts to turn red, flush medium with carbon dioxide, 5 l/min, until pH is restored to 7.2. Otherwise use fresh media.

L-Glutamine
Obtained from M.A. Bioproducts, No. 17-605C; 200 mmol/l solution in 0.85% NaCl solution; 29.23 mg/ml L-glutamine. Store bottles at −20°C. Shelf life at −20°C is 2 years. Thaw once, pipette 2.0-ml aliquots into tubes and refreeze. Shelf life is 2 years at −20°C. Thaw again for use and then discard.

Synchronizing solution
Make a 10^{-4} mol/l solution of methotrexate (Lederle methotrexate sodium parenteral, 2.5 mg/ml by mixing a 2 ml vial (5 mg) of methotrexate with 98 ml of autoclaved Hanks' balanced salt solution). Dilute this stock solution 1:10 with more Hanks' balanced salt solution to obtain a 10^{-5} mol/l working solution.

Use Lederle methotrexate sodium parenteral, 2.5 mg/ml, in a 2.0 ml vial (molarity of 2.5 mg/ml is 5×10^{-3} mol/l). As received from Lederle, solution is stable at room temperature for 1–2 years.

To make stock (dilute 1:50, to 10^{-4} mol/l concentration):

1. Aseptically remove 1.0 ml methotrexate concentrate from sample vial, and pipette the 1.0 ml into 49.0 ml of Hanks' balanced salt solution. Mix well.
2. Aliquot the stock into 1.2-ml portions in screw-top tubes and cap tubes tightly.
3. Label each tube with: the concentration (10^{-4} mol/l), date stock was made, and expiration date of methotrexate.
4. Freeze at −20°C. Thaw only once.

To make working solution:

1. Remove one tube of stock from freezer, and thaw at room temperature (10^{-4} mol/l).
2. Dilute stock 1:10 in Hanks' balanced salt solution (HBSS), to yield 10^{-5} mol/l solution. To do this, aseptically pipette 1.0 ml of 10^{-4} mol/l stock into 9.0 ml of HBSS. Mix well.

3. Aliquot this 10^{-5} mol/l working solution into 1.0-ml portions in small tubes. Cap tightly and freeze. Keep working solutions separate from stock solutions to avoid error in using wrong tube.
4. To use working solution, remove tube from freezer and thaw at room temperature. Do not refreeze.

Thymidine solution
Make a 10^{-3} mol/l solution of thymidine (Sigma) by adding 10 mg of thymidine to 40 ml of autoclaved HBSS.

Thymidine can be obtained from Sigma Cat No. T-9250, molecular weight = 242.2 g/mol. Store at 4°C, dessicated. If properly stored, this powder is stable for 3-4 years.

Working solution is 10^{-3} mol/l in HBSS and stored at -20°C. To make 10^{-3} mol/l thymidine:

1. Weigh carefully 0.012 g thymidine.
2. Add 50.0 ml HBSS.
3. Mix well.

Filter the 10^{-3} mol/l thymidine through a 0.2-m Millipore filter. Pipette 1.0-ml aliquots into freezer tubes. Cap tightly and freeze at -20°C. Thaw for use. May be refrozen and thawed.

Arresting solution
Colcemid stock solution 10 g/ml (Gibco).

Hypotonic solution
0.074 mol/l KCl at 37°C. Add 0.55 g KCl (Sigma) to 100 ml distilled water. Never use a solution over 1 week old.

Fixative
Methanol:acetic acid 3:1. Make fresh and keep at room temperature. Use acetone-free, absolute methyl alcohol (Fisher).

Wright's stain

1. Prepare 1 litre of a 0.25% solution using powdered Wright stain (MCB, Manufacturing Chemists, Norwood, Ohio 95212, USA) and anhydrous acetone free methanol (Fisher).
2. Protect the solution from light and stir with electric stirrer for 60-120 min.
3. Rinse several clean, dark, one-half pint bottles with methanol to aliquot stain.
4. After the Wright's stain is sufficiently mixed, filter it through double No. 1 Whitman filter paper into the precleaned bottles.
5. Wrap the bottles of Wright's stain in aluminum foil and store air-tight for a least 1 month or incubate at 37°C for 2-5 days.

Stain should not be diluted until use and then only in quantities to be used immediately.

Phosphate buffer

1. Prepare a 0.06 mol/l Na_2HPO_4 stock solution by dissolving 8.52 g Na_2HPO_4 (Baker; mol.wt 141.92) in 1 liter of distilled water.
2. Prepare a 0.06 mol/l KH_2PO_4 stock solution by dissolving 8.10 g KH_2PO_4 (Baker; mol. wt 135.05) in 1 liter distilled water. Both stocks should be stored at 4°C.

3. Working buffer is prepared by mixing 51 ml of the KH_2PO_4 solution and 49 ml of the Na_2HPO_4 solution at room temperature. Adjust pH to 6.8, using either the KH_2PO_4 solution or the Na_2HPO_4 solution, and store in a stoppered bottle at 4°C.

OTHER TECHNICS

Bone Core Biopsy

If an aspirate cannot be obtained because of tightly packed cells, or for other reasons, a bone core biopsy can provide successful results in some cases. The amount of material is limited, however, and care must be taken to preserve all cells.

1. The specimen should be placed in a sterile centrifuge tube containing 8 ml RPMI-1640 medium containing 30% fetal calf serum, and 0.5 ml heparin 1000 units/ml. The specimen should be delivered to the laboratory without delay.
2. With sterile technic, the specimen should be processed in a Petri dish, using the same medium as for transport. The core sample should be held with forceps, and very thin sections should be sliced using a scalpel. Disperse as many cells as possible from these sections using fine wire or needle type instruments. Check the contents of the Petri dish under an inverted microscope before discarding fibrous or bony fragments to be certain all cells have been removed.
3. The cell suspension is then placed in culture (unstimulated) for 24–48 hours beginning with step (1) of the short-term culture of bone marrow.

Short-term Culture of Bone Marrow (24 or 48 hours)

1. Add 0.5 ml (or less) of packed bone marrow cells to each culture flask containing 8 ml of RPMI medium with 30% fetal calf serum, and 1 ml of penicillin–streptomycin antibiotic suspension (10 000 units).
2. Culture 24–48 hours at 37°C.
3. At the time of harvest, transfer cells to centrifuge tubes, and follow the direct bone marrow procedure starting with step (2).

Culture of Blasts from Peripheral Blood

This is an alternative procedure, used as a substitute for bone marrow when the bone marrow preparation is inadequate for a valid study. To obtain metaphases, blasts (or other early cells capable of spontaneous division) must be present in the blood. No mitogens are used.

Avoid centrifugation by collecting blood in a chromosome separation vial. Allow red cells to separate. Dispense plasma (containing white cells) into culture bottles according to the total WBC count as follows:

WBC ($\times 10^9/l$)	Plasma/bottle (ml)
6–30	1
30–72	0.5
72–150	0.2
>150	0.1

Add cells to 8–10 ml of RPMI-1640 medium (or MEM) containing 30% fetal calf serum. Use the sterile technic. Allow to incubate overnight at 37°C. The range of hours during which satisfactory numbers of metaphases may be obtained is 18–48 hours. From three to six bottles should be prepared depending on the number of cells available.

Technic for Pleural or Peritoneal Fluid

Centrifuge cells at 900 rev./min for 10 minutes, and discard fluid to obtain a cell button.

Resuspend cells in 8 ml of RPMI-1640 medium with 30% fetal calf serum, and colchicine for 45 min.

Centrifuge at 900 rev./min for 10 min, discard supernatant, and proceed with step (2) of the 72-hour peripheral blood harvest procedure.

Technic for spinal fluid

This sample should be received by the laboratory immediately, otherwise the cells may deteriorate rapidly. The method will depend upon the number of cells per millilitre in the sample. If there are less than 6000 an overnight culture is appropriate. If there are 6000 or more, both a direct and an overnight culture may be carried out, if the total sample is adequate. The sample received should be rinsed with culture medium (RPMI-1640) with extreme care (in siliconized tubes) to avoid cell loss, and resuspended in 3 ml of fresh culture medium. If the sample received is in culture medium, proceed to the method of choice.

Direct method

1. To 7 ml medium per tube, add approximately 1 ml of cell suspension and colcemid 0.05 ml (10 µg/ml) for 45 minutes. (Times for colcemid and KCl may be adjusted as needed.)
2. Centrifuge for 10 min at 900 rev./min.
3. Do *not* rinse with Hanks' solution.
4. Add slowly, with mixing, 3 ml of KCl hypotonic solution (0.075 mol/l) to the tube, and allow to stand for 10 min with gentle mixing two to three times.
5. Centrifuge 10 min at 900 rev./min and discard supernatant.
6. Fix for 15 minutes with methanol/acetic acid (3:1, v/v).
7. Make slides with edging–flaming technic.

Overnight cultures (preferred method)

1. Centrifuge sample and rinse with culture medium; resuspend cells in 3 ml of fresh culture media.
2. Transfer the cell suspension to culture flasks, adding approximately 1 ml per 7 ml/medium.
3. Incubate for 24 or 48 hours.
4. Process as described for the direct method above, except that the time in colcemid should be 60 minutes, and the time in hypotonic KCl should be 20 minutes (standing time).

Technic for lymph node cell suspension

If the specimen is received as solid tissue the following steps are recommended:

1. Place the tissue in a Petri dish in RPMI-1640 medium with 30% fetal calf serum.
2. Remove all capsular tissue by carefully separating it from the other tissue with tweezers and scalpel, or other suitable fine instrument.
3. Using two no. 10 scalpels in a crossing motion, slice the tissue until it is very fine. Do not use scissors since they are not as sharp and tend to mash the tissue. Place all the material and the medium in a centrifuge tube and allow the tissue fragments to settle to the bottom. Pipette the loose cell suspension into another tube. If only a small amount of material is received, one may elect to re-slice the sedimented material in an attempt to obtain additional cells. The cells are centrifuged, resuspended in

fresh medium with colcemid 0.05 ml (10 μg/ml), and remain in the colcemid for 45 min. The harvesting process is then continued using 25 min for KCl exposure.

C-banding technic for bone marrow (modification of the method of Sumner[14])

1. The slides may be fresh or destained. All slides must be oil free (to remove the oil without leaving a film on the slide add pure xylene drop by drop, next to a sink with water running).
2. Place the slides in a Coplin jar containing 0.2 mol/l HCl (10 ml 1mol/l HCl:40 mg H_2O) for 15–30 min at room temperature.
3. Rinse in distilled water.
4. Treat the slides in a saturated solution of $Ba(OH)_2$ (2.5 g $Ba(OH)_2$:100 ml water) starting at 45 s at room temperature. Gently agitate the slide so that barium will not adhere to it.
5. Different timings for the $Ba(OH)_2$ treatment may be adjusted as needed, i.e. from 20 to 120 seconds for fresh unstained or fresh trypsin–Wright's banded slides, or from 1 to 4 seconds for about 1-month-old unstained, or previously trypsin–Wright's banded slides.
6. Rinse with running tap water.
7. Dip once in HCl to remove the barium film.
8. Rinse with running tap water.
9. Place in 2 × SSC (1.75 g NaCl + 0.88 g sodium citrate: 100 ml water) for 30 min to 1 hour.
10. Rinse in running tap water.
11. Blow-dry slides (to prevent uneven staining).
12. Place them on the staining rack.
13. Stain with 8% Giemsa in 0.06 mol/l Sorensen's buffer pH 6.8.
14. Make stain fresh each time (approximately 2 ml per slide).
15. To make 15 ml: 13.8 ml of 6.8 Sorensen's buffer + 1.2 ml of Giemsa.
16. Staining time – 15 min.

C-banding tips

A good starting time is 45 s in $Ba(OH)_2$, at room temperature. If the chromosomes seem pale and 'ghost-like' they are undertreated. Destain and try again, increasing the time by 5–10 s; it can be carried out several times starting with HCl each time.

Instructions For Shipping Specimen

Specimens received from a distance require careful regulations in order to obtain consistently good results. The senders should be informed that this is extremely important. The system described here has been used under supervision for a number of years with nearly 100% success both in obtaining an analyzable preparation and in identifying the chromosomally abnormal clone.

1. At least 1 ml of bone marrow should be shipped.
2. Shipping should be in a way that will allow *delivery* within 24 hours or less.
3. *Ship bone marrow* in 8 ml media which contains the following:

5.6 ml	RPMI-1640 medium
2.4 ml	fetal calf serum
0.1 ml	fresh L-glutamine (29.2 mg/ml)
0.1 ml	preservative-free heparin (1000 units/ml)
0.1 ml	Pen-Strep antibiotic (5000 units/ml)

Substitutions for any of the above products may be made if the product is of equivalent quality and quantity.

Instructions for Laboratory Handling Of Shipped Specimen

1. Pre-prepared medium similar to the above should be available (see special note below).
2. Place 7 ml of the pre-prepared medium in each of eight sterile 50 ml flasks. Add 1 ml of the uncentrifuged, well-mixed bone marrow suspension to each flask. If the suspension appears very dilute, with only a minimum amount of bone marrow cells, a larger amount of suspension may be added to each flask used, or the suspension may be centrifuged and appropriately divided.
3. Culture the preparation for 24 hours (37°C). If desired, part of the culture may continue to 48 hours.

Special note: The above medium mixture contains amounts for one centrifuge tube. In practice, the medium is pre-prepared in 50 or 100 ml lots, using the same proportions. Pre-prepared medium is kept only 3 weeks, if not used.

THE CYTOGENETICS OF ACUTE LYMPHOBLASTIC LEUKEMIA IN CHILDREN

Recent improvement of ALL preparations[11] has made possible the identification of new chromosome subgroups and, in turn, their biological and clinical correlations.[15-17] In the past, about 66–80% of cases had a clonal abnormality identified.[18-20] The ability to identify the abnormal clone in more than 90% of cases is now revealing new information related to the cytogenetic complexity and heterogeneity of ALL. Currently, approximately two-thirds of the structural abnormalities found in ALL are recurring or non-random abnormalities,[9] and this number is increasing. Non-random numerical abnormalities are also found but occur primarily in cases with more than 50 chromosomes. Chromosome 21 is the most frequent addition overall,[18] and a subgroup with a missing 20 is found in the hypodiploid group.[21] The approximate frequency, immunophenotype specificity and relative prognosis (if known), of the non-random chromosomal abnormalities in ALL are presented in Table 11.1.

PLOIDY

The number of cases in the normal group is decreasing, whilst the number in the pseudodiploid group is increasing. Other ploidy groups have remained about the same. This suggests that the majority of cases read as normal in the past were really pseudodiploid. However, occasional cases containing other numbers could have been completely missed. Frequencies (percentage) of the ploidy groups from the first 245 banded cases of our current ALL protocols were: hypodiploid 6.9, pseudodiploid 41.6, normal 8.6, 47–50 17.6, and >50 25.3. Figure 11.2 presents the distribution of modal numbers found in this consecutive series. There is a bimodal pattern with peaks at 46 (pseudodiploid) and 55. Cases with 50 or 51 chromosomes are infrequent at diagnosis. The group with more than 50 has a unique pattern of chromosomal additions. These form trisomies most frequently with numbers 4, 6, 10, 14, 17, 18, 20, 21, and X, with 21 added twice in many cases. This non-random addition of at least nine different chromosomes contributes to the peak of 55 chromosomes shown in Figure 11.2.

Translocations are most frequent in the pseudodiploid and hypodiploid groups, and least frequent in the >50 group. This correlates with the poor prognosis of the pseudodiploid

Table 11.1 Non-random chromosomal abnormalities in acute lymphoblastic leukemia

Chromosome abnormality	Primary lineage/or specificity	Relative prognosis[a] (if known)	Approximate frequency (%)[b]
t(8;14)(q24.1;q32.3)	B, FAB L3	Poor	2
t(8;22)(q24.1;q11.2)	B, FAB L3	Poor	0.4
t(2;8)(p11.1;q24.1)	B, FAB L3	Poor	Rare
t(9;22)(q34;q11)	B	Poor	4
t(4;11)(q21;q23)	Mixed[c]	Poor	0.8
t(1;19)(q23;p13.3)	Pre-B	–	7
t(7;12)(q11;p12)	B	–	0.8
tdic(9;12)(p1?1;p1?2)	B	–	1
t(12;V)(p;V)	B	–	9
t(11;V)(q;V)	B, cALLA-	Poor	3
dup(1q)	B, FAB L3 and 50 ploidy[d]	–	6
del(12p)	B	–	7
del(9p)	B or T	–	8
del(6q)	B or T	Good	13
del(11q)	Undifferentiated or T	–	2
t(11;14)(p13;q11)	T	–	0.4
t(10;14)(q24;q11)	T	–	0.8
t(8;14)(q24;q11)	T	–	0.4
t(7;V)(q32 or q36;V)	T	–	3
inv(14)(q11q32)	T	–	0.8

[a]Many of the abnormalities listed in this table have been identified as subgroups only recently. Additional cases and longer follow-up will be needed to determine the prognosis.
[b]The frequencies in this table are based on 239 consecutive completely banded cases in the recent ALL protocol (Total XI) at St Jude Hospital, with the exception of the B-cell cases who are treated on a separate protocol. During the same period of time six cases were entered on the B-cell protocol, with five having a t(8;14), and one having a t(8;22).
[c]Contains both lymphoid and myeloid characteristics.
[d]Duplication (1q) is considered to be a non-random secondary abnormality occurring in B-cell, FAB L3 cases. It is also specifically associated with the >50 ploidy group. In both instances, its influence on prognosis, if any, is unknown.

group, and the better prognosis of the >50 group. However, translocations are more frequent in the >50 group than first recognized (up to 20% of cases). But, those known to carry a bad prognosis, especially the t(8;14), t(4;11) and t(9;22) are rarely found in this group, occurring most often in the pseudodiploid group. The hypodiploid group is the smallest and, until recently, the prognosis has been in question. Recent studies from St Jude Hospital reveal that patients in this group have a poor prognosis, with a high frequency of translocations and other high-risk factors. Prognosis of the ploidy groups can be summarized as follows: best = >50; intermediate = 47–50 and normal; poor = pseudodiploid and hypodiploid.[21,22,23]

TRANSLOCATIONS

For details of frequencies see Table 11.1 and Figs 11.3–11.6. In St Jude Total XI data, translocations have occurred in 46% of the first 239 banded cases. In addition, four B-cell cases, treated on a separate protocol, all had translocations. Previously recognized translocation subgroups in ALL (all with poor prognosis), include t(9;22)(q34;q11), t(4;11)(q21;q23), and the t(8;14)(q24;q32) associated with B-cell (FAB L3) ALL.[18] Recently,

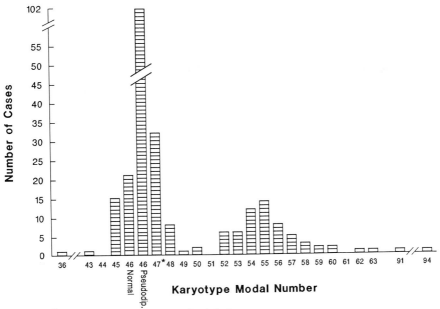

Fig. 11.2 Distribution of modal chromosome numbers in childhood ALL. This graph presents the modal numbers in the stemline of 245 consecutive banded cases in recent ALL protocols at St Jude Hospital. There is a bimodal pattern with a major peak at 46 (pseudodiploid), and a smaller peak at 55. Cases with 50 or 51 chromosomes occur infrequently. No other leukemia has this unique distribution of numbers.

new translocation subgroups have been identified and include the t(1;19)(q23;p13.3) associated with a pre-B phenotype,[15] the t(11;14)(p13;q11)[15] and t(10;14)(q24;q11)[24] with T-cell phenotypes, the t(7;12)(q11;p12)[25] and dic(9;12)[26] in B-lineage phenotypes, and translocations involving 7q32-q36 which are specific for T-cell ALL.[27] The prognosis of these new translocation subgroups must await greater numbers and longer follow-up. The t(2;8)(p11.1;q24.1) and the t(8;22)(q24.1;q11.2), which are variants of the t(8;14)(q24;q32) in lymphoma[28,29] are also found in B-cell ALL. Other translocations occur in large numbers, appearing to be random. However, as more cases are studied, more subgroups are being recognized. In time, many more specific subgroups may be found. Figures 11.3–11.6 illustrate some of the translocations discussed above, as well as many other abnormalities. These examples were chosen to illustrate: (1) varying chromosome numbers (up to 93), (2) the complexity of some karyotypes, and (3) the varying morphologic quality of the DNA. Yet, in each case the numerical and structural abnormalities could be identified, even in very complex cases. Also it should be noted that there are no chromosome 'crossovers'. These examples were obtained from the direct bone marrow method described in this chapter.

OTHER NON-RANDOM CHROMOSOMAL ABNORMALITIES IN ALL

Recent data from ALL Total XI, confirm that other *structural* abnormalities occurring non-randomly include translocations or deletions involving 6q, 9p, 11q and 12p, and duplication (1q), inversion (14) and isochromosome (17q). In the translocations and deletions the breakpoints may vary, but tend to cluster near one point especially 6(q21), 12(p12), 9(p21) and 11(q23). The inv 14 is specifically associated with T-cell disease, and

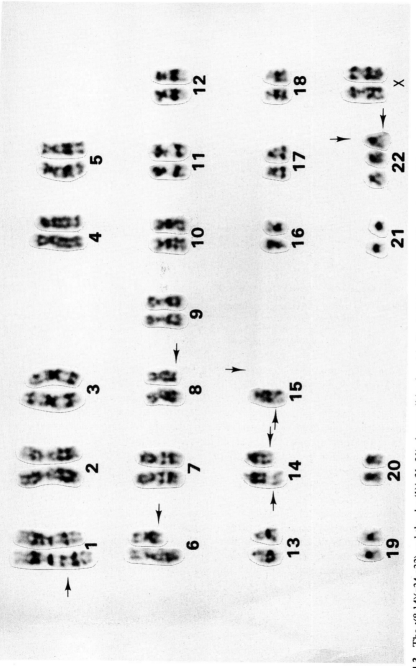

Fig. 11.3 The t(8;14)(q24;q32) and the dup(1)(q21q31) abnormalities found in B-cell ALL (FAB L3). These abnormalities are included in a complex pseudodiploid karyotype found at diagnosis. The karyotype includes three translocations and is as follows: 46,XX, −15, −14, +der(14), t(14;15)(q32;q22)+der(22),t(22;?)(q13;?),t(8;14)(q24;q32). (Reprinted in different (karyotype) form from Cancer Genetics and Cytogenetics, 13:239–257, 1984, with permission of the publisher Elsevier Science, New York, USA, and the Editor, Dr Avery Sandberg.[11])

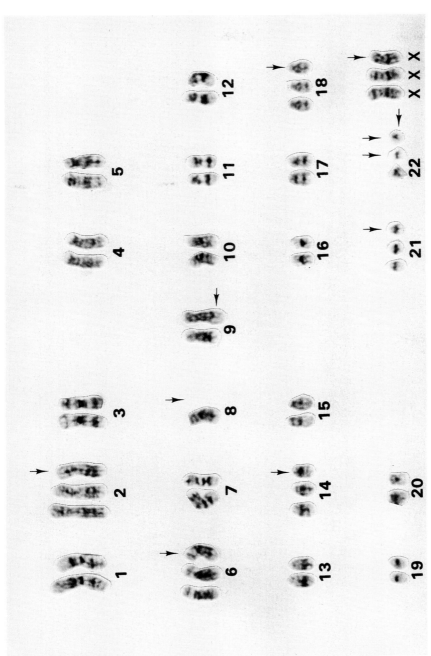

Fig. 11.4 The t(9;22)(q34;q11) (Philadelphia chromosome) in ALL. This appears most often in the pseudodiploid group, but occasionally in other groups including the >50. Duplication of the 22q− portion of the translocation has occurred. The karyotype is: 52,XX, +X, +2, +6, −8, +14, +18, +21, +del(22)(q11),t(9;22)(q34;q11). The trisomies involving chromosomes 6, 14, 18, 21, 22, and X are typical of the >50 ploidy group. The missing 8 was random loss in this metaphase, since the modal number in this case was 53, and included two normal chromosomes 8.

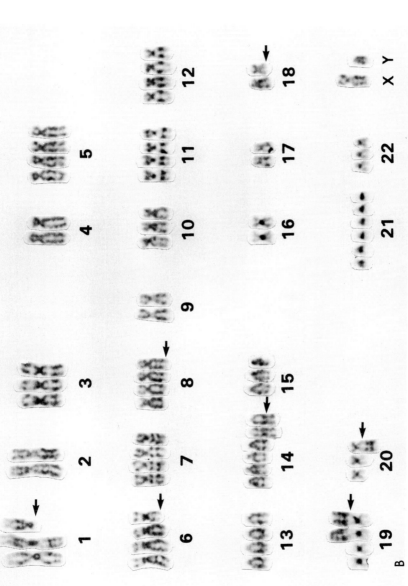

Fig. 11.5 The t(1;19)(q23;p13.3) in a complex karyotype at relapse. At diagnosis only the t(1;19) was present in a pseudodiploid karyotype. The 19q+ portion of the translocation has been duplicated but not the 1q− portion. This karyotype contains 30 additions and 10 structural abnormalities, all of which can be identified. The numbers representing each chromosome pair vary, and include two, three, four and six copies. This represents marked clonal evolution. Such number patterns are not characteristic of either the >50 group or tetraploidy. The karyotype is: 76,XY, +1, +3, +5, +5, +6, +del(6)(q23), +7, +7, +8q+, +8q+, +10, +11, +11, +12, +12+13, +13, +14, +14, +dup(14)(q13→q32), +dup(14)(q13→q32), +15, +der(19),t(1;19)(q23;p13.3), +der(20), t(20;?)(q13;?), +21, +21, +21, +21, +22,t(1;19)(q23;p13.3),del(18)(q21). (This karyotype is reprinted from Cancer Genetics and Cytogenetics, 13:239–257, 1984, with permission of the publishers Elsevier Science, New York, USA, and the Editor Dr Avery Sandberg[11])

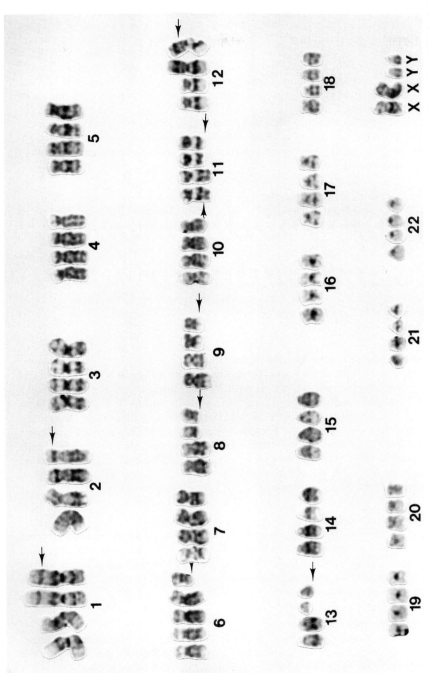

Fig. 11.6 Near-tetraploid side-line at diagnosis in ALL. This karyotype has 93 chromosomes and is a duplication of a pseudodiploid stemline which had the following karyotype: 46,XY, −1, +der(1),t(1;?)(p36;?),del(2)(p22),del(8)(q11;q22),del(9)(q11;q22), −11, +der(11),t(11;?)(q24;?), del(11)(q22;q23),t(12;13)(p13;q14) The del(6)(q16) in the near-tetraploid line was not present in the pseudodiploid stemline and is indicative of clonal evolution in the tetraploid sideline. Except for chromosome 6, the number representing each chromosome pair is 4 (tetrasomy) which is typical of tetraploidy.

both the t(11;14)(p13;q13) and the inversion 14 split the alpha T-cell receptor gene. The dup(1q) is associated with the >50 ploidy group and with B-cell leukemia, usually as a secondary abnormality (clonal evolution). The i(17q) in ALL is almost exclusively associated with the >50 group, and the author's early findings suggest it may be associated with a higher risk of failure. Abnormalities of 11q are associated with higher risk in infants younger than 1 year, where it occurs in about 50% of patients and is characteristically a translocation.[30] Deletions 6q, 12p and 9p may occur alone or with other abnormalities, and the true effect is difficult to determine. Translocations also frequently involve 6q, 12p and 9p. Current studies indicate that structural abnormalities involving 12p are the most frequently occurring in ALL

Non-random additions occur primarily in the >50 group. There is a hypodiploid subgroup with a missing 20, and near-haploid cases have non-random numerical changes. Chromosome 21 is the most frequently added, overall, even after accounting for patients with Down's syndrome with trisomy 21.

Association of Chromosome Abnormalities with Morphology
The t(8;14) and variants t(2;8) and t(8;22)[28,29] are associated with FAB L3 morphology in ALL. However, so far, there are no clearly defined cytogenetic or immunologic correlations with FAB types L1 or L2.[9]

Association of Chromosome Abnormalities with Immunophenotype
Most of the non-random structural abnormalities are closely associated with specific immunologically defined stages in the maturation sequence of either B-lineage leukemia, or T-lineage leukemia. The type of lineage is listed in Table 11.1. Exceptions do occur, but in small numbers.

Molecular Studies related to Chromosome Abnormalities
Molecular studies in ALL show that the oncogene *myc* and the IgH genes are rearranged and expressed abnormally in t(8;14)-positive ALL,[31] as found previously in Burkitt's lymphoma.[31] Two recent studies[16,33] in T-cell ALL revealed that the T-cell receptor locus at band q11 of chromosome 14 is split as a result of the translocation 11;14, suggesting oncogene deregulation similar to that in Burkitt's lymphoma. An additional study has shown that Ph + ALL is different from Ph + chronic myeloid leukemia (CML).[34] Ph + ALL cells express unique *abl*-derived tyrosine kinase active proteins of 185 kilobases and 180 kilobases, which are distinct from the *bcr-abl*-derived p210 protein of CML. This may help to distinguish between Ph + ALL, and Ph + CML in lymphoblastic crisis.

First MIC Cooperative Study Group
The combined use of cytomorphology, immunology and chromosome analysis should serve as the basis for diagnosis, prognosis and treatment in ALL. To this end, the First MIC Cooperative Study Group[9] meeting in Leuven, Belgium, set up initial guidelines for the classification of the acute leukemias according to these disciplines. In time, other disciplines may be added, such as molecular analysis.

Mixed Lineage Leukemia
Approximately 12% of cases that appear to be typical ALL will have surface markers common to the myeloid lineage, and conversely about 18% of cases diagnosed as myeloid will express lymphoid-associated antigens.[2,3,35,36] Although chromosome analysis has not yet been carried out in a large number of cases, results indicate that: (1) nearly all patients with mixed lineage leukemia have an abnomal karyotype, (2) only one abnormal clone is present,

and (3) the chromosome abnormalities are more characteristic of ALL (with only very rare exceptions). Patients with t(4;11) often have mixed lineage leukemia.[37] Translocations involving 14g32 are associated with mixed lineage expression.[38]

Lineage Switch

A lineage conversion occurs between diagnosis and relapse in 8.6% of ALL and AML patients relapsing in the bone marrow.[2,39] Initially it was thought that lineage switch did not reflect the induction of a new malignancy. Recent findings[39] indicate, however, that in the majority of cases, the original blast cell karyotype is replaced by an entirely different (independent) karyotype. This suggests that a second leukemogenic event may occur.[2]

PROGNOSTIC SIGNIFICANCE OF CHROMOSOME ABNORMALITIES IN ACUTE LYMPHOBLASTIC LEUKEMIA IN CHILDREN

The poor response and short survival of patients with the t(9;22) or Philadelphia chromosome has been confirmed by multiple studies.[18,41-44] The t(4;11), and the t(8;14) in B-cell ALL were also found to predict a poor response and short survival.[18]

The chromosome number of the predominant abnormal line (stemline) was found to have prognostic significance in ALL by Secker-Walker et al, in 1978.[45] This was confirmed by the Third International Workshop on Chromosomes in Leukemia (1980)[18] and by others.[46,47] Hyperdiploid karyotypes (>50 chromosomes) have the best prognosis and those with pseudodiploid karyotypes (46 chromosomes with any abnormality) have the poorest prognosis.

Chromosome abnormalities and others presenting clinical and laboratory features were analyzed for a subset of 161 children with ALL who had complete G-banding of all chromosomes and a maximum 6-year follow-up.[48] Eight major types of chromosome abnormalities and 11 clinical and laboratory variables of known prognostic value in ALL were studied. A Cox proportional hazards model[49] indicated that translocation was the strongest single predictor of treatment outcome ($P<0.0001$). The model indicated that translocation increased by six times the risk of treatment failure by comparison with the absence of this feature. Patients with a translocation who relapsed or failed to respond did so early in the disease course. The frequency of translocations was highest among patients with pseudodiploid karyotypes and lowest in the group with 51 or more chromosomes, which correlated with the previous prognostic data on ploidy. Most patients who had the t(9;22), the t(4;11) and the t(8;14) were in the pseudodiploid subgroup, and these translocations are associated with a poor prognosis.[18] Our most recent data analysis indicates that the translocation subgroups with the worst response are the t(9;22) or variant, and the t(8;14) or variant associated with B-cell ALL. Although translocations as a group, in childhood ALL, indicate a poor prognosis, the author's studies suggest that only a moderate proportion of the possible translocation subgroups has as yet been identified. Further studies may disclose some heterogeneity of response as additional new translocation subgroups are identified. Likewise, new therapies may modify the correlation between translocations and prognosis.

The author's observations indicate that 20% of cases in the >50 subgroup may have translocations. These occasionally involve the Philadelphia chromosome, but rarely, *if ever*, involve the t(8;14) or t(4;11) abnormalities. The specific effect of translocation in the hyperdiploid > 50 group is not known. However, we have demonstrated that patients with concurrent structural chromosomal abnormalities generally have a less favourable prognosis than those with only numerical abnormalities.[22]

Studies at St Jude Hospital[21] found that the hypodiploid group (<46) has a poor prognosis. These cases had an increased frequency of known high-risk features including translocations. The translocations, however, did *not* include the t(9;22), the t(8;14) or the t(4;11). Most cases had 45 chromosomes, with a small number ranging from 40 to 44. Chromosome 20 appears to be preferentially lost in some cases in the hypodiploid group.

In the pseudodiploid group alone, a significant difference in response has been found between those with a translocation and those without a translocation with most failures occurring in the translocation group.[48] This has also been observed in the 47–50 group, but not in the hypodiploid group, as yet. The normal group is becoming gradually smaller, and the response of these cases, *as a group*, will eventually have less significance. Many of the normal cases have a T-cell immunophenotype and may have translocations, but T-cell mitogens or other methods are necessary to obtain the malignant metaphases (see Technics).

In regard to specific abnormalities the poorest responders include: the t(8;14) and variants t(2;8) and t(8;22), associated with B-cell ALL with FAB L3 morphology; the t(9;22) or a variant; the t(4;11); and near-haploidy. In time, the influence of each of the newer translocation subtypes will be determined. Also, many of the translocations now appearing to be 'random' will be found to cluster, forming new subgroups.

CLINICAL APPLICATION AND USEFULNESS OF CHROMOSOME INFORMATION IN CHILDHOOD ALL

In general, chromosome studies are important in childhood ALL in order to help: (1) differentiate leukemia from non-malignant conditions; (2) classify the ALL subtypes; (3) determine the degree of progression; (4) test for remission; (5) establish relapse; (6) characterize changes in the course of the disease; and (7) monitor transplant cases.

More specifically, the recognition that certain presenting clinical and biological features help predict the outcome of treatment is very significant. Efforts are continuing to better define prognostic features, so that individualized thereapy may eventually be realized. Whilst the effect of cytogenetic features may vary with the effectiveness of a particular treatment program the *relative* prognostic strength of specific chromosome features tends to remain intact, the very worst features being the most difficult to overcome by different treatment programs.

Three cytogenetic features which have strong prognostic significance in childhood ALL are:

1. The presence of specific abnormalities, such as the t(9;22).
2. The presence of any translocation.
3. The chromosome number of the predominant abnormal line (stemline).

The DNA index has been shown to have strong prognostic significance.[50] This is the ratio of the *modal DNA content* of G_0/G_1 cells to that of normal cells and is obtained by flow cytometric methods. It can be used to separate the better-risk patients (refinement of the cytogenetic >50 group) from those with a relatively worse risk. The DNA index used in combination with complete chromosome analysis can provide much valuable information. However, the DNA index alone does not provide information related to structural chromosome abnormalities, such as translocations. It can provide the DNA content (approximate chromosome number) in cases where chromosomal analysis is unsuccessful or not available.

Cytogenetic and DNA features may be used as risk factors along with clinical and other biological features. At the author's institution, the presence of a translocation, the DNA index, the WBC count, age and race have been used as risk factors for allocation of patients to discrete treatment groups.[51]

THE CYTOGENETICS OF ALL IN ADULTS

ALL is the predominant leukemia of childhood, but also accounts for almost 15% of cases of acute leukemia in adults.[52] It is infrequent in young adults, but increases progressively after the age of 40 years. The presenting clinical features are largely similar to those found in childhood ALL.

Studies of chromosome ploidy indicates some variation between adults and children. In adults the response related to the ploidy groups is, in decreasing complete remission rate and survival: >50 group (best) > normal > hypodiploid > pseudodiploid > 47–50.[18] The number of cases with >50 chromosomes is very small in comparison to the number found in children.

Four kinds of translocations have been shown to have a poor prognosis in adults: the t(9;22), the t(8;14), other 14q+ translocations, and t(4;11). The Philadelphia chromosome is two to three times more frequent in adults than in children and its prognostic value is independent of other factors such as age and WBC count.[18,53] Factors indicative of a poor prognosis are, in order of decreasing importance:[52]

1. Any structural abnormality or translocation.
2. The 47–50 group or pseudodiploidy.
3. B-cell ALL (if chromosome analysis not available).
4. Older age >30 or 35? and high WBC count >50? >20 × 10^9/l.

In adult ALL, bone marrow transplant in first complete remission is being done. Cytogenetic risk factors used to support the use of HLA-matched allogeneic BMT are the presence of translocations: t(9;22), t(8;14) and t(4;11) or the presence of a hypodiploid karyotype.[42]

MULTIPLE ABNORMAL LINES IN ALL

Two or more abnormal lines indicate that clonal evolution has occurred if the karyotypes are related, or that two independent events have apparently occurred if the karyotypes are unrelated. Clonal evolution occurs in stepwise (sequential) fashion. In childhood ALL, multiple abnormal lines have been identified at diagnosis in 25% of cases. Nearly all of these are derived from stepwise clonal evolution. Independent (unrelated) lines are relatively rare (<1% of cases). Many of the karyotypes with clonal evolution are very complex. The prognosis of these cases (as a group) is unknown, but is currently being studied. An additional phenomenon observed in ALL is the doubling of a lower number usually involving pseudodiploid (46) and tetraploid (92) numbers, but occasionally involving near-haploid numbers (i.e. 26 and 52). Doubling appears to be of little consequence clinically, as treatment usually eradicates the high numbers, even if the patient relapses.

THE CYTOGENETICS OF ACUTE MYELOID LEUKEMIA

Standard chromosome technics in AML have in the past generally provided an 80–85% rate of successful preparations, and recognition of the abnormal clone in 75–80% of these cases. With high resolution chromosome analysis Yunis[7,8] has attained a 94% rate of successful growth with elongated mitoses containing 400–850 bands per haploid set. Ninety-three per cent of these show a chromosomal defect. Since 1984, the author's group has used, in AML, the direct method developed for bone marrow preparations in ALL, supplemented in selected cases by unstimulated overnight cultures of bone marrow or circulating blasts. This has yielded a 98% rate of successful studies, and an 82% identification of the abnormal clone, which is quite improved from earlier studies.[54] The direct technic combined with overnight culture may be especially useful in cases where the cytogenetic information is urgently needed. High resolution technics, on the other hand, may allow better clarification of subtle abnormalities and marker chromosomes and are less likely to miss the abnormal clone. The high resolution method is the technic of choice for AML, but the direct method is a reliable option, and at times one may elect to use both. The approximate frequency, primary FAB morphology or other association, and relative prognosis (if known) of the non-random chromosome abnormalities in AML are presented in Table 11.2.

PLOIDY

Chromosome number (ploidy) in AML varies from that in ALL, primarily by the *lack* of a second peak involving cases with more than 50 chromosomes. Occasional cases do occur and the modal numbers are random. In contrast, the >50 group in ALL represents approximately 30% of all ALL patients. Near-haploid cases have not been reported in AML.

NON-RANDOM CHROMOSOMAL ABNORMALITIES IN AML

Table 11.2 lists the reported non-random abnormalities with their approximate frequency, associations with FAB morphology, and relative prognosis, if known.

Whilst in ALL many chromosomal abnormalities are associated with the immunophenotype, in AML they are more closely associated with the morphology of the leukemic cell as classified by the French–American–British (FAB) system.[55] Therefore, in both AML and ALL non-random abnormalities are associated with the laboratory parameter primarily involved in providing the diagnosis and the subtype of the leukemia.

Table 11.2 Non-random chromosomal abnormalities in acute myeloid leukemia

Chromosome abnormality	Primary FAB morphology or other association	Relative prognosis (if known)	Approximate frequency (%)	Reference
t(9;22)(q34;q11)	M1	?Poor	0.4–9.9	FIWCL,[4] Yunis et al,[76] Sasaki[77]
t(8;21)(q22;q22)	M2	Good	6.7	FIWCL[4]
t(15;17)(q22;q21.1)	M3	Good	6.5	FIWCL[4]
t(16;16)(q13;q22.1)	M4 Abnormal and/or increased BM eosinophils	Good	1	Larson et al[69]
inv(16)(p13q22.1)	M4 Abnormal and/or increased BM eosinophils	Good	5–9	Larson et al[69] Yunis et al[68]
del(16)(q22)	M4 abnormal and/or increased BM eosinophils	Good	1	Arthur and Bloomfield[67] Larson et al[69]
t(11;V)(q;V)	M5, M4	Poor	3	FIWCL,[4] Kaneko et al[73]
del(11q)	M5, M4	Poor	2	FIWCL[4]
t(6;9)(p22.2;q34.1)	Increased BM basophils	?Poor	1	FIWCL,[4] Bitter et al[76]
t(3;3)(q26;q21q26)	Abnormal thrombopoiesis	?Poor	1	Bitter et al,[78] Pintado et al[82]
inv(3)(q21q26)	Abnormal thrombopoiesis	?Poor	1	Bitter et al,[78] Pintado et al[82]
del(5q), or −5	–	Poor	4	FIWCL[4]
del(7q), or −7	–	Intermediate	4	FIWCL[4]
+8	–	Intermediate	5.5	FIWCL[4]
+21	–	Good	1.2	FIWCL[4]
−X	M2, with t(8;21)	b	1	FIWCL[4]
−Y	M2, with t(8;21)	b	3	FIWCL[4]

[a]FIWCL = Fourth International Workshop on Chromosomes in Leukemia 1982 (1984) BM (bone marrow)
[b]The FIWCL[4] presented evidence that patients with a missing sex chromosome and having t(8;21) did not appear to have a poorer prognosis than the others.

t(8;21)(q22;q22) in AML (M2)
Rowley[56] first characterized this translocation between chromosomes 8 and 21. Sakurai and Sandberg suggested that this cytogenetic abnormality might define a specific subset of AML.[57] The t(8;21) occurred in 6.7% of AML de novo cases with abnormal karyotypes at the Fourth International Workshop on Chromosomes in Leukemia.[4]

The t(8;21) is found primarily in FAB M2 (myeloblastic leukemia with maturation) but is also observed in FAB M4, and FAB M1.[4] Chromosomes 8 and 21 can also participate in three-way rearrangements similar to the 9 and 22 in CML.[4] It is often accompanied by the loss of either X or Y, which does *not* appear to be associated with a poor prognosis.

The oncogene *c-mos* has been mapped to band q22 on chromosome 8[58] and the oncogene *Hu-ets-2* is located at 21q22,[59] the same breakpoints as found in the t(8;21). The *Hu-ets-2* oncogene moves in the translocation from 21q22 to 8q22.[59,60]

t(15;17)(q22;q21.1) in acute promyelocytic leukemia (M3)[61]
Larson et al[62] reported that this translocation was present in 100% of cases of acute promyelocytic leukemia (APL). The t(15;17) has been identified in 10 of 11 cases in children at St Jude Hospital. It appears to be exclusively associated with FAB M3.

The FAB cooperative group,[63] and others[64] recognized and described a morphologic variation of granules in APL. In some cases, the granules in leukemia promyelocytes are too small to be seen by light microscopy, but are visible by electron microscopy. Therefore, a category called the M3 variant was defined; the t(15;17) is present in the variant.

Disseminated intravascular coagulation (DIC) occurs in a high percentage of cases of AML M3. Chromosome analysis may help to confirm the diagnosis and subtype of these cases by rapid identification of the t(15;17) abnormality.

The t(15;17) may be involved in complex translocations.[65] The study of complex or variant translocations could help determine which chromosome junction is the critical one (15q22 or 17q21).

Structural abnormalities of chromosome 16 in acute myelomonocytic leukemia (M4)
A correlation between abnormal eosinophils and structural rearrangements of 16 has been observed in several studies.[4,66,67] Three non-random abnormalities have been identified. The most frequent is the paracentric inversion 16 (p13;q22.1). A del(16)(q22) and a translocation 16;16 (p13;q22.1) are less frequently found. The inversion 16 and the t(16;16), which have the same breakpoints, are associated with eosinophils that may or may not be increased in number, but have an admixture of large basophilic granules. The del(16) is usually associated with an increase in the number of *marrow* eosinophils ($\geq 6\%$), but not circulating eosinophils. These abnormalities are associated primarily with FAB M4, but have also been observed in M2 and M5. The inversion 16, occurs in approximately 9% of patients with de novo AML.[68] Larson et al[69] recently reported the inv(16) and the t(16;16) as a specific subset of AML with a favorable prognosis. This variant of M4 with abnormal eosinophils has been designated M4E0 by the FAB Cooperative Group.[70] A complex translocation involving 16 and a t(3;16)(q21;q22) has been reported in patients who had eosinophilia and either acute myelomonocytic leukemia or a myelodysplastic syndrome.[71,72] Larson et al[69] have suggested that all of these reported cases with 16 involvement appear to have several things in common: (1) a breakpoint at 16q22, (2) a malignant disease of myeloid origin and (3) an associated qualitative or quantitative abnormality of the eosinophil.

Structural Abnormalities of 11q in acute myeloid leukemia
Thirty-three cases at the Fourth Workshop[4] had some structural abnormality of 11q. Most (63.9%) were classified as M5. When all patients with M5 leukemia were considered, 22% had an abnormality involving 11q.

The breakpoint usually involves 11q23-24, but can occur in 11q13-14. Most involve translocations, but terminal deletions are also frequent. The most common translocation is t(9;11)(p21;q23), but other involved chromosomes include 1,4,10,11,17 and 19. Frequent involvement of 11q occurs in both AML and in ALL. In the author's studies abnormalities of 11q23-24 have occurred in 13% of AML cases and 5% of ALL cases, and have been found in 50% of infant leukemia[30] (<1 year old). Kaneko et al[73] concluded that acute leukemia with 11q23 translocations was characterized by the young age of the patients, hyperleukocytosis and protean morphologic and immunologic phenotypes. Mirro has demonstrated that cases with t(4;11) may have mixed lineage leukemia.[37] The 11q23 band is the location of the C-ets-1 oncogene.[74] Figure 11.7 presents a complex karyotype in a patient with acute monocytic leukemia (M5). The abnormalities include involvement of the 9 and 11 chromosomes but not in the classic 9;11 translocation found in monocytic (M5) leukemia. This karyotype was obtained by the direct bone marrow procedure.

The t(6;9)(p22.2;q34.1) in AML with increased basophils
Rowley and Potter first described this translocation in 1976.[75] It accounts for fewer than 1% of patients with AML de novo. There is an increase in basophils in the bone marrow, but the basophils appear to be morphologically normal. No unique clinical features have been described. Most cases have been classified as M2.

The t(9;22)(q34;q11) in AML
The Philadelphia chromosome occurs in AML with breakpoints identical to those found in CML. However, it is not yet known if the molecular rearrangements are similar. The reported frequency of this translocation has varied from 0.4% to 9.9%.[4,76,77] It appears to be very rare in children. The Ph in AML is thought to have a poor prognosis, but very few cases have been critically analyzed.[78] In AML, it is most often associated with M1 in the FAB classification.

Abnormalities Involving Chromosome 7 (See also secondary leukemia)
The Fourth Workshop[4] recognized monosomy 7 as the most frequent abnormality involving chromosome 7. Deletion 7q was the second most frequent abnormality. The comon segment deleted involved 7q32 to 7q34. Translocations of 7 were identified, including a t(7;17) appearing to be centromeric, which was observed in four cases. The most common abnormalities associated with −7 and 7q− were −5 or 5q−, and monosomy 17. In children, the author's studies show that monosomy 7 and 7q− are infrequent (approximately 1-2% each). Translocations are only slightly more frequent, most involving the short arm of 7. Monosomy 7 is often associated with preleukemia in the pediatric patient.

Deletion of 5q and −5
Deletion of the long arm of 5 or monosomy 5 has been associated with AML or myelodysplastic syndromes following occupational or therapeutic mutagen exposure,[79,80] as well as in AML and preleukemia apparently arising de novo. However, they occur infrequently in children. Different breakpoints may be involved in the deletion, but in all cases examined by the Fourth Workshop[4] the deletion was interpreted as interstitial. Three breakpoint positions were recognized: (type A1) q11 or q12 and q33 or q34; (type A2) q14 or q15 and q33 or q34; and (type B) q22 and q33 or q34. The smallest consistently deleted region was q22 to q33 or q34 which is the critical region for this abnormality. Almost half of the cases with deletion 5 were FAB M2. The 5q− and −5 are often associated with abnormalities of chromosome 7.

Chromosome 3 Abnormalities and Thrombocytosis in AML
An association of abnormalities of chromosome 3 and thrombocytosis in AML patients has been confirmed by several studies.[81,82] Three specific abnormalities have so far been

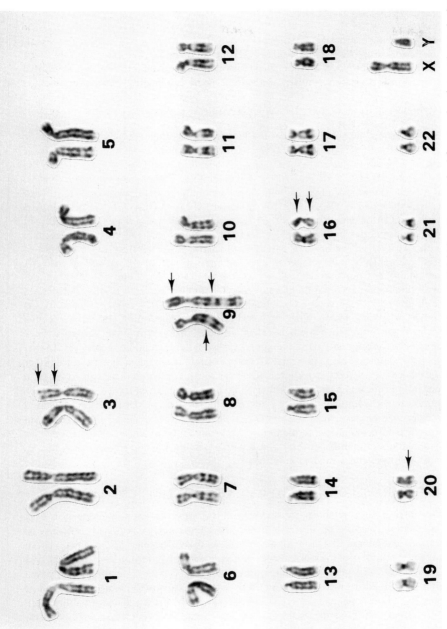

Fig. 11.7 Complex karyotype in acute monocytic leukemia (M5) at diagnosis. This pseudodiploid karyotype contained four translocations and several other abnormalities. Although at least two of the translocations involved chromosomes 9 and 11, neither was the classic t(9;11)(p21;q23) often associated with FAB M5. This example was obtained from the direct bone marrow method described in this chapter. The karyotype is 46,XY, −9, + der(9),t(9;11)(q34;q12), [−9, + der?dic(9),t?dic(9;11)(q34;?p11),t(?dic9;?)(p24;?)], −20, + der(20),t(20;?)(q13;?),del(3)(p25),inv del(3)(p13;p25),inv(16)(p13;q22).

reported: (1) inv(3)(q21;q26), (2) t(3;3)(q21;q26) and (3) ins(5;3)(q14;q21;q26). All involve bands 3q21 and 3q26 simultaneously. Significant thrombocytosis may be present with platelet counts up to 1731 × 10^9/l. There is an increase in the number of megakaryocytes, with numerous micromegakaryocytes.

Other numerical abnormalities in AML
At the Fourth Workshop the +8 in de novo AML occurred in 5.5% of cases[4] and the +21 in 1.2%.[4] Patients with a trisomy 8 often have a history of preleukemia. The +8 is associated with an intermediate prognosis, whilst cases with +21 have a slightly better prognosis.[4]

PROGNOSTIC SIGNIFICANCE OF CHROMOSOME ABNORMALITIES IN AML

The Fourth Workshop[4] demonstrated that the karyotype, classified according to 12 specific chromosome abnormalities, significantly correlated with responses to treatment and survival. With regard to response to initial chemotherapy, the best responses (>65%) were seen in the following subgroups: t(15;17), t(8;21), +21 and hypodiploid. The poorest responses (<50%) were seen in patients who were hyperdiploid or pseudodiploid, or had abnormalities in both 5 and 7, or had −5 or 5q−. Cases with +8, an abnormal 11q, −7 or 7q−, or only normal chromosomes, had an intermediate response. Remission duration and survival were short in patients with abnormalities in 5, 5 and 7, and 11q. The longest median survivals were seen in those with t(15;17), −7 or 7q−, or hypodiploid karyotypes. The presence or absence of abnormal metaphases (NN = normal only; AN = combination of abnormal and normal; AA = abnormal only) did not correlate with response to initial induction therapy, but did correlate with first remission duration and survival. When other risk factors were considered, however, only the specific karyotype classification (not the NN, AN, AA classification) was an independent prognostic factor. With improved chromosome technics, and more effective chemotherapy in the future, such subdivisions of chromosomally normal and abnormal cases may not be relevant as originally used. Certainly, such a system would be second best to that of identifying the abnormal clone in nearly all cases. Yunis[68] has studied a sufficient number of patients in three well-defined chromosomal groups to conclude that these categories have independent prognostic importance. The first is the group with an *inversion 16*, who had a uniform and sustained complete remission and median survival of 25 months. The second group was composed of cases who had *complex chromosomal abnormalities*. This group had a bad prognosis. Efforts to achieve remission in this group failed in almost all instances with a median survival of 2.5 months. A third group with a *trisomy 8* as the single defect, had an intermediate prognosis and a median survival of 10 months.

ACUTE LEUKEMIA SECONDARY TO RADIATION AND/OR CHEMOTHERAPY

Leukemia occurring after previous treatment with radiation or chemotherapy is a very serious complication, because of the resistance to the chemotherapy presently available for these secondary leukemias. The Fourth Workshop[4] analyzed the data on 56 cases. There were almost equal numbers of male and female patients, ages ranged from 18 to 90 years, and the AML occurred 1–17 years after the original diagnosis, with a median of 5 years. Chromosome abnormalities were present in 75% of cases. Numerical changes consisted of −7, −5, and −17 in decreasing frequency. The most frequent structural abnormalities were del(5q), t(17;V) and del(7q) in decreasing order. Translocations occurred in 34% of cases. Survival was shorter for the cases in which chromosomes 5 and 17 were involved.

Multiple Abnormal Lines in AML
The Fourth Workshop[4] studied 81 cases with multiple abnormal lines in AML. The frequency in AML de novo was 10.8% and, in secondary leukemia, was 17.9%. Seventy-eight

cases had related lines and only three cases had unrelated lines. The most frequent primary chromosome changes were -5 or $5q-$, -7 or $7q-$, $+8$, t(8;21) and t(15;17). Additional changes observed in the clonal evolution involved many different chromosomes in a variety of abnormalities. Survival was 3.4 months for patients with de novo leukemia and 3.8 months for patients with secondary leukemia.

THE CYTOGENETICS OF NON-HODGKIN'S LYMPHOMA

Major steps in the identification and classification of the non-Hodgkin's lymphomas (NHLs) were the development of (1) a working formulation of histopathologic classification for clinical usage,[83] (2) immunologic cell surface and cytoplasmic markers to characterize lymphoma,[84] and (3) methotrexate cell synchronization (high resolution) technics for chromosome analyses.[85]

Yunis has observed a chromosomal abnormality in 137 of 144 NHL patients (97%).[85-87] He found that one of 10 *specific* chromosome defects was found in 65% of all patients and those defects were observed to predominate in certain histologic subtypes. The presence of a t(14;18)(q32.3;q21.3) translocation in 87% of follicular lymphomas was a very important finding. Follicular lymphomas constitute 40% of all NHLs. In a study of 71 patients with follicular lymphoma, Yunis[88] found 15 types of non-random chromosomal abnormalities. When sequential cytogenetic studies were carried out, 10 of these types appeared to influence the histopathologic findings, the clinical course or response to treatment.

The Fifth International Workshop on chromosomes in Leukemia-Lymphoma[89] (Japan, 1984), considered the chromosome abnormalities present in NHL in 260 cases. These findings confirmed the close association of particular chromosome abnormalities with histology, and identified a number of new associations. These include: (1) abnormalities of 14q11-13 were correlated with T-cell disease, (2) abnormalities of 1p and trisomy 3 were significantly associated with the T-cell phenotype, and trisomy 12 with B-cell phenotype, (3) clonal chromosome abnormalities were found in 85% of cases of NHL, (4) of patients with an 8q24 translocation, 87% had small non-cleaved cell lymphoma, and (5) of 57 NHL patients with a t(14;18)(q32;q21) abnormality, 65% had a follicular lymphoma and at least another 23% had a diffuse lymphoma of follicular center cell origin.

Burkitt's lymphoma is a disease of B-lymphoid cells with L3 FAB morphology, and may be Epstein-Barr virus (EBV) positive or negative.[90] A reciprocal translocation t(8;14)(q24.1;q32.3) is found in about 80% of cases.[91,92] Molecular technics revealed that the *c-myc* oncogene moves from its normal location at band 8q24.1, becoming deregulated when rearranged with the constant genes of the immunoglobulin heavy chain (IgH) at band 14q32.3.[93] In about 20% of cases *myc* rearranges with the κ (5%) or λ (15%) immunoglobulin light chain genes of a chromosome 2 or 22 in the variant translocations t(2;8)(p11.1;q24.1) and t(8;22)(q24.1;q11.2).[92] In the variant translocations, *myc* remains on chromosome 8 and the κ and λ genes translocate from their normal position in chromosomes 2 and 22, respectively, to a chromosome region distal to the *myc* oncogene.[94]

CONCLUSION

Chromosome analysis may play a very valuable and sometimes critical role in the diagnosis, prognosis and management of blood malignancies. When chromosome analysis is combined with cell morphology in AML, and with cell morphology and immunophenotype in ALL and lymphoma, its clinical application and value are greatly enhanced. Such multidisciplinary approaches will help identify the important characteristics of these heterogeneous diseases, and recognize the risk factors which are closely associated with outcome. There should be continued efforts to define prognostic groups, so that the goal of individualized therapy can eventually be realized.

New technics in cytogenetics are now available that provide consistent and reliable results. Much new cytogenetic information is now known and much more will be forthcoming in the near future in all of these diseases, but especially in ALL. Such information will be useful primarily to the clinician, but also to the molecular biologist. Therefore, all large institutions should make a major effort to develop this capability for the potential contribution it may make to improved patient care and treatment.

ACKNOWLEDGEMENTS

I wish to thank Dr Susana Raimondi, and technologists Terri Huddleston, Ann Harris, Susan Ragsdale and Patsy Mardis for assistance and for outstanding work which contributed to this chapter; Jerry Luther for contributions and consultations related to photography; Peggy Vandiveer for expert word processing; and Shawn Chambers for excellent photographic dark room work. Studies carried out in our laboratory which are referred to in this paper were supported in part by grants from the National Institutes of Health Leukemia Program Project Grant PO1-CA-20180 and CA-21765 and by the American Lebanese Syrian Associated Charities.

REFERENCES

1. Yunis J J 1986 Chromosomal rearrangements, genes, and fragile sites in cancer: clinical and biologic implications. In: DeVita V, Hellman S, Rosenberg S (eds) Important advances in oncology. Lippincott, Philadelphia, pp 93–128
2. Stass S A, Mirro J 1986 Lineage heterogeneity in acute leukemia: acute mixed-lineage leukemia and lineage switch. Clinics in Haematology 15: 811–827
3. Mirro J, Kitchingman G R 1989 The morphology, cytochemistry, molecular characteristics and clinical significance of acute mixed-lineage leukemia. In: C S Scott (ed.) Leukemia cytochemistry and diagnosis: Principles and practice. Ellis Horwood Limited, Chichester, pp 155–179
4. Fourth International Workshop on Chromosomes in Leukemia 1982, 1984 Cancer Genetics and Cytogenetics 11: 251–360
5. Brodeur G M, Dahl G V, Williams D L, Tipton R E, Kalwinsky D K 1980 Transient leukemoid reaction and trisomy 21 mosaicism in a phenotypically normal newborn. Blood 55: 691–693
6. Williams D L, Raimondi S, Rivera G, George S, Berard C W, Murphy S B 1985 Presence of clonal chromosome abnormalities in virtually all cases of acute lymphoblastic leukemia. New England Journal of Medicine 313: 640–641
7. Yunis J J 1984 Recurrent chromosomal defects are found in most patients with acute nonlymphocytic leukemia. Cancer Genetics and Cytogenetics 11: 125–137
8. Yunis J J, Bloomfield C D, Ensrud K 1981 All patients with acute nonlymphocytic leukemia may have a chromosomal defect. New England Journal of Medicine 305: 135–139
9. First MIC Cooperative Study Group 1986 Morphologic, immunologic, and cytogenetic (MIC) working classification of acute lymphoblastic leukemias. Report of the Workshop held in Leuven, Belgium, April 22–23, 1985. Cancer Genetics and Cytogenetics 23: 189–197
10. Yunis J J 1986 Refined chromosomal analysis should be used routinely in acute leukemias and myelodysplastic syndrome. New England Journal of Medicine 315: 322–323
11. Williams D L, Harris A, Williams K J, Brosius M J, Lemonds J W 1984 A direct bone marrow technique for acute lymphoblastic leukemia. Cancer Genetics and Cytogenetics 13: 239–258
12. Burkholder S W, Grujic S, Barr M, Jackson L 1986 A simple banding technique for in situ cultured amniotic fluid cells. Association of Cytogenetic Technologists Eleventh Annual Meeting
13. Yunis J J 1982 Comparative analysis of high-resolution chromosome techniques for leukemic bone marrows. Cancer Genetics and Cytogenetics 7: 43–50
14. Sumner A T 1972 A simple technique for demonstrating centromeric heterochromatin. Experimental Cell Research 75: 304–306
15. Williams D L, Look A T, Melvin S L et al 1984 New chromosomal translocations correlate with specific immunophenotypes of childhood acute lymphoblastic leukemia. Cell 36: 101–109

16 Erikson J, Williams D L, Finan J, Nowell P C, Croce C M 1985 Locus of the α-chain of the T-cell receptor is split by chromosome translocation in T-cell leukemias. Science 229: 784–786
17 Pui C-H, Williams D L, Kalwinsky D K et al 1986 Cytogenetic features and serum lactic dehydrogenase level predict a poor treatment outcome for children with pre-B-cell leukemia. Blood 67: 1688–1692
18 Third International Workshop on Chromosomes in Leukemia 1980, 1981 Cancer Genetics and Cytogenetics 4: 96–137
19 Bloomfield C D, Lindquist L L, Arthur D et al 1981 Chromosomal abnormalities in acute lymphoblastic leukemia. Cancer Research 41: 4838–4843
20 Kaneko Y, Rowley J D, Variakojis D, Chilcote R R, Check I, Sakurai M 1982 Correlation of karyotype with clinical features in acute lymphoblastic leukemia. Cancer Research 42: 2918–2929
21 Pui C-H, Williams D L, Raimondi S C et al 1987 Hypodiploidy is associated with a poor prognosis in childhood acute lymphoblastic leukemia. Blood 70: 247–253
22 Pui C-H, Raimondi, S. C., Dodge R. K. et al 1989. Prognostic importance of structural chromosomal abnormalities in children with hyperdiploid (>50 chromosomes) acute lymphoblastic leukemia. Blood 73: 1963–1967
23 Pui C-H, Williams D L, Raimondi S C et al 1987 Blast cell hypodiploidy confers a poor prognosis in childhood acute lymphoblastic leukemia (ALL). Proceedings of the American Society of clinical Oncology 6, Abstract 145
24 Dubé I D, Raimondi S C, Pi D, Kalousek D K 1986 A new translocation, t(10;14)(q24;q11), in T cell neoplasia. Blood 67: 1181–1184
25 Raimondi S C, Williams D L, Callihan T, Peiper S, Rivera G K, Murphy S B 1986 Nonrandom involvement of the 12p12 breakpoint in chromosome abnormalities of childhood acute lymphoblastic leukemia. Blood 68: 69–75
26 Carrol A J, Raimondi S C, Williams D L et al 1987 dic(9;12): A nonrandom chromosome abnormality in childhood B-cell precursor acute lymphoblastic leukemia. A Pediatric Oncology Group Study. Blood 70: 1962–1965
27 Raimondi S C, Pui C-H, Behm F G, Williams D 1987 7q32–q36 translocations in childhood T-cell leukemia: cytogenetic evidence for involvement of the T-cell receptor β-chain gene. Blood 69: 131–134
28 Van den Berghe H, Parloir A, Gosseye S, Englebienne V, Cornu G, Sokal G 1979 Variant translocation in Burkitt lymphoma. Cancer Genetics and Cytogenetics 1: 9–14
29 Berger R, Bernheim A, Weh H J et al 1979 A new translocation in Burkitt's tumor cells. Human Genetics 53: 111–112
30 Pui C-H, Raimondi S C, Murphy S B et al 1987 An analysis of leukemic cell chromosomal features in infants. Blood 69: 1289–1293
31 Peschle C, Mavilio F, Sposi N M et al 1984 Translocation and rearrangement of c-myc into immunoglobulin alpha heavy chain locus in primary cells from acute lymphocytic leukemia. Proceedings of the National Academy of Sciences of the USA 81: 5514–5518
32 Taub R, Kirsch L, Morton C et al 1982 Translocation of the c-myc gene into the immunoglobulin heavy chain locus in human Burkitt's lymphoma and mouse plasmacytoma cells. Proceedings of the National Academy of Sciences of the USA 79: 7837–7841
33 Lewis W H, Michalopoulos E E, Williams D L, Minden M D, Mak T W 1985 Breakpoints in the human T-cell antigen receptor α-chain locus in two T-cell leukemia patients with chromosomal translocations. Nature 317: 544–546
34 Clark S S, McLaughlin J, Crist W M, Champlin R, Witte O N 1987 Unique forms of the *abl* oncogene tyrosine kinase distinguish Ph positive CML from Ph positive ALL. Science 235: 85–88
35 Mirro J, Pui C-H, Zipf T F et al 1985 Acute mixed lineage leukemia: clinicopathologic correlations and prognostic significance. Blood 66: 1115–1123
36 Pui C-H, Dahl G V, Melvin S et al 1984 Acute leukemia with mixed lymphoid and myeloid phenotype. British Journal of Haematology 56: 121–130
37 Mirro J, Kitchingman G, Williams D et al 1986 Clinical and laboratory characteristics of acute leukemia with the 4;11 translocation. Blood 67: 689–697
38 Hayashi Y, Pui C-H, Behm F G, Fuchs A H, Raimondi S C, Kitchingman G R, Mirrow J Jr, Williams D L 1990 Mixed-lineage expression in childhood acute leukemia. Blood 76: 150
39 Stass S, Mirro J, Melvin S, Pui C-H, Murphy S, Williams D 1984 Lineage switch in acute leukemia. Blood 64: 701–706
40 Pui C-H, Behm F G, Raimondi, S C et al 1989 Secondary acute myeloid leukemia in children treated for acute lymphoid leukemia. New England Journal of Medicine 321: 136–142

41 Bloomfield C D, Peterson L C, Yunis J J, Brunning R D 1977 The Philadelphia chromosome (Ph^1) in adults presenting with acute leukemia: a comparison of Ph^1+ and Ph^1- patients. British Journal of Haematology 36: 347-358
42 Bloomfield C D, Brunning R D, Smith K A, Nesbit M E 1980 Prognostic significance of the Philadelphia chromosome in acute lymphocytic leukemia. Cancer Genetics and Cytogenetics 1: 229-238
43 Sandberg A A, Kohno S, Wake N, Minowada J 1980 Chromosomes and causation of human cancer and leukemia. XLII. Ph^1-positive ALL: an entity within myeloproliferative disorders. Cancer Genetics and Cytogenetics 2: 145-174
44 Ribeiro R C, Abromowitch M, Raimondi S C, Murphy S B, Behm F, Williams D L 1987 Clinical and biologic hallmarks of the Philadelphia chromosome in childhood acute lymphoblastic leukemia. Blood 70: 948-953
45 Secker-Walker L M, Lawler S D, Hardisty R M 1978 Prognostic implications of chromosomal findings in acute lymphoblastic leukemia at diagnosis. British Medical Journal 2: 1529-1530
46 Williams D L, Tsiatis A, Brodeur G M et al 1982 Prognostic importance of chromosome number in 136 untreated children with acute lymphoblastic leukemia. Blood 60: 864-871
47 Kalwinsky D K, Roberson P, Dahl G et al 1985 Clinical relevance of lymphoblast biological features in children with acute lymphoblastic leukemia. Journal of Clinical Oncology 3: 477-484
48 Williams D L, Harber J, Dahl G V et al 1986 Chromosomal translocations play a unique role in influencing prognosis in childhood acute lymphoblastic leukemia. Blood 68: 205-212
49 Cox D R 1972 Regression models and life tables. Journal of the Royal Statistical Society 34: 187-220 Series B
50 Look A T, Roberson P K, Williams D L et al 1985 Prognostic importance of blast cell DNA content in childhood acute lymphoblastic leukemia. Blood 65: 1078-1086
51 Rivera G K, George S L, Williams D L et al 1986 Early results of intensified remission induction chemotherapy for childhood acute lymphocytic leukemia. Medical and Pediatric Oncology 14: 177-181
52 Prentice H G, Grob J-P 1986 Acute lymphoblastic leukemia in adults. In: Clinics in hematology (acute leukemia) WB Saunders Company, London, p 755
53 Third International Workshop on Chromosomes in Leukemia 1983 Chromosomal abnormalities and their clinical significance in acute lymphoblastic leukemia. Cancer Research 43: 868-873
54 Brodeur G M, Williams D L, Kalwinsky D K, Williams K J, Dahl G V 1983 Cytogenetic features of acute nonlymphoblastic leukemia in 73 children and adolescents. Cancer Genetics and Cytogenetics 8: 93-105
55 Bennett J M, Catovsky D, Daniel M T et al 1976 Proposals for the classification of the acute leukemias. British Journal of Haematology 33: 451-458
56 Rowley J D 1973 Identification of a translocation with quinacrine fluorescence in a patient with acute leukemia. Annals of Genetics 16: 109-112
57 Sakurai M, Sandberg A A 1976 Chromosomes and causation of human cancer and leukemia. XI. Correlation of karyotypes with clinical features of acute myeloblastic leukemia. Cancer 37: 285-299
58 Diaz M O, LeBeau M M, Rowley J D et al 1985 The role of the c-mos gene in the 8;21 translocation in human acute myeloblastic leukemia. Science 229: 767-769
59 Sacchi N, Watson D K, Geurt van Kessel A H M et al 1986 Hu-ets-1 and Hu-ets-2 genes are translocated in acute leukemia with (4;11) and (8;21) translocations. Science 231: 379-382
60 LeBeau M M, Rowley J D, Sacchi N, Watson D K, Papas T S, Diaz M O 1986 Hu-ets-2 is translocated to chromosome 8 in the t(8;21) in acute myelogenous leukemia. Cancer Genetics and Cytogenetics 23: 269-274
61 Rowley J D, Golomb H M, Dougherty C 1977 15/17 translocation, a consistent chromosomal change in acute promyelocytic leukemia. Lancet 1: 549-550
62 Larson R A, Kondo K, Vardiman J W, Butler A E, Golomb H M, Rowley J D 1984 Evidence for a 15;17 translocation in every patient with acute promyelocytic leukemia. American Journal of Medicine 76: 827-841
63 Bennett J M, Catovsky D, Daniel M et al 1976 Proposals for the classification of the acute leukemias: French-American-British (FAB) Co-operative group. British Journal of Haematology 33: 451-453
64 Golomb H M, Rowley J D, Vardiman J W, Testa J R, Butler A 1980 'Microgranular' acute promyelocytic leukemia: a distinct clinical, ultrastructural and cytogenetic entity. Blood 55: 253-259
65 Bernstein R, Mendelow B, Pinto M R, Marcom G, Bezwoda W 1980 Complex translocations involving chromosomes 15 and 17 in acute promyelocytic leukemia. British Journal of Haematology 46: 311-314
66 LeBeau M M, Larson R A, Bitter M A, Vardiman J W, Golomb H M, Rowley J D 1983 Association of an inversion of chromosome 16 with abnormal marrow eosinophils in acute myelomonocytic leukemia. New England Journal of Medicine 309: 630-636

67 Arthur D C, Bloomfield C D 1983 Partial deletion of the long arm of chromosome 16 and bone marrow eosinophilia in acute nonlymphocytic leukemia: a new association. Blood 61: 994-998
68 Yunis J J, Brunning R D 1986 Prognostic significance of chromosomal abnormalities in acute leukemias and myelodysplastic syndromes. In: Gale R P and Hoffbrand A V (eds) Acute leukemia. Clinics in Haematology 15: 597-620
69 Larson R A, Williams S F, LeBeau M M et al 1986 Acute myelomonocytic leukemia with abnormal eosinophils and inv(16) or t(16;16) has a favorable prognosis. Blood 68: 1242-1249
70 Bennett J M, Catovsky D, Daniel M T et al 1985 Proposed revised criteria for the classification of acute myeloid leukemia: a report of the French-American-British Cooperative Group. Annals of Internal Medicine 103: 620-625
71 de la Chapelle A, Lahtinen R 1983 Chromosome 16 and bone marrow eosinophilia. New England Journal of Medicine 309: 1394
72 Neri G, Daniel A, Hammond N 1985 Chromosome 16, eosinophilia and leukemia. Cancer Genetics and Cytogenetics 14: 371-372
73 Kaneko Y, Maseki N, Takasaki N et al 1986 Clinical and hematologic characteristics in acute leukemia with 11q23 translocations. Blood 67: 484-491
74 De Taisne C, Gegonne A, Stehelin D, Bernheim A and Berger R 1984 Chromosomal localization of the human proto-oncogene c-ets. Nature 310: 581-583
75 Rowley J D, Potter D 1976 Chromosomal banding patterns in acute nonlymphocytic leukemia. Blood 47: 705-721
76 Yunis J J, Brunning R D, Howe R B, Lobell M 1984 High-resolution chromosomes as an independent prognostic indicator in adult acute nonlymphocytic leukemia. New England Journal of Medicine 311: 812-818
77 Sasaki M, Kondo K, Tomiyasu T 1983 Cytogenetic characterization of ten cases of Ph[1]-positive acute myelogenous leukemia. Cancer Genetics and Cytogenetics 9: 119-128
78 Bitter M A, Le Beau M M, Rowley J D, Larson R A, Golomb H M, Vardiman J W 1987 Associations between morphology, karyotype, and clinical features in myeloid leukemias. (Progress in Pathology) Human Pathology 18: 211-225
79 Golomb H M, Alimena G, Rowley J D et al 1982 Correlation of occupation and karyotype in adults with acute nonlymphocytic leukemia. Blood 60: 404-411
80 Rowley J D, Golomb H M, Vardiman J W 1981 Nonrandom chromosome abnormalities in acute leukemia and dysmyelopoietic syndromes in patients with previously treated malignant disease. Blood 58: 759-767
81 Golomb H M, Vardiman J W, Rowley J D et al 1978 Correlation of clinical findings with quinacrine-banded chromosomes in 90 adults with acute nonlymphocytic leukemia: An eight year study (1970-1977) New England Journal of Medicine 299: 613-619
82 Pintado T, Ferro M T, Roman C S, Mayayo M, Tasana J G 1985 Clinical correlations of the 3q21;q26 cytogenetic anomaly: a leukemic or myelodysplastic syndrome with preserved or increased platelet production and lack of response to cytotoxic drug therapy. Cancer 55: 535-541
83 The Non-Hodgkin's Lymphoma Pathologic Classification Project 1982 National Cancer Institute sponsored study of classifications on non-Hodgkin's lymphomas. Summary and description of a working formulation for clinical usage. Cancer 49: 2112-2135
84 Foon K A, Schraff R W, Gale R P 1982 Surface markers on leukemia and lymphoma cells: Recent advances. Blood 60: 1-19
85 Yunis J J, Oken M M, Kaplan M F, Ensrud K M, Howe R B, Theologides A 1982 Distinctive chromosomal abnormalities in histologic subtypes of non-Hodgkin's lymphoma. New England Journal of Medicine 307: 1231-1236
86 Yunis J J, Oken M M, Theologides A, Howe R B, Kaplan M E 1984 Recurrent chromosomal defects are found in most patients with non-Hodgkin's lymphoma. Cancer Genetics Cytogenetics 13: 17-28
87 Yunis J J 1986 Chromosomal rearrangements, genes and fragile sites in cancer: clinical and biologic implications. In: DeVita V T, Hellman S, Rosenberg S A (eds) Important advances in oncology. 93-127
88 Yunis J J, Frizzera G, Oken M M, McKenna J, Theologides A, Arnesen M 1987 Multiple recurrent genomic defects in follicular lymphoma. New England Journal of Medicine 316: 79-84
89 Fifth International Workshop on Chromosomes in Leukemia-Lymphoma. 1987 Correlation of chromosome abnormalities with histologic and immunologic characteristics in non-Hodgkin's lymphoma and adult T-cell leukemia-lymphoma. Blood 70: 1554-1564
90 Hecht F, Kaiser-McCaw B 1981 Chromosome 14: A step in the development of lymphoid malignancies. In: Burchenal J H, Oettgen H F (eds) Cancer 1, Grune & Stratton, New York, pp 433-444
91 Zech L, Haglund U, Nilsson K et al 1976 Characteristic chromosomal abnormalities in biopsies and lymphoid-cell lines from patients with Burkitt and non-Burkitt lymphomas. International Journal of Cancer 17: 47-56

92 Berger R, Bernheim A 1985 Cytogenetics of Burkitt's lymphoma-leukemia: a review. In: Burkitt's lymphoma: A human cancer model. Oxford University Press, London, 65–80
93 Leder P, Battey J, Lenoir G et al 1983 Translocations among antibody genes in human cancer. Science 222: 765–771
94 Erikson J, Nishikura K, ar-Rushdi A et al 1983 Translocation of an immunoglobulin K locus to a region 3′ of an unrearranged c-myc oncogene enhances c-myc transcription. Proceedings of the National Academy of Sciences of the USA 80: 7581–7585

12
Cytogenetic Abnormalities of Mature T-cell Malignancies

Vasantha Brito-Babapulle

Malignancies resulting from the proliferation of T-cells with a mature post-thymic phenotype (TdT −, CD1a −, CD2 + +, CD3 + CD5 − / +, CD7 − / +) can be broadly classified as follows:

1. Adult T-cell lymphoma/leukemia (ATLL), where at least 95% of the cases are associated with the human T-cell leukemia virus I (HTLV-I).
2. Peripheral T-cell lymphoma (PTL), all of which are diffuse and represent a spectrum of cytological subtypes that include all non-lymphoblastic T-cell lymphomas other than mycosis fungoides and Sézary syndrome (SS).
3. Cutaneous T-cell lymphoma (CTCL) which includes mycosis fungoides and SS.
4. T-prolymphocytic leukemia (T-PLL), resulting from a proliferation of prolymphocytes.
5. T-chronic lymphocytic leukemia (T-CLL), where there is an expansion of large granular lymphocytes (LGLs).[1,2]

Cytogenetic studies on mature T-cell malignancies have been facilitated by the use of T-cell mitogens such as phytohemagglutinin (PHA), concanavalin A (ConA), 12-O-tetradecanoylphorbol-13-acetate (TPA) in combination with purified T-cell growth factor or interleukin 2 (IL-2) or conditioned medium containing IL-2 from cultures of normal T-cells stimulated by PHA. In the author's laboratory mature B-cells are stimulated to divide by TPA, pokeweed mitogen (PWM) and Epstein–Barr virus (EBV).

Interest in the cytogenetics of T-cell disorders has increased recently, and the mapping of the T-cell receptor (TCR) α-chain gene to chromosome 14q11,[3] β-chain gene to 7q35–36[4] and the δ-chain gene to 7p14,[5] has given added incentive for the investigation of chromosome abnormalities which may be associated with functionally significant genes in the T-cell.

METHODS

Cell separation
Mononuclear cell fractions are isolated sterile on a Lymphoprep (Nyegaard Oslo, Norway) gradient from peripheral blood, bone marrow and cells from lymph nodes, spleen or any other tumor tissue by teasing the tissue with sterile scalpel and needle. Cells are washed three times, to remove the Lymphoprep, in sterile Hanks' balanced salt solution (Gibco Ltd, Paisley, Scotland, UK).

Preparation of conditioned medium
The mononuclear fraction from normal peripheral blood is seeded in 25 cm^3 tissue culture flasks (Becton Dickinson, Switzerland) at a concentration of 1.2×10^6 cells/ml in culture medium RPMI-1640 with 25 mmol/l HEPES buffer and L-glutamine (Gibco) with 20% fetal calf serum (Gibco) and 0.2 mg/ml PHA (Wellcome Laboratories, Dartford, England;

lyophilized; rehydrate to 5 ml with sterile distilled water), and cultured at 37°C. Cultures are harvested at 72 hours by centrifugation of cells at 1800 rev./min. The culture medium is collected and passed through a 0.45-mm millipore filter and aliquoted in 2-ml quantities and stored at −20°C.

Setting up cultures
The mononuclear fraction containing the malignant cells are seeded at 1.2×10^6 cells/ml in 10 ml RPMI-1640 containing 20% fetal calf serum in 25 cm^3 tissue culture flasks. Cultures are set up without mitogens for 24 and 48 hours and with PHA only at 0.2 mg/ml and PHA (0.1 mg/ml) together with TPA (Sigma, St Louis, USA) at a final concentration of 10^{-7} mol/ml for 3, 5 and 7 days at 37°C. Conditioned medium is added at a concentration of 1 ml/10 ml culture. Cultures were harvested after adding colcemid (Gibco, Ohio, USA; 10 mg/ml lyophilized in phosphate-buffered saline; rehydrate with 10 ml sterile distilled water) at a final concentration of 0.05 mg/ml for 1 hour. Cells are collected by centrifugation at 1800 rev./min. and treated with 0.075 mol/l potassium chloride solution for 8 min. The cells are pelleted by centrifugation (1800 rev./min.) and fixed in 3 parts methanol : 1 part glacial acetic acid. Cells are washed twice in fixative, dropped on a glass slide and air dried. Slides are allowed to age for a week and trypsin–Giemsa banding is carried out to identify individual chromosomes.

Trypsin–Giemsa banding
Incubate slides in 2 × SSC (0.3 mol/l sodium chloride + 0.03 mol/l trisodium citrate) at 60–65°C in a water bath for 1 hour. Rinse in physiological saline. Dip for 1–3 seconds in Bacto trypsin solution at 4°C (Difco, Detroit Michigan, USA; lyophilized powder rehydrated with 10 ml and diluted to 100 ml with Ca^{2+} and Mg^{2+} free Hanks' balanced salt solution and stored in fridge). Rinse well in physiological saline. Leave slides in buffer pH 6.8 for 1 min (M1 Sorensen's buffer concentrate pH 6.8; Mercia Brocades, West Byfleet, Surrey, UK) and stain with Gurr's Giemsa (6% in buffer pH 6.8) for up to 1 min, rinse in buffer pH 6.8 and air dry.

ADULT T-CELL LYMPHOMA/LEUKEMIA (ATLL)

ATLL is a distinct T-cell disorder associated with HTLV-I,[6,7] although few cases have been reported where there is no evidence for the involvement of HTLV-I.[8] Presumably in these cases a different oncogenetic mechanism affects the same target cell. This disorder is prevalent mainly in south-western Japan and the Caribbean basin,[9,10] with sporadic clusters in other parts of the world. The leukemic cells in ATLL are morphologically pleomorphic with a mature T-cell helper phenotype (CD4) but show suppression in vitro of PWM-induced B-cell differentiation.[11] ATLL may have an acute or subacute clinical course with a typical feature being hypercalcemia with or without lytic bone lesions.[1,12]

The author's studies in two Caribbean patients with ATLL revealed, in one, a 1q+, del6(q21), t(11,14)(q13;q22-24), i(17q), together with trisomy for chromosome 3 and partial trisomy for chromosome 7, whilst the other had partial trisomy for chromosome 7 resulting from an extra chromosome 7 with deletion of part of the short arm.[13,14] Some of the important abnormalities of ATLL reported in the literature are summarized in Table 12.1.

Chromosome studies on 105 cases of Japanese ATLL[15-21] and 19 cases of non-Japanese ATLL[14,22,23] with HTLV-I have been reported. An abstract from the USA reports a further 12 cases, but discusses only one specific abnormality and has therefore been excluded from Table 12.1 but it will be referred to in the subsequent discussion.

Trisomy or partial trisomy for chromosomes 3 and 7 and a 6q− are the most frequent abnormalities reported in ATLL. Breakpoints for 6q− vary from q11 to q24 with some being

Table 12.1 Chromosome abnormalities in ATLL

	Total no. of cases	inv(14)(q11q32)	t(14;14)(q11;q32)	14+	14q11–13	14q32	6q–	Trisomy or partial trisomy 7	Trisomy partial trisomy 3	10p	Reference
Japanese ATLL	15	–	–	–	–	2	–	5	1	–	15
	8	–	–	–	–	3	1	1	1	–	16
	30	1	–	–	–	7	16	2	10	2	17
	18	–	–	–	1	–	1	5	5	–	18
	15	1	–	–	–	2	3	3	3	–	19
	11	1	–	4	2	1	1	1	2	3	20
	8	2	1	–	4	–	1	–	2	–	21
Subtotal	105	5	1	4	7	15	23	17	24	5	
Non-Japanese ATLL	11	–	–	–	–	–	6	–	–	1	22
	6	–	–	–	–	–	2	2	4	–	23
	2	–	–	–	–	–	1	2	1	–	14
Subtotal	19	–	–	–	–	–	9	4	5	1	
Total	124	5	1	4	7	15	32	21	29	6	

interstitial deletions. The above abnormalities are common both in Japanese and non-Japanese (mainly Caribbean) ATLL.

Of the abnormalities of chromosome 14, involvement of band q32 was observed in 15/105 Japanese ATLL and inv(14)(q11q32) in five of them. The 14q+ observed in the Caribbean patient studied in this laboratory had a breakpoint at q22-24. The overall incidence of abnormalities involving the 14q11 region to which the TCR α-chain gene maps appears to be low in ATLL (Table 12.1). However, one report describes 14q11 involvement in six out of eight cases of ATLL investigated.[21] The reason for this difference is not clear at the present time.

Abnormalities of 10p have been described in 11 cases and in a recent report 5 out of 12 cases had abnormalities of 10p.[24]

The chromosome abnormalities in three cases of ATLL not associated with HTLV-I are similar to those of HTLV-I-associated ATLL. Partial trisomy 3 was observed in one case, partial trisomy 7 and del10(p13) in the second case and del10(p13) in the third case.[8]

Although relatively consistent non-random chromosome abnormalities have been described in ATLL there is no evidence of a specific abnormality characteristic of this disease.

PERIPHERAL T-CELL LYMPHOMA (PTL)

This is a relatively rare form of non-Hodgkin's lymphoma. The proliferating cell in PTL is often CD4+, but CD8+ cases have also been observed. The majority of PTL cases are classified histologically as diffuse mixed cell type or diffuse large cell, usually of an immunoblastic subtype of non-Hodgkin's lymphoma. Less than 2% are classified as well differentiated or small cell lymphocytic and these may be the tissue equivalent of T-CLL.[12]

Investigation of one such a case during its leukemic phase revealed that the proliferating lymphocyte was a CD8+ large granular lymphocyte coexisting with immunoblasts which also had azurophil granules as the LGL.[25] Forty-five of the 50 cells analysed had a t(1;22)(q12;q13), dup(1)(q31 q32), t(8;14)(q24;q32), t(9;14)(p11;q32) (Fig. 12.1). Three cells had t(1;22)(q12;q13) dup(1)(q31 q32); t(8;14)(q24;q32). One cell had t(1;22)(q12;q13) and dup(1)(q31 q32); this presumably was the stemline. The t(8;14)(q24;q32) was cytogenetically indistinguishable from that seen in Burkitt's lymphoma and appears to have arisen during clonal evolution. The spleen cells revealed, in addition, a t(1;3)(p34;q22) and other abnormalities.[25] The t(8;14)(q24;q32) may have been associated with the aggressive behaviour of this T-cell disorder compared to other proliferations of LGL. Interestingly, the appearance of a t(8;14)(q24;q32) as a secondary abnormality in a low grade follicular lymphoma with t(14;18) (q32;q21) is also usually associated with change to a more aggressive clinical course (Croce C, personal communication).

A diffuse mixed cell lymphoma of T-cell origin has been described with t(14;18)(q32;q21) — an abnormality cytogenetically similar to that seen in B-cell follicular lymphoma.[26] Two out of six cases of T-lymphoma with 14q32 breakpoint, one of which was t(10;14)(q22;q32), have also been described.[27] An inv(14)(q11;q32) has been reported in one case of PTL[29] and in a cell line SUP-T$_1$ derived from a T-lymphoma.[29] A t(4;14)(q26;q32) and a t(6;14)(q23;q32) were observed in two lymphoepithelioid (Lennert's) lymphomas.[30]

Recent reports on cytogenetic abnormalities of PTL suggest that abnormalities of chromosome 3 may occur with high incidence. In five cases of PTL investigated by Lakkala-Paranko et al,[31] three were T-zone lymphomas and all three had trisomy 3; in one it was the only abnormality. One case of Lennerts' lymphoma, out of eight PTLs studied by Sanger et al,[30] also had trisomy for chromosome 3. Investigation of eight cases of Lennert's lymphoma revealed five with trisomy 3 and 2 with abnormalities of 3q22,[32,33] whilst in six cases of other T-lymphomas, two had trisomy 3 and two had abnormalities of 3q21.[34]

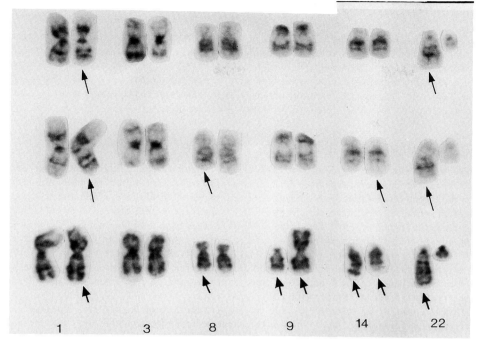

Fig. 12.1 T-lymphoma of CD8 + large granular lymphocytes. Partial karyotypes from two cells from the spleen (top and middle row) and one cell from peripheral blood (bottom row) showing sequential appearance of chromosomal abnormalities. Top row: dup(1)(q31;q32), t(1;22)(q12;q13). Middle row: dup(1)(q31;q32), t(1;22)(q12;q13), t(8;14)(q24;q32). Bottom row: dup(1)(q31;q32), t(1;22)(q12;q13), t(8;14)(q24;q32), t(9;14)(p11;q32). A 9p+ was found only in peripheral blood cells. (Reproduced from Brito-Babapulle et al[25] with permission of the publishers.)

Another chromosome region which appears to be non-randomly involved in PTL is the short arm (p) of chromosome 6. An ins(6;11)(q22;q21q25) has been reported in a case of PTLs[35] and a 6p+q+, 6p+ and del(6)(p23-p24) have been reported in three cases of T-lymphoma.[36]

Further studies on more cases of PTLs are required to see whether chromosome abnormalities specific for different subtypes of PTL are present.

CUTANEOUS T-CELL LYMPHOMA (CTCL)

Sézary syndrome (SS) and mycosis fungoides are two related disorders which are included in the group of CTCL.[37] The cytogenetic studies carried out so far on CTCL show that chromosomal abnormalities are often complex and non-clonal with variation in ploidy.[38-42] Where clonal abnormalities are present they are thought to be associated with a more aggressive clinical course.[37] The study of eight cases of Sézary syndrome in the author's laboratory revealed clonal chromosome abnormalities in 6[14] (unpublished observations). One had only tetraploid cells whereas one case had tetraploid and diploid cells. A del(6)(q21) was seen in two cases and a del(6)(q23) in one case. Abnormalities of chromosome 2p were frequent with a del(2)(p14-15), a 2p+ with break point of p23 and a t(2;7)(p11-12;q35-36). Chromosome 7 was involved in four cases. Trisomy or partial trisomy for 7 was observed in two cases resulting from t(7;7;7)(p14;q11-q35;q11-q32) and an i(7q). One case had a t(7;22)(p14-15;q13). The cases 7q35-36 and 7p14-15 are chromosomal bands to which TCR β- and δ-chain genes are mapped.[4,5]

A 6q - has been described in six cases of CTCL with clonal abnormalities;[38,40,42] break points were 6q21 or 6q23. A t(2;14)(p24;q11) and a t(14;14)(q12;q31) have been reported in two cases of Sézary syndrome.[41,43]

The author's studies of Sézary syndrome were carried out on peripheral blood. Nowell et al[43] observed the same chromosome abnormality in cells from blood, lymph node and skin suggesting that the same clone was present in all three tissues.

T-PROLYMPHOCYTIC LEUKEMIA (T-PLL)

Prolymphocytic leukemia is characterized by marked splenomegaly, high WBC count and minimal lymph node enlargement. Diagnosis is made by identification of the prolymphocyte in peripheral blood films. With the advent of cell marker studies, a form of the disease where the leukemic cell is of T-cell origin (T-PLL) has been recognized and represents a distinct clinicopathological entity.[44] Two-thirds of T-PLL cases have a CD4 + , CD8 - membrane phenotype whilst others may be CD4 - , CD8 + or co-express CD4 and CD8.[45] T-PLL is an aggressive disease and the mean survival in a series of 50 patients from the author's institution was found to be 7 months. From our experience T-PLL cells are best stimulated by a combination of TPA and PHA and clonal chromosome abnormalities have been observed in 15 out of 16 cases studied.

Eleven out of 16 cases of T-PLL investigated in this laboratory had chromosome abnormalities involving 14q11 which is the chromosomal band to which the TCR α-chain gene is localized.[3] Ten had inv(14)(q11q32) (Fig. 12.2) and one had der11t(11;14)(14;14)(p13;q11q32;q11). Thus in 11 cases 14q11 was juxtaposed to 14q32. Other translocations involving 14q11 were observed in two cases.[46]

Trisomy or partial trisomy or multisomy for 8q (Fig. 12.2) was observed in 10 out of 16 T-PLL patients. In all such cases trisomy, partial trisomy or multisomy for 8q resulted from

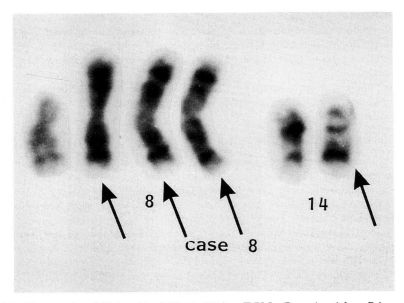

Fig. 12.2 Three copies of i(8q) and inv(14)(q11;q32) in a T-PLL. (Reproduced from Brito-Babapulle et al[46] with permission of the publishers.)

an i(8q) or t(8;8)(p12;q11) except in one case where two copies of t(8;21)(p12;q11), in addition to a normal chromosome 8, were present in a subclone.[46]

Of two cases of T-PLL reported in the literature[47,48] one had inv(14)[47] and the other t(14;14)(q11;q32). Another patient was described as having T-helper CLL.[49] However, splenomegaly, a WBC count of 39×10^9 with 84% non-granular lymphocytes with indented nuclei, an aggressive clinical course with poor response to therapy and short survival suggest that this patient may also have had T-PLL. An inv(14)(q11;q32) was observed in two out of three cases described as chronic T leukemia but without the clinical details,[50] and an inv(14)(q11;q32) was observed in seven cases and i(8q) or t(8;8)(p12;q11) in five cases in a series of eight cases reported under the diagnosis of T-CLL.[51] In the absence of morphological information it is not possible to exclude a diagnosis of T-PLL in some of these cases.

T-CELL CHRONIC LYMPHOCYTIC LEUKEMIA (T-CLL)

T-CLL results from the expansion of large granular lymphocytes usually identified as Tγ lymphocytes. The most common membrane phenotype is CD4 – , CD8 + . This disorder is characterized by moderate blood and bone marrow lymphocytosis, absence of lymphadenopathy and usually splenomegaly, polyclonal hypergammaglobulinemia and a relatively chronic clinical course.[43] Twelve such cases have been studied using PHA as mitogen in 3- and 5-day cultures, and obtained mitoses in eight of them. The following clonal rearrangements were observed: t(11;15)(q13;q22–24) and del(6)(q21) in a CD8 + T-CLL, int del(14)(q22q24) in another CD8 + case, t(1;5)(q12;q35) in a CD4 + , CD8 + case and t(4;17)(p15–16;q23) in a CD4 + , Leu7 + T-CLL. Random numerical changes were observed in one CD8 + case whilst three other CD8 + cases had normal karyotypes[14] (unpublished observations). The following clonal chromosome abnormalities have been reported by others in T-CLL/LGL proliferations: 47 XX + C;[52] trisomy 8 and trisomy 14 in two out of three cases;[53] and 46, Y, – X, – 14, del(2)(p13), der(X)t(X;14)(q22;q11)) + Mar, t(?;2)(?;p11) in one out of four cases.[54] Clonal abnormalities in the latter case were detected only in cultures stimulated with phorbol myristate acetate. No consistent abnormality characteristic of T-CLL resulting from LGL proliferations has yet been described.

DISCUSSION

The investigation of mature T-cell malignancies and those of others show that certain chromosome abnormalities occur non-randomly. Their incidence has been summarized in Tables 12.2 and 12.3.

Trisomy for chromosome 3 appears to be characteristic of ATLL and PTL (Table 12.2). The genes of significance on chromosome 3 are the oncogene *raf-1* on p25, the transferrin

Table 12.2 Incidence of + 3, 6q – and + 7 in mature T-cell malignancies

	Trisomy or partial trisomy 3 (%)	6q – (%)	Trisomy or partial trisomy 7 (%)
ATLL (124)	29 (23.4)	31 (25)	18 (14.5)
PTL (40)	11 (27.5)	1	—
CTCL (44)[a]	—	9 (20.5)	2
T-PLL (19)	—	3 (15.8)	2
T-CLL (12)[a]	—	1	—

[a]Many cases with non-clonal abnormalities have been reported. These have been excluded from this analysis.

Table 12.3 Incidence of chromosome 14 abnormalities involving q11 and q32 in mature T-cell malignancies

Disease	(No. of cases)	Inv(14)(q11q32) (%)	Tandem rearrangement of 14q11 and 14q32	Other translocations involving 14q32 (%)	Other rearrangements involving 14q11 (%)
ATLL	(124)	5(4)	1	15(12)	7 (5.6)
PTL	(40)	1	–	6	–
SUP T1 (cell line)	(1)	1	–	–	–
CTCL	(44)[a]	–	1	–	1
T-PLL	(19)	12(63)	1	–	3(15)
'Chronic T-cell leukemia'	(12)[b]	9	1	–	–
T-CLL (LGL)	(12)[a]	–	–	–	1

[a] Many cases with non-clonal abnormalities have been reported. These have been excluded here.
[b] Several of these cases have clinical and hematological features suggestive of T-PLL but no detailed morphological findings were available (see text).

gene on q21 and the transferrin receptor gene on q26.[55] The oncogene c-raf has been reported to be expressed in rapidly proliferating, yet not transformed, T-cell lines derived from autoimmune mice.[56] In addition it has been reported that the cooperation of the oncogenes v-rafI and v-myc results in the induction of murine immunoblastic lymphomas of T and B lineage.[57] The expression of the transferrin receptor, on the other hand, is thought to be significant in T-cell proliferations.[58]

6q – has been reported in all five types of mature T-cell malignancies which have been discussed. The oncogene mcf3 which is probably the same as c-ros has been mapped to 6q16–q22, whilst c-myb has been mapped to 6q22.[55] Recent evidence indicates that c-myb may play a role in thymic lymphocyte differentiation.[59]

Although trisomy is common in ATLL and PTL, trisomy 7 occurs frequently in ATLL but not in PTL, and partial trisomy 7 has been observed both in T-PLL and CTCL (Table 12.2). In ATLL the presence of trisomy 3 or 7 or both has been associated with clinical severity of the disease.[18] Since partial trisomy of chromosome 7 usually results in trisomy for 7q, the presence of the c-met oncogene on 7q22–q23[55] is of interest, and may be pathogenically important.

Trisomy for 8q (see Fig. 12.1), resulting from i(8q) or t(8;8)(p12;q11), which is an abnormality characteristic of T-PLL, is particularly interesting in view of recent studies on the expression of c-myc in a case of T-PLL.[60] A high level of c-myc expression was observed although the vast majority of cells were quiescent, as was shown by the lack of histone H3 expression and the very low number of cells in S phase as assessed by microfluorimetric analysis. It has been suggested that the cells were arrested outside of G_0. Cells with high levels of c-myc might not necessarily be proliferating but simply advanced into the G_1 phase of the cell cycle to a stage of 'competence'. The morphology of the prolymphocyte with diffuse chromatin and a prominent nucleolus, similar to normal lymphocytes undergoing blastic transformation in response to mitogens, supports such an interpretation. Treatment with cytosine arabinoside at high doses leads to a marked decrease in c-myc expression possibly by inhibiting DNA polymerase and interfering with the progression of cells through the S phase of the cell cycle. Chemotherapy selectively enriches the peripheral blood lymphocytes of the patient under study of truly G_0 cells.[60]

CYTOGENETIC ABNORMALITIES OF MATURE T-CELL MALIGNANCIES 335

Another interesting finding was the involvement of 10p in 5 out of 12 cases of ATLL.[24] Since the gene for the IL2 receptor is mapped to 10p14–15[55] the presence of an extra restriction fragment homologous to the IL2-2R probe in two cases with 10p abnormalities is intriguing.

Abnormalities of chromosome 14 in the T-cell disorders are of particular interest. Since the TCR α-chain gene is mapped to 14q11[3] and the gene is transcriptionally active in the T-cell, chromosome rearrangements involving this locus could be considered analogous to those involving immunoglobulin loci in B-cell disorders, where an oncogene or putative oncogenic sequence is activated or deregulated by being brought adjacent to a transcriptionally active gene.[61] Although such translocations have been described in mature T-cell disorders (Table 12.3), rearrangements of 14q32 with 14q11 or other chromosomes are of special interest. The involvement of 14q32 in B-cell disorders is understandable due to the localization of the immunoglobulin heavy chain gene (IgH) to this band.[55] Since the IgH gene is not functionally significant in T-cells the involvement of 14q32 in T-cell disorders deserves special attention. The inv(14)(q11q32) in the cell line SUP-T1 derived from a T-lymphoma results from a site-specific recombination event between an IgH variable gene (IgV_H) and the TCR chain joining segment (TCR α J) which gives rise to an Ig–TCR hybrid gene. This suggests that there are common signal sequences present in both TCR and IgH loci that make them susceptible to the same recombinases. In a few cases of T-PLL the breakpoint in 14q32 in the inv(14)(q11q32) (see Fig. 12.1) was 3' of the IgH locus and may involve a oncogenic sequence such as AK-T1[62] or a putative oncogene tcl-1[16] localized to 14q32 which could be activated by becoming juxtaposed to the TCR α-chain gene on 14q11 (Fig. 12.3).[3] ATLL and PTL are

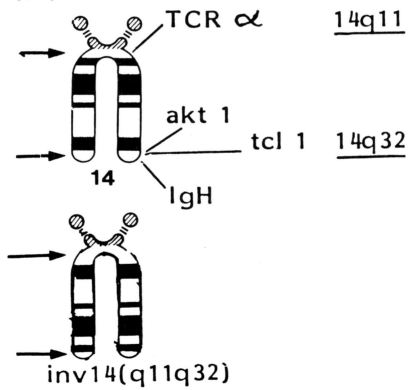

Fig 12.3 Schematic diagram of the normal and inverted homologue of chromosome 14 with the location of TCR α-chain gene (14q11) and the IgH gene, and *AK-T1* and *tcl-1* oncogenes.

often characterized by chromosome rearrangements between 14q32 and other chromosomes similar to those seen in B-cell disorders (Table 12.3).

In PTL some of the translocations involving the 14q32 described are: t(8;14)(q24;q32), t(14;18)(q32;q21), t(4;14)(q26;q32) and t(6;14)(22;q32). *c-myc* is mapped to 8q24, *bcl-2* and *c-yes* to 18q21, IL2 gene to 4q26 and *c-myb* to 6q22.[55] It still has to be clarified whether these oncogenic sequences are being activated by translocation to a yet unidentified or unlocalized gene on 14q32 that is transcriptionally active in the T-cell. Interestingly segments of V_H genes are known to be transcribed in T-cells (T.H. Rabbitts, personal communication). Further molecular investigations are required before the role of genes on 14q32 which are significant in T-cell neoplasia can be elucidated.

REFERENCES

1 Jaffe E S 1984 Pathologic and clinical spectrum of post-thymic: T-cell malignancies. Cancer Investigation 2: 413-426
2 Catovsky D, Matutes E 1987 The classification of T-cell leukemias. In: Gale R P, Rai K (eds) UCLA symposia on chronic lymphocytic leukemia: Recent advances, future directions, New York, Liss, pp. 163-176
3 Croce M, Isobe M, Palumbo A et al 1985 Gene for α chain of human T-cell receptor. Location on chromosome 14 region involved in T-cell neoplasms. Science 227: 1044-1047
4 Isobe M, Erikson J, Emanuel B S, Nowell P C, Croce C M 1985 Location of gene for β submit of human T-cell receptor at band 7q35, a region prone to rearrangements in T-cells. Science 228: 580-582
5 Murre C, Waldmann R A, Morton C C, Bongiovanni K F, Waldmann T A, Shows T B, Seidman J G 1985 Human β-chain genes are rearranged in leukemic T-cells and map to the short arm of chromosome 7. Nature 316: 549-552
6 Blattner W A, Kalyanaraman U S, Robert-Guroff et al 1982 The human type C retrovirus HTLVI in blacks from the Caribbean region and relationship to adult T-cell leukemia/lymphoma. International Journal of Cancer 30: 257-264
7 Haynes B F, Miller S E, Polker Th J et al 1983 Identification of human T-cell leukemia virus in a Japanese patient with adult T-cell leukemia and cutaneous lymphomatous vasculitis. Proceedings of the National Academy of Sciences of the USA 80: 2054-2058
8 Shimoyama M, Abe T, Miyamoto K, Minato K et al 1987 Chromosome alterations and clinical features of adult T-cell leukemia-lymphoma, not associated with human T-cell leukemia virus type I. Blood 69: 984-989
9 Catovsky D, Greaves M F, Rose M et al 1982 Adult T-cell lymphoma leukemia in blacks from the West Indies. Lancet i: 639-643
10 Hanaoka M, Sasaki M, Matsumoto H et al 1979 Adult T-cell Leukemia H: Histological classification and characteristics. Acta Pathologica Japonica 29: 723-738
11 Matutes E, Brito-Babapulle V, Catovsky D 1985 Clinical, immunological, ultrastructural and cytogenetic studies in black patients with adult T-cell lymphoma/leukemia. In: Miwa M et al (eds) Retrovirus in human lymphoma/leukemia. In: Japan Science Society press, Tokyo/VNU Science Press, Utrecht 59-70
12 Blayney D W, Jaffe E S, Fisher R I et al 1983 The human T-cell leukemia/lymphoma virus (HTLV), lymphoma, lytic bone lesions and hypercalcemia. Annals of Internal Medicine 98: 144-150
13 Brito-Babapulle V, Matutes E, Hegde M, Catovsky D 1984 Adult T-cell lymphoma/leukemia in a Caribbean patient: cytogenetic immunologic and ultrastructural findings. Cancer Genetics and Cytogenetics 12: 343-357
14 Brito-Babapulle V, Matutes E, Parreira L, Catovsky D 1986 Abnormalities of chromosome 7q and Tac expansion in T-cell leukemias. Blood 67: 516-521
15 Ueshima Y, Fukuhara S, Hattori T, Uchiyama T, Takatsuki K, Uchino H 1981 Chromosome studies in adult T-cell leukemia in Japan: Significance of trisomy 7. Blood 58: 420-425
16 Shiraishi Y, Taguchi T, Kubonishi I, Taguchi H, Miyoshi I 1985 Chromosome abnormalities, sister chromatid exchanges and cell cycle analysis in phytohaemagglutinin-stimulated adult T-cell leukemia lymphocytes. Cancer Genetics and Cytogenetics 15: 65-67
17 Miyamoto K, Tomita N, Ishii A et al 1984 Chromosome abnormalities in leukemia cells in adult patients with T-cell leukemia. Journal of the National Cancer Institute 73: 353-361

18 Sanada I, Tanaka R, Kumagai E et al 1985 Chromosomal aberrations in adult T-cell leukemia: Relationship to clinical severity. Blood 65: 649–654
19 Fujita K, Yamasaki Y, Sawada H, Izumi Y, Fukuhara S, Uchino H 1988 Cytogenetic studies on adult T-cell leukemia in Japan. Personal communication
20 Fujita K, Fukuhara S, Nasu K et al 1986 Recurrent Chromosome abnormalities in adult T-cell lymphomas of peripheral T-cell origin. International Journal of Cancer 37: 517–524
21 Sadamori N, Nishino K, Kusano M et al 1986 Significance of chromosome 14 anomaly at band 14q11 in Japanese patients with adult T-cell leukemia. Cancer 58: 2244–2250
22 Whang-Peng J, Bunn P A, Knutsen T et al 1985 Cytogenetic studies in human T-cell lymphoma virus (HTLV) positive leukemia/lymphoma in the United States. Journal of the National Cancer Institute 74: 357–369
23 Rowley J D, Haren M J, Wong-Staal F, Franchini G, Gallo R C, Blattner W 1984 Chromosome pattern in cells from patients positive for human T-cell leukemia/lymphoma virus. In: Gallo R C, Essex M E, Gross L (eds) Human T-cell leukemia/lymphoma viruses. Cold Spring Harbor Laboratory, New York, pp. 85–89
24 Szabo P, Macera M J, Verma R S, Weksler M E, Dosik H 1987 The abnormality of chromosome 10p and interleukin-2 receptor (IL-2R) gene in adult T-cell leukemia (ATL). American Journal of Human Genetics 39 (Supplement): A222
25 Brito-Babapulle V, Matutes E, Foroni L, Pomfret M, Catovsky D 1987 A t(8;14)(q24;q32) in a T-lymphoma/leukemia of CD8+ large granular lymphocytes. Leukemia 1: 789–794
26 Takeuchi J, Ochi H, Minowada J, Barcos M, Ozer H, Henderson E S, Sandberg A A 1985 Cytogenetic studies of a diffuse mixed cell lymphoma of T-cell origin. Cancer Genetics and Cytogenetics 14: 257–266
27 Bloomfield C D, Arthur D C, Frizzera G, Levine E G, Peterson B A, Gajl-Peczalska K J 1983 Non random chromosome abnormalities in lymphoma. Cancer Research 43: 2975–2984
28 Clare N, Boldt D, Messerschmidt G, Zeltzer P, Hansen K, Manhoff L 1986 Lymphocyte malignancy and chromosome 14: Structural alterations involving band q11. Blood 67: 704–709
29 Denny C T, Yoshikai Y, Mak T W, Smith S D, Hollis G F, Kirsch I R 1986 A chromosome 14 inversion in a T-cell lymphoma is caused by site specific recombination between immunoglobulin and T-cell receptor loci. Nature 320: 549–551
30 Sanger W G, Weisenburger D D, Armitage J O, Purtilo D T 1986 Cytogenetic abnormalities in non-cutaneous peripheral T-cell lymphoma. Cancer Genetics and Cytogenetics 23: 53–59
31 Lakkala-Paranko, Franssira K, Lappalainen K et al 1987 Chromosome abnormalities in peripheral T-cell Lymphoma. British Journal of Haematology 66: 451–460
32 Godde-Salz E, Feller A C, Lennert K 1986 Cytogenetic and immunohistochemical analysis of lymphoepithelioid cell lymphoma (Lennert Lymphoma): Further substantiation of its T-cell nature. Leukemia Research 10: 313–323
33 Godde-Salz E, Schwarze E W 1984 Biclonal trisomy 3 in a case of epitheloid cellular lymphogranulomatosis (Lennerts' Lymphoma). Cancer Genetics Cytogenetics 13: 337–341
34 Yunis J J, Oken M M, Theologides A, Howe R B, Kaplan M E 1984 Recurrent chromosomal defects are found in most patients with non-Hodgkin's lymphoma. Cancer Genetics and Cytogenetics 13: 17–28
35 Donti E, Falini B, Bordoni S, Rosetti A, Carloni I, Donti G V 1987 ins(6;11) in a case of peripheral T-cell lymphoma. Cancer Genetics and Cytogenetics 27: 367–369
36 Mecucci C, Michaux J L, Tricot G, Louwagie A, Van den Berghe H 1985 Rearrangements of the short arm of chromosome No. 6 in T-cell lymphomas. Leukemia Research 9: 1139–1148
37 Lutzner M, Edelson R, Schein R, Green I, Kirkpatrick C, Ahmed A 1975 Cutaneous T-cell lymphomas: The Sézary syndrome, mycosis fungoides and related disorders. Annals of Internal Medicine 83: 534–552
38 Whang-Peng J, Bunn P A, Knutsen T, Mathews M J, Schechter G, Minna J D 1982 Clinical implications of cytogenetic studies in cutaneous T-cell lymphoma (CTCL). Cancer 50: 1539–1553
39 Warburton D, Shapiro P E, Berger C L, Edelson R L 1987 Rearrangements of chromosome 10 in cutaneous T-cell lymphoma (Abstract 319). Ninth international workshop in human gene mapping, Paris
40 Johnson G A, Dewald G W, Strand W R, Winkelmann R K 1985 Chromosome studies in 17 patients with Sézary syndrome. Cancer 55: 2426–2433
41 Berger R, Bernheim A 1987 Cytogenetic studies of Sézary cells. Cancer Genetics and Cytogenetics 27: 79–87
42 Shah-Reddy I, Mayeda K, Mirchandani I, Koppitch F C 1982 Sézary syndrome with a (14;14)(q12;q31) translocation. Cancer 49: 75–79

43 Nowell P C, Finan J B, Vonderheid E C 1982 Clonal characteristics of cutaneous T-cell lymphomas: Cytogenetic evidence from blood, lymph nodes and skin. Journal of Investigative Dermatology 78: 69–75

44 Catovsky D 1984 Chronic lymphocytic prolymphocytic and hairy cell leukemias. In: Goldman J M, Preisler H D (eds) Leukemias. London, Butterworths, pp. 266–298

45 Matutes E, Garcia Talavera J, O'Brien M, Catovsky D 1986 The morphological spectrum of T-prolymphocytic leukemia. British Journal Haematology 64: 111–124

46 Brito-Babapulle V, Pomfret M, Matutes E, Catovsky D 1987 Cytogenetic studies on prolymphocytic leukemia II T-cell prolymphocytic leukemia. Blood 70: 926–931

47 Corwin J D, Kadin M E, Andres T L 1983 T-cell prolymphocytic leukemia: 2 cases having a post thymic helper phenotype with complement receptors and 14q+ chromosome abnormality. Acta Haematologica 70: 43–49

48 Turchini M F, Geneix A, Travade Ph et al 1984 Studies in a case of T-cell prolymphocytic leukemia. Cancer Genetics and Cytogenetics 12: 171–174

49 Pasqualetti D, Cafaro A, Gastaldi R et al 1987 T-helper phenotype chronic lymphocytic leukemia (Thp-CLL): Characterisation of an Italian case with particular biological findings. Blut 54: 289–298

50 Ueshima Y, Rowley J D, Variakojis D, Winter J, Gordon L 1984 Cytogenetic studies on patients with chronic T-cell leukemia/lymphoma. Blood 63: 1028–1038

51 Zech L, Godal T, Hammarstrom L et al 1986 Specific chromosome markers involved with chronic T lymphocyte tumours. Cancer Genetics and Cytogenetics 21: 67–77

52 Brody J L, Burnigham R A, Nowell P C, Rowlands D T, Frieburg P, Daniele R P 1975 Persistent lymphocytosis with chromosomal evidence of malignancy. American Journal of Medicine 58: 547–552

53 Loughran Jr. T P, Kadin M E, Starkebaum G et al 1985 Leukemia of large granular lymphocytes: association with clonal chromosomal abnormalities and autoimmune neutropenia and hemolytic anaemia. Annals of Internal Medicine 102: 169–175

54 McKenna R W, Arthur D C, Gajl-Peczalska, Flynn P, Brunning R D 1985 Granulated T-cell lymphocytosis with neutropenia: malignant or benign chronic lymphoproliferative disorder? Blood 66: 259–266

55 Human Gene Mapping 8 1985 Eighth International Workshop on Human Gene mapping. Cytogenetics and Cell Genetics 40: 1–823

56 Rosenberg Y J, Malek T R, Schaeffer D E et al 1985 Unusual expression of IL2 receptors and both the c-myb and c-raf oncogenes in T-cell lines and clones derived from autoimmune MRL-1pr/1pr mice. Journal of Immunology 134: 3120–3123

57 Rapp U R, Cleveland J L, Fredrickson T N et al 1985 Rapid induction of hemopoietic neoplasms in new born mice by a raf(mil)/myc recombinant murine retrovirus. Journal of Virology 55: 23–33

58 Neckers L M, Cossman J 1983 Transferrin 1983 Receptor induction in mitogen stimulated human T lymphocytes is required for DNA synthesis and cell division and is regulated by interleukin 2. Proceedings of the National Academy of Sciences of the USA 80: 3494–3498

59 Thompson C B, Challoner P B, Neiman P E, Groudine M 1986 Expression of the c-myb and c-fes onc genes during cellular proliferation. Nature 319: 374–380

60 Kaczmarek L, Elfenbein I B, Narni F, Vonderheid C E, Barry W E, Calabretta B 1987 The effect of cytosine – arabinoside treatment on the over expression of c-myc proto-oncogene in a case of prolymphocytic leukemia. Cancer Genetics and Cytogenetics 27: 89–99

61 Croce C M 1987 Role of chromosome translocations in human neoplasia. Cell 49: 155–156

62 Testa J R, Huebner K, Croce C M, Stall S 1985 AKT-1 gene, the human homologue of a retroviral oncogene is located on chromosome 14 at band q32 (abstract). Cytogenetics and Cell Genetics 40: 761

13
Immunoglobulin and T-cell Receptor Gene Analysis for the Investigation of Lymphoproliferative Disorders

L Foroni, P Mason, L Luzzatto

INTRODUCTION

Immunoglobulins (Ig) and T-cell receptors (TCR) are the molecules responsible for antigen recognition by lymphoid cells.[1-3] They are synthesized by B- and T-lymphocytes respectively and they may be regarded as their most characteristic products. Ig molecules are tetrameric and they are composed of a pair of identical heavy (H) chains and a pair of identical light (L) chains.[4,5] They exist in both a membrane-bound and a circulating form in the plasma. TCR molecules are heterodimers of a β- and an α-chain and they are always membrane bound.[6-8] Another form of TCR consists of a similar heterodimer called γδ.[9,10] Both Ig and TCR molecules have regions which vary in primary structure; this variability accounts for the ability of Ig and TCR molecules to recognize a large number of different antigens. At the same time molecules within each group must have regions in common (constant regions) because they share effector pathways.[11-13]

The means by which molecules of similar, but not identical, structure are produced is now known.[14-17] The process involves the joining of a limited number of DNA segments in an orderly fashion.[18,19] Once a particular rearrangement of DNA has taken place in a cell it will be characteristic of that cell and of its progeny, i.e. of that clone of T- or B-cells. In addition, the nature of the gene (Ig or TCR) that has undergone rearrangement will reflect the B- or T-cell nature of the clone. The coding genes for each of the Ig and TCR polypeptide chains are clustered in specific chromosomal regions (Table 13.1). The configuration of each cluster before the rearrangement is referred to as 'germline' because that is the form in which it is inherited.[35]

GENE CLUSTERS

Immunoglobulin genes
Current nomenclature, localization and actual or estimated number of DNA regions coding for each portion of the H and L chains are summarized in Table 13.1. Three major separate

Table 13.1 Chromosomal localization and gene organization of Ig and TCR genes

Gene locus	Chromosome and band	Variable region			Constant region	Reference
		V	D	J		
IgH	14 q32	100–150[a]	12	6	9	16, 20,21,36–41
Ig κ	2 p12	60[a]	–	5	1	22,23,42–50
Ig λ	22 p11	20–30[a]	–	6–9	6	24,25,51–55
TCR α	14 q11	20[a]	–	60–70[a]	1	26–29, 34,56,57
TCR β	7 p35	150[a]	2	7	2	30,31,58,59
TCR γ	7 p15	14[a]	–	3	2	32,60,61
TCR δ	14 q11	?	2	2	1	33,34

[a] The final correct number has yet to be determined.

sets can be identified for each polypeptide chain: segments coding for the variable (V), joining (J) and constant (C) regions respectively.

The general organization of the germline configuration of the three Ig loci is similar, but several features are distinctive, and not all details are yet known. The reader is referred to some recent reviews[35,62,63] for a more thorough discussion. Here only a few points that are specifically relevant to the study of gene rearrangements in leukemia are listed.

1. For the H chain genes (Fig. 13.1 and Table 13.2) a fourth set of DNA regions, named diversity (D), contributes to the structure of the terminal part of the variable region.[16,38,41,64] Another distinctive feature of the H genes is the multiplicity of C regions, of which there are nine.[36,37] They exibit considerable structural differences, and they underly the various Ig classes and subclasses. V_H genes are located 5' with respect to the J–C region,[39] but the exact distance between the V and D, and between the D and J–C clusters is not yet known. A physical link between these regions has been recently established by chromosomal walking.[67a] The first V_H gene has been located at 75 kilobases (kb) upstream of the J_H, with approximately 15–20 D_H segments present within the intervening DNA region.

2. In the κ-chain locus the estimated number of V genes is about 50–60[43–50] (as against more than 300 in the mouse[68]). It is generally assumed that the V_κ cluster is located 5' to the J–C region, and this has now been formally supported by the finding that at least some V_κ segments are located at about 25 kb from the J–C region on chromosome 2.[69,70]

3. In the λ-chain locus (unlike κ) there are 6 C_λ genes[52–54] but, unlike H, these are all nearly identical.[51,55] Each C_λ gene segment is preceded by a J segment located 1.5 kb upstream of the C region.[53–55] V_λ genes are very few: not more than two in some inbred species[71], 12 or 13 in the chicken,[72] but probably between 20 and 30 in human.[73–75] Thus, there are considerable differences in the structure of the two L chain loci among species. It is not yet known how this relates to the ratio of mature B-cells that produce κ- and λ-chain respectively (normally about 2:1 in human) and to the nature of the antibodies (Ab) that are produced.

TCR genes

The best characterized TCR molecule is a heterodimer of two polypeptide chains designated α and β.[6–8] The αβ TCR is expressed on the cell membrane of 95% of peripheral blood

Table 13.2 Probes used in the study of the Ig and TCR gene configuration in lymphoproliferative disorders.

Name	Region		Size(kb)	Reference
J_H	Joining	H chain	2.5	36
C_μ	Constant	μ H chain	1.2	36
C_γ	Constant	γ H chain	1.8	37
C_κ	Constant	κ L chains	0.6	43
C_λ	Constant	λ L chains	8.0	65
C_β	Constant	β TCR chain	0.7	86
$J_\alpha BX$	Joining	γ TCR chain	0.68	66
$J_\alpha BX$	Joining	α TCR chain	2.1	167
$J_\alpha BS$	Joining	α TCR chain	1.3	67
$J_\alpha HE$	Joining	α TCR chain	3.3	67
J_δ	Joining	δ TCR chain	2.5	34

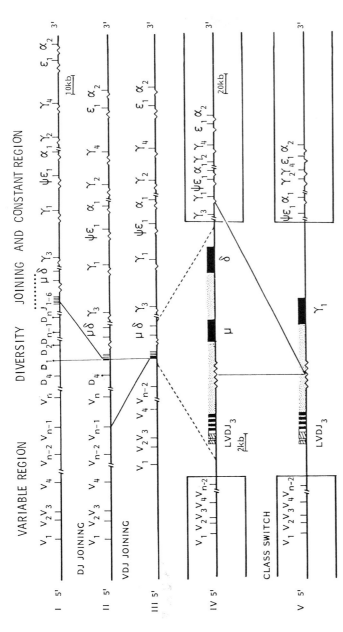

Fig.13.1 Rearrangement events at a heavy (H) chain immunoglobulin (Ig) locus. The top diagram (I) is a map of a DNA segment belonging to chromosome 14 band q32. The individual vertical bars are the V_H, D_H, J_H, and C_H regions, respectively. The broken lines symbolize unknown distances. Zig-zag lines indicate switch regions between the C_H regions. The total number of V_H and D_H segments is still incomplete. Unpublished data from the laboratory of TH Rabbitts suggest that the number of D_H segments may be larger than the current estimate of 12 and the distance between V_n and J is approximately 75 kb. Diagrams II and III illustrate how part of the map is changed after DJ and VDJ joining respectively. At each of these two successive stages, the length of DNA comprised between the intersecting cross-lines is deleted. Diagram IV is a blown-up diagram of a small region of III, illustrating the configuration of rearranged heavy chain gene. Individual blocks symbolize, from left to right, the leader sequence (L) the V_H and D_H segments and J_H, the μ and δ (C_H) segments. The primary transcript will extend from L to either the end of μ or the end of δ; the dotted segments between L and V, from J_3 to μ, and the entire VDJ complex is the introns. Diagram V is a diagram of a rearranged gene after class switch. The blocks symbolize various regions as in diagram IV. The diagonal cross-line was drawn across S regions to indicate that these are same as in diagram IV, but now γ_1, instead of μ, has become adjacent to it. The diagonal cross-line was drawn across S regions to indicate that these are involved in the class switching. Framed areas on both sides of diagrams IV and V are on a different scale from the central portions.

T-lymphocytes.[76-78] On the remaining 5% of T-cells a rarer type of TCR has been identified, which is called γδ.[79-82] The nomenclature currently used for the different TCR genes, the estimated or known number of coding DNA segments and their chromosomal localization is summarized in Table 13.1 whilst a diagram of their structure is shown in Fig. 13.2.

The β and γ loci are similar, in that they have two separate J-C clusters in tandem[83-86] (Fig. 13.2). The rearrangement process will bring a V region next to either the J_1-C_1 or the J_2-C_2 region (in which case the J_1-C_1 is deleted). However, the number of V segments is very different, with an estimated 150 V_β[58,59] but only 15-20 V_γ (some of which are non-functional, or pseudogenes).[60,61] Therefore, the number of potential rearranged genes is much smaller at the γ than at the β locus.[60,87] The physical organization of the human V_β cluster and its evolutionary relationship to the mouse homologue has been recently worked out.[88] The structure of the α TCR locus is different. Here it is estimated that there are up to 60-70 J_α regions,[34,56,89] with about 15-20 V_α regions. It is not yet clear whether a V_α can skip J regions in the course of the α rearrangement process. Very recently, it has been found that the δ locus is physically adjacent to α and partly interspersed with it, inasmuch as the V segments for both genes are located upstream to J_α-C_α,[33,34,90] Therefore, an α rearrangement, which entails V_α-$J\alpha$ joining, leads to an obligatory deletion of C_δ (Fig. 13.2). Apart from the fact that the great majority of T-cells bear an αβ receptor, rather than γδ, the functional significance of these two types of TCR molecules is not yet known.

GENE REARRANGEMENT

A process known as gene rearrangement precedes, and is an absolute requirement for, the production of each type of Ig or TCR polypeptide chain.[16-18,35] The change in the DNA configuration associated with the assembly of a functional Ig gene is shown diagrammatically in Fig. 13.1. For the H chains the process consists of the physical juxtaposition, first of one of the many D_H segments present in the germline DNA and one of the J_H segments (DJ joining) and secondly of a V_H segment to the newly formed DJ segment (VDJ joining). The enzymatic reactions and the various steps required for this process have not yet been fully elucidated, but they may involve some or all of the following: changes in chromatin structure, binding of nuclear factors[91] to sequences adjacent to the DNA segments to be rearranged, DNA deletions (looping-out/deletion mechanism[92-97]), sister chromatid exchange events[94,98] or the looping out–excision–reintegration model.[99,100] Such unique genetic events in somatic cells may be either the cause or the effect of an early lymphoid cell becoming committed to the B- or to the T-cell lineage. Before showing how DNA analysis can help in the characterization of leukemic cell populations several aspects of the DNA rearrangement process must be considered that will enable a lymphocyte to produce ultimately a functional Ig or TCR molecule.

Hierarchy in gene rearrangement
Since each Ig or TCR molecule consists of two types of polypeptide chains, at least one allele for each chain must be productively rearranged before a complete molecule can be synthesized.[101] It has been found, without exception so far, that the IgH chain genes rearrange before IgL chain genes,[102-104] and that TCR γ- and δ-gene rearrangement precedes β, which precedes α-gene rearrangement.[105-107] With respect to the IgL chain genes, in the majority of cases the rearrangement of the κL chains precedes λ-chain gene rearrangement.[102,103]

Complexity of the rearrangement process
The rearrangement of the H chains is more complex than that of L chains because it requires at least two successive steps: DJ joining takes place before VDJ joining which completes the

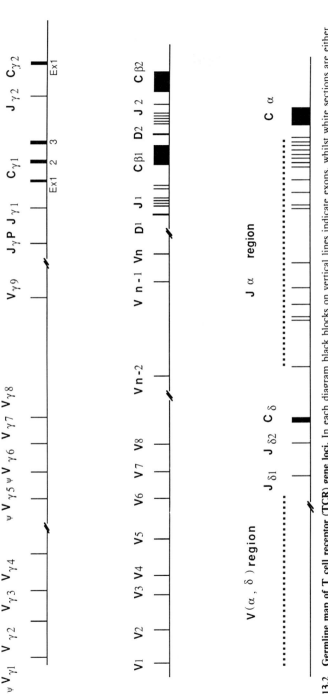

Fig.13.2 Germline map of T cell receptor (TCR) gene loci. In each diagram black blocks on vertical lines indicate exons, whilst white sections are either introns or non-transcribed DNA regions. Breaks in the horizontal line indicate that the distance between the respective regions is unknown. *Top:* The γ-gene locus is characterized by having only a limited number of V regions (numbered), three of which are pseudogenes (ψ). *Middle:* The β-gene locus includes D regions (like IgH) located proximal to each J-C region. The estimated number of V regions is approximately 100–150. Both γ- and β-chain loci have two separate C regions in tandem, either of which can participate in assembly of a functional gene. Rearrangements involving the γ₂ or the β₂ regions respectively will entail deletion of the β₁ and γ₁ regions. *Bottom:* The TCR α and δ loci characterized by the fact that the latter is contained within the former. The dotted line at the left symbolizes an unknown number of V_α and V_δ genes. It can be inferred from the diagram that joining of any of the V segments to any J will be associated with δ deletion (see text). The number of V regions is not yet known. It is possible, but not proven, that the same V regions may be involved alternatively in the assembly of either a δ- or an α-gene.

rearrangement process.[38,41] (A two-step process takes place also in the rearrangement of the TCR β-chain genes.[108,109]) Since the VDJ complex is generated next to an IgH C_μ segment, the first type of H chain produced is always a C_μ chain.[110] (δ chains are also produced by a mechanism of alternative splicing at the RNA level). The H chain gene cluster includes additional C_H segments which are used to generate molecules of different Ig classes (or isotypes). This process, known as class switching[14,40,111–115] requires that C_μ, and sometimes other C regions, must be deleted, so that the already existing rearranged VDJ becomes juxtaposed to another C region. This deletion event is dependent upon the presence, between C regions, of repeat sequences, known as switching (Sw) sequences (see Fig. 13.1). A class switch may also occur by changes in RNA processing rather than as a result of DNA deletions.[115,116]

Not all gene rearrangements are productive
The assembly of the DNA segments mentioned is necessary, but not sufficient, by itself, for the production of a polypeptide chain. The rearrangement sometimes 'misfires', presumably because the rearranged DNA sequence does not fulfil all the requirements for efficient transcription and processing, or because it contains a translation termination signal within the coding sequence.[117] If rearrangement of one allele is unproductive then the cell will proceed to rearrange the second allele. On the other hand, a second rearrangement is avoided if the first one is productive: this phenomenon is known as allelic exclusion.[98,118] Although the precise mechanism of the allelic exclusion is unknown, its biological importance is clear in that it prevents a B-cell from producing multiple or hybrid Ig molecules with different antigen specificities. Although the κ- and λ-chains are not allelic, an operationally similar process of exclusion ensures that an individual B-cell produces only one type of light chain.

ANTIBODY DIVERSITY

As discussed above the random joining of any V to any D and J segment (combinatorial joining) is an extremely important source of diversity in the human immune system, but additional mechanisms generate further diversity in the antibody repertoire. Some of these are listed briefly and others are given more comprehensive reviews for a thorough discussion.

1. Junctional diversity (flexibility in the VJ/VDJ joining).[92,93]
2. Somatic hypermutation affecting the variable but not constant region DNA segments of a rearranged gene.[119–121]
3. Insertion of single or multiple base pairs (N-region insertion) by terminal transferase (TdT) in the Ig or TCR genes of rearranged alleles in lymphoid cells.[122]

RATIONALE FOR ANALYSIS OF IG AND TCR GENE ARRANGEMENT

The presence of a rearranged Ig or TCR gene in a particular DNA sample can be inferred from the finding, upon hybridization with a particular probe, of a restriction fragment differing in size from that revealed by the same probe in non-rearranged germline DNA. This is due to the change in the position of restriction sites by the joining in a 5′ position of the D and/or V segments to the J region, as mentioned above. The new restriction fragment containing the rearranged gene will only be detectable if the cell in which it has occurred has expanded to comprise a significant proportion of the DNA being analysed. This change in DNA fragment size can be revealed by Southern blot analysis.[123] In the main body of this chapter the techniques used for this analysis are described. Also the technical problems involved and the interpretation of the resulting data are examined.

DESCRIPTION OF TECHNIQUES

In this section some of the procedures currently in use in the authors' laboratory are reported step by step. Whenever appropriate the column on the right supplies comments regarding the respective steps printed in the left column. At the end, commonly encountered technical problems will be discussed before proceeding to the interpretation of results.

Solutions used throughout this and the following sections are described in detail in Appendix I.

PREPARATION OF CELLS

Depending on the material supplied and on what cell type is to be analysed cells are prepared in one of the following ways.

From peripheral blood

Blood is best collected using a sterile technique in a sterile container with citrate dextrose phosphate (CDP), acid citrate dextrose (ACD) or heparin. However, any anticoagulant is acceptable if the sample is to be processed immediately (see below).

Sample size

With a normal white blood cell (WBC) count, 10 ml of blood should yield at least 125 μg of DNA (this is based on 5 pg of DNA per cell, and 50% recovery). This amount will be sufficient for most analyses. However, making allowances for possible losses or need for additional digestions, it is advisable to start with 20 ml of blood if possible. If the WBC count is abnormal, the amount of blood needed will be proportionately more or less.

Sample storage

Whenever possible, samples should be processed within 4 hours of collection. However, satisfactory results have been obtained with samples collected up to 24 hours before processing: unfortunately in such cases success is not guaranteed! In general it is recommended that if the sample can be processed within 12 hours of collection it can be kept at room temperature (RT). If it has to wait longer it is probably better to freeze it (see below).

The following description is for the processing of 20 ml of blood. For smaller or larger amounts proportional adjustments of reagent volumes will have to be made.

Analysis of total WBC

This is more usually carried out for analysing DNA with probes other than Ig and TCR.

1. Freeze the sample at $-80°C$	Samples can be kept at $-80°C$ probably indefinitely
2. After at least 4 hours thaw the sample in a water bath at $37°C$	Thawing can be done also at room temperature
3. Spin the sample at 2000 rev./min for 10 min in a bench centrifuge at RT to collect total WBC	The supernatant will be dark red because the red cells have been lysed by freezing
4. Pour off the supernatant and gently shake the white cell pellet	The pellet will also contain red cell stroma: this does not matter; this pellet is often loose and gelatinous; take care in pouring off the supernatant
5. Depending on the size of the pellet, add between 5 and 20 ml of PBS and gently resuspend the pellet with a plastic pipette	With a normal WBC count 5 ml will be sufficient; cells will form visible clumps: this does not matter

6. Spin at 2000 rev./min for 10 min at RT
7. Repeat steps (5) and (6) twice
8. Pour off the supernatant   A small amount of PBS will be left behind by surface tension
9. Spin again for 2 min and remove residual supernatant by using a fine Pasteur pipette; the cells can now be processed immediately or stored at $-20°C$ or $-80°C$ Samples kept at $-20°C$ have been successfully processed after as long as 2 years

Analysis of mononuclear cells

1. Dilute blood sample 1:1 (v/v) with PBS or Ca^{2+}/Mg^{2+} free medium
2. To a 50 ml conical tube, add 20 ml of Lymphoprep (Nyeegard) and then layer carefully onto it 20 ml of diluted blood   For 20 ml of blood two tubes will be required; smaller tubes must be used if less than 10 ml of blood is used
3. Spin for 30 min at 1500 rev./min in a bench centrifuge at RT   Mononuclear cells will form a layer at the interface between the plasma and the Lymphoprep; granulocytes and red cells will be at the bottom below the Lymphoprep
4. Transfer the mononuclear cell layer to another 50 ml tube using a Pasteur pipette   With normal blood about 5–10 ml will be transferred
5. Make up to 50 ml with PBS   Other similar saline media such as Hanks' solution can be used
6. After resuspending cells for the last time do a cell count with an electronic counter or a counting chamber
7. Continue as from steps (6)–(9) for analysis of total WBC

Analysis of mononuclear cells and granulocytes separately

1. Prepare a solution of Fycoll-Hypaque (F/H) to a final density of 1.100
2. Dilute blood as above (step (1))
3. Add to a 50 ml tube 15 ml of the F/H solution
4. Layer very carefully on top of it 15 ml of Lymphoprep using a Pasteur pipette
5. On top of the previous two layers carefully layer 20 ml of diluted blood
6. Spin for 30 min at 1500 rev./min at RT in a bench centrifuge   Mononuclear cells will form a layer between plasma and Lymphoprep; granulocytes will form a layer between Lymphoprep and F/H
7. Collect each cell layer into a separate tube and proceed as from step (5) to (7) for mononuclear cells   The granulocyte layer will be usually contaminated by reticulocytes and some red cells — this does not matter

Analysis of tissue specimens (spleen, lymph nodes or other biopsy material)
Samples must be either fresh or snap-frozen in liquid nitrogen. No satisfactory results have ever been obtained from paraffin-embedded samples in particular when picric acid or mercuric chloride had been used as fixatives.

1. Place the sample or a portion of it into a suitable sterile container such as a Petri dish and allow it to thaw if necessary
2. Add 5-10 ml of Hanks' medium
3. Cut the sample into small pieces and mince them using forceps and/or a razor blade and/or crush the tissue with blunt end of a syringe plunger
4. Transfer the fluid (now containing as many as possible teased out cells) to a 50 ml tube
5. Continue as from steps (3)-(9) for analysis of total WBC

The procedure described here is meant for handling 10-100 mg of material

This step is meant to tease out as many cells as possible from the solid tissue

Leave behind coarse pieces; when dealing with solid tumors the sample can be homogenized by using a glass Dounce device
During the washes clumps of material are often seen but proceed anyway

PREPARATION OF CELLULAR DNA

Remember that you want to obtain *high-molecular-weight DNA*. Therefore be careful to avoid mechanical shearing as much as possible.

Procedure

1. Thaw the sample at RT if previously stored at $-20°C$ or $-80°C$
2. Break the cell pellet by shaking gently
3. Add one by one, 0.5 ml aliquots of lysis buffer

   The final volume needed will depend upon the total number of cells; use 2.5 ml for $<10^7$ cells, 5 ml for 5×10^7 cells and up to 20-25 ml for 10^8 or more cells

4. Mix vigorously by shaking or pipetting with a wide-mouthed pipette or teasing with a blunted siliconized Pasteur pipette

   A homogeneous clear and moderately viscous suspension should be obtained; at this stage the cells' cytoplasm has been largely disintegrated and the suspension consists mainly of naked nuclei

5. Add 100 μl of 20% sodium dodecylsulfate per ml of lysis buffer

   Solution will become more viscous because all the DNA is now released from the nuclei

6. Mix thoroughly by gently inverting the tube
7. Incubate at 37°C for at least 10 min, to a maximum of overnight; then transfer the DNA mixture to a polypropylene tube

   Select the size of the tube to be about three times the volume of your DNA solution; many plastics other than polypropylene cannot be used because they are attacked by chloroform

8. Add 1 volume of phenol and 1 volume of chloroform

   Wear gloves and use a glass pipette when working with chloroform and phenol

9. Mix by shaking vigorously for a few seconds

   The mixture will appear as a milky emulsion

10. Spin at 2000 rev./min for 20 min in a bench centrifuge at RT

    Two phases will separate: an upper aqueous phase consisting of the DNA solution and a lower phase consisting of phenol-chloroform; at the interface between the two phases a white layer consists of precipitated protein

11. Collect the upper aqueous phase with a wide-mouthed plastic pipette leaving the white interphase behind and transfer the aqueous phase to a new polypropylene tube

    Leaving all of the protein interphase behind is not always easy at this stage; do not worry if a little is transferred to begin with; if the aqueous phase is much too viscous dilute it with lysis buffer

12. To the lower phase add 1/2 volume of lysis buffer; repeat steps (9)–(11)
13. Combine the aqueous phases and repeat steps (9)–(11) at least twice

    Repeat more than twice if interface is still thick

14. Add, to the aqueous phase, 1 volume of chloroform
15. Repeat steps (9)–(11)
16. Add two volumes of cold ($-20°C$) absolute ethanol to the aqueous phase
17. Mix by gently inverting the tube
18. If the DNA precipitate forms immediately, use a yellow tip to transfer it to an Eppendorf tube (1.5–1.9 ml) containing 70% ethanol and go to step (21); if no precipitate is seen go to step (19)

    Whether a precipitate is seen or not depends mainly on the amount of DNA, but also on its average molecular weight

19. If the DNA precipitate has not appeared after step (17) leave the sample at $-20°C$ overnight; then transfer the mixture to a siliconized Corex tube and spin at 10 000 rev./min at $5°C$ for 10 min in a Sorvall centrifuge
20. Remove the supernatant by using a Pasteur pipette; to the DNA pellet add 1 ml of 70% ethanol; by shaking gently remove the pellet and transfer it to a siliconized Eppendorf tube
21. Collect the DNA precipitate by centrifugation in a bench microfuge at maximum speed (14 000 rev./min) for 5 min
22. Remove ethanol completely

    Use a yellow tip or a very finely drawn out Pasteur pipette to remove the ethanol; it is important that as little ethanol as possible remains with the DNA pellet

23. Dissolve the pellet in 50–400 µl of TE

    Use 50 µl per 2.5 ml of lysis buffer (see step (3))

24. Leave at RT overnight or for longer if necessary to allow the DNA to dissolve completely

    The DNA can be helped into solution by sucking it in and out of a yellow tip with its end snipped off

25. Measure the concentration of solution by reading its absorbance in a spectrophotometer at 260 nm after appropriate dilution (usually 1:20 to 1:40) in TE buffer

    A DNA solution of 50 µg/ml the DNA has an absorbance at 260 nm of 1.0; read also at 280 nm: the ratio $A_{260/280}$ should be about 1.7

26. Assess that high-molecular-weight DNA has been obtained by running 0.5 µg of the DNA sample on a 0.5% agarose gel (see below — Gel electrophoresis)

    Use lambda phage DNA for comparison; 'good' DNA will migrate as a thick single band just behind lambda DNA (Fig. 13.3)

Assessment of the quality of the DNA

Evaluation of high molecular weight of the DNA samples

A DNA sample is regarded as of high molecular weight (HMW) when a single thick band is observed on a 0.5% agarose gel, having a size similar to or larger than that of undigested bacteriophage lambda DNA (approximately 48 kb — Fig. 13.3). Of course this DNA is not homogeneous and its fragments (arising during extraction by mechanical breakage of the much larger molecules present originally in chromosomes) range in size from about 50 to

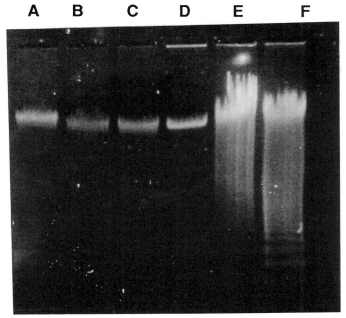

Fig.13.3 Assessment of quality of DNA preparations.I: Gel electrophoresis of undigested DNA.
Various samples of undigested total genomic DNA were applied (lanes A,B,C,E,F,) to 0.5% agarose gel (containing 0.5 µg/ml of ethidium bromide) in a minigel apparatus. Electrophoresis was carried out at 50 V for approximately 1½ h. Lane D contains 0.2 µg of intact bacteriophage lambda DNA (approximate mol. wt = 48 000). Samples A–C display, after the run, an appearance similar to the DNA marker (a single discrete high mol. weight band), whilst a large proportion of the DNA in samples E and F migrates faster than the marker DNA, indicating that these contain a substantial proportion of degraded DNA. Thus, as discussed in the text, samples A–C are probably suitable for Southern blot analysis, whereas E and F are definitely not suitable. A low agarose concentration was deliberately used as a more stringent test, because degraded DNA may not produce a smear in a more concentrated gel.

100 kb. This appears as a single band because a 0.5% agarose gel has poor resolving power in this range. The DNA sample can be regarded as partially or totally degraded when a significant proportion of the DNA can be seen migrating as a smear in front of the 48-kb lambda DNA marker. Only HMW DNA can be used for gene rearrangement analysis. Data obtained from partially or totally degraded DNA samples are not reliable.

DIGESTION OF DNA

For Southern blot analysis a typical DNA digestion mixture contains 10 µg of DNA, an appropriate buffer and a restriction enzyme, in a final volume suitable for subsequent gel electrophoresis. Smaller amounts (1–2.5 µg of DNA) can be used for a test digestion, if necessary. Digestion of DNA is often helped by the addition of spermidine which probably makes the polynucleotide chain of the DNA more accessible to the restriction enzyme by binding to the phosphate groups. However, spermidine should not be added with enzymes requiring a NaCl concentration of less than 50 mmol/l in the buffer (see below).

Some restriction enzymes are very labile: some are very expensive and some are both. They must be stored at −20°C and removed from the freezer for as short a time as possible. When outside the freezer they must be kept on ice.

Composition of digestion mixture

Components of stock solutions		Volume
10 μg of DNA*		4–40 (μl)
Buffer	10 ×	6 (μl)
Enzyme†	10 U/μl	6 (μl)
Spermidine	300 mmol/l	0.6 (μl)
Double distilled water to a final volume of 60 μl		

*From the DNA concentration measured as described in the section above, step (25), work out the volume containing 10 μg.
†Volume will depend on the concentration of enzyme as provided by the manufacturer.
(Restriction enzymes can be obtained from England Biolabs, New England Nuclear, or Amersham, UK.)

The following restriction enzymes are recommended if Southern blot analysis is carried out for Ig and TCR genes: EcoRI, HindIII, BamHI, BglII, SacI. All these restriction enzymes, except SacI, work at medium salt concentration (final working concentration: 50–100 mmol/l NaCl) and spermidine can be added to the mixture. For detailed information about the probes used and size of the germline fragments revealed by Southern blot analysis see Tables 13.2 and 13.3.

Assessment of DNA digestion

After each DNA digestion, run 0.5 μg of DNA on a 0.8% agarose minigel. Digestion can be regarded as satisfactory to a first approximation if a smear of DNA fragments is seen ranging in size from 30 to 30 000 base pairs (Fig. 13.4). Each restriction enzyme generates its own particular pattern depending upon the frequency of the respective cleavage sites in the genome. Within the DNA smear produced by digestion with some enzymes, discrete bands are visible, and called satellites. They are generated when a restriction enzyme cuts within repeat sequences.

GEL ELECTROPHORESIS OF DNA

For the type of DNA analysis described in this chapter electrophoresis of DNA is carried out in agarose. At neutral pH values, DNA is negatively charged so that fragments loaded into a sample well at the cathode end of the gel will migrate towards the anode. The rate of migration will depend on fragment size. Fragments varying in size between a few hundred base pairs to several thousand base pairs can be resolved by this method.

Equipment

Tanks, gel plates and slot formers of different types, sizes and capacity are commercially available (see Appendix II).

Buffers

Tris-borate (TBE) and Tris-acetate (TAE) buffers are both commonly used (TE). Tris-acetate (1 ×) gives higher current and sharper bands and therefore is recommended for Southern blot analysis. Tris-borate (0.5 ×) gives lower current and therefore higher voltage can be used. Tris-borate is convenient for quick analysis of DNA (see Preparation of DNA, step (26)), or for analysis of pilot digests (see above, Digestion of DNA).

Preparation of the gel

The following instructions are for a 0.8% agarose gel of about 8 mm thickness on a 18 × 13 cm plate.

Table 13.3 Restriction enzymes commonly used for the analysis of gene rearrangements and approximate size of corresponding germline fragments detected by Southern blot analysis

Probe	Restriction enzyme	Germline fragment (kb)	Other alleles	Reference
Ig J_H	HindIII	10.5[a]	HPVR	124
	BglI	4.0		
	BamHI	18.0[a]		
	EcoRI	19.0[a]	HPVR	124
	SacI	13.0		
Ig C_μ	BamHI	18.0[a]	HPVR	124
Ig $C\kappa$	BamHI	10.5		
	BglII	10.5		
Ig $C\lambda$	EcoRI	16;[a] 14;[a] 8;	23;18;13;5	51, 52
	HindIII	13; 11; 9		
Ig C_γ	BamHI	25[a]; 13.5[a]; 12.5; 9.0; 10; 8.8	11.8; 9.4	125
	EcoRI	28; 23; 19; 11;[a] 9[a]		
TCR C_β	EcoRI	12.0; 4.0		
	HindIII	7.8; 6.0; 3.5		
	BamHI	24.0		
	Sac I	6.0; 5.5		
	BglII	10.5[a], 0.8;	9.5	126
TCR J_γ	BamHI	18; 12		
	HindIII	1.8[a]	5.4	127
	EcoRI	3.5; 1.5		
TCR J_α BS	BamHI	3.8		
TCR J_α BX	HindIII	8.0; 2.0		
	BglII	4.8; 3.7		
TCR J_α HE	SacI	8.0; 2.0		
	HindIII	5.5		
TCR_δ	BamHI	23.0		
	BglII	4.7		
	HindIII	6.0		
	EcoRI	6.0; 5.5		

These enzymes are recommended because the size of the germline restriction fragment is expected to be altered whenever a gene rearrangement takes place. Note that the same enzyme (e.g EcoRI) is informative with several probes, and therefore a blot of DNA samples digested with it can be hybridized in sequence with different probes. For each probe, restriction enzymes are listed in the order in which their usage is recommended. As stated in the text, at least two enzymes must be always used with each individual probe. HPVR: hypervariable regions.[a]
The size of these fragments varies due to RFLP.

Most standard agarose gels take from 12 to 20 lanes. In setting up the gel necessary controls, economy and efficiency should be thought of. With respect to the former one lane should always be reserved for a size marker and at least one lane for a 'control' germline DNA from normal granulocytes.

1. Assemble the apparatus as described below; if commercially available equipment is used, follow manufacturers' instructions
2. Wrap the plate edges with autoclave tape or plastic tape and make sure that the tape makes a tight seal so that no leakage will occur during the setting of the gel
3. Place the plate on a level surface

352 THE LEUKEMIC CELL

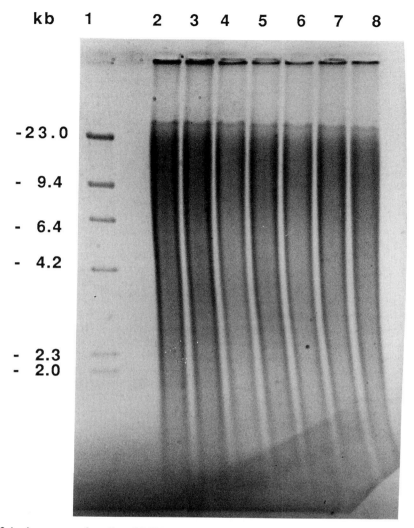

Fig.13.4 Assessment of quality of DNA preparations. II: Gel electrophoresis of digested DNA.
Lanes 2–8 contain DNA samples digested with the restriction enzyme EcoRI. Electrophoresis on a 0.8% agarose gel run at 30 V overnight on a horizontal gel apparatus, and visualized on an ultraviolet transilluminator after ethidium bromide staining. Lane 1 contains 0.5 μg of bacteriophage lambda DNA digested with HindIII. Fragment sizes of the bacteriophage lambda molecular weight marker are given along the side and the distances in millimetres from the origin was measured by a ruler. The right-end corner of the gel has been cut as an orientation mark. This trick is particularly useful when dealing with more than one gel at the time: cut a different corner from each gel in order to distinguish them from each other. The DNA appears well digested in all lanes, although further analysis may sometimes reveal that this was not so (see Fig. 13.7).

4. Place the slot former about 1 cm from one end of the gel and with its bottom end 3 mm above the glass plate surface

5. Weigh out 1.6 g of agarose and add to 200 ml of TAE (1 ×) buffer

Adjust volume for gels of different size or thickness

6. Dissolve the agarose/buffer mixture by heating in a boiling water bath, or on a bunsen burner, or a hot plate or in a microwave oven until fully dissolved
7. Cool the solution to about 50°C and pour it onto the glass plate — Avoid formation of air bubbles in the agarose solution and between the slot former and the plate
8. Allow the gel to set at RT for about 1 hour
9. Carefully remove the slot former and the tape
10. Place the gel into the electrophoresis tank, which has been filled with enough 1 × buffer to barely cover the gel (2 mm depth above the gel); the wells must be at the cathode end

Loading the gel with the DNA samples

Add one-tenth volume of tracking dye to each sample, mix and carefully layer the sample under the buffer into the well. This is conveniently performed using yellow micropipette tips.

The use of molecular weight standards

In order to measure the size of DNA fragments which will be revealed by Southern blot analysis, each gel should include molecular weight standards, usually obtained by the digestion of lambda phage DNA with *HindIII*. This is also commercially available (Biolabs). Use 0.5-1 µg per gel in one slot (Table 13.4).

Other molecular size markers are also commercially available, but in general range of size marker fragments is selected on the basis of resolution required and range of hybridizing fragments expected.

Electrophoretic run

The voltage and duration must be selected based on a number of criteria. With a 0.8% agarose gel of the size described above, to be used for Southern blot analysis, the recommended voltage is 35 V for 16 hours. For minigels, 50-100 V for ½-1 hour is usually adequate. If ethidium bromide is added to the minigel at a final concentration of 0.5 µg/ml,

Table 13.4 Bacteriophage lambda DNA molecular weight markers commonly used for Southern blot analysis[a]

HindIII	EcoRI	KpnI	BglII
23.130[b]	21.226[b]	29.942[b]	22.010
9.416	7.421	17.057[b]	13.286
6.557	5.804	1.503	9.688[b]
4.361[b]	5.643		2.392
2.322	4.788		651
2.027	3.530[b]		415[b]
0.564			60
0.125			

See Minter et al.[128] [a]The native molecule is double stranded and 48.502 base pairs in length. Heating at 65°C for 10 min, in TE 1 ×, followed by rapid cooling causes separation of the cohesive ends at the 'cos' site. This generates a linear molecule with single-stranded 'sticky' ends 12 nucleotides long. [b]Indicates which lambda bacteriophage fragments have cos ends.

migration of DNA fragments can be followed on an ultraviolet transilluminator and timing of the run can be adjusted according to the length of migration required. For Southern blot analysis the following general guidelines might be useful:

1. Fragments of large size (above 10 kb) are better resolved in a low percentage agarose gel (0.6–0.7%) when low voltage (20–30 V) is applied for a long period of time (24–36 hours). This approach is recommended particularly when fragments larger than 10 kb are to be resolved.
2. Fragments of small size (below 5 kb) are better resolved in a high percentage agarose gel (0.9–1.2%). Voltage between 40 and 50 V can be applied overnight. But if the expected fragments are smaller than 1 kb, 20–30 V overnight for 16 hours, might be safer. In general, too high voltage can cause over-heating of the gel resulting in distortion of DNA bands.

Visualization of DNA bands

1. Wear plastic disposable gloves
2. Lift the gel on the supporting plate out of the tank and place it on the bench on a sheet of Saran Wrap
3. Pour the buffer from the electrophoretic tank into a plastic tray
4. Add ethidium bromide (EtBr) to a final concentration of 0.3–0.5 µg/ml and mix well

   EtBr is highly toxic and mutagenic; keep bottle or container wrapped in aluminium foil, since EtBr is decomposed by prolonged exposure to light
5. Transfer the gel to the tray and allow to stain for about 30 min

   Handle gels with care as they are easily broken especially if the agarose concentration is less than 0.8%
6. Visualize the DNA on an ultraviolet transilluminator

   EtBr is an intercalating agent which renders DNA highly fluorescent under ultraviolet light; use goggles or an ultraviolet facial mask
7. Place a ruler alongside the gel and photograph the gel; label the picture with a serial number (see Fig. 13.4)

Measurement of the restriction fragment length

On each gel one lane should contain a set of size markers such as lambda DNA digested with HindIII or EcoRI (fragment lengths are given in Table 13.4) so that the sizes of the DNA fragments revealed later by hybridization can be accurately measured. The size of a band can be worked out as follows:

1. Plot the size of each molecular weight marker band against distance of migration from the origin, onto semilog graph paper.
2. Join the positions of the fragments with a line.
3. The size of bands subsequently detected by autoradiography can be read off the curve.

SOUTHERN BLOTTING PROCEDURE

In order to carry out the hybridization with the desired probe the DNA must first be transferred to a suitable material.

The following protocol applies to gels 13 × 18 cm size. Suitable adjustments will be required for different gels.

Treatment of the gel

1. Place the gel in a plastic tray slightly larger than the size of the gel
2. Add enough 0.25 mol/l HCl to completely cover the gel (about 500 ml) and place the tray onto a horizontal shaker for 15-20 min

   The acid treatment partially depurinates the DNA and thereby improves the transfer of large DNA fragments (above 8-10 kb); this treatment is not essential if fragments smaller than 5 kb are to be transferred

3. Aspirate off the solution and replace it with denaturing solution (0.5 mol/l NaOH, 1.5 mol/l NaCl) to cover completely and shake the gel gently for 30 min

   This treatment denatures the DNA, i.e. it separates the two strands; this is absolutely critical for the subsequent transfer; for this reason two changes of NaOH are often recommended; this is not necessary, provided the volume of solution used and conditions are as described

4. Aspirate off the solution and add the neutralizing solution (0.5 mol/l Tris-HCL pH 8.0, 1.5 mol/l NaCl)

   This treatment removes excess alkali; the final pH of the gel is around 9; keep in mind that if the pH is too high the transfer will not be so good, but if the gel is left at near-neutral pH for too long the DNA will renature and the transfer of single-stranded DNA could be less efficient

The gel is now ready for DNA transfer.

Transfer of DNA

Several kinds of nitrocellulose or nylon filters are in use. Good results have been obtained using Hybond-N from Amersham. With other filters some pre-treatment may be necessary according to the manufacturers' instructions.

1. Cut the filter to the size of the gel
2. Set up an apparatus consisting of a solid support which bridges the two ends of a tray (as in Fig. 13.5)
3. Place two layers of Whatman 3MM paper saturated with $20 \times$ SSC across the solid support dipping into the reservoir containing at least 500 ml of $20 \times$ SSC
4. Place the neutralized gel, face down, on top of the 3MM paper
5. Remove any air bubbles trapped between gel and 3MM paper

   A convenient way is to gently roll a 10 ml plastic pipette across the surface of the gel

6. Cover the gel with Saran Wrap and using a razor blade cut out a window exactly the size of the gel, and remove it

   In this way the capillary action of the paper towels (step (9)) is exerted entirely on the gel, and not elsewhere

7. Place the dry Hybond-N filter on top of the gel

   Other filters will have been presoaked (see introduction to this section)

8. Cut three pieces of Whatman 3MM paper to the same size as the gel; soak them in $3 \times$ SSC and place on top of the filter; roll a plastic pipette on top of the 3MM paper to make sure that no air bubbles are trapped between the filter and the 3MM paper
9. Stack dry paper towels on top of the 3MM paper, 5-10 cm high

   Dry towels exert capillary action thus driving DNA transfer from the gel to the filter

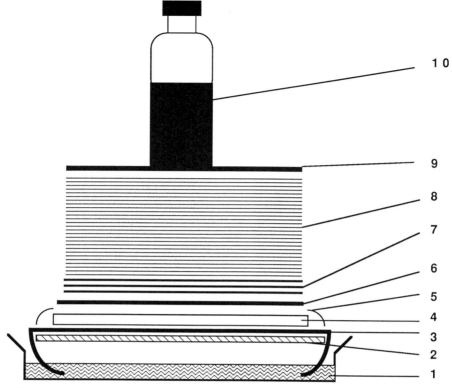

Fig.13.5 Southern blotting: cross-sectional diagram of details of the transfer apparatus. (1) Tray filled with 20 × SSC. (2) Glass plate supported between two sides of the tray. (3) Wick consisting of two sheets of Whatman 3MM paper or one sheet of 17MM. (4) Gel. (5) Saran Wrap lining all four sides of the gel. (6) Nylon or nitrocellulose filter. (7) Three sheets of Whatman 3MM paper. (8) Paper towels. (9) Glass plate. (10) Weight (a popular choice is a half-filled 500 ml glass bottle).

10. Place a glass plate (about the same size as the gel) on top of the towels and a weight (approx. 0.5 kg) on top of the plate

    This ensures good contact between the towels and gel throughout the blotting process

11. Leave overnight to transfer
12. Remove the weight, the glass plate and the paper towels
13. Invert the sandwich consisting of the filter between the 3MM paper and the gel onto a sheet of 3MM paper on your bench
14. Using a soft pencil or a biro, mark the position of the gel slots by piercing through the agarose slots onto the filter; also mark onto the filter the number previously assigned to the gel picture (see above, Visualization of DNA bands, step (7))
15. Remove the gel and transfer the filter to a tray containing 3 × SSC and leave the filter for 5–10 min to soak

    This step will wash the filter free of excess 20 × SSC and agarose debris

16. Remove the filter using flat-end millipore forceps; drain excess fluid and place on top of a dry 3MM sheet DNA side up, for 20–30 min at RT
17. Place the filter between two sheets of dry 3MM paper and bake it for 2 hours at 80°C in an oven

This step serves to immobilize the DNA onto the filter; with other types of filter a vacuum oven may be necessary; some protocols involve exposing nylon filter to ultraviolet light for 5 min before, or instead of, baking

The filter is now ready for hybridization.

NUCLEIC ACID LABELING

Ig and TCR gene analysis is carried out by using probes for different segments of the constant and joining regions of the respective loci. Each probe corresponds to a specific DNA segment of the region under investigation. When this probe is made radioactive by DNA labeling and then denatured by boiling, it is able to form a hybrid with the denatured DNA fixed onto the filter during the hybridization step. The location of the homologous sequence to which the probe has hybridized will then be revealed by autoradiography. A list of the most commonly used probes for Ig and TCR gene analysis are given in Table 13.2. The sizes of the germline fragments revealed by these probes by Southern blot analysis are shown in Table 13.3. A description of the techniques used for the isolation and amplification of DNA probes is beyond the scope of this chapter and therefore the reader is referred for these techniques to Maniatis et al[129] (pp. 86–96).

DNA probes are labeled with ^{32}P-labeled dCTP by nick-translation or by priming with oligonucleotides. The template for the labeling reaction can be either total recombinant plasmid DNA or a purified DNA fragment excised from the plasmid and purified on either an agarose or an acrylamide gel[129] (pp. 174–178). Better results are obtained when the probe has been prepared from a purified DNA fragment. If the fragment has been purified from an agarose gel (use Ultrapure Agarose from BRL), it is advisable to pass it through a Sephadex G-50 column prior to labeling (this precaution is not necessary for acrylamide-purified fragments). A Sephadex G-50 column is prepared as follows.

1. Mix 8 g of Sephadex G-50 (Sigma) with 100 ml of TE (1 ×) buffer and leave overnight at RT
2. Make the suspension 0.02% in sodium azide to prevent bacterial growth

The suspension is now ready to use.

3. Take a 1 ml disposable syringe and remove the plunger. Place a plug of polymer wool (filtration wool, see Appendix II) at the bottom of the syringe
4. Fill the syringe with Sephadex G-50 slurry using a Pasteur pipette. Allow excess TE to drain from the column and add more slurry until the level of packed Sephadex reaches the top

The TE buffer will pass through the syringe while the Sephadex will be retained by the plastic wool

5. Transfer the syringe into a 10 ml capless tube so that it is supported by the rim of the tube, and spin in a bench centrifuge for 5 min at 1800 rev./min

The length of the Sephadex column will be shorter and it will appear more packed within the syringe

6. Add TE buffer to fill completely the syringe and repeat step (5) twice; pour off or remove TE from the tube using a vacuum pump

   These steps remove the azide from the column

7. Place a clean 0.5 ml capless tube into the bottom of the 10 ml tube and replace syringe above it; add the DNA solution in a volume of at least 50 µl to the top of the Sephadex column in the syringe and repeat step (5)
8. Transfer the eluate collected in the 0.5 Eppendorf tube to a new Eppendorf tube and check the DNA concentration as described above (Preparation of cellular DNA, step (25))

Now the DNA probe is ready for radioactive labeling. Two methods are described for this purpose.

Nick-translation

The nick-translation (NT) procedure makes use of two *E. coli* enzymes, DNAase I and DNA polymerase I.[130] DNAase I creates single-strand nicks in double-stranded DNA. DNA polymerase I, which has both 5' to 3' exonuclease activity and 5' to 3' DNA polymerase activity, then initiates at the nicks the replacement of the old strand of DNA with a newly synthesized strand. Since the solution contains a ^{32}P-labeled nucleotide triphosphate the newly synthesized strand is radiolabeled. In the following protocol ^{32}P-labeled dCTP is the radiolabeled nucleotide and a nick-translation kit available from Amersham is used.

1. Wear gloves and keep solutions in ice; use a Geiger counter (able to detect beta emission) to monitor any radioactive contamination
   (solutions and amount in µl are given as for the Amersham NT kit)
2. In an Eppendorf tube mix:

	volume (µl)
DNA	1–10 (100–200 ng)
Alpha ^{32}P-labeled dCTP (3000 Ci/mmol or III TBq/mmol)*	1 (10 µCi or 0.37 MBq)
Nucleotide/Buffer solution	4
Enzyme solution (DNase I, DNA polymerase I)	2
Double distilled water	to a final volume of 20 µl

*The amount of radiolabeled dCTP to be used must be adjusted according to the quoted activity on a particular date. A reference table is provided by the manufacturers.

3. Spin tube briefly at maximum speed in a bench microfuge and then incubate in a water bath at 15°C for 1½ hours
4. At the end of the incubation add 100 µl of TE buffer/0.1% SDS

   This step inactivates the enzymes

5. Separate unincorporated nucleotides from the labeled DNA by passing the DNA through a Sephadex G-50 column prepared as previously described

6. Collect the eluate into a new Eppendorf tube and check total counts in a scintillation counter; calculate specific activity as follows: specific activity = total counts/μg of DNA

Ideally the specific activity should be around 10^8 counts/min per μg (= 3×10^8 dis./min per μg)

Oligolabeling procedure[131]

This procedure makes use of the hybridization of short random sequence oligonucleotides to homologous sequences of denatured DNA. The oligonucleotides act as primers for the synthesis of a radiolabeled complementary strand by the Klenow fragment of the DNA polymerase I in the presence of a nucleoside triphosphate mix. Kits from Amersham and Pharmacia are available.

1. 25–50 ng of DNA is made up in 10 μl double distilled water and denatured by incubation in a boiling water bath for 5 min and then cooled on ice

2. In an Eppendorf tube at RT combine: (the protocol given is for an Amersham kit; follow manufacturers' recommendations if other kits are used)

H₂O	to a final volume of 50 μl
Heat-denatured DNA (25 ng)	10 μl
Nucleotide/buffer mix	10 μl
Primer solution	5 μl
Alpha ^{32}P-labeled dCTP (3000 Ci/mmol or 110 TBq/mmol)	2 μl (20 μCi or 0.74 MBq)
(Enzyme) Klenow (1 U)	2 μl

3. Incubate for 2 hours at 37°C or overnight at RT
4. At the end of the incubation add 100 μl of TE buffer/0.1% SDS to terminate the reaction
5. Remove unincorporated nucleotides using a Sephadex G-50 spun column prepared as described above
6. Check specific activity as described above

The specific activity will be usually five to eight times higher than that obtained using a nucleotide labeling technic

When the DNA probe has been labeled to a satisfactory final specific activity you may proceed to the following section. As a general rule $15-20 \times 10^6$ counts/min should be added to each bag (see below) containing a maximum of two or three filters.

FILTER HYBRIDIZATION

The purpose of this procedure is to produce a hybrid between the radioactively labeled probe and the filter-bound DNA. The hybrid will be subsequently visualized by autoradiography.

This procedure can be divided into four stages: prehybridization, hybridization, washing and autoradiography.

Prehybridization

The purpose of this step is to reduce non-specifically bound background radioactivity, by exposing the filter to denatured (carrier) DNA from herring or salmon sperm. Subsequently, during the hybridization step, the denatured radioactively labeled probe competes with the bound carrier DNA for hybrid formation and it should only successfully hybridize to a complementary sequence.

1. Transfer the dry filter to a plastic freezer bag that is about 1 cm wider and 3 cm longer than the filter; heat-seal the fourth side of the bag and then snip off one corner

    Two or three filters can be hybridized in the same bag; for filters other than N-Hybond prewetting may again be necessary

2. Introduce through the opening 10–15 ml of hybridization solution; remove air bubbles by rolling a glass pipette on top of the bag and squeezing out air bubbles through the corner

    Air bubbles may prevent contact between filter and solution, thus eventually causing 'spotting'

3. Heat seal the bag completely and make sure there are no leaks

4. Incubate the bag in a shaking water bath at 65°C for 1–6 hours

    Longer prehybridization may result in further reduction of background

Hybridization

During this step the denatured radiolabeled probe is allowed to hybridize to the denatured filter-bound DNA.

5. Take the required volume of radiolabeled probe (see above, Nucleic acid labeling) into an Eppendorf tube and place it into a boiling water bath for 10 min; cool in ice immediately for 5 min

    Boiling denatures the probe; quick cooling is essential to prevent renaturation

6. Cut off one corner of the bag and pour off the prehybridization solution

7. Introduce into the bag 15 ml of hybridization solution (i.e. approximately 1 ml per 10 cm^2 of filter)

    As a general rule use as little hybridization solution as possible but enough to permit the filters to move about freely (about 10 ml per filter)

8. Add denatured probe by using a Gilson pipette to a final concentration of $0.5–1.0 \times 10^6$ counts/min per ml of hybridization solution; the specific activity of the probe should be at least 10^8 counts/min per µg

    This will mean adding 10^7 counts/min in 100 ng of probe DNA

9. Remove air bubbles avoiding leakage of radioactive solution

    See above, Pre-hybridization, step (2)

10. Heat seal the corner of the bag

    For any radioactive contamination use a Geiger monitor

11. Mix the contents of the bag thoroughly by massaging it in all directions, in order to achieve complete and homogeneous distribution of the probe

12. Incubate the bag at 65°C in a shaking water bath overnight

Washing

The aim of this procedure is to remove all unbound probe as well as any non-specifically hybridized molecules of the probe. This is achieved by washing the filters under conditions of salt concentration and temperature which will denature non-specific hybrids. It is critical that no part of the filter should dry out during the entire procedure.

13. Prepare a plastic sandwich box or a tray containing at least 500 ml of 1 × SSC, 0.2% SDS prewarmed to 65°C
14. Take the bag containing the filter from the shaking water bath and cut a corner of the bag; pour off as much solution as possible into a sink suitable for disposal of radioactive liquid waste
15. Cut three sides of the bag and promptly deliver the filter into the box; submerge immediately
16. Place the box into a shaking water bath at 65°C for 10 min
17. Pour off the solution and do two more washes of 30 min each, in the same solution always with shaking at 65°C — These are two 'low stringency' washes
18. Repeat twice, each time for 30 min, using 0.1 × SSC, 0.2% SDS under the same conditions — These are two 'high stringency' washes

When changing washing solution always make sure that no part of the filter ever dries out. For this purpose, make sure that you always have the container with the replacement solution ready by your side.

19. Remove filter from the box with forceps and blot on filter paper; allow to dry at RT for 15–30 min

Autoradiography

20. Wrap the filter in Saran Wrap — Wrapping should be tight so that the filter has no room for play within the wrapping
21. With radioactive ink make very small spots on two sticky labels; when they are perfectly dry stick them on Saran Wrap one at the top right and one at the bottom centre of the wrapping — Cover radioactive labels with cellulose tape to prevent the radioactive ink from marking the screens
22. Place the filter and a sheet of XAR-5 Kodak film into a cassette; include an intensifying screen on top of the film — This step should be carried out in a dark room with a safe light

The length of exposure time required to obtain a good signal depends mainly on the total amount of DNA applied to the original gel and the specific activity of the probe. Thus the time is quite variable (1–15 days) and must often be decided empirically. As an example, using 10 μg of DNA and a probe of specific activity 10^8 dis./min per μg a 48-hour exposure may give good signals.

DEHYBRIDIZATION PROCEDURE

It is sometimes convenient to hybridize the same filter with several different probes in sequence. For example a HindIII filter can be used with a J_H, C_β and J_γ probe. Dehybridization is absolutely necessary when it is required to rehybridize a filter with the same probe. It is not necessary if a different probe is used. However, if the intensity of the signal obtained from the previous hybridization is still very strong it might be necessary to remove it in order not to confuse the result obtained with the new probe.

Three different methods for dehybridization are given below.

1. Boil filters in a large volume (1–1.5 l) of 2 × SSC for 2 min. Then transfer to a tray at RT containing 3 × SSC and leave for 5 min. Then proceed with prehybridization and continue with hybridization with a new probe as described above. This method results in efficient removal of signals or background, but it also causes some loss of the DNA from the filter. Therefore, it is advisable only if the signals of the previous hybridization were particularly intense or if only one or two subsequent hybridizations are required.
2. Transfer filter to a tray containing a prewarmed solution (65 °C) of 0.01 × SSC, 0.2% SDS and incubate in a 65 °C water bath for 2–3 hours with shaking. Change buffer twice during the procedure.
3. Transfer filter to a tray containing 50 mmol/l NaOH and shake at RT for 30 min, rinse well in distilled water and prehybridize as described above.

The procedures (1) and (2) result in a less efficient removal of previous signals but also reduce loss of DNA from the filter.

After these procedures continue with prehybridization and hybridization directly or dry the filter and expose with an X-ray film (to ensure complete removal of pre-existing signals, or at least strong reduction in intensity) or store the filter in a plastic bag in a drawer.

ANALYZING SOUTHERN BLOTS

The final result of a DNA analysis, as described above, is an autoradiography film. If good technique is adhered to, the developing tank will deliver a good picture.

However, occasionally things can go wrong, even in the most experienced hands. Because the procedure is somewhat laborious, it is not always easy to determine which step (or steps) has failed. Many horrendous disappointments may be due to relatively trivial causes. In Table 13.5 and in the accompanying figure (Fig. 13.6) a list has been included of some of these, together with rather obvious remedies. Some individual problems require more detailed discussion.

INCOMPLETE DNA DIGESTION

As described above, the extent of digestion ought to be assessed routinely on an aliquot of every DNA sample to be blotted. However, this is a relatively crude test and incomplete digestion is unfortunately one of the most common pitfalls of Southern blot analysis. More specifically, by reference to the restriction map of the respective locus, the suspicious band will have the size of the fragment generated by the cleavage at a restriction site adjacent to the normal one, on either side of the probe (Fig. 13.7). In simple terms, it is as though the restriction enzyme has skipped a cleavage site. Fragments generated by partial digestion are of course always larger than the true germline (G) fragments, and partial digestion should be always considered as a possibility, especially when a full restriction map is not available.

Technical factors contributing to the risk of partial digestion include: (1) quality of DNA; (2) insufficient amount of enzyme due to error in amount added or inadequate storage, or faulty batch received from manufacturers; (3) conditions of digestion–these include time, temperature and type of buffer, especially salt concentration and concentration of Mg^{2+}.

Digestion of DNA that is not very pure can be helped sometimes by the addition of spermidine (see above, Digestion of DNA); and for the last two causes the respective remedies are obvious. However, in some cases individual restriction sites in the DNA are truly much more resistant than average to digestion. This is proved by the fact that bands

Table 13.5 Troubleshooting of faults in Southern blots*

Lane	Symptoms	Likely cause	Suggested remedies
1	Film black over the filter area but not outside	Poor washing of filter	Check entire washing procedure, particularly salt and SDS concentration
		Incorrect handling of the filter (especially initial wetting)	Always read manufacturers' recommendations for the filters you are using
2	Film entirely blank	Poor/expired film	Replace
		Probe not added	Always test bag with Geiger monitor tube
		Probe not denatured	
		Washing temperature too high	
		Bag leaked	Check the bag before replacing it in the water bath overnight
		Low specific activity of the probe	
3	Black spots or patches all over the filter	Partial drying of the filter during hybridization or washes	Always make sure that filters are completely submerged while washing
		Too short exposure	
4	Band seen but very faint	Probe too dilute	
		Low specific activity	
		Exposure too short	
		Too little DNA	Check concentration
		Poor transfer of DNA	
5	Expected bands on heavy background	Degraded DNA	Review DNA preparation procedure or storage
		Probe contains repeat sequences	Check structure of the probe
6	Multiple extra bands (in addition to expected) on background smear	Stringency too low	Check buffers used for hybridization and washes particularly salt concentration
		Also check temperature of water bath	
7	Extra band(s) of size larger than expected	Incomplete DNA digestion	See text
8	Extra bands of size 2–9 kb	Contamination of DNA by plasmid	See text

*A wealth of experience has been acquired by the authors.

resulting from incomplete digestions are seen with one probe but not with others. A very important example is that of the EcoRI and HindIII sites between J and C regions of the TCRβ [132](Fig. 13.7). In these cases the intensity of the signal corresponding to the 'partial' fragment is usually different (frequently weaker) from that of the signal corresponding to the completely digested fragment (see also lane 7 in Fig. 13.6). Even in these cases attention to the points listed above can usually overcome the problem.

INADEQUATE RESOLUTION OF GEL ELECTROPHORETIC ANALYSIS

A rearranged gene might yield a seemingly germline pattern simply because it happens to yield a restriction fragment of the same or of very similar size (Fig. 13.8), and is therefore difficult to resolve from the G fragment.

In this respect it is important to note that, in general, the resolution of Southern blot anlaysis, given a constant set of electrophoretic conditions, is a function of fragment size. Using the gel electrophoresis system described in the previous part, the resolution is rather poor for fragments above 20 kb in size, which are also transferred less efficiently. In order to improve resolution of large fragments it is advisable to modify the technique as follows:

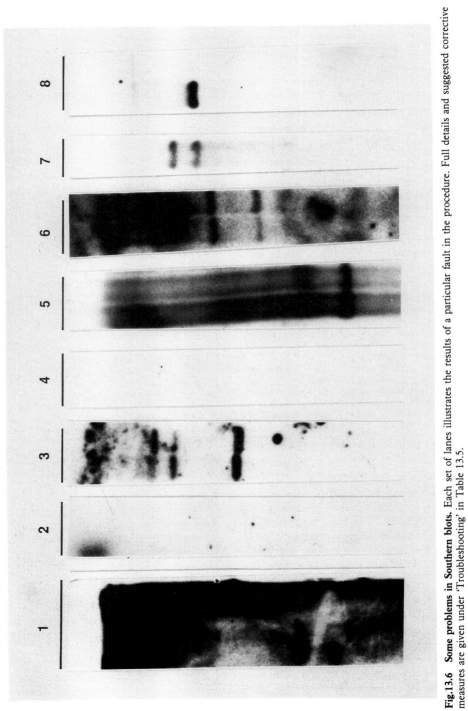

Fig. 13.6 Some problems in Southern blots. Each set of lanes illustrates the results of a particular fault in the procedure. Full details and suggested corrective measures are given under 'Troubleshooting' in Table 13.5.

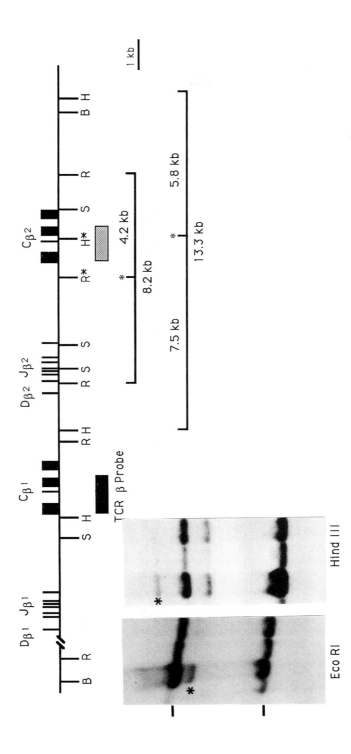

Fig. 13.7 Southern blot analysis may reveal unsuspected incomplete DNA digestion The germline restriction map of the TCR β genes is illustrated at the top of the figure (see Fig. 13.2). Restriction sites are indicated as follows: B: BamHI, R: EcoRI, S: SacI, H: HindIII. The probe used is shown by a bar and the cross-hybridizing region of the Cβ2 is indicated by a dotted bar. The positions of the EcoRI and HindIII sites, which are more resistant to cleavage by the respective restriction enzymes, are indicated by asterisks. The fragments normally expected and the abnormally large restriction fragments resulting from failure of cleavage at these sites are shown below. On the left is an illustrative Southern blot. The positions of germline fragments are indicated by short lines along the side of the DNA lanes. The bands marked by asterisks in one lane of each blot, which could be mistaken for gene rearrangements, arise through failure of cleavage at the sites described above.

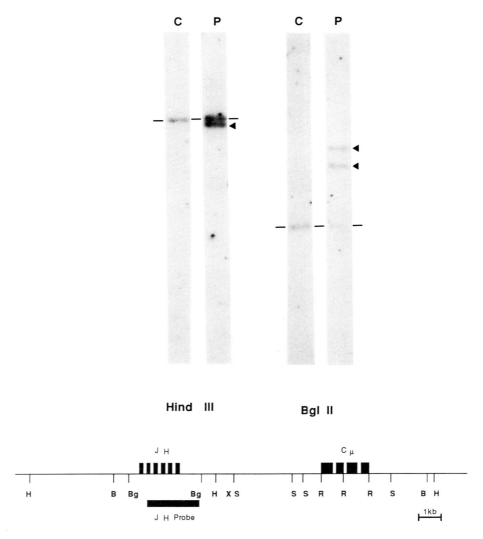

Fig.13.8 Variable resolving power of Southern blot analysis. DNA from control granulocytes (C) and from peripheral blood white cells from a patient with a lymphoproliferative disorder (P) were digested with the restriction enzymes as indicated below each set of lanes. Positions of germline DNA fragments are indicated by thin lines. Fragments in position other than germline are indicated by an arrow. In the patient's HindIII DNA digest two bands were detected, one of which appeared to be in germline configuration. However, digestion with BglII revealed two bands, both of which are clearly in different positions from that of the respective germline fragment, indicating that not only one, but both, alleles are rearranged. In the restriction map at the bottom, germline J_H (1-6) and C_μ IgH chain gene regions are illustrated by black boxes. The position of the genomic J_H probe used is indicated by a bar. Abbreviations are as from Fig.13.7. In addition, X: Xba I, Bg: BglII.

1. Electrophoresis (see above, Gel electrophoresis of DNA) should be carried out for a longer time (up to 48 hours instead of 16 hours) and at a lower voltage (25–30 V instead of 35–40 V).
2. Depurination treatment (see above, Treatment of the gel) can be prolonged up to 45 minutes.

In practice these adaptations should be applied to BamHI digests when they are to be hybridized with the probes J_H, C_μ, C_γ, TCR C_β and J_γ and to EcoRI digests when hybridized with J_H and C_γ and C_λ probes (see Table 13.3). In this way it is possible to resolve rearranged (R) fragments even if they are very similar in size to germline (G) fragments. However, if R and G fragments are identical in size, then no technical refinement can separate them. This is one of the reasons why it should be regarded as imperative to always use at least two restriction enzymes in this type of analysis.

CONTAMINATION BY NON-GENOMIC DNA

A dangerous pitfall in the interpretation of bands smaller than G, is the presence of contaminating DNA sequences that hybridize with the probe. The most common sources are plasmid or bacteriophage with or without the probe insert. Usually contamination of this sort (in jargon 'parachute bands') can be suspected with bands ranging in size from about 2.7 kb (the size of a pUC vector) to 6 kb (the size of pBR322 with an insert of 2 kb). A common feature is a band in the size range present in more than one lane and/or of unusual intensity (often much stronger than the G or another R band in the same lane; see Fig. 13.6, lane 8). It is worth bearing in mind that as little as 5 pg of DNA will be sufficient to generate a 'parachute band'. The source of contamination can include any reagent from the tracking-dye to the buffer used to dissolve and resuspend the DNA after precipitation. The culprit is often the end of the Gilson automatic pipette which has been promiscuously used for plasmid and genomic DNA manipulation. Prevention consists of cleaning the pipettes periodically by soaking overnight in 0.1% SDS, or using separate sets of pipettes for genomic and plasmid DNA.

GENETIC VARIATION IN DNA (RESTRICTION FRAGMENT LENGTH POLYMORPHISM)

Even excluding the problems described above, a band which is not in the expected G position should not be automatically assumed to reflect a gene rearrangement because genetic variation in the germline gene may occur. This possibility can be ruled out by testing DNA from non-leukemic cells (e.g. granulocytes) from the patient as previously described. This is yet another reason why at least two restriction enzymes should be used. If both digests produce a pattern different from any expected germline pattern, genetic polymorphism is highly unlikely. A number of genetic polymorphisms involving restriction sites which are also affected by gene rearrangement in the Ig and TCR loci are already known and listed in Table 13.3 as 'other alleles'.[51,52,124-127]

INTERPRETATION OF RESULTS

Having avoided or overcome most of the pitfalls discussed so far, a good autoradiograph will finally have been obtained, but just as with diagnostic X-ray films, correct interpretation is now necessary. Problems may be encountered when facing the remaining task, namely to derive as much information as possible on the biological and clinical significance of the data.

368 THE LEUKEMIC CELL

It is of course impossible to discuss all eventualities. Here some basic principles and some illustrative results are given.

BASICS

How is a germline band recognized?
It is of course always essential to know the restriction map of the region under investigation and the position on the map of the DNA probe used. The maps which are most commonly used for reference are shown in Figs 13.7, 13.8, 13.11 and 13.13, and the expected sizes of the G fragments are listed in Table 13.3. A band of the size predicted by the germline map is normally regarded as G. If the correct technique has been followed, those bands in the control lane (C) containing DNA prepared from granulocytes will be seen.

How is a rearranged band recognized?
Two situations can be encountered:

1. The hybridization reveals two bands, one corresponding to the size of the germline fragment and one in a different position. If the intensity of the two bands is comparable it can be assumed that one allele is in a germline configuration (G) and one allele is rearranged (R) (Fig. 13.9, lane 3).
2. The hybridization reveals two bands, neither of which corresponds to the germline fragment. Again if the intensity of the two bands is comparable, it can be assumed that both alleles are rearranged and this configuration is referred to as R_1/R_2 (Fig. 13.9).

Other patterns corresponding to a combination of (1) and (2) or more complex ones may be encountered, and they will be discussed below.

Presence and size of a clone
As briefly outlined in the introduction, gene rearrangements are a normal ontogenetic event required for the diversification of B- and T-cells. Because of the vast heterogeneity of potential rearrangements, and because of the limited size of normal individual B- and T-cell clones, in a normal B- or T-cell lymphoid population, the proportion of DNA having a particular R band will not be detectable by Southern blot analysis. Thus, the very finding of a clearly visible R band directly indicates that the corresponding clone has expanded to comprise a significant proportion of the DNA being analysed. In the authors' experience, a clone must be at least 5% of the total cell population for a discrete rearranged band to be reliably detected. Sometimes less can be detected but not as little as 0.1% as others have claimed.[133]

Nature of the clone
A band on an autoradiograph cannot by itself be synonymous with leukemia. On the other hand, if a B- or T-cell clone has expanded to a substantial fraction of the total, it is difficult to call it anything other than neoplastic.[134] In practice, therefore, rearranged Ig bands tend to be diagnostic of B-cell malignancies[103,133-146] and rearranged TCR bands tend to be diagnostic of T-cell malignancies.[60,66,67,86,127,137,147-170] Several exceptions and caveats are mentioned in the next section.

RESULTS OF DNA ANALYSIS FROM LEUKEMIC PATIENTS WITH INDIVIDUAL PROBES

Ig heavy chain genes
Rearrangements at this locus are analysed using probes for the respective regions: joining (J_H), constant μ (C_μ) and constant γ (C_γ). The most informative digests are obtained with the

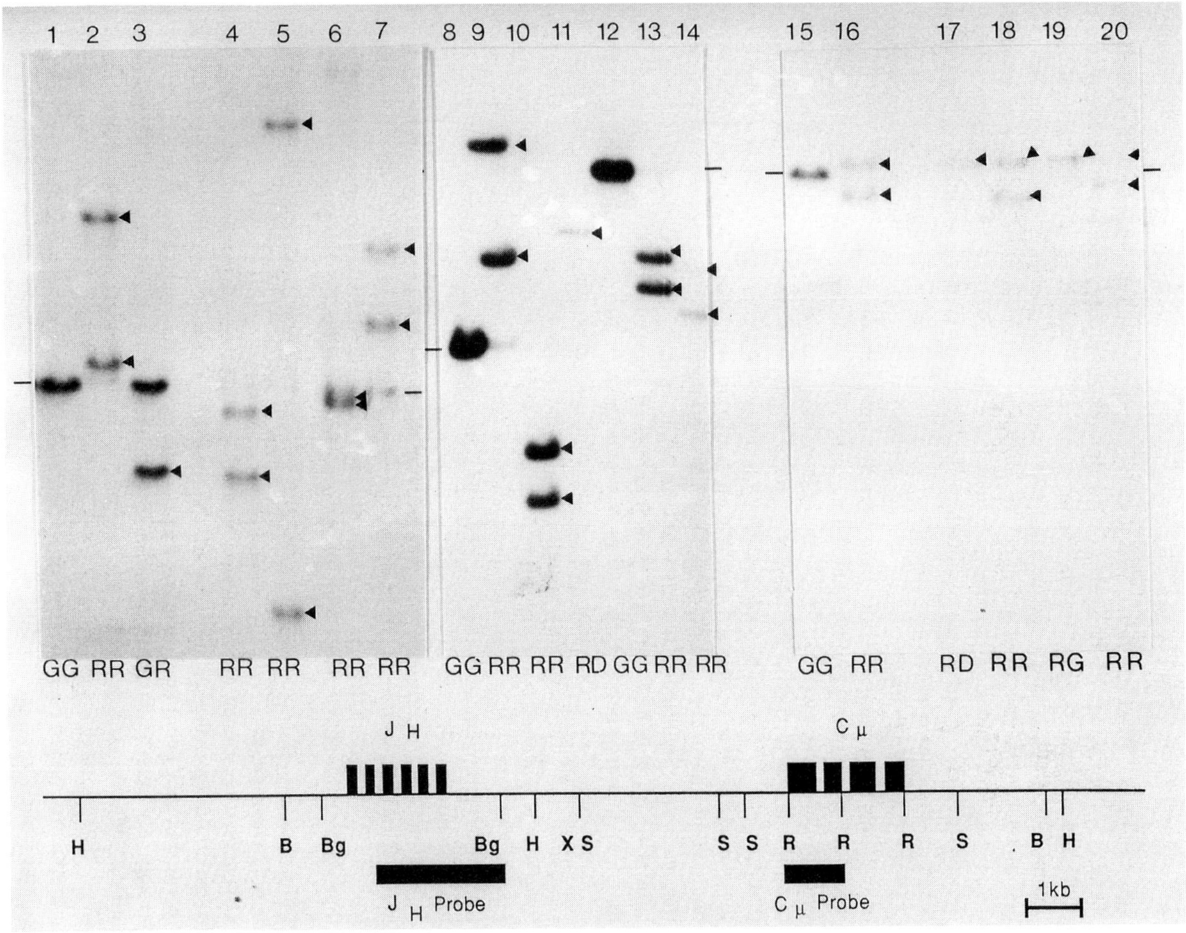

Fig. 13.9 Southern blot analysis of the heavy chain gene region in leukemic patients: illustrative examples. Individual lanes contain DNA samples from purified leukemic cells, except for lanes 1,8,12 and 15, which contain DNA prepared from granulocytes obtained from normal donors. DNA samples were digested with BglII (lanes 1–11), HindIII (lanes 12–14) and BamHI(lanes 15–20). Position of G fragments is indicated by a thin line whilst R fragments are marked by an arrow. The pattern observed is given in shorthand notation at the bottom of each lane. GG: both genes are in germline configuration; RG: one gene is rearranged and the other is in germline configuration; RR: both genes are rearranged. D stands for deletion. Lanes 11 and 17 are labeled RD because the absence of G implies that one allele is deleted. The faint G band in lanes 2,4,5,6,7,9, and 13, is attributed to a mixture of leukemic and normal cells. These cells, unlike granulocytes, do not separate from leukemic cells by the conventional lymphoprep technic. The probes used were Ig J_H (lanes 1–14) and C_μ (lanes 15–20). At the bottom is a map of the J_H and C_μ germline region with the restriction enzyme sites abbreviated as in Figs 13.7 and 13.8. Position of the probes used is marked by bars.

enzymes EcoRI, Hind III, BglII, SacI, BamHI (see Table 13.3 for the germline patterns and the size of the G fragments revealed by the different Ig probes; and Fig. 13.9 for examples of Southern blots). There is some minor variation in the sizes reported from different laboratories, probably due to technical differences in measurements. It is wise to run, on each gel, one DNA sample from granulocytes as an internal control for the size of germline fragments. The restriction enzymes mentioned and listed in Table 13.4 have been selected because they are most capable of differentiating germline versus rearranged configuration, based on the criteria previously stated.

In the authors' laboratory the J_H and C_μ probes have been tested against a large number of leukemic samples and results have been reported previously.[140,141,146,147,167,168,171-174] With rare exceptions, germline patterns are seen only in patients with T-cell disorder and with myeloid leukemia.[146,147,167,168] In some cases of acute and chronic lymphoid leukemia classified as B-cell type on the basis of phenotypic markers, one allele only was rearranged (R/G pattern);[141] but in the vast majority of patients, two rearranged bands were found, and the two alleles were rearranged in a different way from each other (R_1R_2 pattern). So far, no two patients have been found with identical rearrangements. Sometimes two rearranged fragments were seen together with a faint germline band R_1/R_2 + G pattern (see Fig. 13.9 lanes 2,4,5,6,7,9 and 13). In these cases it can be assumed that the G band originated from the normal mononuclear cells which co-separated with the leukemic cells; granulocyte contamination was excluded by microscopic observation of cells separated on Lymphoprep.[140] Indeed, this pattern was more frequently encountered in B-chronic lymphocytic leukemia and hairy cell leukemia in which normal lymphocytes and monocytes are likely to constitute a significant proportion of total mononuclear cells. An IgH C_γ probe showed a rearrangement of the γ Ig genes in a few cases of IgG-producing leukemias. With this particular probe, because of the high degree of restriction length polymorphism in the C_γ region, true rearrangement versus genetic variation can be proved only by testing a non-B-lymphoid source of DNA from the same patient (Fig. 13.10). In C_γ-producing leukemias, absence of the C_μ DNA segments can be demonstrated in agreement with the fact that class switch is associated with deletion of the C_μ region.[111-113]

Ig κ L chain genes
This analysis is carried out by using a constant κ-chain gene (C_κ probe). BamHI and BglII restriction enzyme digests are most informative. Both enzymes have sites flanking the J–C_κ region and they generate a germline fragment of approximately 10.5 kb. A germline pattern was usually detected in acute lymphoblastic leukemias in the authors' laboratory and in others.[135,140] At least one allele was rearranged in κ-producing leukemias and both alleles were deleted in the vast majority of λ-producing leukemias.[135-141] In a few cases of λ-producing leukemic cells at least one rearranged C_κ chain gene was retained in a germline configuration.

Ig λ-chain genes
C_λ probes give more complex patterns than those seen with C_μ or C_κ because six C_λ regions are present in germline DNA. Therefore, in EcoRI digests at least three fragments are seen but different patterns are found in different subjects, due to a high degree of restriction fragment length polymorphism (RFLP) (see Table 13.3 and Fig. 13.11, lanes 1 and 2).[52-55] Again, gene rearrangement versus RFLP can be differentiated only by testing, side by side, the leukemic and non-leukemic DNA from the same patient (for instance from granulocytes). Because control DNA from the same patient is not always available, a particular pattern can be regarded tentatively as rearranged if it does not correspond to any one of the polymorphic patterns previously described.

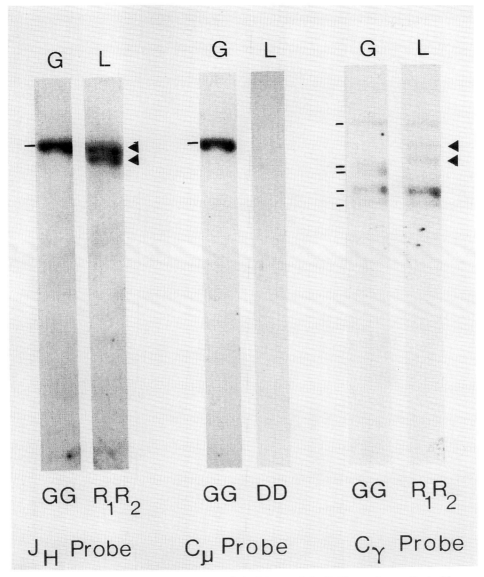

Fig.13.10 Southern blot analysis reveals a 'switched' heavy chain (IgG) gene in a patient with hairy cell leukemia. DNA was prepared from granulocytes (G) and mononuclear cells (L) separated on a Lymphoprep gradient from the peripheral blood of the patient. After digestion with BamHI, and blotting, the filter obtained was hybridized successively to a J_H, C_μ and C_γ probe, as indicated at the bottom of each set of lanes. Multiple bands in the C_γ hybridization is due to the cross-hybridization of the probe used with four different $C\gamma$ regions (see Table 13.3). Position of the germline band in the G sample is marked by a line whilst rearranged bands in the L lanes are marked by arrows. The final interpretation of the observed patterns for the three DNA regions investigated is shown at the bottom of each set of lanes.

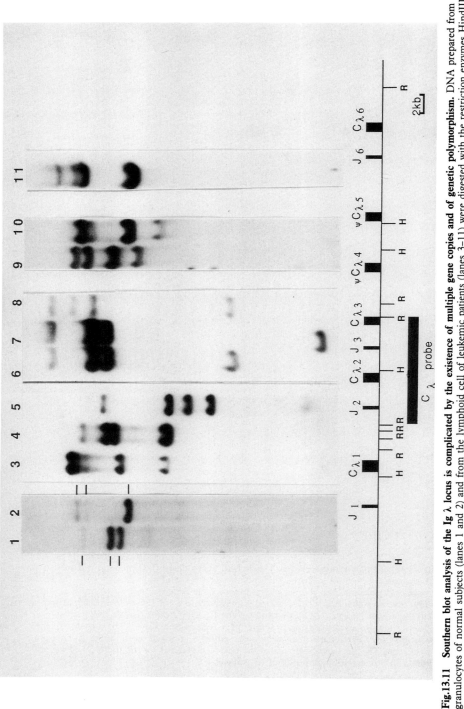

Fig.13.11 Southern blot analysis of the Ig λ locus is complicated by the existence of multiple gene copies and of genetic polymorphism. DNA prepared from granulocytes of normal subjects (lanes 1 and 2) and from the lymphoid cell of leukemic patients (lanes 3–11) were digested with the restriction enzymes HindIII (lane 1,4,6,7 and 9) and EcoRI (lane 2, 3,5,8, and 10) and hybridized, after Southern blotting, to a C_λ probe. Positions of the germline fragments are marked by lines along the side of lanes 1 and 2. A restriction map of the C_λ region in its germline configuration is illustrated at the bottom of the figure. Abbreviations are as from Fig.13.7. Position of the six C_λ DNA segments is indicated by black boxes. Position of the probe used is marked by a bar.

TCR α-chain genes

As already mentioned in the Introduction, the TCR α locus[34,56,57,169] includes one C region which is located 3' to a large and not yet completely characterized region of DNA containing probably more than 70 J_α segments, any of which may be involved in gene rearrangement (see Fig. 13.2). Therefore, unless probes for all J_α genes are used, rearrangements in leukemic patients can only be revealed in a limited number of cases.[34,67,169] Restriction enzymes to be used are selected on the basis of the specific J_α probes that are available.[43,67] In the authors' laboratory the three probes described in Table 13.3 have been tested on a total of 21 T-cell leukemias. A J_α deletion, indicating gene rearrangement downstream, was detected in only one case which has been fully reported elsewhere.[167] At first sight this would suggest that TCR β- and γ-genes, (rearranged in the same patient), normally rearrange before α. Alternatively, these findings may simply mean that, in the majority of cases, α-gene rearrangement has probably involved J_α segments upstream to those tested (as demonstrated in other studies[67]). It must be concluded that, at least at the present state of understanding, TCR α-gene analysis yields little information, relative to the labor involved, in analysis of leukemic DNA.

TCR β-chain genes

The β-chain genes were the first TCR genes to be cloned and more is known about their structure in both normal and leukemic cells than about the α- and β-genes. This DNA region is complex (see map in Fig. 13.2 and see Table 13.1). Each of two highly homologous DNA segments ($C_{\beta 1}$ and $C_{\beta 2}$), are flanked at the 5' position by seven J_β segments.[86] A D segment has been identified 5' to each cluster of J segments. Rearrangement can involve either J region on each allele. A rearrangement of the β_1 cluster on one allele leaves the $C_{\beta 2}$ cluster on the same allele in a germline configuration. As the same set of V_β is involved in either type of rearrangement, $C_{\beta 1}$ is deleted when the rearrangement involves $C_{\beta 2}$. Different combinations are seen when both alleles are rearranged. Probes for the C and J DNA regions are available. Due to the homology of the DNA sequences, cross-hybridization between the two C and J regions is observed. EcoRI, BamHI and HindIII are the restriction enzymes most commonly used for the analysis of the C_β gene configuration. With BamHI the C_β probe identifies a single germline band of approximately 24 kb containing both TCR clusters. The size of this band will be altered by a rearrangement irrespective of which cluster has been involved. However, DNA fragments in rearranged configuration are difficult to resolve from germline fragments because of the large size. If BamHI digests are used, it is better to modify the standard protocol and carry out gel electrophoresis for 48 hours at 25–30 V, in order to favor separation of large fragments, as previously mentioned.

More precise information on the gene configuration of each C region can be obtained from EcoRI and HindIII DNA digests. Using a C_β probe against an EcoRI digest, a germline DNA sample shows two fragments of 12 and 4 kb. The larger fragment contains the $C_{\beta 1}$ region, whilst the smaller fragment contains the $C_{\beta 2}$ DNA segment (see map in Fig. 13.7). The rearrangement of $C_{\beta 1}$ on either one or both alleles causes the disappearance of the corresponding germline 12-kb fragment and the appearance of a new band representing the rearranged $C_{\beta 1}$. The rearrangement of the $C_{\beta 2}$ region does not modify the 4-kb fragment because the EcoRI sites are 3' to the $J_{\beta 2}$ segments and are not modified by the gene rearrangement (Fig. 13.12, P1). It should be recalled that rearrangement of the β_2 region involves the deletion of the β_1 region. For this reason, in a clonal T-cell population the rearrangement of both $C_{\beta 2}$ regions is associated with a complete disappearance of the 12-kb EcoRI fragment (Fig. 13.12, P2). Analysis of a HindIII digest of a control DNA sample (granulocytes) will reveal three fragments: a fragment of 3.5 kb corresponding to the $C_{\beta 1}$ segments, a 7.8-kb segment corresponding to the 5' portion of the $C_{\beta 2}$ DNA segment, and a 5.8-kb fragment corresponding to the remaining 3' portion of the $C_{\beta 2}$ region (see Fig.13.7)

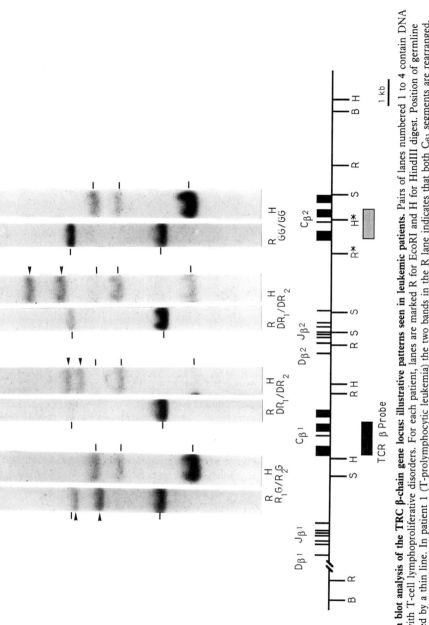

Fig.13.12 Southern blot analysis of the TRC β-chain gene locus: illustrative patterns seen in leukemic patients. Pairs of lanes numbered 1 to 4 contain DNA from four patients with T-cell lymphoproliferative disorders. For each patient, lanes are marked R for EcoRI and H for HindIII digest. Position of germline fragments is indicated by a thin line. In patient 1 (T-prolymphocytic leukemia) the two bands in the R lane indicates that both $C_{\beta 1}$ segments are rearranged, whilst the H lane shows only G bands. Therefore the conclusion is, in shorthand, R_1G/R_2G. In patient 2 (T-acute lymphoblastic leukemia) the absence of the 12-kb band in R lane indicates that both $C_{\beta 1}$ segments are deleted, whilst the H lane shows two rearranged bands. The conclusion is DR_1/DR_2. In patient 3 the interpretation is the same as in patient 2 (DR_1/DR_2), but a faint G band in R lane at 12 kb and in the H lane at 3.5 kb, which should not be misleading, is probably due to the presence of non-leukemic mononuclear cells. Patient 4 (T-chronic lymphocytic leukemia/lymphocytosis) shows only G bands in both lanes.

When the $C_{\beta 1}$ segment is involved in the rearrangement, no change in the 3.5-kb HindIII fragment is observed, because it does not include any of the $J_{\beta 1}$ segments. When rearrangement involves one of the $C_{\beta 2}$ region, the 7.8-kb fragment will be modified in association with the disappearance of the 3.5-kb $C_{\beta 1}$ segment on the same allele. In conclusion, in the large majority of cases, analysis of both EcoRI (showing the rearrangement of the $C_{\beta 1}$ regions) and HindIII (showing the rearrangements of the $C_{\beta 2}$ regions) will provide complete information on the configuration of the TCR β-gene locus. Configuration of the β_2 region can also be studied by testing XbaI DNA digests, in particular if further information about the $C_{\beta 2}$ region is needed.[132] Examples of different DNA patterns obtained, are given in Fig. 13.12.

It is worth a mention at this point that TCR β-gene analysis has been initially used to demonstrate clonal versus polyclonal T-cell proliferation in a number of T-cell disorders otherwise incompletely characterized.[132,157,160-164,167,168,170] At the DNA level a polyclonal T-cell population differs from a monoclonal T-cell proliferation because no discrete rearranged bands can be demonstrated in the first case. Although a deletion of the 12-kb fragment, or a strong reduction in its intensity, is noted in a polyclonal population (due to the great variability of the β-gene rearrangements–see Introduction), a HindIII digest fails to demonstrate a discrete rearranged band. It is still possible that a clonal population, accounting for less than 5% of the total cells, is present, but the techniques available will fail to detect a discrete band because this is below the threshold of the technique.

TCR γ-chain genes
This DNA region has been also studied extensively in various laboratories.[66,127] Although the general organization of the locus is similar to that of the TCR β, the number of V segments is smaller. As a result, a nearly complete map of the γ-chain gene locus is available.[127] DNA samples are analysed with probes for the J or C regions (Fig. 13.13) after digestion with BamHI, HindIII or EcoRI, or all of these. BamHI alone already provides extensive information with respect to the gene configuration (Fig. 13.13). In germline DNA two fragments are detected of 18 and 12 kb, which correspond to the $J_\gamma P$, $J_\gamma/C_{\gamma 1}$ region and to the $J_\gamma/C_{\gamma 2}$ region respectively. A rearrangement involving $C_{\gamma 1}$ region will entail a change in the 18-kb fragment. A rearrangement involving $C_{\gamma 2}$ is associated with deletion of γ_1, disappearance of the 18-kb fragment on the same allele, and the presence of a new DNA fragment, containing the rearranged γ_2 region, in lieu of the 12-kb fragment (Fig. 13.13). Rearrangement of the γ_1 or γ_2 region can be also revealed in HindIII digests. The germline DNA will show either two fragments of 5.4 and 1.8 kb, corresponding to the two J_γ regions, or only the 1.8-kb fragment, because a polymorphic HindIII restriction site in the $J_{\gamma 2}$ region which generates a fragment identical in size to the $J_{\gamma 1}$ HindIII fragment (H in brackets in the map of Fig. 13.13).

Rearranged patterns can be worked out by analogy to what has been described for the α and β DNA region. The V_γ DNA segments are not more than 15–20, and for most of them the positions of individual HindIII sites associated with them have been mapped.[67] Therefore, every TCR γ rearrangement generates a HindIII segment of predictable length. The limited V_γ repertoire, and consequent limited range of gene rearrangement, has provided a useful tool for the recognition of a clonal versus a polyclonal T-cell population. In the latter situation a set of multiple rearranged fragments is seen (Fig. 13.14, P4). In fact although each T-cell has its own γ-gene rearrangement, because the pattern is restricted in its repertoire by the limited number of available V segments, a limited number of possible rearranged fragments are generated even in a normal polyclonal T-cell population. By contrast, in a monoclonal population only one of these rearranged fragments will be seen. Sometimes all fragments are seen but one of them gives a much stronger signal. This is

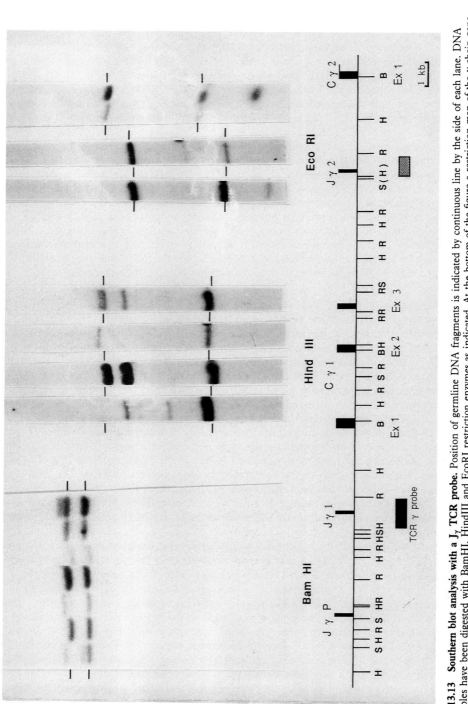

Fig.13.13 Southern blot analysis with a J_γ TCR probe. Position of germline DNA fragments is indicated by continuous line by the side of each lane. DNA samples have been digested with BamHI, HindIII and EcoRI restriction enzymes as indicated. At the bottom of the figure a restriction map of the γ-chain gene region containing the two C_γ DNA segments is partially illustrated (for a complete map see Lefranc et al[127]). Blocks indicate position of the C_γ and J_γ DNA segments. The probe used is indicated by a bar. The region homologous to the $J\gamma$ probe, upstream of the $C_{\gamma 2}$ is indicated by a dotted bar. A polymorphic HindIII site is indicated in brackets.[127]

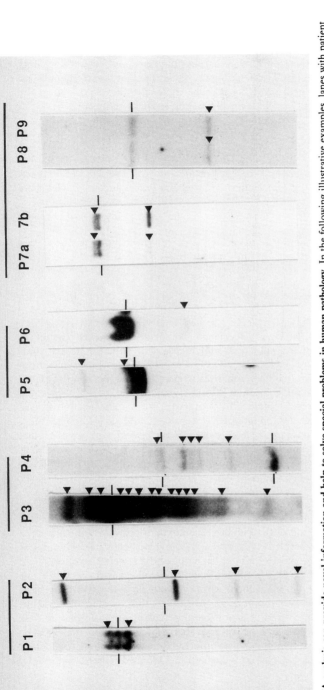

Fig.13.14 DNA analysis can provide novel information and help to solve special problems in human pathology. In the following illustrative examples, lanes with patient DNA are labeled P1 to P9. Positions of germline fragments are marked by thin lines. Rearranged bands detected by the J_H probe (P1–3, P5–9) and by the TCR Jγ probe (P4) are marked by arrows. For the germline restriction map of the heavy chain locus see Fig.13.8. For discussion and comments see text. (a) **Evidence for two expanded clones:** P1 was a patient with myelofibrosis in blastic transformation; P2 was a patient with B-ALL. (b) **Evidence for multiple clones:** P3 was a patient with B-cell lymphocytosis. A multiple-band pattern was detected suggesting the presence of multiple B-cell clones, each one sufficient size to yield a visible band. P4 is a patient with a T-cell lymphoproliferative disorder whose peripheral blood mononuclear cells were monoclonal on grounds of a uniform chromosomal abnormality. Multiple bands presumably represent subclones with different TCR γ-gene rearrangements which have taken place after leukemic transformation.[176] (c) **Very small clone:** P5 and P6 were two patients with type II essential mixed-type cryoglobulinemia. Each one of these shows a faint discrete rearranged band indicating the presence of a relatively small but expanded B-cell clone (see text). (d) **The same clone from different sources:** P7 was a patient who presented with lymph node enlargement and lymphocytosis in his peripheral blood. Lane **a** is DNA from a bone marrow biopsy and lane **b** is from a tonsil biopsy. Both samples show the presence of discrete rearranged bands (R_1/R_2 pattern) which migrate in exactly the same position. The same rearrangements were also found in the patient's tongue biopsy and their identity was confirmed by using another restriction enzyme (data not shown). These findings suggest that the same leukemic clone infiltrates different tissues. P8 and P9 are two Siamese twins who developed ALL at the age 7 months, 2 months after surgical separation. Southern blot analysis shows the presence of the same rearranged band in the two samples suggesting a common origin of the leukemic proliferation, which must therefore have risen before the twins were separated. A similar result was obtained after digestion with EcoRI.[180] As stated in the text, identical R bands have never been seen in two different patients, with this single exception.

characteristic of a predominant clone on a background of normal T-cells. This pattern is most frequently detected in cases of T-cell lymphocytosis.[168,169]

Analysis of the TCR δ locus is not covered here because the respective probes were only just becoming available at the time this was first written. The principles and techniques are exactly the same as for the other genes and the δ probe showed to be very useful in the analysis of certain T-cell disorders,[34,147] presumably arising from an early stage of T-cell ontogeny.

SOME SPECIAL USES OF GENE REARRANGEMENT ANALYSIS

After briefly reviewing the most common principles in the study of a variety of leukemias with different probes, some less common findings are listed and miscellaneous problems are illustrated by 'real life examples'.

Hidden gene rearrangement

As explained earlier an R band may just lie by chance at or very near the G position. As a result what appeared to be a G/R pattern in one enzyme digest could turn out to be R_1/R_2 (see Fig. 13.8)

Location, size and number of clones

Evidence for two clones
In some cases (rather rare in the authors' experience) the patterns observed cannot be accounted for by the presence of a single neoplastic clone. For instance, three bands $(G/R_1/R_2)$ of similar intensity are seen (Fig. 13.14, P1). This occurrence has been encountered in a patient with transformed myelofibrosis who at the time had a WBC of 100 $\times 10^9/l$ with 90% blasts: therefore the contribution from contaminating normal cells could be regarded as insignificant. The result obtained by Southern blotting indicates that at least two sizeable clones coexisted (either G/G and R_1/R_2, or G/R and G/R_2 respectively). Sometimes the evidence for two clones can be even more straightforward, with a pattern that could be called R_1/R_2, R_3/R_4 (see Fig. 13.14, P2). Of course the size of the two clones does not necessarily need to be the same and it is not certain that there is an evolutionary relationship between them.

Evidence for multiple clones
Another rare finding is that of numerous discrete bands. The obvious interpretation is that of several expanded clones. Again, it is difficult to be certain of their origin. On the one hand it should be recalled that, if a number of B-cells were to undergo vigorous proliferation (for instance in response to an immunological stimulus), each one of them would be of sufficient size to make its own R band detectable by Southern blot analysis–there is no proof for this possibility, which is reminiscent of the 'oligoclonal' serum protein patterns which have been described for instance in patients with rheumatoid arthritis;[175] this may be the case for patient 3 in Fig. 13.14. On the other hand, it is possible that leukemic transformation took place in a primitive (prearrangement) cell which was able subsequently to undergo the regular gene rearrangement process, thus generating different R genes belonging to different subclones. This may be the case for patient 4 in Fig. 13.14 as discussed more fully elsewhere.[176]

A very small clone
Type II essential cryoglobulinemia represents another situation in which it is not certain whether a minor R band indicates a malignant process or simply an expanded B-cell clone. It has been proved in a number of cases that the IgM produced by these patients is

monoclonal.[177-179] In two cases (kindly referred to the authors by Dr C. Winnearls) an R band could not be detected, presumably belonging to the B-cell clone involved (Fig. 13.14C).

The same clone in different tissues
Gene rearrangement study offers a unique tool for analysis of special cases in which evidence of neoplastic proliferation is seen in different areas (for instance blood and in lymph nodes, or even in non-hemopoietic organs). Phenotype markers may be the same but this does not prove by itself a common origin. On the other hand, if the same R bands are found it seems reasonable to infer that cells from one and the same population have 'infiltrated' organs or 'spilled' into the blood respectively (see Fig. 13.14, P7a and P7b). A rather exceptional example of 'spillover' demonstrated by the same approach is the finding of the same pattern (R/G) in two Siamese twins who developed acute lymphoblastic leukemia at the age of 7 months (see Fig. 13.14, P8 and P9). It was inferred that leukemic transformation must have taken place before birth in one of the twins and the resulting clone had spread to the other through the common circulatory system.[180]

Analysis of solid tissues
The authors have less experience with solid hematological malignancies as opposed to leukemias. The principles of analysis and interpretation are, in fact, exactly the same. The main difference is that contamination by non-neoplastic cells will be the rule rather than the exception (Fig. 13.14, P7a and P7b). As for leukemias, where gene analysis will usually confirm the diagnosis and classification based on conventional markers, the DNA analysis will usually confirm the diagnosis in lymphomas based on conventional histology and immunocytochemistry. However, the value of DNA analysis has been rather prominent in a heterogeneous group of disorders in which the neoplastic versus inflammatory nature has been controversial. Examples of such disorders are lymphomatoid papulosis,[181,185] histiocytic cytophagic panniculitis[183,184] and lymphomatoid granulomatosis.[182,183]

Genetic markers in cell lines
Cell lines from patients with leukemia are very useful tools in studying this disease. Obtaining such cell lines is not easy and, moreover, once a cell line is obtained, it is not always certain that it is derived from the original leukemic clone, especially since the phenotype may change in culture.[186,187] Clearly the finding of the same R bands in an established cell line and in the original leukemic cells will prove that the former has originated from the latter (Fig. 13.15).

'Clonal infidelity', 'marker promiscuity' or 'molecular chimerism'
In a minor although not negligible proportion of cases, gene rearrangements are seen that are inconsistent with what is inferred from the phenotype (i.e. T-cell receptor gene rearrangement in B-cells and Ig gene rearrangement in T-cells). Space does not permit a full discussion of this phenomenon which has been described by some of the phrases used to head this section, and the reader is referred to a number of recent publications.[152,188-189] These cases could be regarded as falling into two groups:

1. In one group the phenotypic features of the leukemic cells are such as to make their classification straightforward, and there is no reason to change the diagnosis because of the finding of an unexpected rearrangement. In general, such unexpected rearrangements are rare in chronic leukemias although examples have been reported.[152,191] There is no evidence yet that this finding correlates with particular clinical or prognostic features.

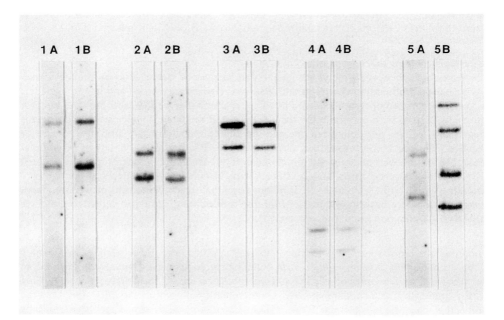

Fig.13.15 Gene rearrangement used as markers in cell lines. Samples from five patients (1–4 with B-PLL and no.5 with HCL) were analysed. For each patient, lane A contains DNA from fresh peripheral blood leukemic cells; lane B contains DNA from a long-term culture.[186,187] Restriction enzymes used were HindIII (for patients 1–3) and BglII (for patients 4 and 5). Note that in cases 1–4 the position of the rearranged bands is the same in the two lanes.

2. The other group consists mostly of cases of acute leukemias often with an unusual combination of markers, and sometimes difficult classification.

Although in some of these cases the taxonomic designation may be somewhat arbitrary, it will be important to determine which of the rearranged genes are productive and whether their expression, or lack of it, has clinical correlations.

CONCLUDING REMARKS

The methods whereby the DNA of leukemic cells can be tested have been described in some detail in order to find out the configuration of those genes that are characteristically rearranged in lymphoid cells. The methods are simple, but attention to detail is essential. As with so many other methods, even if the protocol is followed carefully, it may be found that the initial results leave a lot to be desired; but after a few attempts, perhaps without knowingly having done anything different, things improve until decent Southern blots become reproducible, and almost routine (it is to be hoped that the troubleshooting section of this chapter may help towards this goal).

What should never become routine is the biological interpretation of the results. In one way, gene rearrangements are the ultimate markers. Indeed, morphological features of leukemic cells result from the additive effects of the expression of entire sets of genes; cytochemical and immunochemical markers are often the products of individual genes, but their expression may be influenced by a variety of factors, which sometimes interfere with their 'ideal' lineage-specificity. By contrast, gene rearrangements, because they consist of and are revealed by structural changes in the DNA itself, are the only markers that do not depend on gene expression in order to provide information about cell lineage (with the only limitations referred to above). It is quite remarkable that this unique kind of marker is available mainly for lymphoid malignancies, because in lymphoid cells gene rearrangements fulfil a physiological role: indeed, it has been suggested that the relatively high prevalence of lymphoid neoplasms may be related to this phenomenon,[191] as is apparent especially in those instances in which a cytogenetically visible translocation may have a molecular basis analogous to an Ig or to a TCR gene rearrangement. From the diagnostic point of view, it can be seen that in the majority of cases the taxomony of leukemias, as assessed by conventional phenotypic markers, is merely confirmed by the genotypic markers that DNA analysis provides. However, in a minority of cases, the latter approach yields information that is not obtained through conventional markers. So far, a comparable approach is not available for myeloid leukemias, or for other malignancies. Although other gene rearrangements do of course take place regularly in chronic myeloid leukemia, and they are likely to turn up in other leukemias as well, they are fundamentally different from those described here, because they are intrinsically pathological. As far as is known, it is only in lymphoid cells that gene expression requires gene rearrangement, because it is only the TCR and the Ig systems that need somatic diversification in order to generate the vast repertoire of antigen-recognizing structures.

Of course a gene rearrangement found to be present in a discrete quantity in genomic DNA, also gives the information that the cell in which it has taken place has undergone a major clonal expansion. In this respect a gene rearrangement is a marker in quite a different way from any other conventional phenotypic feature. In general, it could be said that cytochemistry and immunochemistry give information about cell lineage, a consistent chromosomal abnormality indicates a clone, and a discrete gene rearrangement can give away both at once. It is for this reason that we have dwelt at some length not only on the technique for demonstrating gene rearrangements, but also on the interpretation of the findings obtained in common and less common situations.

Since this chapter was written, numerous papers have been published describing in detail the organisation of the TCR α–δ and how it is involved in translocations in neoplastic disorders of T-cells. Some references to this work have been added (192–202).

APPENDIX I: SOLUTIONS

A list of the most commonly used solution described in this chapter is given. Order is according to the sequential order of use.

PBS (10 × stock solution): dissolve NaCl 85 g/l, $Na_2 HPO_4$ 11.15 g/l, KH_2PO_4 2 g/l.

Lymphoprep from Nijegard (density 1.077).

Ficoll-Hypaque – mix 3 parts of 20% Ficoll (w/v) with 2 parts of 34% Hypaque (w/v). Using a hydrometer (Gallenkamp) adjust density to 1.100 by adding slowly double distilled water. Sterilize by filtration. (Do not autoclave.)

Hanks' medium supplied by Gibco.

Lysis buffer (10 × stock solution). Mix NaCl 175.2 g/l (3 mol/l), EDTA 37.2 g/l (100 mmol/l), Tris-HCl pH 7.5 12.1 g/l (100 mmol/l). Dilute in seven volumes of double distilled water prior to use and add urea (Analar grade, BDH) 42 g/100 ml (7 mol/l).

20% SDS – add 20 g of Sodium dodecylsulfate to about 70 ml double distilled water. Leave overnight to dissolve or at 65°C for a few hours. Bring the volume up to 100 ml when completely dissolved.

Phenol – for each 500 ml of water-saturated phenol (BDH) add 250 ml of 1 mol/l Tris-HCl pH 9.0 into the bottle. Shake and leave until the layers separate. Remove the top layer and repeat. Add 0.1 mol/l Tris-HCl pH 8. Shake, stand and repeat as above.

Add twice 250 ml of TE × buffer and repeat as above. This solution can be kept for as long as 2 weeks with TE (see below), but will be slowly oxidized and begin to appear slightly pink. The phenol should not be used after this stage.

Chloroform – mix with isopropanol 24:1 (v/v)

Absolute ethanol from BDH (Analar).

70% ethanol – mix 70 ml of absolute ethanol with 30 ml of double distilled water.

Siliconizing solution – dimethylchlorosilane solution from BDH.

TE – (10 × stock solution). Mix Trizma base 12.1 g/l (100 mmol/l) and EDTA 3.72 g/l (10 mmol/l) in 700 ml of double distilled water. Bring pH to 8 using concentrated HCl and bring volume to 1 l.

Tris-borate (TBE 10 × stock solution). Dissolve Trizma base 102 g/l, EDTA 6 g/l, boric acid 32 g/l. Final pH of the soultion is approximately pH 8.0.

Tris-acetate (TAE 10 × stock solution). Mix Trizma base 48.4 g/l (400 mmol/l), sodium acetate 4.1 g/l (50 mmol/l) and EDTA 3.72 g/l (10 mmol/l). Dissolve in 700 ml of double distilled water and bring the pH to 7.8 with glacial acetic acid.

Tracking dye – mix glycerol to 50% (v/v) with 0.25% bromophenol blue (using a 1% stock solution) and 0.25% xylene cyanol (using a 1% w/v stock solution) in water.

Ethidium bromide – make up a stock solution of 10 mg/ml. Wrap the container with aluminium foil to avoid light exposure.

0.25 mol/l HCl – dilute 50 ml of 5 mol/l HCl in 1 l double distilled water.

Denaturation solution – dissolve NaCl 87.5 g/l and NaOH 20 g/l in 800 ml of water. Increase volume to 1 l. *Neutralization solution*–dissolve Trizma base 60.5 g/l and NaCl 87.5 g/l in 700 ml of double distilled water. Bring the pH to 7.5 with concentrated HCl. Bring volume to 1 l.

20 × SSC – dissolve NaCl 175 g/l and sodium citrate 87.5 g/l in 800 ml of double distilled water. Bring the pH to 7 with citric acid. Bring volume to 1 l.

3 × SSC – mix 150 ml of 20 × SSC in 1 l of double distilled water.

Prehybridization solution for 100 ml mix:

Stock solution	Amount stock added (ml)	Final concentration
20 × SSPE	25	5 × SSPE
20% SDS	0.5	0.1% SDS
100 × Denhardt's solution	5	5 × Denhardt's
10 mg/ml herring sperm DNA	1	100 µg/ml
Water	68.5	–

Denhardt's solution (100 × stock solution)–2% Ficoll, 2% bovine serum albumin (Pentax Fraction V), 2% polyvinylpyrrolidone. Weigh out 10 g of each and make up to 500 ml with double distilled water. Filter and store at −20°C.

Carrier DNA – herring or salmon sperm DNA (Boehringer). Make up a solution 10 mg/ml in double distilled water. Boil for 15 min and then pass it through a 19 gauge needle several times until viscosity decreases and store at $-20°C$.

20 × SSPE – dissolve NaCl 174 g/l, $NaH_2PO_4.H_2O$ 27.6 g/l and EDTA 7.4 g in 800 ml of double distilled water. Adjust to pH 7.4 with NaOH pellets. Make up to 1 l, autoclave and store at RT.

Dextran sulphate – 50% stock solution (w/v). Weight 25 g of dextran sulphate in a 50 ml Falcon or Sterilin tube. Add approximately 20 ml of double distilled water. Leave at 65°C to dissolve, inverting the tube frequently. Adjust the volume to 50 ml. Store at $-20°C$.

Hybridization solution

Stock solution	Volume added (ml)	Final concentration
20 × SSPE	25	5 × SSPE
20% SDS	0.5	0.1% SDS
10 mg/ml herring sperm DNA	1	100 µg/ml
100 × Denhardt's	2	2 × Denhardt's
50 × dextran sulphate	10	5% dextran sulphate
Double distilled water	61.5	

Washing solution – 1 × SSC; 0.2% SDS
     0.1 × SSC; 0.2% SDS

Sephadex G-50–150 µm from Sigma.

2 × SSC dilute 20 × SSC 1:10. (v/v) with double distilled water.

50 mmol/l NaOH – dissolve 2 g of NaOH pellets in a litre of double distilled water.

APPENDIX II: EQUIPMENT

Electrophoresis tanks	BRL, Biorad
Power pack	LKB, Shandon, Biorad
UV transilluminator	Genetic Research Instrumentation (G.R.I)
Gilson pipette	Anachem
Polypropylene tubes	Sarstedt
Millipore forceps	Millipore
Plastic freezer bags	Gelman
XAR-5 Kodak films	Kodak, Fuji
3MM paper	Whatman
Transfer filters	Amersham, UK
Saran wrap	G.R.I.
Geiger monitor	G.R.I.
Filtration wool	Interpet Ltd

ACKNOWLEDGEMENTS

We are grateful to the following colleagues: Dr T. Cox, Professor E.C. Gordon Smith, Dr C. Winnearls, Professor J. Goldman, Dr Gordon Stamp, Dr D. Lampert, Dr M. Leyton, Dr G.J. Mufti, Dr D. Swirsky, Dr P. Sissons and many other hematologists who supplied blood samples from selected patients. We thank Professor D Catovsky and his collaborators for providng most of the leukemic samples and for the immunological studies. We also thank Dr J.V. Melo for supplying material from different lymphoblastoid cell lines.

We are indebted to all members of the Laboratory of Molecular Genetics of this Department for providing technical assistance, helpful scientific criticism and constant support; in particular to N.S. Foulkes, T.J. Vulliamy, Dr M. Laffan, Dr V. Poggi, Dr S. Wittaker, P.P. Pandolfi de Rinaldis, J. Foldi, R. Scurr and M. Gonzalez. We thank Mrs J. Garnet for secretarial assistance and N.S. Foulkes and T.J. Vulliamy for reading the manuscript.

This work received financial support from the Cancer Research Campaign through a project grant.

REFERENCES

1 Miller J F A P 1961 Immunological functions of the thymus. Lancet ii: 748–750
2 Gowans J I, Knight J 1964 The route of recirculation of lymphocytes in the rat. Proceedings of the Royal Society of London (B) 159: 257–282
3 Benacerraf B, Unanue E R 1979 Textbook of immunology. Williams and Wilkins, Baltimore
4 Edelman G M 1970 The structure and function of antibodies. Scientific American 223: 34–42
5 Porter R P 1973 Structural studies of immunoglobulins. Science 180: 713–716
6 Allison J P, McIntyre B W, Bloch D 1972 Tumor-specific antigen of murine T-lymphoma defined with monoclonal antibody. Journal of Immunology 129: 2293–2300
7 Haskins K, Kubo R, White J, Pigeon M, Kappler J, Marrack P 1983 The major histocompatibility complex-restricted antigen receptor in T cells; I: isolation with a monoclonal antibody. Journal of Experimental Medicine 157: 1149–1169
8 Meuer S C, Acuto O, Hussey R E et al 1983 Evidence for the T3-associated 90K heterodimer as the T-cell antigen receptor. Nature 303: 808–810
9 Littman D R, Newton M, Crommie D et al 1987 Characterization of an expressed CD3-associated Tiγ-chain reveals C$_\gamma$ domain polymorphism. Nature 326: 85–88
10 Band H, Hochstenbach F, McLean J, Hata S, Krangel M S, Brenner M B 1987 Immunochemical proof that a novel rearranging gene encodes the T cell receptor subunit. Science 238: 682–684
11 Hilschmann N, Craig L C 1965 Amino acid sequence studies with Bence Jones proteins. Proceedings of the National Academy of Sciences of the USA 53: 1403–1409
12 Wu T T, Kabat E A 1970 An analysis of the variable regions of Bence Jones proteins and myeloma light chains and their implications for the antibody complementarity. Journal of Experimental Medicine 132: 211–250
13 Edelman G M 1969 The covalent structure of an entire G-immunoglobulin molecule. Proceedings of the National Academy of Sciences of the USA 63: 78–85
14 Dreyer W J, Bennett J C 1985 The molecular basis of antibody formation: A Paradox. Proceedings of the National Academy of Sciences of the USA 54: 864–869
15 Hozumi N, Tonegawa S 1976 Evidence for somatic rearrangement for immunoglobulin genes coding for variable and constant regions. Proceedings of the National Academy of Sciences of the USA 73: 3628–3632
16 Early P, Huang H, Davis M, Calame K, Hood L 1980 An immunoglobulin heavy chain variable region is generated from three segments of DNA: V_H, D and J_H Cell 19: 981–992
17 Ellison J W, Hood L E 1983 Human antibody genes evolutionary and molecular genetic perspectives. Advances in Human Genetics 13: 112–147
18 Brack C, Hirama M, Lenhard-Schuller R, Tonegawa S 1978 A complete immunoglobulin gene is created by somatic recombination. Cell 15: 1–14
19 Seidman J G, Max E F, Leder P 1979 A κ-immunoglobulin gene is formed by site-specific recombination without further somatic mutation. Nature 280: 370–375
20 Croce C H, Shander M, Martinis J et al 1979 Chromosomal localisation of the genes for human immunoglobulin heavy chains. Proceedings of the National Academy of Sciences of the USA 76: 3416–3419
21 Kirsch I R, Morton C C, Nakamara K, Leder P 1982 Human immunoglobulin heavy chain genes map to a region of translocations in malignant B lymphocytes. Science 216: 301–303
22 Malcolm S, Barton P, Murphy C, Ferguson-Smith H A, Bentley D L, Rabbitts T H 1982 Localisation of human immunoglobulin kappa light chain variable region genes to the short arm of chromosome 2 by in situ hybridization. Proceedings of the National Academy of Sciences of the USA 79: 4957–4961

23 McBridge O W, Hieter P A, Hollis G F, Swan D, Otey M C, Leder P 1982 Chromosomal localisation of human kappa and lambda immunoglobulin light chain constant region genes. Journal of Experimental Medicine 155: 1480–1490
24 Erikson J, Martinis J, Croce C M 1981 Assignment of the genes for human immunoglobulin chains to chromosome 22. Nature 294: 173–175
25 de la Chappelle A, Lenoir A, Bove G et al 1983 Lambda Ig constant region genes are translocated to chromosome 8 in a Burkitt's lymphoma. Nucleic Acids Research 11: 1133–1142
26 Rabbitts T H, Lefranc M P, Stinson M A et al 1985 The chromosomal localization of T cell receptor genes and a T cell rearranging gene: possible correlation with specific translocations in human T cell leukaemias. EMBO Journal 4: 1461–1465
27 Collins M K L, Goodfellow P N, Spurr N F et al 1985 The human T-cell receptor α chain gene maps to chromosome 14. Nature 314: 273–276
28 Caccia W, Bruns G A P, Kirsch I R, Hollis G F, Bartness V, Mak T W 1985 T cell receptor β chain genes are located on chromosome 14 at 14q11–14q12 in humans. Journal of Experimental Medicine 161: 1255–1260
29 Croce C M, Isobe M, Palumbo A et al 1985 Gene for α chain of human T cell receptor: localisation on chromosome 14 region involved in T cell neoplasms. Science 277: 1044–1047
30 Caccia N, Kronenberg M, Saxe D et al 1984 The T cell receptor β chain genes are located on chromosome 6 in mice and chromosome 7 in humans. Cell 37: 1091–1099
31 Le Beau M M, Diaz M O, Rowley J D, Mak T W 1985 Chromosomal localisation of the human T-cell receptor β-chain genes. Cell 41: 335–336
32 Murre C, Waldmann R A, Morton C C et al 1985 Human β-chain genes are rearranged in leukaemic T-cells and map to the short arm of chromosome 7. Nature 316: 549–552
33 Hata S, Brenner M B, Krangll M S 1987 Identification of putative human T cell receptor δ complementary DNA clones. Science 238: 678–682
34 Baer R, Boehm T, Spits H, Rabbitts T H 1988 Organisation and rearrangements in the human J_δ-C_δ/J_α-C_α locus: restricted V-J segment usage and aberrant recombination between J segments. EMBO Journal 7: 1661–1668
35 Tonegawa S 1983 Somatic generation of antibody diversity. Nature 302: 575–581
36 Flanagan J C, Rabbitts T H 1982 Arrangement of human immunoglobulin heavy chain constant region genes implies evolutionary duplication of a segment containing γ, ε, and α genes. Nature 300: 709–713
37 Flanagan J C, Rabbitts T H 1982 The sequence of a human immunoglobin epsilon heavy chain constant region gene, and evidence for three non-allelic genes. EMBO Journal 1: 655–660
38 Siebenlist V, Ravetch J V, Korsmeyer, S, Waldmann T, Leder P 1981 Human immunoglobulin D segments encoded in tandem multigenic families. Nature 294: 631–635
39 Yancopoulos G D, Desiderio S V, Paskind M, Kearney J F, Baltimore D, Alt F W 1984 Preferential utilization of the most J_H-proximal V_H gene segments in pre-B-cell lines. Nature 311: 727–733
40 Mathyssens G, Rabbitts T H 1980 Structure and multiplicity of genes for the human immunoglobin heavy chain region. Proceedings of the National Academy of Sciences of the USA 77: 6561–6565
41 Ravetch J, Siebenlist U, Korsmeyer S J, Waldmann T, Leder P 1981 Structure of the human immunoglobin κ locus. Characterization of embryonic and rearranged J and D genes. Cell 27: 583–591
42 Bentley D L, Rabbitts T H 1980 Human immunoglobulin variable region genes – DNA sequences of two Vκ genes and a pseudogene. Nature 288: 730–733
43 Bentley D L, Rabbitts T H 1981 Human Vκ Ig gene number: implications for the origin of Ab diversity. Cell 24: 613–623
44 Bentley D L, Rabbitts T H 1983 Evolution of immunoglobin V genes: evidence indicating that recently duplicated human Vκ sequences have diverged by gene conversion. Cell 32: 181–183
45 Bentley D L 1984 Most κ immunoglobulin mRNA in human lymphocytes is homologous to a small family of germ-line V genes. Nature 307: 77–80
46 Hieter P A, Mak E E, Seidman J G, Maizel J V, Leder P 1980 Cloned human and mouse kappa immunoglobulin constant and J region genes conserve homology in functional segments. Cell 22: 197–207
47 Hieter P A, Haizel J V, Jr Leder P 1982 Evolution of human immunoglobulin κ J region genes. Journal of Biological Chemistry 257: 1516–1522
48 Pech M, Zachau H G 1984 Immunoglobulin genes of different subgroups are interdigitated with the Vκ locus. Nucleic Acids Research 12: 9229–9236
49 Pech H, Smola H, Pohlenz H D, Straubinger B, Gerl R, Zachau H G 1985 A large section of the gene locus encoding human immunoglobulin variable regions of the kappa type is duplicated. Journal of Molecular Biology 183: 291–299

50 Pohlenz H D, Straubinger B, Thiebe R, Pech M, Zimmer F J, Zachau H G 1987 The human Vκ locus. Journal of Molecular Biology 193: 241–253
51 Hieter P A, Hollis G F, Korsmeyer S J, Waldmann T A, Leder P 1981 Cluster arrangement of immunoglobulin lambda constant region genes in man. Nature 294: 536–540
52 Taub R, Hollis G, Hieter P, Korsmeyer S, Waldmann T A, Leder P 1983 Variable amplification of immunoglobulin λ light-chain genes in human populations. Nature 304: 172–174
53 Chang H, Dmitrovsky E, Hieter P A et al 1986 Identification of three new Ig λ-like genes in man. Journal of Experimental Medicine 163: 425–435
54 Udey J A, Blomberg B 1987 Human λ light chain locus: organization and DNA sequences of three genomic J λ regions. Immunogenetics 25: 63–70
55 Dariavach P, Lefranc G, Lefranc M P 1987 Human immunoglobulin C lambda 6 encodes the Kern$^+$ O$_z$- lambda chain. Cλ lambda 4 and C lambda 5 are pseudogenes. Proceedings of the National Academy of Sciences of the USA 84: 9074–9078
56 Yoshikai Y, Clark S P, Taylor S et al 1985 Organisation and sequences of the variable, joining and constant region genes of the human T cell receptor α chain. Nature 316: 837–840
57 Yoshikai Y, Kimura N, Toyonaga B, Mak T W 1986 Sequences and repertoire of the human T cell receptor α chain variable region genes in mature T lymphocytes. Journal of Experimental Medicine 164: 90–103
58 Toyonaga B, Yoshikai Y, Vadasz V, Chin B, Mak T W 1985 Organisation and sequences of the diversity, joining and constant region genes of the human T cell receptor β chain. Proceedings of the National Academy of Sciences of the USA 82: 8624–8629
59 Kimura N, Toyonaga B, Yoshikai Y et al 1986 Sequences and diversity of human T cell receptor β chain variable region genes. Journal of Experimental Medicine 164: 739–750
60 Lefranc M P, Forster A, Baer L, Stinson M A, Rabbitts T H 1986 Diversity and rearrangement of the human T cell rearranging γ genes; true germ-line variable genes belonging to two subgroups. Cell 45: 237–246
61 Forster A, Huck S, Ghanem N, Lefranc M P, Rabbitts T H 1987 New subgroups in the human T-cell rearranging V γ gene locus. EMBO Journal 6: 1945–1950
62 Honjo T 1983 Immunoglobulin genes. Annual Review of Immunology 1: 499–528
63 Honjo T, Habu S 1985 Origin of immune diversity: Genetic variation and selection. Annual Review of Biochemistry 54: 803–830
64 Kurosawa Y, Tonegawa S 1982 Organisation, structure and assembly of immunoglobulin heavy chain diversity DNA segments. Journal of Experimental Medicine 155: 201–218
65 Rabbitts T H, Forster A, Matthews J G 1983 The breakpoint of the Philadelphia chromosome 22 in chronic myeloid leukaemia is distal to the immunoglobulin lambda light chain constant region genes. Journal of Molecular Biology and Medicine 1: 11–19
66 Lefranc M P, Rabbitts T H 1985 Two tandemly organised human genes coding the T-cell γ constant region sequences show multiple rearrangement in different T-cell types. Nature 316: 464–466
67 Baer R, LeFranc H P, Minowada J, Forster A, Stinson M A, Rabbitts T H 1986 Organisation of the T cell receptor α-chain gene and rearrangement in human T cell leukaemias. Journal of Molecular Biology and Medicine 3: 265–277
67a Buluwela L, Albertson D G, Sherrington P, Rabbitts P, Spurr N, Rabbitts T H 1988 The use of chromosome translocations to study human immunoglobulin gene organisation: mapping D_H segments within 35 kb of the Cμ gene. EMBO J. 7: 2003–2010
68 Potter M, Newell J B, Rudikoff S, Haber E 1982 Classification of mouse V κ groups based on the partial aminoacid sequence of the first invariant tryptophan: impact of 14 new sequences from IgG myeloma proteins. Molecular Immunology 19: 1619–1630
69 Klobeck H G, Zimmer F J, Combriato G, Zauchau H G 1987 Linking of the human immunoglobulin Vk and JkCk regions by chromosomal walking. Nucleic Acids Research 15: 9655–9665
70 Lorenz W, Straubinger B, Zachau H G 1987 Physical map of the human immunoglobulin k locus and its implications for mechanisms of Vk-Jk rearrangement. Nucleic Acids Research 15: 9667–9676
71 Eisen H N, Reilly E B 1985 Lambda chains and genes in inbred mice. Annual Review of Immunology 3: 337–365
72 Reynaud C, Anquez V, Dahan A, Weill J C 1985 A single rearrangement event generates most of the chicken immuglobulin light chain diversity. Cell 40: 283–291
73 Tsujimoto Y, Croce C M 1984 Molecular cloning of a human immunoglobulin λ chain variable sequence. Nucleic Acids Research 12: 8407–8414
74 Anderson M L M, Szajnert M F, Kaplan J C, McColl L, Young B D 1984 The isolation of human Ig Vλ gene from a recombinant library of chromosome 22 and estimation of its copy number. Nucleic Acids Research 12: 6647–6661
75 Soloman A 1985 Light chains of immunoglobulins. Methods of Enzymology 116: 101–121

76 Kindreol B, Shreffier D C 1972 H-2 dependence of cooperation between T and B cells in vivo. Journal of Immunology 109: 940–943
77 Reinherz E L, Acuto O, Fabbi M et al 1984 Clonotypic surface structure on human T lymphocytes: functional and biochemical analysis of the antigen receptor complex. Immunological Reviews 81: 95–129
78 Royer H D, Acuto O, Fabbi M et al 1984 Genes encoding the Ti$^\beta$ subunit of the antigen MHC receptor undergo rearrangement during intrathymic ontogeny prior to surface T3-Ti expression. Cell 39: 261–266
79 Brenner M B, McLean J, Scheft H et al 1987 Two forms of the T-cell receptor γ protein found on peripheral blood cytotoxin T lymphocytes. Nature 325: 689–694
80 Brenner M B, McLean J, Dialynas D P et al 1986 Identification of a putative second T-cell receptor. Nature 322: 145–149
81 Bank I, DePinho R A, Brenner M B, Cassimeris J, Chess L 1986 A functional T3 molecule associated with a novel heterodimer on the surface of immature thymocytes. Nature 322: 179–181
82 Borst J, Van De Griend R J, Van Oostveen J W et al 1987 A T-cell receptor γ /CD3 complex found on cloned functional lymphocytes. Nature 325: 683–688
83 Hedrick S M, Cohen D T, Nielsen E A, Davis M M 1984 Isolation of cDNA clones encoding T cell-specific membrane-associated proteins. Nature 308: 143–153
84 Hedrick S M, Nielsen E A, Kavaler J, Cohen D T, Davis M M 1984 Sequence relationships between putative T-cell receptor polypeptides and immunoglobulins. Nature 308: 153–158
85 Malissen M, Minard K, Mjolsness S et al 1984 Mouse T cell antigen receptor: structure and organization of constant and joining gene segments encoding the β polypeptide. Cell 37: 1101–1110
86 Sims J E, Tunnacliffe A, Smith W J, Rabbitts T H 1984 Complexity of human T-cell antigen receptor β -chain constant-and variable-region genes. Nature 312: 541–545
87 Kranz D H, Saito H, Heller M et al 1985 Limited diversity of the rearranged T-cell $_\gamma$ gene. Nature 313: 752–755
88 Lat E, Concannon P, Hood, L 1988 Conserved organisation of the human and murine T-cell receptor β-gene families. Nature 331: 543–546
89 Hayday A C, Diamond D J, Tanigawa G et al 1985 Unusual organisation and diversity of T-cell receptor α chain genes. Nature 316: 828–832
90 Chien Y, Iwadhima H, Wettstein D A et al 1987 T cell receptor δ gene rearrangements in early thymocytes. Nature 330: 722–727
91 Sen R, Baltimore D 1986 Multiple nuclear factors interact with the immunoglobulin enhancer sequences. Cell 46: 705–716
92 Max E E, Seidman J G, Leder P 1979 Sequences of five potential recombination sites encoded to an immunoglobulin K constant region gene. Proceedings of the National Academy of Sciences of the USA 76: 3450–54
93 Sakano H, Huippi K, Heinrich G, Tonegawa S 1979 Sequences at the somatic recombination sites of immunoglobulin light chain genes. Nature 280: 288–294
94 Hochtl J, Muller C R, Zachau H G 1982 Recombined flanks of the variable and joining segments of immunoglobulin genes. Proceedings of the National Academy of Sciences of the USA 79: 1383–1387
95 Alt F, Baltimore D 1982 Joining of immunoglobulin heavy chain gene segments: implications from a chromosome with evidence of three D-J_H fusions. Proceedings of the National Academy of Sciences of the USA 79: 4118–4122
96 Lewis S, Rosenberg N, Alt F, Baltimore D 1982 Continuing kappa-gene rearrangement in a cell line transformed by Abelson murine leukaemia virus. Cell 30: 807–816
97 Feddersen R T M, Van Ness B G 1985 Double recombination of a single immunoglobulin k-chain allele: implications for the mechanism of rearrangement. Proceedings of the National Academy of Sciences of the USA 82: 4793–4797
98 Van Ness B G, Coleclough C, Perry R, Weigert M 1982 DNA between variable and joining gene segments of immunoglobulin k light chain is frequently retained in cells that rearrange k locus. Proceedings of the National Academy of Sciences of the USA 79: 262–266
99 Steinmetz M, Altenburger W, Zachau H G 1980 A rearranged DNA segment possibly related to the translocation of immunoglobulin gene segments. Nucleic Acids Research 8: 1709–1720
100 Selsing E, Storb U 1981 Mapping of immunoglobulin variable region genes: relationship of the 'deletion' model of immunoglobulin gene rearrangement. Nucleic Acids Research 9: 5725–5735
101 Coleclough C 1983 Change, necessity and antibody gene dynamics. Nature 303: 23–26
102 Hieter P A, Korsmeyer S J, Waldmann T A, Leder P 1981 Human immunoglobulin κ light-chain genes are deleted or rearranged in λ-producing B cells. Nature 290: 368–372

103 Korsmeyer S J, Hieter P A, Ravetch J V, Poplack D G, Waldman T A, Leder P 1981 Developmental hierarchy of immunoglobulin gene rearrangements in human leukaemic pre-B-cell. Proceedings of the National Academy of Sciences of the USA 78: 7096–7100
104 Korsmeyer S J, Hieter P A, Sharrow S O, Goldman C K, Leder P, Waldmann T A 1982 Normal human B cells display ordered light-chain gene rearrangements and deletions. Journal of Experimental Medicine 156: 975–985
105 Snodgrass R H, Bembic Z, Steinmetz M, von Boehmer H 1985 Expressions of T-cell antigen receptor genes during fetal development in the thymus. Nature 315: 232–233
106 Raulet H D, Garman R D, Saito H, Tonegawa S 1985 Developmental regulation of T-cell receptor gene expression. Nature 314: 103–107
107 Pardoll D M, Fowlkes B J, Bluestone J A et al Differential expression of two distinct T-cell receptors during thymocyte development. Nature 336: 79–81
108 Davis M M, Chien Y, Gascoigne R J N, Hendrick S M 1984 A murine T cell receptor gene complex: isolation, structure and rearrangement. Immunological Reviews 81: 235–258
109 Kronenberg M, Siu G, Hood L E, Shastri N 1986 The molecular genetics of the T-cell antigen receptor and T-cell antigen recognition. Annual Review of Immunology 4: 529–591
110 Mather E L, Nelson K J, Haimovich J, Perry R P 1984 Mode of regulation of immunoglobulin μ- and δ- chain expression varies during B-lymphocyte maturation. Cell 36: 329–338
111 Katoka T, Kawakani T, Kakahashi N, Honjo T 1980 Rearrangement of immunoglobulin γ-1 chain gene and mechanism for heavy-chain class switch. Proceedings of the National Academy of Sciences of the USA 77: 913–923
112 Maki R, Trainecker A, Sakano H, Roeder W, Tonegawa S 1980 Exon shuffling generates an immunoglobulin chain gene. Proceedings of the National Academy of Sciences of the USA 77: 2138–2142
113 Kataoka T, Miyata T, Honjo T 1981 Repetitive sequences in class switch recombination regions of immunoglobulin heavy chain genes. Cell 23: 357–368
114 Rabbitts T H, Forster A, Milstein C 1981 Human immunoglobulin heavy chain genes: evolutionary comparisons of $C\mu$, $C\delta$, $C\gamma$ genes and associated switch sequences. Nucleic Acids Research 9: 4509 4524
115 Shimizu A, Honjo T 1984 Immunoglobulin class switching. Cell 36: 801–803
116 Hirano T, Kumagai Y, Okumura K, Ovary 1983 Regulation of murine IgE production: Importance of a not-yet-described T cell for IgE secretion demonstrated in SJA9 mice. Proceedings of the National Academy of Sciences of the USA 80: 3435–3438
117 Taussing M 1987 The genetics of antibody V regions. Immunology Today 8: 356–359
118 Early P, Hood L 1981 Allelic exclusion and non-productive immunoglobulin gene rearrangements. Cell 24: 1–3
119 Cohn M, Blomberg B, Geckeler W, Raschke W, Riblet R, Weigert M 1974 First order considerations in analysing the generator of diversity. In: E Sercarz, A R Williamson, C F Fox (eds) The immune system genes, receptor, signals. Academic Press, New York, pp 89–117
120 Bernard O, Hozumi N, Tonegawa S 1978 Sequences of mouse immunoglobulin light chain genes before and after somatic changes. Cell 15: 1133–1144
121 Kim S, Davis M, Sinn E, Patten P, Hood L 1981 Antibody diversity: somatic hypermutation of rearranged V_H genes. Cell 27: 573–581
122 Yancopoulos G D, Backwell T K, Suth H, Hood L, Alt F W Introduced T cell receptor variable region segments recombine in pre-B cell: Evidence that B and T cells use a common recombinase. Cell 44: 251–259
123 Southern E M 1975 Detection of specific sequences among DNA fragments separated by gel electrophoresis. Journal of Molecular Biology 98: 503–510
124 Silva A J, Johnson J P, White R L 1987 Characterisation of a highly polymorphic region 5' to J_H in the human immunoglobulin heavy chain. Nucleic Acids Research 15: 3845–3857
125 Lefranc M P, Rabbitts T H 1984 Determination of the immunoglobulin A2m allotype by restriction fragment length polymorphism. Nucleic Acids Research 12: 1303–1311
126 Robinson M A, Kindt T J 1985 Segregation of polymorphic T cell receptor genes in human families. Proceedings of the National Academy of Sciences of the USA 82: 3804–3808
127 Lefranc M P, Forster A, Rabbitts T H 1986 Genetic polymorphism and exon changes of the constant regions of the human T-cell rearranging gene. Proceedings of the National Academy of Sciences of the USA 83: 9596–9600
128 Minter S J, Sealy P G, Arrand J E 1985 Nucleic acid size markers. In: B D Hames, S J Higgins (eds) Nucleic acid hybridization: a practical approach. IRL Press, Oxford, p 216
129 Maniatis T, Fritsch E F, Sambrook J 1982 Molecular cloning. A laboratory manual. Cold Spring Harbor Laboratory, New York
130 Rigby P J, Dillkman M, Rhode C, Berg P 1977 Labelling deoxyribonucleic acid to high specific activity in vitro by nick translation with DNA polymerase I. Journal of Molecular Biology 113: 237–251

131 Feinberg A, Vogelstein 1983 A technique for radiolabelling DNA restriction endonuclease fragments to high specific activity. Analytical Biochemistry 132: 6–13
132 Flug F, Pelicci P O, Bonetti F, Knowles D M II, Dalla-Favera R 1985 T-cell receptor gene rearrangements as markers of lineage and clonality in T-cell neoplasms. Proceedings of the National Academy of Sciences of the USA 82: 3460–3464
133 Cleary M L, Chao J, Warnke R, Sklar J 1984 Immunoglobulin gene arrangement as a diagnostic criterion of B cell lymphoma. Proceedings of the National Academy of Sciences of the USA 81: 593–597
134 Davey M P, Waldmann T A 1986 Clonality and lymphoproliferative lesions. New England Journal of Medicine 315: 509–511
135 Korsmeyer S J, Arnold A, Bakhshi A et al 1983 Immunoglobulin gene rearrangement and cell surface antigen expression in acute lymphocytic leukaemias of T cell and B cell precursor origins. Journal of Clinical Investigation 71: 301–313
136 Korsmeyer S J, Greene W C, Cossman J et al 1983 Rearrangement and expression of immunoglobulin genes and expression of Tac antigen in hairy leukemia. Proceedings of the National Academy of Sciences of the USA 80: 4522–4526
137 Ford A M, Molgaard H V, Greaves M F, Gould H J 1983 Immunoglobulin gene organisation and expression in haemopoietic stem cell leukemia. Journal EMBO Journal 2: 997–1001
138 Bakhshi A, Minowada J, Arnold A et al 1983 Lymphoid blast crises of chronic myelogenous leukaemia represent stages in the development of B-cell precursors. New England Journal of Medicine 309: 826–831
139 Arnold A, Cossman J, Bakhshi A, Jaffe E S, Waldmann T A, Kosmeyer S J 1983 Immunoglobulin-gene rearrangements as unique clonal markers in human lymphoid neoplasms. New England Journal of Medicine 309: 1593–1599
140 Foroni L, Catovsky D, Rabbitts T H, Luzzatto L 1984 DNA rearrangement of immunoglobulin genes correlate with phenotypic markers in B-cell malignancies. Molecular Biology and Medicine 2: 63–79
141 Foroni L, Catovsky D, Luzzatto L 1987 Immunoglobulin gene rearrangements in hairy cell leukemia and other chronic B cell lymphoproliferative disorders. Leukemia 4: 389–392
142 Foa R, Migone N, Saitta M et al 1984 Different stages of B cell differentiation in non-acute lymphoblastic leukaemia. Journal of Clinical Investigation 74: 1756–1763
143 Foa R, Migone N, Basso G et al 1986 Molecular and immunological evidence of B-cell commitment in null acute lymphoblastic leukaemia. International Journal of Cancer 38: 317–323
144 Meyers F J, Cardiff D R, Taylor C R, Zuniga M, Radich J 1984 Hairy cell leukaemia has a B-cell genotype. Haematology and Oncology 2: 145–150
145 Van Dongen J J H, Hooijkaas H, Michiels J J et al 1984 Richter's syndrome with different immunoglobulin light chains and different heavy chain gene rearrangements. Blood 64: 571–575
146 Luzzatto L, Foroni L 1986 DNA rearrangements of cell lineage specific genes in lympholiferative disorders. Progress in Hematology XIV, Grune and Stratton, New York, pp 303–332
147 Foroni L, Laffan M, Boehm T, Rabbitts T H, Catovsky D, Luzzatto L 1989 Rearrangement of the T-cell receptor δ genes in human T cell leukemias. Blood 73: 559–565
148 Aisenberg A C, Kroutins T G, Mak T W, Wilkes B M 1985 Rearrangement of the gene for the beta chain of the T-cell receptor in T-cell chronic lymphocytic leukemia and related disorders. New England Journal of Medicine 313: 529–533
149 Aisenberg A C, Wilkes B M 1985 The genotype and phenotype of non-T, non-B acute lymphoblastic leukemia. Blood 66: 1215–1218
150 Zawderer M, Iwamoto A, Mak T W 1986 Gene rearrangement and expression in autoreactive helper T cells. Journal of Experimental Medicine 163: 1314–1318
151 Minden M D, Toyonaga B, Ha K et al 1985 Somatic rearrangement of T-cell antigen receptor gene in human T-cell malignancies. Proceedings of the National Academy of Sciences of the USA 82: 1224–1227
152 Minden M D, Mak T W 1986 Review: The structure of the T cell antigen receptor genes in normal and malignant T cells. Blood 68: 327–336
153 Greenberg J H, Quertermous T, Seidmann J G, Kersey J H 1986 Human T cell γ-chain gene rearrangements in acute lymphoid and non lymphoid leukemia: comparison with the T-cell receptor beta-chain gene. Journal of Immunology 137: 2043–2049
154 Griesser H, Feller A, Lennert K, Minden M, Mak T W 1986 Rearrangement of the β chain of the T cell antigen receptor and immunoglobulin genes in lymphoproliferative disorders. Journal of Clinical Investigation 78: 1179–1184
155 Griesser H, Feller A, Lennert K 1986 The structure of the T cell gamma chain gene in lymphoproliferative disorders and lymphoid cell lines. Blood 68: 592–594

156 Quertermous T, Murre C, Dialynas D et al 1986 Human T-cell gamma chain genes: organisation, diversity and rearrangement. Science 231: 252–255
157 O'Connor N T J, Weatherall D J, Feller A C et al 1985 Rearrangement of the T-cell-receptor beta-chain gene in the diagnosis of lympholiferative disorders. Lancet i: 1295–1297
158 O'Connor N T J, Feller A C, Wainscoat J S et al 1986 T-cell origin of Lennert's lymphoma. British Journal of Haematology vol 64: 521–528
159 Rabbitts T H, Stinson A, Forster et al 1985 Heterogeneity of T-cell beta chain gene rearrangements in human leukaemias and lymphomas. EMBO Journal 4: 2217–2224
160 Weiss L H, Hu E, Wood S G 1985 Clonal rearrangement of T-cell receptor genes in mycosis fungoides and dermatopathic lymphadenopathy. New England Journal of Medicine 313: 539–544
161 Bertness V, Kirsch I, Hollis G, Johnson B, Bunn P A 1985 T-cell receptor gene rearrangements as clinical markers of human T-cell lymphomas. New England Journal of Medicine 313: 534–538
162 Waldman T A, Avis M M, Bongiovanni K F, Korsmeyer S J 1985 Rearrangements of genes for the antigen receptor of T cells as markers of lineage and clonality in human lymphoid neoplasms. New England Journal of Medicine 313: 776–783
163 Rambaldi A, Pelicci P G, Allavena P et al 1985 T cell receptor beta chain gene rearrangements in lymphoproliferative disorders of large granular lymphocytes/natural killer cells. Journal of Experimental Medicine 162: 2156–2162
164 Foa R, Pelicci P G, Migone N et al 1986 Analysis of T-cell receptor beta chain (T β) gene rearrangements demonstrates the monoclonal nature of T cell chronic lympholiferative disorders. Blood 67: 247–250
165 Feller A C, Griesser G H, Mak T W, Lennert K 1986 Lymphoepitheloid lymphoma (Lennert's lymphoma) is a monoclonal proliferation of helper/inducer T cells. Blood 68: 663–667
166 Asou N, Matsuoka M, Hattori T et al 1987 T cell γ gene rearrangements in hematology neoplasms. Blood 69: 968–970
167 Foroni L, Foldi J, Matutes E et al 1987 α,β and γ T-cell receptor genes: rearrangements correlate with haematological phenotype in T cell leukemias. British Journal of Haematology 67: 307–318
168 Foroni L, Matutes E, Foldi J et al 1988 T-cell leukemias with rearrangement of the γ but not β T-cell receptor genes. Blood 70: 356–362
169 Sangster R N, Minowada J, Suciu Foca N, Minden M, T W Mak 1986 Rearrangement and expression of the α,β and γ chain T cell receptor genes in human thymic leukemia cells and functional T cells. Journal of Experimental Medicine 163: 1491–1508
170 Furley A J, Mizutani S, Weilbaecher K et al 1986 Developmentally regulated rearrangement and expression of genes encoding the T cell receptor–T3 complex. Cell 46: 75–87
171 Brito-Babapulle V, Melo J V, Foroni I et al 1984 Neoplastic κ and λ cells in a B-PLL with chromosome translocations of both light chain gene regions. International Journal of Cancer 34: 769–773
172 Melo J V, Foroni L, Brito-Babapulle V et al 1985 Prolymphocytic leukemia of B cell type: rearranged immunoglobulin (Ig) genes with defective Ig production. Blood 66: 391–398
173 Parreira A, Pombo De Oliveira M S, Matutes E, Foroni L, Morilla R, Catovsky D 1988 Terminal deoxynucleotidyl transferase positive acute myeloid leukaemia: an association with immature myeloblastic leukaemia. British Journal of Haematology 69: 219–224
174 Matutes E, Brito-Babapulle V, Worner I, Sainati L, Foroni L, Catovsky D 1988 T-cell chronic lymphocytic leukaemic: the spectrum of mature T-cell disorders. Nouvelle Revue Française d'Hematologie 30: 347–351
175 Koopman J W, Schrohenloher R E 1985 Rheumatoid factor. In: Utsinger P D, Zvaifler N J, Ehrlich G E (eds) Rheumatoid arthritis. Lippincot, Philadelphia, pp 217–241
176 Brito-Babapulle V, Matutes E, Foroni L, Pomfret M, Catovsky D 1987 A t(8;14) (q24;q32) in a T-lymphoma/leukemia of CD8+ large granular lymphocytes. Leukemia 1: 789–794
177 Fong S, Chen P P, Gilbertson T A, Fox R I, Vaughan J H, Carson D A 1985 Structural similarities in the κ light chains of human rheumatoid factor paraproteins and serum immunoglobulins bearing a cross-reactive idiotype. Journal of Immunology 135: 1995–1960
178 Fong S, Chen P P, Gilbertson T A, Weber J R, Fox R I, Carson D A 1986 Expression of three cross-reactive idiotypes on rheumatoid factor autoantibodies from patients with autoimmune disease and seropositive adults. Journal of Immunology 137: 122–128
179 Radoux V, Chen P P, Sorge J, Carson D A 1986 A conserved human germline Vk gene directly encodes rheumatoid factor light chains. Journal of Experimental Medicine 164: 2119–2124
180 Pombo de Oliveira M S, Awad E L, Seed F E R, Foroni L et al 1986 Lymphoblastic leukemia in siamese twins: evidence for identity. Lancet ii: 969–970
181 Espinoza C G, Erkman-Balis, Fenske N A 1985 Lymphomatoid papulosis: A premalignant T cell disorder. Journal of the American Academy of Dermatology 13: 736–743

182 Whittaker S, Foroni L, Luzzatto L et al 1988 Lymphomatoid granulomatosis – evidence of a clonal T-cell origin and association with lethal middle line granuloma. Quarterly Journal of Medicine 256: 645–655
183 Winkelmann R K, Bowie J W 1980 Haemorragic diathesis associated with benign histiocytic, cytophagic panniculitis and systemic histiocytosis. Archives of Internal Medicine 140: 1460–1463
184 Coupe M, Foroni L, Stamp G et al 1988 Clonal rearrangement of the T cell receptor γ gene associated with a bizarre lymphoproliferative syndrome. European Journal of Haematology 41: 289–294
185 Katzenstein A L A, Carrington C R B, Liebow A 1979 Lymphomatoid granulomatosis. A clinicopathologic study of 152 cases. Cancer 43: 360–373
186 Melo J V, Brito-Babapulle V, Foroni L, Robinson D S F, Luzzatto L, Catovsky D 1986 Two new cell lines from B-prolymphocytic leukemia characterisation by morphology, immunological markers, karyotype and Ig gene rearrangement. International Journal of Cancer 38: 531–538
187 Melo J V, Foroni L, Brito-Babapulle V, Luzzatto L, Catovsky D 1988 The establishment of cell lines from chronic B-cell leukaemias: evidence of leukemic origin by karyotypic abnormalities and Ig gene rearrangement. Clinical and Experimental Immunology 73: 23–28
188 Kitchingman G R, Rovigatti U, Mauer A M, Melvin S, Murphy S B, Stass S 1985 Rearrangement of immunoglobulin heavy chain genes in T-cell acute lymphoblastic leukemia. Blood 65: 725–729
189 Greaves M F, Chan L C, Furley A J W, Watt S H, Molgaard H V 1986 Review: Lineage promiscuity in haemopoietic differentiation and leukemia. Blood 67: 1–11
190 Furley A J W, Chan L C, Mizutani S et al 1987 Lineage specificity of rearrangement and expression of genes encoding the T cell receptor-T3 complex and immunoglobulin heavy chain in leukemia. Leukemia 1: 644–652
191 Norton J D, Pattison J, Hoffbrand A V, Jani H, Yaxley J C, Leber B F 1987 Rearrangement and expression of T cell antigen receptor genes in B cell chronic lymphocytic leukemia. Blood 71: 178–185
192 Takihara Y, Tkachuk D, Michalopoulos E, Champagne E, Reimann J, Minden M, and Mak T W 1988 Sequence and organisation of the diversity, joining, and constant region genes of the human T-cell δ chain locus. Proceedings of the National Academy of Science USA 85: 6097–6101
193 Boehm T, Baer R, Lavenir I, Forster A, Waters J J, Nacheva E, Rabbitts T H 1988 The mechanism of chromosomal translocation t(11;14) involving the T cell receptor Cδ locus on human chromosome 14q11 and a transcribed region of chromosome 11p15. EMBO Journal 7: 385–394
194 Hochstenbach F, Parker C, McLean J, Gieselmann V, Band H, Bank I, Chess L, Spits H, Strominger J L, Seidman J G, Brenner M B 1988 Characterisation of a third form of human T cell receptor γδ. Journal of Experimental Medicine 168: 761–776
195 Saito T, Hochstenbach F, Marusic-Galesic S, Kruisbeek A M, Brenner M B, Germain R N 1988 Surface expression of only γδ and/or αβ T-cell receptor heterodimers by cells with four (α,β,γ,δ) functional receptor chains. Journal of Experimental Medicine 168: 1003–1020
196 Chien Y-h, Iwashima M, Wettstein D A, Kapla K B, Elliott J F, Born W, Davis M M 1987 T-cell receptor δ gene rearrangements in early thymocytes. Nature (London) 330: 722–727
197 Marrack P, Kappler J 1988 The T-cell repertoire for antigen and MHC. Immunology Today 9: 308–315
198 Triebel F, Lefranc M-P, Hercend T 1988 Further evidence for a sequentially ordered activation of T-cell rearranging γ genes during T lymphocyte differentiation. European Journal of Immunology 18: 789–794
199 Bonneville M, Janeway C A, Jr, Ito K, Haser W, Ishida I, Nakanishi N, Tonegawa S 1988 Intestinal intraepithelial lymphocytes are a distinct set of γδ T cells. Nature (London) 366: 479–481
200 Rabbitts T H, Boehm T, Mengle-Gaw L 1988 Chromosomal abnormalities in lymphoid tumours: mechanism and role in tumour pathogenesis. Trends in Genetics 4: 300–304
201 Foroni L, Laffan M, Boehm T, Rabbitts T H, Catovsky D, Luzzatto L 1989 Rearrangement of the T-cell receptor δ genes in human T-cell leukemias. Blood 73: no. 2, 559–565
202 Boehm T, Rabbitts T 1989 The human T cell receptor genes are targets for chromosomal abnormalities in T cell tumors. FASEB Journal 3: 2344–2359

14
The Analysis of Molecular Changes in Leukemia

Bryan D Young   Trivadi S Ganesan   Lynne Hiorns

The development of the leukemic cell from its normal progenitor is often accompanied by chromosomal changes which include translocations, deletions and duplications. In a number of instances these changes have been shown to affect cellular genes that have been identified in other systems as targets for retroviral transduction. The products of such oncogenes have a wide range of involvement in cell growth and proliferation and hence their alteration may play a key role in the generation and evolution of the leukemic cell. Recent advances in molecular genetics offer the opportunity to delineate the extent and nature of such alterations and correlate them with more conventional forms of analysis. Furthermore, in certain instances, it is possible to take advantage of the fact that these changes are restricted to the leukemic cell to detect minimal residual disease in the patient with great sensitivity. This will have important implications for the monitoring of patients after therapy. Two of the currently most productive areas are concentrated on: the *bcr-abl* translocation in CML and the occurrence of *ras* gene mutations. It is also demonstrated how this technology may be used to enhance understanding of the leukemic process.

MOLECULAR ANALYSIS OF CHROMOSOMAL TRANSLOCATION

Cytogenetic changes are becoming increasingly important in understanding the pathogenesis of human malignancies. The chromosomal changes observed in leukemias and lymphomas have been particularly well studied.[1] Although some abnormalities are consistently present in certain malignancies, there are many other well-defined alterations which show only an association with a particular disease as classified by morphological or histopathological criteria. In order to unravel the complex relationship between chromosomal changes and the clinical manifestations of disease, it will be necessary to analyse the genetic nature and consequences of these alterations.

The chromosomal mapping of known oncogenes lead to the hypothesis that some might be directly altered by such changes.[2] This prediction has been borne out for a number of translocations in which breakpoints have been shown to lie in close proximity to certain genes. Although it is suspected that many other documented chromosomal alterations may involve known oncogenes or genes controlling cell growth, direct evidence is lacking.

The involvement of certain genes in chromosomal translocations has been well established and these are listed in Table 14.1. The translocation t(9;22) which generates the Philadelphia chromosome is one of the best studied at both the cytogenetic[3] and molecular level.[4-6] The majority of patients with chronic myeloid leukemia (CML) have the characteristic Philadelphia translocation t(9;22)(q34;q11) in their leukemic cells. The oncogene *c-abl*, which is normally present on chromosome 9, is translocated to chromosome 22 where it comes into juxaposition with the 5′ portion of a gene known as the *bcr* or *phl* gene, whose product has an unknown function in normal cells. The molecular consequence of this

Table 14.1 Involvement of genes in chromosomal translocations

Disease	Translocation	Genes	Reference
CML	t(9;22)	*c-abl/bcr*	4,5
ALL	t(9;22)	*c-abl/bcr*	6
Burkitt's lymphoma	t(8;14)	*c-myc*/IgH	7
	t(2;8)	IgK/*c-myc*	8
	t(8;22)	*c-myc*/IgL	9
Follicular lymphoma	t(14;18)	IgH/*bcl-2*	10,11
CLL	t(11;14)	*bcl-1*/IgH	12
CLL	t(14;19)	IgH/*bcl-3*	13
T-cell lymphoma	inv(14)	IgH/TCRA	14,15
	t(7;9)	TCRB/?	16

translocation is the transcription of chimeric mRNA and the expression of a chimeric *bcr-abl* protein with enhanced in vitro tyrosine kinase activity.[5] Although the breakpoints on chromosome 9 can occur over a 200 kilobase (kb) range the breakpoints on chromosome 22 are clustered within a 5 kb sequence designated the breakpoint cluster region (bcr). However in some Philadelphia-positive acute lymphoblastic leukemias (ALL) the break in the *bcr* gene has been shown to lie further 5' such that only the first exon of *bcr* is included in the chimeric mRNA.[6]

In B-cell leukemias and lymphomas, the immunoglobulin (Ig) genes have been found to be directly involved in certain chromosomal translocations (Table 14.1). It was shown that the *c-myc* oncogene was translocated into the heavy chain (H) locus[7] or, more rarely, into either of the light chain loci in Burkitt's lymphomas.[8,9] More recently, the J_H region of the IgH locus has been shown to be involved in the t(14;18) translocation which is a common feature of follicular lymphoma. This has lead to the identification of a gene of unknown function on chromosome 18 (*bcl-2*) which is directly affected by the translocation.[10,11] Similarly the t(11;14) and the t(14;19) found in B-cell CLL have been shown to involve the IgH locus, and molecular analysis has lead to the cloning of DNA from the breakpoint of the partner chromosomes.[12,13] In T-cell lymphomas an analogous involvement of the T-cell receptor (TCR) genes has been demonstrated for both inv(14) and t(7;9). The inversion inv(14) was shown[14,15] to be a recombination between the TCRA and the IgH loci, whereas the t(7;9) involved a recombination between the TCRB locus and a region on chromosome 9 which is close to, but does not involve, the oncogene *c-abl*.[16]

At the molecular level a reciprocal translocation results in two new junction regions with an abnormal pattern of restriction enzyme sites. Hence, if a DNA probe corresponds to a sequence close to such a junction, Southern analysis of the genomic DNA will reveal an abnormal hybridization pattern. In principle a suitable DNA probe can be used to detect translocation in tumor cells for which karyotype data are lacking. This approach can only be successful if the breakpoints are known to be clustered within a limited range. Some breakpoints have been shown to occur over a wide range (100 kb) and it would therefore be difficult to use a single probe to detect all such translocations.[17] This problem can potentially be solved by using pulsed field gel electrophoresis to provide a much larger range of analysis (150–1000 kb).[18,19] A further problem is that deletions are known to occur around junction regions[20,21] and this could result in loss of sequence homologous to the probe and lack of detection of the rearranged allele. Provided such difficulties are taken into account, this approach to detection of translocation can be used as discussed below to obtain information which cannot readily be acquired by conventional cytogenetics. The molecular detection of the *bcr-abl* rearrangement serves as an example of how this approach can yield extra information on the origin and course of chronic myeloid leukemia. It will be possible to adopt similar approaches in other leukemias as the molecular nature of their alterations becomes understood.

DETECTION OF THE PH TRANSLOCATION IN CML

Genomic DNA was prepared from the myeloid cells of eight patients with Ph + CML and subjected to Southern analysis using a DNA probe to the *bcr* region. As shown in Fig. 14.1 each DNA sample had a germline BamHI fragment (arrowed) representing the normal chromosome 22 and several had aberrant fragments. Those samples which showed only germline fragments with BamHI had aberrant non-germline fragments with other restriction enzymes (data not shown). In practice all Ph + CML samples examined in this way with appropriate *bcr* probes have exhibited rearrangement with a variety of restriction enzymes at the DNA level. If all the cells bear the translocation, the aberrant and germline bands should be of equal intensity. If the Ph + clone is mixed with normal cells the relative intensity of the aberrant band is correspondingly reduced. The lower practical limit of detection of Ph + cells in an excess of normal cells is about 5% by this approach. This is comparable to the detection level obtained by conventional cytogenetics. However, recent advances using the polymerase chain reaction detailed below offer the possibility of much more sensitive detection of Ph + in a background of normal cells.

ANALYSIS OF PH-NEGATIVE CML

About 10% of patients regarded on clinical and hematological grounds as having CML lack the Ph translocation. Some of these patients have a leukemia that is totally indistinguishable

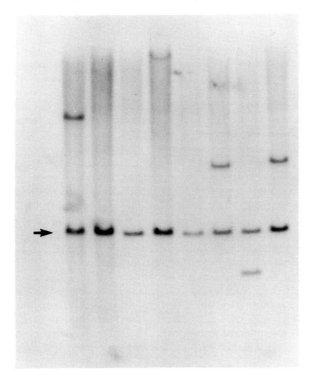

Fig. 14.1 Southern analysis of the Philadelphia translocation. DNA from Philadelphia chromosome positive CML cells from eight patients was digested with BamH1 and probed with the *bcr* intron probe after size fractionation on a 0.7% agarose gel. The germline BamH1 *bcr* fragment is arrowed.

from Ph+ disease in all other respects, whereas in other cases subtle clinical or hematological features suggest the disease is different. In retrospective analysis of the hematological features of 25 patients previously regarded as having Ph− CML showed that all but one case could be better reclassified as examples of the myelodysplastic syndrome or as chronic myeloproliferative disorders other than CML.[22] A similar retrospective study came to the same conclusion.[21] The availability of *bcr* probes which consistently detect rearrangement in Ph+ CML has allowed the existence of Ph− CML to be examined at the molecular level. There have now been several reports of Ph− CML in which a rearrangement of sequence around the *bcr* probe has been detected.[24-26] The extent to which *c-abl* is involved in these alterations in unclear. It has been reported that both *bcr* and *c-abl* have been found to be rearranged in a Ph− CML.[27] However, in another case of Ph− CML, *bcr* rearrangement was detected without apparent translocation involving *c-abl* or expression of novel *abl*-related mRNA species.[28] In a study[29] of seven Ph− CML patients, evidence for *bcr* rearrangement was presented. Although one of the patients had a complex translocation, t(4;9;22), the rest had either a normal karyotype or minor alterations which did not involve chromosome 9 or 22.

The definition of Ph− CML is imprecise because there is no single feature on which the diagnosis can be firmly based. In general Ph− CML patients differ from Ph+ patients in having a smaller spleen at corresponding leukocyte counts, more commonly thrombocytopenia at presentation and a leukocyte differential that may lack a peak of myelocytes, may lack basophilia or eosinophilia or may show monocytosis. There can also be dysplastic changes in the granulocyte series, which are rarely or never seen in Ph+ disease. The observation that at least some Ph− CML patients have a *bcr* rearrangement suggests that these patients should be grouped with Ph+ disease. However, until the molecular basis for these observations is explained it will remain unclear to what extent this group should be regarded as a variant of Ph+ disease.

CLONAL SURVIVAL IN BONE MARROW TRANSPLANTATION FOR CML

Allogeneic bone marrow transplantation (BMT) using HLA-identical siblings is currently a promising form of treatment for patients with CML. In a recent analysis performed for the International Bone Marrow Transplant Registry the actuarial probability for survival in the chronic phase was $55 \pm 5\%$ and the actuarial probability of relapse was $19 \pm 7\%$ at 4 years. Two cases of leukemia recurring in donor cells after BMT for CML have been reported.[30,31] The evidence that the relapse was in donor cells was based on sex chromosome differences demonstrated in dividing cells. It is now possible to address this problem consistently in each patient using the DNA minisatellite probes.[32] A particular minisatellite region was cloned from the intron of the human myoglobin gene and shown to be highly polymorphic. Using such DNA probes it is possible to derive a unique DNA 'fingerprint' of each individual and this has been used in paternity testing and determination of twin zygosity.[33,34] The probability of any two individuals having identical patterns is very low and it is therefore possible to use such an approach to distinguish host versus donor origin of cells after relapse. In a recent study[35] four transplanted patients who had relapsed with Ph+ disease were studied using the fingerprinting probes 15.1.11.4 and 6.3. It was possible to show that the 'fingerprints' for the original leukemias were identical to those of the relapsed leukemias in each patient, thus confirming the relapse to be in the hosts' cells (Fig. 14.2).

Glucose-6-phosphate dehydrogenase (G6PD) analysis of Ph+ CML has suggested that the Philadelphia translocation may be a secondary event which is preceded by clonal expansion of Ph− cells.[36] It is therefore possible that the Ph+ relapse in host cells could have involved a second 9;22 translocation. The molecular rearrangements in the *bcr* gene appear to be unique for each patient, and hence a second independent translocation would

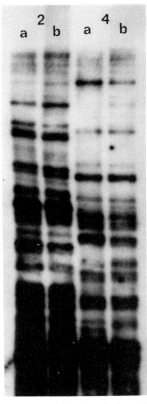

Fig. 14.2 Use of 'mini-satellite' probes[30-32] to identify host origin of relapse following bone marrow transplantation in three patients with CML. DNA from pre-transplant cells (a) and from post-transplant relapse cells (b) was digested with Hinfl and probed with the mini-satellite probe 15.1.11.4.

be expected to result in a different molecular pattern. In the four patients studied, the *bcr* gene rearrangements were identical before and after BMT (Fig. 14.3) and it was concluded that the original Ph + clone was responsible for the relapse in each case. Furthermore, it is clear that in the evolution of the disease no further alteration to the *bcr* gene has taken place following the initial rearrangement.

In this study all four patients unequivocally demonstrated recurrence of the original clone even as late as 4 years in patient 4. Furthermore, it has been reported that Ph + metaphases can appear after BMT without hematological relapse, only to disappear in the course of time.[35] This issue can be addressed by monitoring the presence of the rearrangement after BMT. Similar investigations have been carried out in ALL using immunoglobulin gene rearrangement as a clonal marker[38] (see also Ch. 12). In follicular lymphoma where t(14:18) is observed in the majority of cases, the breakpoints on chromosome 18 cluster within a transcriptionally active region (*bcl-2*).[39,40] Using probes from this region the question of clonality can be addressed in patients with follicular lymphoma who have relapsed after any modality of therapy.

One explanation of recurrence of leukemia in donor cells after BMT is a transfection of a transforming DNA sequence to transplanted stem cells. An alternative hypothesis is that the stroma may be part of the leukemic clone and, being radioresistant, offers an abnormal milieu to donor cells. However, donor cell recurrent leukemia after BMT accounts for less than 5% of relapse.[41] Possibly normal donor stem cells are naturally resistant to the development of leukemia and there is a variable efficiency in transfection. It is now possible to characterize relapse after BMT particularly in CML with a combination of *bcr* and minisatellite probes.

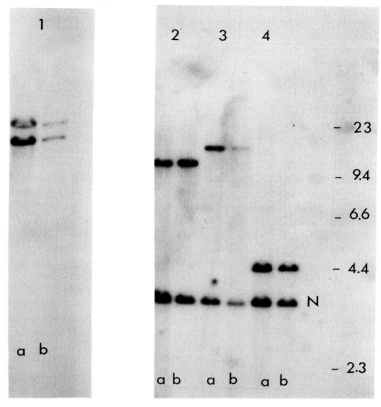

Fig. 14.3 Use of the *bcr* intron probe to determine the origin of leukemic relapse in four CML patients. DNA samples from leukemic cells pre-transplant (a) and from post-transplant relapse (b) were digested with BamH1 and probed with the *bcr* intron probe.

IDENTIFICATION OF A NEW 5' BREAKPOINT IN THE *BCR* GENE

About 20% of cases of adult ALL and about 5% of childhood ALL carry a t(9;22) translocation[42] which appears cytogenetically indistinguishable from the Ph translocation characteristic of CML. It has therefore been difficult to distinguish a de novo Ph+ ALL from a CML in lymphoid blast crisis, which may have had an undetected asymptomatic chronic phase. The observation[43] that in two Ph+ ALL patients the breakpoints of chromosome 22 had occurred outside the *bcr* region normally broken in CML[4] suggested a possible molecular basis for such a distinction. In further studies it was shown that there is a subgroup of Ph+ ALL patients with no observable rearrangements in the immediate vicinity of the *bcr* locus[44] and that the breakpoints on chromosome 22 lie between this region and the more proximal Cλ locus.[45] There appeared to be a correlation between the absence of a detectable rearrangement in the CML specific breakpoint region and the presence of 190 kilodalton (kDa) *abl*-related species in some cases of Ph+ ALL.[46–48] Subsequently, site-directed antibodies were used to demonstrate that the 190-kDa *abl*-related species does have *bcr*-related sequence at its amino terminus.[47] Molecular cloning of the mRNA for this species confirmed that the p190 was a chimeric molecule and that the breakpoint on chromosome 22 was 5' of the previously identified cluster of breakpoints but still within the *bcr* gene.[6] The p190 has so far been identified only in ALL patients whereas the p210 has been found in both CML and ALL. It is not yet clear whether the Ph + ALLs which express the p190 species should be regarded as a subgroup of ALL with lymphoid restriction of leukemic involvement. The subdivision of Ph + ALL on the size of the chimeric *bcr-abl* species and comparison of their clinical course may help to determine whether the precise breakpoint has any diagnostic value.

POINT MUTATIONS OF *RAS* GENES IN LEUKEMIA

In contrast to the disease specificity of the chromosomal translocations discussed above, about 10% of all human tumors are thought to have acquired mutations to members of the *ras* gene family. These changes have been found to occur at certain positions within the coding sequence, resulting in critical changes to the *ras* products. The three members of the *ras* gene family, *H-ras*, *K-ras* and *N-ras* map to chromosomes 11, 12 and 1 respectively. The homologous p21 proteins encoded by this family can bind guanine nucleotides, have intrinsic GTPase activity and are localized at the inner surface of the plasma membrane.[50] They are thought to have a role in the transduction of receptor-mediated external signals into the cell, although the precise biochemical pathway remains to be elucidated. The transforming potential of oncogenic versions of the *ras* genes has been shown to be due to single base substitutions which alter the corresponding amino acid and result in reduced GTPase activity.[51,52] These point mutations have been found in either codon 12, 13 or 61 of members of the *ras* gene family[53,54] in tumor cells and were not found in normal cells from the same patients. In contrast to some of the specific chromosomal rearrangements discussed above, mutations to *ras* genes have been found in a wide variety of human tumors with varying frequency. The highest incidence (25–50%) has been reported in acute myeloid leukemia (AML).

The mutations in *ras* genes which have been identified in hematopoietic malignancies are summarized in Table 14.2. It is clear that, although the majority of mutations have occurred in the *N-ras* gene, both *K-ras* and *H-ras* can be affected. Some of the mutations have been found in cell lines and therefore could have arisen in culture. However, there are clear examples of leukemias in which the mutation was present in the primary tumor material. The high frequency of activation of *N-ras* in AML has not been matched by a similar frequency in other myeloid or lymphoid malignancies.[55] For example, none of 14 myeloid CML blast crises was found to have mutated *ras* genes.[56] It is also apparent that there is no obvious correlation between *ras* mutation and either AML subtype (FAB classification) or karyotypic alteration. It is therefore difficult to establish the role of *ras* mutation in the origin and progression of these tumors. It is of interest that *N-ras* mutations have been demonstrated in three out of eight patients with myelodysplastic syndrome (MDS).[57] Since it is difficult to predict when MDS will evolve into overt leukemia, it would be important to show whether the presence of a *ras* mutation could predict a leukemic transformation.

DETECTION OF MUTATIONS IN *RAS* GENES

The earliest method for the detection of mutated *ras* genes involved the transfection of genomic DNA from the tumor of interest into mouse 3T3 fibroblasts. The formation of foci was taken to indicate that there was a gene of oncogenic potential in the genomic DNA. The identification of the transforming gene required that DNA be prepared from foci and the transfection cycle repeated several times. This approach was used by many laboratories to demonstrate the presence of mutated forms of the various members of the *ras* family in human tumor cell lines and tissue. The time-consuming nature of this method has limited its application to relatively small numbers of tumor samples.

THE ANALYSIS OF MOLECULAR CHANGES IN LEUKEMIA 399

Table 14.2 Mutations of human *ras* genes in hemopoietic malignancies

ras gene	Patient or cell line	Type of tumor	Position 12	Position 13	Position 61	Method of detection	Reference
N-ras	normal		GGT Gly	GGT Gly	CAA Gln	Sequence	58
	LK	Childhood ALL L$_2$	NGT			Oligonucleotide probing	55
	J Vi	Childhood ALL L$_2$	NGT			Oligonucleotide probing	55
	AML	AML M$_2$	GAT Asp			NIH/3T3 assay and sequence	59
	AML	AML	GAT Asp			Oligonucleotide probing	62
	NHL	non HD lymphoma	TGT Cys			NIH/3T3 and oligonucleotide	60
	AML 1	AML	GAT Asp			NIH/3T3 and oligonucleotide	54
	AML 33	AML M$_1$	GAT Asp			NIH/3T3 and oligonucleotide	54
	AML 49	AML M$_5$	GTT Val			NIH/3T3 and oligonucleotide	54
	AML 77	AML M$_4$	GTT Val			NIH/3T3 and oligonucleotide	54
	AML 73	AML M$_2$	GTT Val			NIH/3T3 and oligonucleotide	54
	AML100	AML M$_1$	GTT Val			Oligonucleotide probing	61
	PARA 1	MDS (RA)	CGT Arg			NIH/3T3 assay and sequence	57
	RAEB 1	MDS (RAEB)	CGT Arg			NIH/3T3 assay and sequence	57
	RAEB 2	MDS (RAEB)	CGT Arg			NIH/3T3 assay and sequence	57
	MV 26	AML M$_1$			CGA Arg	Oligonucleotide probing	61
	MV 34	AML M$_4$			CAN His	Oligonucleotide probing	61
	MV 65	AML M$_4$			CGA Arg	Oligonucleotide probing	61
	MV 81	AML M$_1$			CGA Arg	Oligonucleotide probing	61
	MOLT 4	T-ALL cell line	NGT			Oligonucleotide probing	63
	HL 60	AML M$_3$ cell line			CTA Leu	Sequence	64
	31-26-146	AML	N/A			NIH/3T3 assay	65
	MOLT 3	T-ALL cell line	N/A			NIH/3T3 assay	65
	8392	Pre-B-ALL cell line	N/A			NIH/3T3 assay	65
	IM 9	CML cell line	N/A			NIH/3T3 assay	65
	3 patients	AML	N/A			NIH/3T3 assay	66
	AML	AML	N/A			2-D gel electrophoresis	67
	6 samples	Mixed	N/A			NIH/3T3 assay	68
	AW Ramos	Burkitt's lymphoma	N/A			NIH/3T3 assay	64
	T-ALL-1	T-ALL cell line	N/A			NIH/3T3 assay	72
	P-12	T-ALL cell line	N/A			NIH/3T3 assay	72
	RPMI 8402	T-ALL cell line	N/A			NIH/3T3 assay	72
H-ras	normal		GGC Gly	GGT Gly	CAG Gln	Sequence	69
	ALL	ALL		N/A		2-D gel electrophoresis	67
K-ras	normal		GGT Gly	GGC Gly	CAA Gln	Sequence	70
	MV 41	AML M$_4$	GAT Asp			Oligonucleotide probing	61
	MV 71	AML M$_6$	GTT Val			Oligonucleotide probing	61
	LL	LL cell line		N/A		NIH/3T3 assay	68
	CCRF-CEM	T-ALL cell line		N/A		NIH/3T3 assay	65
	BL	Burkitt's lymphoma		N/A		NIH/3T3 assay	71

Recently, a technic of enzymatic amplification of segments of a gene has been developed which allows many more DNA samples to be examined for *ras* gene mutations. This method can be applied to any gene for which the sequence is known and in which mutations might be suspected. The basis of this technic is the polymerase chain reaction (PCR) which allows the enrichment of specific sequences by a factor of 10^6, a level of selection which was previously unobtainable. PCR has been used for the examination of nucleotide sequence variations,[73,74] chromosomal rearrangements,[75] for high efficiency cloning of genomic sequences,[76] for direct sequencing of mitochondrial[77] and genomic DNA,[78,79] and for the detection of viral pathogens.[80]

Oligonucleotide sequences are synthesized flanking the region of interest and complementary to opposing strands. As illustrated in Fig. 14.4 these are annealed to the complementary strands and used to direct the enzymatic elongation by DNA polymerase. This is repeated 25–30 times to amplify the chosen region exponentially by a factor of up to 10^5–10^6. The reaction products are probed with either a wild-type oligonucleotide or a group of oligonucleotides corresponding to mutant sequence (codons 12, 13 or 61 of the *ras* genes). The degree of amplification obtained by the PCR method readily permits the detection of mutants in *ras* genes by simple dot–blot hybridization. DNA from the cell line HT1080 and a series of normal DNA samples was amplified by the PCR method and probed with both the wild-type oligonucleotide and a mixture of mutant oligonucleotides which included the known mutation to *N-ras* in HT1080. As shown in Fig. 14.5 the presence of the known mutation in *N-ras* in HT1080, and its absence in normal DNA, is detected by dot–blot hybridization. A further sophistication of this technic is the direct sequence analysis of the amplified products,[79] which could confirm the mutations found by oligonucleotide hybridization. In diseases such as the hemoglobinopathies, where mutations can occur at a large number of sites, this would be the method of choice for identifying the particular lesion.

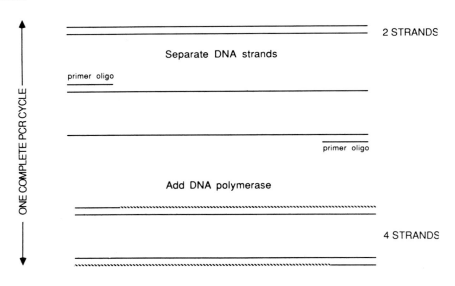

Fig. 14.4 Schematic description of the polymerase chain reaction (PCR) method as described in the Methods section.

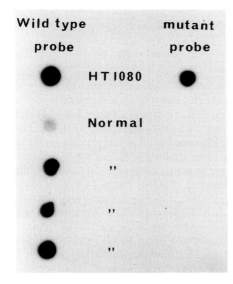

Fig. 14.5 Detection of a point mutation in the *N-ras* gene in the cell line HT1080. The polymerase chain reaction (PCR) was used to amplify the relevant region of the *N-ras* gene with the primers GATTCTTACAGAAAACAAGTG and CTGTAGAGGTTAATATCCGCA from HT1080 and four normal DNA samples. The wild-type probe was GTACTCTTCTTGTCCAGCTG and the mutant probe was the mixed oligonucleotide GTACTCTTCTT[A,C OR T]TCCAGCTG. The amplification and probing was as described in the Methods section.

A potential application of this technic is the detection of residual disease in patients after treatment. In order to establish the level of sensitivity the following mixing experiment was performed. Leukemic DNA with a known mutation was mixed in varying proportions with normal genomic DNA. Each mixed aliquot was subjected to enzymatic amplification and probed with both wild-type oligonucleotide and the appropriate mutant oligonucleotide. It is clear from Fig. 14.6 that tumor DNA remains detectable at a level of about 5%. This approach may be useful for detection of minimal residual disease, provided careful controls are used. An advantage of this method is that it is not necessary for the tumor DNA to be

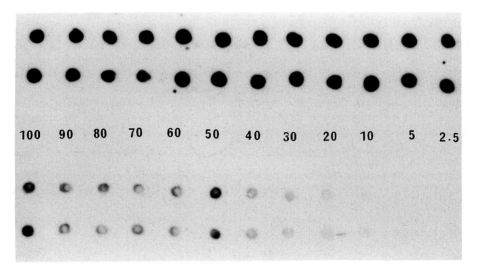

Fig. 14.6 Detection of leukemic cells against a normal cell background. Leukemic cells with a known *N-ras* mutation in codon 13 were mixed with normal cells at the concentration shown. The relevant region of the *N-ras* gene was amplified using the primers ATGACTGAGTACAAACTGGTG and CTCTATGGTGGGATCATATTC. The wild-type probe (a) was TTCCCAACACCACCTGCTCC and mutant probe (b) was the mixed oligonucleotide TTCCCAACA[G,A or T]CACCTGCTCC. The numbers are the percentage leukemic cells.

as large as is required for Southern blotting since relatively small segments (100–200 base pairs) are usually amplified in PCR.

FUTURE APPLICATIONS OF MOLECULAR ANALYSIS IN LEUKEMIA

Although it is difficult to predict the future role of molecular analysis, it is likely to be central to the study and classification of leukemias. Already the unexpected heterogeneity in the *bcr-abl* fusion may offer the possibility of distinction of CML lymphoid blast crisis from de novo Ph + ALL. Although this translocation formed the basis of this study, there could be other unknown molecular lesions required for the full progression of CML as suggested by the cytogenetic evidence. The precise effect of the expression of the *bcr-abl* fusion products remains uncertain, but the development of antibodies which recognize only the junction regions may help to elucidate their role. In addition to those in Table 14.1 there are a number of well-defined chromosomal translocations which await molecular analysis. As the physical mapping of the human genome progresses it is likely that the genes involved will be identified and subjected to the kind of analysis described above for the *bcr-abl* fusion.

The polymerase chain reaction has already been used to analyze the follicular lymphoma translocation t(14;18) and it was shown that one cell in 10^5 could be detected.[75] Oligonucleotide primers were chosen on either side of the breakpoint and therefore only rearranged DNA can be amplified, resulting in a very low background and high sensitivity. The large variation in the breakpoint position in the *c-abl* gene in the t(9;22) translocation would make this approach difficult. However, it is possible to apply the PCR technic to a cDNA copy of the chimeric mRNA and thus it will be possible to detect the Ph + cells with similar levels of sensitivity. The ability to detect such low levels of residual disease post-treatment is likely to influence the long-term management of such patients.

METHODS

DETECTION OF MUTATIONS IN *RAS* GENES

The following protocols have been used to detect point mutations in members of the *ras* gene family. The technics can be adapted for amplification and examination of any DNA sequence for which sequence information is available. Although two methods of polymerase chain reaction are described, the use of the Taq polymerase is preferable because the higher temperatures used give greater specificity in the amplification and the protocol is less labor intensive. Primer oligonucleotides are usually chosen to lie 100–200 base pairs apart on opposite strands, although amplification of larger fragments (up to 3 kb) has been reported.

Isolation of genomic DNA

High-molecular-weight DNA can be prepared from leukemic cells by the following method. Such DNA would be suitable for Southern analysis or for the polymerase chain reaction, but would be too small for pulsed field gel analysis. It is important to avoid shearing the DNA by using wide bore pipettes and micropipette tips with the ends cut off. Use of a vortexer or a fast shaker should be avoided.

Materials
PBS: 8 g NaCl, 0.2 g KCl, 1.5 g NaH_2PO_4, 0.2 g K_2HPO_4 dissolved in 1 l
EDTA/Tris solution: 0.1 M EDTA, 50 mmol/l Tris-HCl pH 7.4
SDS stock: 10% sodium dodecylsulpfate
20 mg/ml proteinase K stock solution

Buffer-saturated redistilled phenol
24:1 chloroform:isoamyl alcohol
TE buffer:1 mmol/l EDTA, 10 mmol/l Tris-HCl pH 7.4
RNAase at 500 µg/ml (pre-boiled for 10 min)
Water bath at 37°C
Low speed centrifuge

Method

1. Harvest cells by low speed centrifugation (or disrupt tissue fragments by stirring at 4°C in 4% EDTA, 0.15% Tris).
2. Wash cells by centrifugation several times with PBS.
3. Resuspend cell pellet in 20 volumes of EDTA/Tris solution and add SDS to 0.5% final concentration, mixing gently.
4. Add proteinase K to 100 µg/ml. Mix and incubate 37°C for 4 hours.
5. Add NaCl to 0.1 mol/l and extract twice with an equal volume of phenol. Carefully remove the aqueous phase.
6. Extract the aqueous phase with an equal volume of chloroform.
7. Add 2 volumes of ethanol and leave overnight at $-20°C$. Recover DNA either by spooling out with a sterile glass rod or by centrifugation.
8. Air dry the pellet and redissolve in TE buffer.
9. Add RNAase to 50 µg/ml and incubate for 6 hours at 37°C.
10. Repeat steps (5)–(8).

Polymerase Chain Reaction

Using Klenow polymerase

Materials

10 × Klenow buffer { 0.5 mol/l NaCl
0.1 mol/l $MgCl_2$
0.1 mol/l Tris pH 7.5 }

20 µmol/l primer 1
20 µmol/l primer 2
40 mM dNTPs (10 mmol/l of each)
Dimethyl sulfoxide (DMSO) 100%
Sterile distilled water
Genomic DNA

Klenow enzyme (sequencing grade Boehringer Manheim)
Eppendorf tubes
Microfuge
Hot block/water bath at 37°C
Hot block/water bath at 95°C
Clock

Method

1. Make up reaction mixture as follows: in a 1.5 ml Eppendorf tube:
   1 µg DNA
   10 µl 10 × Klenow buffer
   15 µl 40 mmol/l dNTPs

5 μl primer 1
5 μl primer 2
10 μl DMSO
Distilled water to a final volume of 100 μl.
2. Close the tubes and heat at 95°C for 10 min to denature
3. Zero clock
4. Spin for 10 s at 10 000 rev./min
5. Transfer to 37°C for remainder of 2 min
6. Add 1 unit of Klenow enzyme (in 1 μl)
7. Mix well and incubate at 37°C for 2 min
8. Transfer to 95°C for 2 min
9. Repeat steps (3)–(8) a further 29 times

The final stage is denaturation at 95°C leaving single-stranded DNA which can be stored at −20°C until required.

Using Taq polymerase

Materials

10 × Taq Buffer {	500 mmol/l KCl 100 mmol/l Tris pH 8.4 5 mmol/l $MgCl_2$
Gelatin (Sigma)	2 mg/ml
dNTPs	40 mmol/l (10 mmol/l each)

Primer 1 (20 μmol/l)
Primer 2 (20 μmol/l)
Sterile distilled water
Taq polymerase (Cetus Corporation)
Genomic DNA
Eppendorf tubes
Hot block/water bath at 55°C
Hot block/water bath at 70°C
Hot block/water bath at 95°C
Clock

Method

1. Make up reaction mixture as follows: in a 1.5 ml Eppendorf tube:
   1 μg DNA
   10 μl Taq buffer (10 ×)
   2 μl dNTPs
   5 μl primer 1
   5 μl primer 2
   10 μl gelatin
   Distilled water to a final volume of 100 μl
2. Close the tubes and heat to 95°C for 10 min to denature
3. Transfer the tubes to 55°C for 2 min
4. Add 2 units of Taq polymerase (in 1 μl)
5. Transfer the tubes to 70°C for 2 min
6. Transfer the tubes to 95°C for 2 min
7. Transfer the tubes to 55°C for 2 min
8. Repeat steps (5)–(7) a further 29 times

Note: it may be necessary to add fresh Taq polymerase after 10 cycles, depending on the stability of the batch used.

Application of amplified DNA to filters
The amplified fragments can be visualized after agarose gel electrophoresis and then blotted to filters. Alternatively, the following protocol can be used to dot–blot the amplified framents to filters.

Materials

2 × denaturing solution $\begin{cases} 0.8 \text{ mol/l NaOH} \\ 0.05 \text{ mol/l EDTA} \end{cases}$

Gene Screen filter (Dupont/NEN)
Saran Wrap (Dow)
Ultraviolet transilluminator.

Method

1. A 5 µl aliquot of each amplified DNA sample is denatured with an equal volume of denaturing solution and mixed.
2. The denatured sample is applied to Gene Screen filters in 2-µl aliquots allowing the filter to dry between additions.
3. The dry filter is wrapped in Saran Wrap and exposed to mid-range ultraviolet illumination for 5 min.

Kinase end labeling
A second series of oligonucleotides is synthesized to be complementary to the region of interest, containing single base substitutions, corresponding to possible mutations. These oligonucleotides are radioactively labeled in the following protocol to use as probes against the amplified DNA.

Materials

Oligomeric (n = 20) oligonucleotide probes

10 × kinase buffer $\begin{cases} 0.75 \text{ mol/l Tris pH 9.5} \\ 12.5 \text{ mmol/l spermidine} \\ 1.25 \text{ mmol/l EDTA} \\ 0.1 \text{ mol/l MgCl}_2 \\ 50.0 \text{ mmol/l DTT} \\ 50\% \text{ glycerol.} \end{cases}$

^{32}P-labeled ATP in aqueous solution (PB10218 Amersham) T$_4$ kinase (Boehringer Manheim)
Sterile distilled water

1 × SSPE $\begin{cases} 0.01 \text{ mol/l NaPO}_4 \text{ pH 7.0} \\ 0.18 \text{ mol/l NaCl} \\ 1.0 \text{ mmol/l EDTA} \end{cases}$

1.5 ml Eppendorf tubes
37°C water bath

Method

1. 250 ng oligonucleotide is dispensed into an Eppendorf tube (1.5 ml) and the following solutions added:
   5 µl kinase buffer
   250 µCi (9.25 MBq) [^{32}P] ATP
   20 units T$_4$ kinase
   Distilled water to a final volume of 50 µl

2. The tube is incubated at 37°C for 30 min.
3. A Bio-gel P4 column is prepared in 1 × SSPE packed into a 1-ml syringe, with glass wool at the bottom, and spun at 15 000 rev./min for 3 min to pack the column.
4. 50 µl 1 × SSPE is added to the reaction mixture and the 100 µl total is loaded on top of the bio-gel column and spun at 15 000 rev./min for 5 min with the tip of the column resting in an Eppendorf tube. The eluate is collected and used in the hybridization. The column containing unincorporated dNTPs is disposed of as solid waste.

Oligonucleotide probe hybridization

The labeled oligonucleotide probes are hybridized to the filter, and washed under conditions which permit only perfectly matched sequences to remain stable. After hybridization the filters can be stripped of signal and re-hybridized many times.

Materials

10 × SSPE (see Kinase end labeling)
20% sodium dodecylsulfate
100 × Denharts { 2% BSA
2% Ficoll
2% Polyvinylpyrrolidone
Distilled water

Method

1. Hybridization solution is made up as follows:
    50 ml 10 × SSPE
    5 ml 100 × Denharts
    2.5 ml 20% SDS
    32.5 ml distilled water
    Note: total volume 90 ml
2. 20 ml hybridization solution is dispensed into a Perspex chamber and the filters are immersed individually, and left at 48°C to prehybridize for 1–6 hours.
3. The labeled oligonucleotide probes are added to 10 ml of hybridization solution, and the filters transferred to this solution and incubated for 16 hours at 48°C.

Note: all filters for each position are probed together including the normal probe, so that intensities can be compared.

Washing the filters

The following washing conditions have been carefully developed, so that by the addition of 3 mol/l $(CH_3)_4NCl$ the melting temperature of the oligonucleotides is independent of their base composition and thus the same conditions can be used for all positions of all three *ras* genes.

Materials

Wash buffer 1: { 2 × SSPE (see Kinase end labeling)
20% SDS

Wash buffer 2 { 3 mol/l $(CH_3)_4NCL$
50 mmol/l Tris pH 8.0
2 mmol/l EDTA
0.1% SDS

Method

1. The filters are removed from the hybridization buffer (which can be stored at −20°C for re-use) and rinsed briefly in wash buffer 1.

2. The filters are washed thoroughly in wash buffer 1 for 2 × 20 min at room temperature.
3. The filters are rinsed in wash buffer 2 and washed for 20 min at room temperature.
4. Wash buffer 2 is heated to 63°C and the filters are washed at this temperature for 15 min.
5. The filters are wrapped while damp in Saran Wrap and exposed to Fuji RX X-ray film as required.

ACKNOWLEDGEMENTS

The authors would like to thank Dr J M Goldman and Dr T A Lister for valuable discussions and for provision of patient material. This work is supported by the Imperial Cancer Research Fund.

REFERENCES

1 Rowley J D, Testa J R 1983 Chromosome abnormalities in malignant hematologic disease. In: Advances in cancer research, Academic Press, New York, pp 103-148
2 Rowley J D 1983 Human oncogene locations and chromosome aberrations. Nature 301: 290-291
3 Rowley J D 1986 The Philadelphia chromosome translocation. In: Genetic rearrangements in leukemia and lymphoma, Churchill Livingstone, New York, pp 82-99
4 Groffen J, Stephenson J R, Heisterkamp N, de Klein A, Bartram C R, Grosveld G 1984 Philadelphia breakpoints are clustered within a limited region, bcr, on chromosome 22. Cell 36: 93-99
5 Ben-Neriah Y, Daley G Q, Mes-Masson A M, Witte O N, Baltimore D 1986 The chronic myelogenous leukemia-specific P210 protein is the product of the bcr/abl hybrid gene. Science 233: 212-214
6 Hermans A, Heisterkamp N, von Lindern M et al 1987 Unique fusion of bcr and c-abl genes in Philadelphia chromosome positive acute lymphoblastic leukemia. Cell 51: 33-40
7 Battey J, Moulding C, Taub R et al P 1985 The human c-myc oncogene: structural consequences of translocation into the IGH locus in Burkitt's lymphoma. Cell 34: 779-787
8 Taub R, Kelly K, Battey J, Latt S, Lenoir G M 1984 A novel alteration in the structure of an activated c-myc gene in a variant t(2;8) Burkitt lymphoma. Cell 37: 511-520
9 Hollis G F, Mitchell K F, Battey J, Potter H, Taub R 1984 A variant translocation places the immunoglobulin genes 3' to the c-myc oncogene in Burkitt's lymphoma. Nature 307: 752-754
10 Tsujimoto Y, Croce C M 1986 Analysis of the structure, transcripts and protein products of bcl-2, the gene involved in human follicular lymphoma. Proceedings of the National Academy of Sciences of the USA 83: 5214-5218
11 Tsujimoto Y, Finger L R, Yunis J, Nowell P C, Croce C M 1985 Cloning of the chromosome breakpoint of neoplastic B cells with the t(14;18) chromosome translocation. Science 226: 1097-1099
12 Tsujimoto Y, Jaffe E, Cossman J, Gorham J, Nowell P C, Croce C M 1985 Clustering of breakpoints on chromosome 11 in human B-cell neoplasms with the t(11;14) chromosome translocation. Nature 315: 340-343
13 McKeithan T W, Rowley J D, Shows T B, Diaz M O 1987 Cloning of the chromosome translocation breakpoint junction of the t(14;19) in chronic lymphocytic leukemia. Proceedings of the National Academy of Sciences of the USA 84: 9257-9260
14 Baer R, Chen K C, Smith S D, Rabbitts T H 1985 The mechanism of chromosome 14 inversion in a human T cell lymphoma. Cell 43: 705-713
15 Denny C H, Hollis G F, Hecht F et al 1986 Common mechanism of chromosome inversion in B and T cell tumours: Relevance to lymphoid development. Science 234: 197-200
16 Reynolds T C, Smith S D, Sklar J 1987 Analysis of DNA surrounding the breakpoints of chromosomal translocations involving the β T cell receptor gene in human lymphoblastic neoplasms. Cell 50: 107-117
17 Leibowitz D, Schaefer-Rego K, Popenhoe D W, Mears J G, Bank A 1985 Variable breakpoints on the Philadelphia chromosome in chronic myeloid leukemia. Blood 66: 243-245
18 Schwarz D C, and Cantor C R 1984 Separation of yeast chromosome sized DNA by pulsed field gradient gel electrophoresis. Cell 37: 67-75

19. Westbrook C A, Rubin C M, Le Beau M M et al 1987 Molecular analysis of TCRB and ABL in a t(7;9)- containing cell line (SUP-T3) from a human T-cell leukemia. Proceedings of the National Academy of Sciences of the USA 84: 251-255
20. de Klein A, van Agthoven T, Groffen C, Heisterkamp N, Groffen J, Grosveld G 1986 Molecular analysis of both translocation products of a Philadelphia-positive CML patient. Nucleic Acids Research 14: 7071-7082
21. Popenhoe D W, Schaefer-Rego K, Mears J G, Bank A, Leibowitz D 1986 Frequent and extensive deletion during the 9.22 translocation in CML. Blood 68: 1123-1128
22. Pugh W C, Pearson M, Vardiman, J W, Rowley J D 1985 Philadelphia chromosome-negative chronic myelogenous leukemia: a morpological reassessment. British Journal of Haematology 60: 457-468
23. Travis L B, Pierre R V, Dewald G W 1986 Ph1-negative chronic granulocytic leukemia: a nonentity. American Journal of Clinical Pathology 85: 186-193
24. Morris C M, Reeve A E, Fitzgerald P H, Hollings P E, Beard M E J, Heaton D C 1986 Genomic diversity correlates with clinical variation in Ph1-negative chronic myeloid leukemia. Nature 320: 281-283
25. Bartram C R, Carbonell F 1986 Bcr rearrangement in Ph1-negative CML. Cancer Genetics and Cytogenetics 21: 183-184
26. Wiedemann L M, Karhi K, Chan L C 1987 Similar molecular alterations occur in related leukemias with or without the Philadelphia chromosome. In: Modern trends in human leukemia VII, Springer-Verlag, Berlin, pp 149-152
27. Bartram C R, Kleihauer D, de Klein A et al 1985 C-abl and bcr are rearranged in a Ph1-negative CML patient. EMBO Journal 4: 683-686
28. Bartram C R 1985 Bcr rearrangement without juxtaposition of c-abl in chronic myelocytic leukemia. Journal of Experimental Medicine 162: 2175-2179
29. Ganesan T S, Rassool F, Guo A P et al 1986 Rearrangement of the bcr gene in Philadelphia chromosome negative chronic myeloid leukemia. Blood 68: 957-960
30. Marmont A, Frassoni F, Bacigalupo A et al 1984 Recurrence of Ph positive leukemia in donor cells after marrow transplantation for chronic granulocytic leukemia. New England Journal of Medicine 310: 903-906
31. Thomas E D, Clift R A, Fefer A et al 1986 Transplantation for the treatment of chronic myelogenous leukemia. Annals of Internal Medicine 104: 155-166
32. Jeffreys A J, Wilson V, Thein S L 1985 Hypervariable minisatellite regions in human DNA. Nature 314: 67-73
33. Jeffreys A J, Wilson V, Thein S L 1985 Individual specific fingerprints of human DNA. Nature 316: 76-79
34. Hill A V S, Jeffreys A J 1984 Use of minisatellite DNA probes for determination of twin zygosity at birth. Lancet ii: 1394
35. Ganesan T S, Min G L, Goldman J M, Young B D 1987 Molecular analysis of relapse in chronic myeloid leukemia after allogeneic bone marrow transplantation. Blood 70: 873-876
36. Fialkow P T, Martin R J, Najfeld V, Penfold G K, Jacobson R J, Hansen J A 1981 Evidence for the multistep pathogenesis of chronic myelogenous leukemias. Blood 58: 158-164
37. Apperley J F, Jones L, Arthur C et al 1986 Incidence of relapse after T-cell depleted marrow transplant for chronic granulocytic leukemia in 1st chronic phase. Blood 68:5, supplement 1, 270a
38. Swansong H W E, Hu E, Sklar J, Levitt L J 1985 A prospective assessment of residual clonal disease in adult ALL utilising immunoglobulin gene rearrangement. Blood 66:5, Supplement 1 246a
39. Cleary M L, Sklar J 1985 Nucleotide sequence of a t(14:18) chromosomal breakpoint in follicular lymphoma and demonstration of a breakpoint-cluster region near a transcriptionally active locus on chromosome 18. Proceedings of the National Academy of Sciences of the USA 82: 7439-7443
40. Cleary M L, Gallili N, Sklar J 1986 Detection of a second t(14:18) breakpoint cluster region in human follicular lymphomas. Journal of Experimental Medicine 164: 315-320
41. Boyd C N, Ramberg R C, Thomas E D 1982 The incidence of recurrence of leukemia in donor cells after allogeneic bone marrow transplantation. Leukemia Research 6: 833-837
42. Third International Workshop on chromosomes in leukemia 1981 Cancer Genetics and Cytogenetics 4: 95-142
43. Rodenhuis S, Smets L A, Slater R M, Behrendt H, Veerman A J P 1985 Distinguishing the Philadelphia chromosome of acute lymphoblastic leukemia from its counterpart in chronic myelogenous leukemia. New England Journal of Medicine 313: 51-52
44. De Klein A, Hagemeijer A, Bartram C R et al 1986 bcr rearrangement and translocation of the c-abl oncogene in Philadelphia positive acute lymphoblastic leukemia. Blood 68: 1369-1375

45 Erikson J, Griffin C A, Rushdi A A et al 1986 Heterogeneity of chromosome 22 breakpoint in Philadelphia-positive (Ph+) acute lymphocytic leukemia. Proceedings of the National Academy of Sciences of the USA 83: 1807–1811
46 Clark S S, McLaughlin J, Crist W M, Champlin R, Witte O 1987 Unique forms of the abl tyrosine kinase distinguish Ph'-positive CML from Ph'-positive ALL. Science 235: 85–88
47 Kurzrock R, Shtalrid M, Romero P et al 1987 A novel c-abl protein product in Philadelphia-positive acute lymphoblastic leukemia. Nature 325: 631–635
48 Chan L C, Karhi K K, Rayter S I et al 1987 A novel abl protein expressed in Philadelphia chromosome positive acute lymphoblastic leukemia. Nature 325: 635–637
49 Walker L, Ganesan T S, Dhut S et al 1987 A novel protein in Philadelphia chromosome positive acute lymphoblastic leukemia. Nature 329: 851–853
50 Varmus H E 1984 Molecular genetics of cellular oncogenes. Annual Review of Genetics 18: 553–612
51 McGrath J P, Capon D J, Goeddel D V, Levinson A D 1984 Comparative biochemical properties of normal and activated human ras p21 protein. Nature 310: 644–649
52 Gibbs J B, Sigal I S, Poe M, Scolnick E M 1984 Intrinsic GTPase activity distinguishes normal and oncogenic ras p21 molecules. Proceedings of the National Academy of Sciences of the USA 81: 5704–5708
53 Pierce J H, Eva A, Aaronson S A 1986 In: Acute leukemia, Gale R P, Hoffbrand A V (eds) Clinics in hematology, Saunders, London, vol 15 pp 573–596
54 Bos J L, Toksoz D, Marshall C J et al 1985 Amino acid substitutions at codon 13 of the N-ras oncogene in human acute myeloid leukaemia. Nature 315: 726–730
55 Rodenhuis S, Bos J L, Slater R M, Behrandt H, van't Veer M, Smets L A 1986 Absence of oncogene amplifications and occasional activation of N-ras in lymphoblastic leukemia of childhood. Blood 67: 1698–1704
56 Janssen J W G, Steenvoorden A C M, Lyons J et al 1987 RAS gene mutations in acute and chronic myelocytic leukemias, chronic myeloproliferative disorders, and myelodysplastic syndromes. Proceedings of the National Academy of Sciences of the USA 84: 9228–9232
57 Hirai H, Kobayashi Y, Mano H et al 1987 A point mutation at codon 13 of the N-ras oncogene in myelodysplastic syndrome. Nature 327: 430–432
58 Taparowsky E, Shimizu K, Goldfarb M, Wigler M 1983 Structure and activation of the human N-ras gene. Cell 34: 581–586
59 Signer E, Moroni C, Gambke C 1985 Activation of N-ras genes in bone marrow cells of a female patient with acute myeloid leukemia. Montasschrift für kinderheilkunde 133: 602
60 Wodnar-Filipowicz A, Senn H P, Jiricny J, Signer E, Moroni C 1987 Glycine–cysteine substitution at codon 13 of the N-ras proto-oncogene in a human T-cell non-Hodgkins lymphoma. Oncogene 1: 457–462
61 Bos J L, Verlann de Vries M, van der Eb A J et al 1987 Mutations in N-ras predominate in acute myeloid leukemia. Blood 69: 1237–1241
62 Tran-Thang C, Senn H P, Wikstram L, Jiricny J, Moroni C 1986 Probing of N-ras mutations in acute leukemia DNA using synthetic oligonucleotides. Leukemia Research 10: 100
63 Verlaan de Vries M, Bogaard M E, van den Elst H, van Boom J H, van der Eb A J, Bos J L 1986 A dot-blot screening procedure for mutated ras oncogenes using synthetic oligodeoxynucleotides. Gene 50: 313–320
64 Murray M J, Cunningham J M, Parada L F, Dautry F, Lebowitz P, Weinberg R A 1983 The HL60 transforming sequence: A ras oncogene co-existing with altered myc genes in haematopoietic tumours. Cell 33: 749–757
65 Eva A, Tronick S R, Gol R A, Pierce J H, Aaronson S A 1983 Transforming genes of human hematopoietic tumors: Frequent detection of ras-related oncogenes whose activation appears to be independent of tumor phenotype. Proceedings of the National Academy of Sciences of the USA 80: 4926–4930
66 Needleman S W, Kraus M H, Srivastava S K, Levine P H, Aaronson S A 1986 High frequency of N-ras activation in acute myelogenous leukemia. Blood 67: 753–757
67 Shen W V, Furth M E, Franza R 1986 Expression of ras proteins in human leukemia. Proceedings of the American Association for Cancer Research 27: 429–434
68 Winkler-Gol R, Eva A, Yuasa Y, Needleman S, Tronick S, Aaronson S 1984 Detection of activated ras oncogenes in human tumours and search for gross modification of these genes in tumours and patients at high cancer risk. Archives of Dental Physiology 29: 1371–1372
69 Premkumar-Reddy E, Reynolds R K, Santos E, Barbacid M 1982 A point mutation is responsible for the aquisition of transforming properties by the T24 human bladder carcinoma oncogene. Nature 300: 149–152
70 Shimizu K, Birnbaum D, Ruley M A et al 1983 Structure of the Ki-ras gene of the human lung carcinoma cell line Calu-1. Nature 304: 497–500

71 Lenoir G M, Land H, Parada L F, Cunningham J M, Weinberg R A 1984 Activated oncogenes in Burkitt's lymphoma. Current Topics in Microbiology and Immunology 113: 6–14
72 Souyri M, Furth M E, Fleissner E 1984 Role of N-ras oncogenes in human T-cell leukemias. Genes and Cancer 399–411
73 Saiki R K, Bugawan T L, Horn G T, Mullis K B, Ehrlich H A 1986 Analysis of enzymatically amplified β-globin and HLA-DQα DNA with allele-specific oligonucleutide probes. Nature 324: 163–166
74 Bos J L, Fearon E R, Hamilton S R et al 1987 Prevalence of ras mutations in human colorectal cancers. Nature 327: 293–297
75 Lee M S, Chang K S, Cabanillas F, Freireich E J, Trujillo J M, Stass S A 1987 Detection of minimal residual cells carrying the t(14;18) by DNA sequence amplification. Science 237: 175–178
76 Scharf S J, Horn G T, Ehrlich H A 1986 Direct cloning and sequence analysis of enzymatically amplified genomic sequences. Science 233: 1076–1078
77 Wrischnik L A, Higuchi R G, Stoneking M, Ehrlich H A, Arnheim N, Wilson A C 1987 Length mutations in human mitochondrial DNA: Direct sequencing of enzymatically amplified DNA. Nucleic Acids Research 15: 529–542
78 McMahon G, Davis E, Wogan G N 1987 Characterisation of c-KI-ras oncogene alleles by direct sequencing of enzymatically amplified DNA from carcinogen- induced tumours. Proceedings of the National Academy of Sciences of the USA 84: 4974–4978
79 Wong C, Dowling C E, Saiki R K, Higuchi R G, Ehrlich H A, Kazazian H H 1987 Characterisation of β-thalassaemia mutations using direct genomic sequencing of amplified single copy DNA. Nature 330: 384–386
80 Kwok S, Mack D H, Mullis K B et al 1987 Identification of human immunodeficiency virus sequences by using in vitro enzymatic amplification and oligomer cleavage detection. Journal of Virology 61: 1690–1694

Index

Page numbers in *italics* refer to figures and tables; 'pl' refers to colour plate number

Abelson virus, 279
Aberrant leukemic features detection, 185-6
Acid α-naphthyl acetate esterase (ANAE) method, 37-8
Acid phosphatase, 5
  chronic lymphoid leukemias, 32-3
Acid phosphatase method, 24
  acute lymphoblastic leukemia (ALL), 30-1
  acute monocytic leukemia, 27
Acquired immune deficiency syndrome (AIDS), bone marrow biopsy, 84
Acute early erythroblastic leukemia (AEL), 110-19
  blast ultrastructural investigation, 111, *112*
  diagnosis, 111
  ferritin at blast surface, 111
  Golgi zone of blast, *112*
  incidence, 111
  phenotypes, 111, 113
  PPO detection, *113*
Acute granulocytic leukemia, cytochemistry, 25-7
Acute leukemia
  ADA in, 221-2
  analysis of nuclear TdT by flow cytometry, 188-90
  APAAP technic, 205, 207
  B-cell associated markers, 174
  bone marrow biopsy, 60-2
  cCD22 and CD19 as markers for B-lineage commitment, 179
  chromosomal abnormalities, 288
  classification and subtyping, 288
  common-ALL markers, 174
  cytocentrifuge preparations and smears of cells, 177-85
  cytogenetics, 288
  detection of aberrant leukemic features, 185-6
  diagnosis, 62
  disease evolution, 61-2
  gene rearrangement inconsistent with phenotype, 380
  gene rearrangements, 183
  immunological staining with colloidal gold, 186-8

  inability to differentiate into mature non-dividing populations, 188
  J5 membrane labeling, *116*
  markers in, 7-8
  markers of maturity, 175-6
  membrane immunofluorescence IF staining in diagnosis, 171-2, 174-6
  microplate method for McAbs in diagnosis, 171-2, 174-6
  morphology, 2
  myeloid associated markers, 174
  phenotypes, 180
  with proliferation of eosinophil and basophil precursors, 117-18
  proliferative capacity, 187
  secondary to radiation and chemotherapy, 320-1
  subclassification, 215
  T- and B-cell precursors, 181
  T-cell associated markers, 174
  TdT levels, 218
  transcriptional and translational event control, 183
  triple immunofluorescence using flow cytometry, 190-2
  two-colour immunofluorescence method, 176-7
  undifferentiated, 185
Acute lymphoblastic leukemia (ALL), 2, 12-13
  ADA in, 222
  antigen expression, pl 29
  APAAP technic in diagnosis, 205
  asynchrony in subgroup, 185
  B progenitor malignancies, 30
  B-ALL, 30
  B-lineage, 179
  biphenotypic acute leukemia, 8
  blast cells, pl 29
  bone marrow transplant, 315
  chromosome 11q structural abnormalities, 318
  chromosome 9p deletions, 12
  chromosome abnormalities, 11, 31, 305-6
  chromosome abnormality with breakpoint at 11q23, 12
  chromosome number of stemline, 313

411

Acute lymphoblastic leukemia (ALL) (contd)
  clonal abnormality identification, 305
  co-expression of lymphoid and myeloid
    antigens, 8
  coexistence of t(14;18) and t(8;14), 14
  common-ALL, 30, 179, *181*, 183, 186, 189,
    205
  cytochemistry, 30-1
  cytogenetic technics, 288, 289
  cytogenetics, 314-15
  diagnosis, 181
  direct cytogenetic procedure for bone marrow
    aspirate, 293-4
  double immunofluorescence assays, 186
  FAB L3 morphology and chromosome
    abnormalities, 312
  fidelity of differentiation, 183
  fidelity of markers, 181
  germline patterns, 370
  heterogeneity, 12
  hyperdiploidy, 12
  Ig rearrangement, 16
  immunoglobulin gene rearrangement
    investigation, 396
  immunophenotype and chromosome
    abnormalities, 312
  isochromosome 17q, 12
  karyotype in survival prediction, 12
  lineage designation, 215
  lineage switch, 313
  maturation block, 183
  meningeal relapse, 7
  molecular studies, 312
  multiple abnormal lines, 315
  non-random chromosome abnormalities, 307,
    308-11, 312
  non-T-ALL, 215
  null-ALL, 30, 179, *182*
  Ph+, 397, 398
  phenotype of intermediate thymocyte, pl 30
  phenotypes in non-lymphoid leukemias, 215
  phenotypic switch, 9
  Philadelphia chromosome, *309*, 315
  Philadelphia-positive, 393
  ploidy, 305-6, 315, 316
  pre-B-ALL, 179, *182*, 183, 184, 185, *186*,
    205
  prognosis, 8, *11*, 306, 313-14
  ras mutations, 16
  relapse prediction by TdT, 218, 220
  Siamese twins, 379
  t(9;22) translocation, 397
  T progenitor malignancies, 30
  T-ALL, 30
  TCR rearrangement, 16
  TdT activity, 7
  TdT levels, 218
  TdT as prognostic factor, 218, 220-1
  translocation, 305-7, 315
Acute lymphoblastic leukemia (ALL), childhood
  clinical applications of chromosome
    information, 314
  cytogenetics, 305-13, 314
  DNA index, 314

G-banding of chromosomes, 313
hyperdiploidy, 313-14
modal chromosome numbers, *307*
Philadelphia chromosome, 313
ploidy, 305-6
prognostic significance, 313-14
pseudodiploidy, 314
translocation, 305-7, 313, 314
Acute megakaryoblastic leukemia, 106-10
  APAAP in diagnosis, 205
  classification, 106
  diagnosis, 106
  heterogeneity, 110
  incidence, 108, 110
  phenotypes of blasts, 106, *109*
  platelet marker detection, 106
  PPO technic, 106
  prognosis, 110
  trisomy association, 110
Acute monoblastic leukemia, 118-19
Acute monocytic leukemia
  bone marrow, pl 11, pl 14
  chloroacetate esterase reaction, pl 16
  cytochemistry methods, 27-8
  α-naphthyl butyrate esterase reaction, pl 15
  NASDA esterase reaction, pl 14
  peripheral blood, pl 10
Acute myeloblastic leukemia, 113-16
  abnormal granule formation, 113
  Auer rod formation, 113
  blast crisis, 117
  blast with myeloperoxidase activity, 113
  buffy coat preparation of peripheral blood, pl
    7-8
  chromosome rearrangement, 116
  giant granule formation, 113, *114*
  light-chain immunoglobulin gene
    rearrangement, 116
  MPO detection, 114
Acute myelofibrosis, 68
Acute myelogenous leukemia
  ADA in, 222
  TdT in, 220
Acute myeloid leukemia (AML), 2
  5q syndrome, 279
  +21 chromosome abnormalities, 321
  +8 chromosome abnormalities, 320
  abnormal metaphase, 320
  ADA in, 222
  ALL phenotypes, 215
  analysis on FACScan, *191*, 192
  antibody Y1/82A preferential reaction, 205
  APAAP in diagnosis, 205
  biphenotypic acute leukemia, 8
  blast cell culture technic, 268-9
  blast cell subsets, *183*
  buoyant density separation, 272-3
  CD11c expression, pl 25
  CD34 marker, 184
  cell culture, 271-5
  chromosome 3 abnormalities, 318, 320
  chromosome abnormalities, 11, 13, 320
  circulating micromegakaryocytes, 204
  clonogenic cells, 273

Acute myeloid leukemia (AML) (contd)
  cluster-forming cells, 272, 274
  co-culturing of normal and leukemic cells, 274
  co-expression of lymphoid and myeloid antigens, 8
  coarse fibrosis, 62
  colony formation of cells, 272, 274
  colony stimulating activity, 278
  complex chromosomal abnormalities, 320
  complex karyotype in M5, 319
  CSF production, 278
  CSF-stimulated agar cultures, 273
  culture patterns, 271–2
  cytogenetics, 315–16
  deletion of 5q and, −5 318
  diagnosis with McAb anti-MPO, 8
  direct cytogenetic method for bone marrow preparations, 315
  disseminated intravascular coagulation (DIC), 317
  expression of CD13, class II and CD7 antigen, 190
  FAB classification, 205
  high resolution cytogenetic technic, 289, 295, 315
  HLA-DR +, pl 25
  Ig rearrangement, 16
  immunological phenotype, 205
  initiating cell, 255
  inversion, 16, 320
  lineage switch, 313
  long-term cultures, 275
  maturation block, 183
  mixed lineage membrane markers of blast cells, 255
  MPO positivity, 26
  multiple abnormal lines, 320
  myeloid leukemic cell characteristics, 277
  naphthol AS-D acetate esterase reaction, 26
  naphthol AS-D chloracetate esterase reaction, 26
  non-random chromosomal abnormalities, 316–20
  normal progenitor absence from marrow, 274
  PAS reaction, 27
  phenotypic features, 184
  phenotypic switch, 9
  Philadelphia chromosome, 318
  ploidy, 316, 320
  prognosis, 13, 117, 320
  prognostic significance of chromosome abnormalities, 320
  ras gene mutations, 16, 398
  remission, 275
  secondary in children, 13
  structural abnormalities of chromosome 11q, 317–18
  T11, pl 25
  t(6;9)(p22.2;q34.1) chromosome translocation, 318
  t(8;21)(q22;q22) chromosome translocation, 317
  t(9;22)(q34;q11) chromosome translocation, 318
  TCR rearrangement, 16
  TdT expression, 7, 207
  terminal transferase expression, 207
  thrombocytosis, 318, 320
  treatment, 13
  triple labelled cells, 191–2
  trisomy, 8, 320
Acute myelomonocytic leukemia
  abnormal eosinophil component, pl 16–17
  chromosome 16 structural abnormalities, 317
  cytochemistry, 28
  eosinophil precursors, pl 17
  NASDA esterase reaction, pl 12
Acute non-lymphoblastic leukemia, blast cells, pl 25, pl 26
Acute promyelocytic leukemia, 116
  Auer bodies, 116
  naphthol AS-D acetate esterase reaction, 26
  t(15;17)(q22;q21.1) chromosome translocation, 317
Acute undifferentiated leukemia (AUL), ALL phenotypes, 215
Adenosine deaminase (ADA)
  abnormal expression of activity, 217
  biochemical parameters, 217
  chemotherapeutic targets, 223–4
  deficiency, 223
  enzyme activity variation in leukemic cells, 217
  functional immune system relationship, 216
  human gene coding, 217
  immune function development, 215
  inhibitors, 223, 224
  isolation, 217
  in leukemia, 221–2
  lymphopenia in deficiency, 216
  methods for detection, 226
  monoclonal antibodies, 226
  polyclonal antibody, 226
S-Adenosylhomocysteine hydrolase, 216
Adult T-cell leukemia (ATL)
  cytochemistry, 31
  mature post-thymic phenotype, 327
Adult T-cell leukemia/lymphoma (ATLL), 4, 160–2, 328–9
  Caribbean patients, 328
  chromosome 14 abnormalities, 330
  chromosome abnormalities, 328, 329, 330
  circulating lymphocytes, 161
  convoluted lymphocyte similarities, 143
  functional analysis, 243
  HTLV-1 pathogenic role, 160
  IL-2 receptor expression, 160
  Japanese patients, 328, 329, 330
  suppressor function of cells, 162
  trisomy for chromosomes 3 and 7 and 6q, 328, 330
Agar culture
  CSF-stimulated for AML leukemic cells, 273
  efficiency, 266
  interpretation, 266–7
  preculture procedures, 267–9
  scoring, 265
  system, 254
  time of scoring, 266–7

INDEX

Aggressive myelomatosis, 14
AK-TI oncogene, 335
Alkaline phosphatase, 10
Alkaline phosphatase method, 24, 34-5
  reactions, 35
Alkaline phosphatase-anti-alkaline phosphatase (APAAP) technic, 198
  acute leukemia diagnosis, 205, 207
  advantages, 203-5
  antigen expression pattern, 206
  applications, 205, 207-8
  chronic leukemia diagnosis, 207
  detection of rare cells, 204-5
  hairy cell leukemia diagnosis, 207
  incubation cycle, 209
  intracellular antigens, 203
  light microscopy compatibility, 203
  method, 211
  multiple myeloma diagnosis, 207-8
  non-hemopoietic neoplasms, 208
  permanence of preparations, 204
  principle, 208, 209
  with rabbit antisera, 208, 210
  reagents, 210-11
  sample preparation, 209-10
  sample size, 205
  semi-automated procedures, 208
  three layer sequence of reagents, 208
Allelic exclusion, 344
3-Aminocarbazole method, 23
Angioimmunoblastic lymphadenopathy, bone marrow biopsy, 84, 85
Anti-B-cell McAbs, 135
Anti-BrDU McAb, 187
Anti-idiotype antibodies and B-cell growth, 245
Anti-IL-2R McAbs, 234
Anti-MPO, 8
Anti-TdT reagents, 179
Anti-white cell antibodies, 196
Antibody diversity in lymphoproliferative disorder investigation, 344
Araldite resin, 129
Asynchrony in ALL subgroup, 185
ATP, 216
  deoxycoformycin (dCF) administration, 223
Auer rods, 113, 116, pl 7-8
Autocrine hypothesis of cancer, 275-6
Azurophil granules, 26
  fusion, 113
  in large granular lymphocytes, 140
  in lymphocytes, 133

B-cell
  activation and proliferation, 240-1
  allelic exclusion in light chain production, 344
  antigens, 171
  antisera, 168
  associated markers for acute leukemia, 174
  binding of antigen to receptor, 240
  cCD22 expression, 181
  CD22 expression, 204
  characterization, 234
  chromosome breakpoint in tumours, 11
  chronic leukemia morphology, 3-4
  differential antigens, 241
  differentiation, 181, 241-2
  differentiation factor (BCDF), 241
  differentiation stage identification, 234
  effect on helper activity on IgM and IgG production, 237
  electron microscopy of disorders, 5
  Epstein-Barr virus-transformed lines, 241, 245
  functional properties of subpopulations, 234
  functional studies with neoplastic, 244-5
  growth factor HMW-BCGF, 241
  growth factors, 245
  heterogeneity of malignancies, 168
  IgM presence on neoplastic cells, 197
  LFA-1 positive small lymphocytic lymphoma, 17
  lymphoma and Ig genes, 393
  malignancy and Ig expression, 177
  non-Hodgkin's lymphomas, 3-4
  pokeweed mitogen stimulation, 235
  precursors in bone marrow, 180
  sequence of antigen expression during maturation, 203
  T-cell-derived factors in proliferation, 241
  uncontrolled proliferation in malignancy, 245
B-cell acute lymphoblastic leukemia (B-ALL), 185
  childhood, 314
  chromosome abnormalities, 308
  pre-B-ALL, 185
  TdT activity, 218
B-cell leukemia
  Ig genes, 393
  markers in, 9-10
B-cell prolymphocytic leukemia (B-PLL)
  14q+ abnormality, 14
  cytochemistry, 31, 32
B-cell-derived B-cell growth factors, 245
B-chronic lymphocytic leukemia (B-CLL), 143, 146
  cell lack of LFA-1, 17
  clonality, 15
  cytochemistry, 31, 32
  functional studies, 244
  more than ten percent prolymphocytes (CLL/PL), 148
  PMA induction of IL-2 receptors, 244
  trisomy in, 14
B-lineage cells, CD22 antigens, 171
B-lineage-ALL, cCD22 in diagnosis, 179
B-ly7, 9
B-lymphocytes
  FMC4 labeled, 136
  functional gene rearrangement, 15
  functional studies, 242-5
  HLA-DR expression, 135
  McAb FMC7 labeled, 138
  morphological types, 135
  mouse red blood cell rosettes, 127
  nucleolated, 136, 138
  peripheral blood, 137
  subpopulation, 134-5
  ultrastructure, 134-40

B-lymphoid
  cell characterization, 2
  development in bone marrow, *182*
  differentiation, *134*
B-prolymphocytic leukemia (B-PLL), 244
BamHI, 394
Basophil granules, 118
Basophilic leukemia, 117
  cytochemistry, 29
bcr
  intron probe, *397*
  new 5' breakpoint on gene, 397–8
  rearrangement, 395, 396
bcr-abl fusion, 402
Benign T-cell leukemia, 243
Benzidine base technic, 23
Biphenotypic acute leukemia, 2, 8–9
  therapy, 9
Blast cells
  acute monocytic leukemia, pl 11
  bone marrow in poorly differentiated leukemia, pl 5–6
  colony culture technic, 268–9
  culture, 254
  culture from peripheral blood, 302
  membrane labeling with McAbs, 91
  myeloblastic leukemia, pl 1–4
  recognition, 5
  with small peroxidase granule, *115*
  ultrastructure in bone marrow, *105*
  unusual membrane phenotypes, *116*
Blast crisis, 29, 117, 118, 221
  in ALL phenotypes, 215
Bone marrow
  analysis on FACScan, *191*
  antigens in ALL, 186–7
  blast ultrastructure, *105*
  C-banding technic, 304
  direct cytogenetic procedure (Williams' method), 289–95
  gated population, 191–2
  high resolution chromosome technic of Yunis, 295–305
  high resolution cytogenetic technic, 289
  histology, 6, 56–8, 60
  hypercellular infiltration, 60
  hypocellular, 60
  immunocytochemistry, 6
  lymphocyte preparation, 127–8
  malignant infiltration, 54, *55*
  morphology, 47
  myeloid cell colony counts, 266
  preparation for electron microscopy, 91
  stroma, 55
  TdT + cells, 190
  trabecular bone, 54, *55*
  transplant, 315
  triple labelled cells, 191–2
Bone marrow biopsy, 47–54
  AIDS-patterns, 84
  angioimmunoblastic lymphadenopathy, 84, *85*
  chronic lymphocytic leukemia (CLL), 70, 72–4
  chronic myeloid leukemia (CML), 66–7

  evaluation, 53–4, *55*
  hairy cell leukemia, 74, *75*
  histologic parameters in diagnosis, 84
  histomorphometry, 48, *49*
  Hodgkin's disease, 82–4
  indications, 52–3
  instruments, 48–50
  multiple myeloma, 77, 79–81, *82*
  myelodysplastic syndromes, 54–60
  myelofibrosis/osteomyelosclerosis, 67–70
  non-Hodgkin's lymphoma, 77
  polycythemia vera, 62–3
  primary thrombocythemia, 63–6
  processing, 50, *51*, *52*
  sites, 47–8
  staining, 50
  Waldenström's macroglobulinemia, 74, *76*, 77
Bone marrow transplantation
  allelogenic, 395–6
  bcr gene rearrangements, 396
  in CML, 395–6
  recurrence of leukemia, 396
Bordier needle, *48*, 49–50
Bromodeoxyaridine (BrdU), 187
Burkhardt drill, *48*, 49–50, *52*
Burkitt's lymphoma
  c-myc oncogene translocation, 393
  chromosome breakpoint, 11
  reciprocal translocation, 321
  t(8;14), 14
Burst colony-forming units-erythroid (BFU-E), 104, 105, 254
Burst-erythroid colonies, 264

c-abl oncogene, 392
  rearrangement, 395
C-banding technic for bone marrow, 304
c-mos oncogene, 317
c-myb oncogene, 334
c-myc oncogene, 334
  in Burkitt's lymphoma, 321
  translocation in Burkitt's lymphoma, 393
c-myc protein detection, 188
c-raf oncogene, 334
Ca^{2+}, intracellular, 235
Carcinoembryonic antigen, McAbs against, 208
Carcinogenesis, autocrine concepts, 275–6
Catalase localization by immunoelectron microscopy, 105–6
cCD3
  expression in T-ALL, 181
  as marker for T-ALL, 179–80
  in non-T-ALL, 187
cCD22 in diagnosis of B-lineage ALL, 179
CD2, expression in B-cells, 204
CD3, on thymic blasts, *182*
CD4 + T-cell malignancies
  ATLL, 243
  Sézary syndrome, 242–3
  T-chronic lymphocytic leukemia (CLL), 243
  T-prolymphocytic leukemia (T-PLL), 243
CD7 in myeloid malignancies, 184

CD19 as B-lineage acute leukemia marker, 179
CD34
  marker for AML, 184
  marker for pre-B-ALL, 184
Cell
  kinetics, 17
  lines as genetic markers, 379, *380*
  markers, 6–10
Cell smear labeling technic, 196–9, 203
  antigens for, 199
Cell smears
  immunoenzymatic staining, 199, *200–2*
  phenotyping, 199
Cellular immunohematology, 168
Cerebriform mononuclear cell, 140
Chediak-Higashi syndrome, 113
Chemotherapy and chromosome abnormalities in AML, 320
Chloracetate esterase (NASDCA) method, 38–9
Chromatin
  hairy cell variant cells, 150
  prolymphocytic leukemia (B-PLL), *147*
  splenic lymphoma with circulating villous lymphocytes (SLVL), 150
Chromosome 3
  abnormalities and thrombocytosis in AML, 318, 320
  trisomy in mature T-cell malignancies, 333–4
Chromosome 5 long arm deletion, 13
Chromosome 6q- in mature T-cell malignancies, *333*, 334
Chromosome 7
  abnormalities, 318
  in mature T-cell malignancies, *333*, 334
Chromosome 8q in mature T-cell malignancies, 334
Chromosome 9
  abnormalities in AML, *319*
  deletions, 12
Chromosome 10p in mature T-cell malignancies, 335
Chromosome 11 abnormalities in AML, *319*
Chromosome 11q23 breakpoint incidence in children, 12, 13
Chromosome 11q structural abnormalities in acute myeloid leukemia, 317–18
Chromosome 14 mature T-cell malignancies, 335
Chromosome 16 structural abnormalities in myelomonocytic leukemia, 317
Chromosome abnormalities, 10–12
  in acute leukemia, 288
  acute lymphoblastic leukemia (ALL), 12–13
  acute myeloid leukemia (AML), 13, *319*
  biphenotypic acute leukemia, 8
  with breakpoint at 11q23, 12, 13
  breakpoints, 11
  childhood acute lymphoblastic leukemia (ALL), 305–13
  clinical information in childhood ALL, 314
  complex in AML, 320
  inv(16), 13
  lymphoproliferative disorders, 14–15
  methods of identification, 12
  non-random in AML, 316–20
  t(8;21), 13
Chromosome analysis in acute leukemia, 288
Chromosome translocation
  genes in, *393*
  molecular analysis, 392–4
Chronic granulocytic leukemia (CGL), 3, 10
Chronic leukemia diagnosis with APAAP technic, 207
Chronic lymphocytic leukemia (CLL), 3, 9
  ADA in, 221
  antigen expression, pl 27, pl 28
  bone marrow biopsy, 70, 72–4
  clonality, 15–16
  colony formation capacity, 278
  deoxycoformycin (dCF) administration, 224
  growth patterns, *72*
  histological subdivisions, 73
  histology, 70, 73
  immunocytochemical staining reactions, *207*
  proliferative cell systems, *73*
  terminal transformation, 73
Chronic lymphoid leukemias, 31–3
  cytochemical profile, *32*
Chronic myeloblastic leukemia
  basophil granules, 118
  blast crisis, 117, 118
  mast cell granules, 118
  myeloperoxidase reaction, 117
  Philadelphia chromosome, 118
Chronic myelogenous leukemia
  ADA in, 221
  in blast crisis (CML/BC), 221
  leukemic cells with lymphoid features, 215
  TdT in, 220
Chronic myeloid leukemia (CML)
  acute transformation, 270–1
  bcr intron probe, *397*
  blast crisis, 29
  bone marrow biopsy, 66–7
  bone marrow transplantation, 395
  cell culture, 269–71
  colony formation capacity, 278
  colony-forming cells, 269, 271
  cytochemistry, 29
  eosinophil progenitor cells, 269
  eosinophil to GM colony ratio, 269
  gene rearrangements, 381
  granulocytic precursors in blood, 269
  granulocytic type, 66, *67*
  initiating clonogenic cell, 255
  leukemic clone, 270
  light density fractions, 270
  megakaryocytic/granulocytic type, 66, *67*
  morphology, 3
  myeloid leukemic cell characteristics, 277
  myleran therapy, 270
  Philadelphia translocation, 392, 394–5, 397
  progress monitoring, 271
  ras mutations, 16
  relapse, 395, 396
  spontaneous colony formation, 269
Chronic myelomonocytic leukemia (CMML), 58
  ras mutations, 16

Class switching, *341*, 344
Clonality, 15
Clones
  evidence for two, 378
  in gene rearrangement, 368
  infidelity, 379–80
  location, size and number, 278–9
  markers, 15–16
  multiple, 378
  same in different tissues, 379
  very small, 378–9
Clonogenic cell, 276
Cluster-forming cells, 267
Clusters of differentiation (CD), 6–7
  classification, 168, *169–70*, 171
  membrane markers, *173*
C probes, 368, *369*, 370
CNS relapse, 7
Colony formation stimulation, 278
Colony forming unit cell-granulocyte macrophage (CFU-GM), 26
Colony stimulating factor (CSF), 10, 253, 254
  action on responding normal granulocyte-macrophage populations, 80
  co-factor in initiation and progression of myeloid leukemia, 281
  control of granulocyte-monocyte population, 256
  dependency in human myeloid leukemia, 277–8
  dose response curve in cultures, 257
  gene location, 279
  human marrow assays, 278–9
  levels of production, 277–8
  microbial infection and synthesis, 277
  mouse marrow assays, 278
  murine, 280
  myeloid leukemia development, 279
  myeloid leukemia suppression, 280
  production derangement in myeloid leukemia, 279
  provision in semisolid cultures, 262–3
  receptor status of leukemic cells, 281
  recombinant human, 264
  in semi-solid cultures, 262
  signalling pathway derangement in myeloid leukemia, 279
Colony-forming cells, 253
Colony-forming unit-erythroid (CFU-E), 104, 105, 254
Common-ALL, 179, *181*, 183
  APAAP technic in diagnosis, 205
  markers in acute leukemia, 174
  positive TdT staining, 189
Common-ALL antigen, 171, 186
  antisera, 168
Concanavalin A (ConA), 234
  cytogenetic studies on mature T-cell malignancies, 327
Cryptic erythroleukemia, 29
Cutaneous T-cell lymphoma (CTCL)
  cytogenetics, 331–2
  deoxycoformycin (dCF) administration, 224
  mature post-thymic phenotype, 327

Cytocentrifuge preparations and smears of cells method for McAbs, 177–85
  controls, 179
  equipment, 178
  materials, 178
  method, 197
Cytochemistry, 5
  in acute monocytic leukemia, 27–8
  classification of leukemias, 23, 25–33
  methods, 23–5, 27–8
  standardization of procedures, 23
Cytochemistry, ultrastructural, 5–6, 91, 93–6
  Anderson technic, 94–5
  catalase staining, 95–6
  fixation technic, 95
  glycogen staining, 96
  Graham and Karnovsky technic, 94
  peroxidase method, 93–4
  Roels technic, 94
Cytogenetic technics, 288
  bone marrow high resolution, 289
  direct procedure for bone marrow aspirate (Williams' method), 289–95
  G-banding technic, 292–3
  high resolution chromosome technic of Yunis for bone marrow aspirate, 295–305
Cytogenetics, 288
  acute lymphoblastic leukemia (ALL) in children, 305–13
  methods, 288–305
  non-Hodgkin's lymphoma, 321
  see also cytogenetic technics
Cytokeratin, McAbs against, 208
Cytoplasmic antigen detection, 6
Cytoplasmic granules in T-prolymphocytic leukemia (T-PLL), *155*, 156
Cytoscan, 2
Cytotoxic activities
  antibody-dependent cellular cytotoxicity, 238–40
  killer cell activity and natural killer activity, 238–40

DAB-tetra-HCl, 94
Dehybridization procedure, 361–2
Deoxyadenosine, 216
Deoxycoformycin (dCF), 223
3,3'diaminobenzidine (DAB), 93–4, 95
Diaminobenzidine (DAB) method, 23
Differentiation antigens, 171
Differentiation inducing factor (DIF), 280
Dipeptidylaminopeptidase IV
  acute lymphoblastic leukemia (ALL), 30–1
  chronic lymphoid leukemias, 32–3
  method, 25, 39–40
Disseminated intravascular coagulation (DIC), 317
DNA
  application of amplified to filters, 405
  assessment of quality, 348–9, *352*
  contamination, 367
  digestion, 349–50

DNA (contd)
  evaluation of high molecular weight samples, 348–9
  filter hybridization, 359–61
  fingerprinting, 395
  fragment size change, 344
  gel electrophoresis, 350–4
  genetic variation, 367
  genomic in *ras* gene mutation detection, 398, 402–3
  germline, 342
  germline fragment position, *366*
  immunological markers and probes, 188
  incomplete digestion, 362–3, *365*
  index, 314
  polymerase 1, 358
  preparation of cellular, 347–8
  probe for chromosomal translocation, 393
  probes, 357
  rearranged Ig gene, 344
  rearranged TCR gene, 344
  rearrangement, 342, 344
  transfer for Southern blot analysis, 354–7
  visualization of bands, 354
DNA analysis, *1*, 1, 15–16
  clonal markers, 15
  genotypic markers, 381
  ras mutations, 16
  of solid tissues, 379
DNA analysis results in leukemia, 368, 370, 373, 375, *377*, 378
  Ig heavy chain gene probes, 368, *369*, 370, *371*
  Ig κ L chain genes, 370
  Ig λ-chain genes, 370
  TCR α-chain genes, 373
  TCR β-chain genes, 373, *374*, 375
  TCR γ-chain genes, 375
DNAase 1, 358
Donor cell recurrent leukemia, 396
Down's syndrome
  acute leukemia, *111*
  acute megakaryoblastic leukemia in, 110
Drills for bone marrow biopsy, *48*, 49–50
DuoCHROME, 188

Electron microscopy, 5, 91–3
  contributions to study of leukemic cells, *93*
  methods, 91–3
Endocrine hormones, 275
Endogenous peroxide activity, 199
Endopeptidase, 7
Endoplasmic reticulum
  peroxidase activity, 103
  platelet peroxidase in, 101
  T-prolymphocytic leukemia (T-PLL), 156
Enzyme-linked immunoassay (ELISA), 237
Eosinophil colonies, 264
  in CML, 269
  scoring, 265
  time of scoring, 267
Eosinophil-colony-stimulating factors (EO-CSF), 264

Eosinophilic leukemia
  cytochemistry, 29
  diagnosis, 117
Eosinophils, peroxidase, 99
EPICS PROFILE, 188
Epithelial membrane antigen, 208
Epstein-Barr virus (EBV), 327
Epstein-Barr virus-transformed B-cell, 245 lines, 241
Erythroid colonies, 264
Erythroid progenitors, 104–5
Erythroleukemia
  cryptic, 28
  cytochemistry, 28
Erythrons, 56
Erythropoietin, 254
Essential cryoglobulinemia, type II, 378

Fa6-152, 105, *106*
  in acute early erythroblastic leukemia diagnosis, 111
FACScan, 188
Fast garnet GBC method, 35
Ferritin
  in acute early erythroblastic leukemia diagnosis, 111
  entry to cytoplasm, 105
  lymphocyte immunolabeling, 131
  as marker molecule, 131
  in theta-granules, 111, *112*
Fetal calf serum, 258
Fetal circulation, maternal red cells in, 204–5
Fibrinogen, 104
Fibroblast
  clonogenic, 279
  colony formation (F-CFC), 279
Fibronectin, 104
Ficoll-Isopaque, 127
Filter hybridization, 359–61
Flow cytometry, 2, 7, 168, 188–90
  analysis of DNA content, 12
  triple immunofluorescence, 190–2
Fluorescein-activated cell sorting (FACS), 267, 268
Follicular lymphoma
  aggressive transformation, 14
  clonality, 396
  electron microscopy, 5
  translocation t(14;18), 11, 14
Fourth International Workshop on Leukocyte Differentiation Antigens, 6
French-American-British (FAB) working group, 57
  classification of acute non-lymphocytic leukemias, 60

G-banding
  of chromosomes in childhood acute lymphoblastic leukemia (ALL), 313
  cytogenetic technic, 292–3
  photography of preparations, 299
Galton D, 3

GCT conditioned medium, 263
Gel electrophoretic analysis inadequate resolution, 363, 367
Gene clusters in lymphoproliferative disorder investigation, 339–40, 342
Gene rearrangement, 342, 344, 380–1
 clone presence and size, 368
 DNA quality for analysis, 349
 hierarchy in, 342
 inconsistent with phenotype, 379–80
 lymphoid cells, 381
Gene rearrangement analysis, 378–80
 restriction enzymes for, *351*
Genetic markers in cell lines, 379, *380*
Genomic probes, 234
Germline, 339, 340
 band, 368
 fragments, 367
 patterns, 370, *372*
Gey's medium, 95
Glucose-6-phosphate dehydrogenase (G6PD), 395
β-Glucuronidase
 chronic lymphoid leukemias, 32–3
 method, 25, 39
β-Glycerophosphate, 130
Glycogen localization by immunoelectron microscopy, 105–6
Glycoproteins in promegakaryoblasts, 108
Gold, colloidal, 133
 electron-dense, 96, 97
 immunological staining, 186–8
 as marker molecule, 131
 see also Immunogold
Golgi region
 hairy cell variant cells, 150
 hairy cells, *149*, 150
 large granular lymphocyte leukemia, 157
α-Granules, 103, 104
θ-Granules, 105, *106*
 ferritin in, 111, *112*
 Golgi zone in acute early erythroblastic leukemia, 111
Granulocyte analysis, 346
Granulocyte colony-stimulating factor (G-CSF), 10
 assays, 278
 in myeloid leukemia, 277, 281
 WEHI-3B population suppression, 280
Granulocyte-macrophage colony
 adherent cell removal, 260–1
 crude conditioned media, 263
 culture preparation, 261–2
 culture technics, 260–4
 density separation, 260
 growth stimulation, 262–3
 preculture fractionation, 267
 purified colony-stimulating factors, 263–4
 recloning of CML, 270
 scoring, 265–6
 staining, 265
 stimulation of colony formation by other cell types, 264
 technical procedures, 257–60

Granulocyte-macrophage colony-forming cells (GM-CFC), 253, 256
Granulocyte-macrophage colony-stimulating factor (GM-CSF), 10
 assays, 278
 in myeloid leukemia, 277
Granulocyte–monocyte
 population control by colony-stimulating factors, 256
 progenitors, 254–5
Granulocytic cells
 colony-stimulating factor receptors, 256
 double esterase staining, pl 13
Growth factor-receptor binding, 276
Growth factors, 1
 in autocrine hypothesis of cancer, 276
 B-cell, 245
 encoding genes, 13
 hemopoietic, 10
 imbalance, 276
 receptors, 276
 recombinant, 10
Guanosine triphosphate (GTP), 216
 activity of codons, 16

H chain genes, 339, 340
H-ras gene, 398
Hairy cell leukemia, 3
 acid phosphatase diagnosis, 24
 antigen expression, pl 31
 B-cell origin neoplastic cells, pl 31
 B-ly7 McAb, 10
 BCGF-induced proliferation, 244
 bone marrow biopsy, 74, *75*
 cell recognition, 127
 cell subtypes, *76*
 cytochemistry, 31, 32
 deoxycoformycin (dCF) administration, 223–4
 diagnosis with APAAP technic, 207
 functional studies, 244
 α_2-interferon therapy, 244
 McAb reactivity, 9
 neoplastic B-cells, 244
 peripheral blood buffy-coat preparation, pl 22
 surface IgM staining, 198
 switched heavy chain gene, *371*
 ultrastructure, 148–50
 variant form, 3, 150, *151*
Helper activity, 237, *238*
Hemopoiesis, 53, 56
 cellular events, 253
 myelodysplastic syndromes, 56
Hemopoietic cells
 granulocyte-monocyte colony growth, 254–5
 liquid culture systems, 253
 megakaryocyte colony culture, 254
 regulators controlling populations, 255–7
Hemopoietic growth factors, *1*, 10
Heterochromatin, 133, 143, 147
 in prolymphocytes of CLL/PL, 148
 splenic lymphoma with circulating villous lymphocytes (SLVL), 150

Heterologous anti-human B- and T-cell sera tests, 127
Hexa-azotized pararosaniline, 24
Hidden gene rearrangement, 378
Histology, 6
HL60 cells, 280
HLA-DR, 134
Hodgkin's disease
  bone marrow biopsy, 82–4
  chemotherapy, 84
  Hodgkin cells, 83, 84
  Reed-Sternberg cells, 83, 84
Horseradish peroxidase, 96
  as marker molecule, 131
  substrate conditions, 199
Hu-ets-2 oncogene, 317
Human granulocyte culture, 254
Human multi-CSF, 256
Human myeloid leukemia
  clonal culture of cells, 253
  CSF dependency, 277–8
  CSF membrane receptor expression, 281
Human placental conditioned medium (HPCM), 263
Human T-cell leukemia virus 1 (HTLV-1), 143
  anti-Tac (CD25) reactivity, *145*
  association with ATLL, 160, 243, 327, 328
  infection, *145*
  infection of CD4+ polylobed lymphocytes, 143
  leukemia induced by, 276
Humphrey's stain, 129
Hybridoma technic, 17, 127
Hydroxyurea, 267
Hyperdiploidy in childhood acute lymphoblastic leukemia (ALL), 313–14
Hypergranular promyelocytic leukemia, 26

Ig-TCR hybrid gene, 335
IgM
  on surface human white cells, 198
  suppression of pokeweed mitogen-induced synthesis, 239
  see also Immunoglobulin (Ig)
Iliac crest, 47–8, 49
Immunocytochemical labeling of leukemia samples, 196
Immunoelectron microscopy, 96–7, 99–106
  catalase localization, 105–6
  controls, 97
  erythroid progenitor and precursor characteristics, 104–5
  glycogen localization, 105–6
  immunoperoxidase method, 97
  localization of platelet proteins, 103–4
  of lymphocytes, 130–3
  method, 96–7
  myeloperoxidase localization, 97, *98*, 99, 101
  platelet peroxidase localization, 101–3
  results, 97, 99–106
Immunoferritin labeling of lymphocytes, 131
Immunofluorescence, 7
  in cytospins, 177–8

Immunoglobulin genes, 339–40
  analysis probes, *340*, 357
  arrangement analysis, 344
  chromosomal localization, *339*, 340
  germline configuration, 340
  H chain rearrangement events, *341*, 342
  L chain rearrangement, 342
  organization, *339*, 340
  probes, *340*
  rearrangement investigation, 396
  solutions for analysis, 381–3
Immunoglobulin heavy chain gene (IgH), 335
  probes, 368, *369*, 370, *371*
Immunoglobulin heavy and light chain antisera, 168
Immunoglobulin (Ig)
  coding genes for polypeptide chains, 339
  detection of cytoplasmic, 131
  in investigation of lymphoproliferative disorders, 339
  κ L chain genes, 370
  λ-chain genes, 370, *372*
  production quantitation, 237
  surface expression of hairy cells, 148
  T-cell-dependent synthesis, 235
Immunogold, 96–7
  interpretation of labeling, 187–8
  labeling, 5, 186–8
  labeling of membrane antigens, 132–3
  lymphocyte characterization, 127
  membrane labeling of leukemic blasts, 91
  see also Gold, colloidal
Immunolabeling of lymphocytes, 130–3
  immunoferritin method, 131
  immunogold technic, 132
  immunoperoxidase method, 131
Immunological staining with colloidal gold *see* Immunogold
Immunoperoxidase labeling of lymphocytes, 131
Immunophenotyping, 5
[^{45}C]Inosine, 226
α_2-Interferon therapy, 244
Interleukin, 10
Interleukin-2 (IL-2), 234, 235
  growth of malignant B-cells, 244
  in HTLV-1-induced leukemia, 276
  humoral and cellular immune response role, 236
  pokeweed mitogen induced production, 235
Interleukin-2 (IL-2) receptors
  expression, 243
  expression in adult T-cell leukemia lymphoma (ATLL), 160
  induction by HTLV-1, 143
  on polylobed lymphocytes, 143
Interleukin-5 (IL-5), 264
Interleukin-6 (IL-6), 241
International Committee for Standardization in Haematology (ICSH), 23
International Workshop on Chromosomes in Leukemia, 12
Intracytoplasmic inclusions
  chronic lymphocytic leukemia (B-CLL), 143
  prolymphocytic leukemia (B-PLL), 147

INDEX   421

Inversion 16 in AML, 320
Isochromosome 17q, 12

Jamshidi needle, *48*, 49, *50*, *52*
J$_H$ probes, 368, *369*, 370
Junctional diversity, 344

K-ras gene, 398
K-ras gene mutations, 16
Ki67, 187
Killer cell activity, 239–40
Kinase end labeling, 405–6

L3 morphology, 14
Large granular lymphocyte leukemia, 4, 156–7
  clonality, 15
  cytoplasmic features, 157
  granular structures, 157
  peripheral blood buffy-coat preparation, pl 23
Large granular lymphocyte (LGL), 140–2
  and cells from T-chronic lymphocytic leukemia (T-CLL), 141–2
  cytoplasmic organelles, 140
  expansion in T-CLL, 333
  Fc γ receptor bearing, 140
  in Leu7 cell population, 140
  natural killer function, 140, 141
  reactive with McAb Leu7, *142*
  in T-chronic lymphocytic leukemia (T-CLL), 327
  T-lymphoma of CD8+, *331*
Lead nitrate in acid phosphatase preparations, 130
Lectin, 234, 235
  gold labelled, 96
Lennert's lymphoma *see* Lymphoepithelioid lymphoma
Leu7 cell population, 140
Leukemic blast cell culture technic, 268–9
Leukemic colony cells, 267
Leukemic transformation in CSF production, 279
Leukocyte alkaline phosphatase (LAP) in CML, 29
Leukocytes
  Anderson technic, 92
  buffy coat, 91, 92, 94
  embedding, 93
  fixation, 92
  peripheral blood, 91–2
LFA-1 molecule expression, 17
Lineage switch in AML and ALL, 313
Lymph node histology, 6
Lymphoblastic lymphoma, 220
Lymphocyte functional assays
  B-cell activation and proliferation, 240–1
  B-cell differentiation, 241–2
  cytotoxic activities, 238–40
  helper T-cell activity, 235–7
  suppressor T-cell activity, 237–8
  suppressor-inducer activity, 238
  T-cell proliferation tests, 234–5

Lymphocytes
  acid phosphatase technic, 130
  chronic lymphocytic leukemia (B-CLL), *146*
  cytochemical technic, 130
  cytoplasm, 133
  dehydration, 128–9
  embedding, 129
  fixation, 128
  homing receptor, 17
  immunoelectron microscopy, 130–3
  immunolabeling, 130–3
  non-nucleolated, *136*
  normal villous, *136*, *138*, *139*
  nucleus, 133
  polylobed, 143, 160, *161*
  sample preparation, 127–8
  staining, 129–30
  subset identification, 133–4
  ultrastructural features, 133–43
  villous in SLVL, *152*
Lymphoepithelioid lymphoma, 330
Lymphoid antigen co-expression, 8
Lymphoid cells
  heterogeneity, 133
  methods of study, 127
  ultrastructure, 127
Lymphoid leukemias of B-cell type, 143, 146–53
  chronic lymphocytic leukemia (B-CLL), 143, *146*
  hairy cell leukemia, 148–50
  hairy cell variant, 150, *151*
  plasma cell leukemia, 151–2, *153*
  prolymphocytic leukemia (B-PLL), 147
  splenic lymphoma with circulating villous lymphocytes (SLVL), 150
Lymphoid tissue, lymphocyte preparation, 128
Lymphokines, 10
Lymphomas, TdT in, 220–1
Lymphoplasmacytic lymphoma, 14
Lymphoplasmacytoid cell, *137*
  in plasma cell leukemia, *153*
Lymphoproliferative disorder, 70–84
  angioimmunoblastic lymphadenopathy, 84, *85*
  chromosome abnormalities, 14–15
  chronic lymphocytic leukemia (CLL), 70, 72–84
  growth patterns, *72*
  hairy cell leukemia, 74, *75*
  Hodgkin's disease, 82–4
  multiple myeloma, 77, 79–81, *82*
  non-Hodgkin's lymphoma, 77
  Waldenström's macroglobulinemia, 74, *76*, 77
Lymphoproliferative disorder investigation, 339
  antibody diversity, 344
  cell preparation, 345–7
  cellular DNA preparation, 347–9
  dehybridization procedure, 361–2
  DNA analysis results, 368, 370, 373, 375, 378
  DNA digestion, 349–50
  filter hybridization, 359–61
  gel electrophoresis, 350–4
  gel electrophoretic analysis inadequate resolution, 363
  gene clusters, 339–40, 342

Lymphoproliferative disorder investigation (contd)
  interpretation of results, 367–80
  nucleic acid labeling, 357–9
  Southern blot analysis, 354–7
  technics, 345–62
Lysosomal granules
  chronic lymphocytic leukemia (B-CLL), *146*
  hairy cell variant cells, 150
  hairy cells, *149*, 150
  large granular lymphocyte leukemia, 157
  prolymphocytic leukemia (B-PLL), 147

M1 leukemia, 280
M4EO, 29
M-CSF assays, 278
McAb *see* Monoclonal antibodies
Major histocompatibility
  antigens (HLA-DR), 134
  complex (MHC), 234
Malignant lymphoma, bone marrow biopsy, 77, *78*, *79*
Malignant myelosclerosis, 61
Marker
  of maturity for acute leukemia, 175–6
  molecules for immunolabeling, 130–1
  promiscuity, 379–80
Marrow particles
  embedding, 93
  fixation, 92
Mast cell
  granules, 118
  leukemia, 29
Mature T-cell leukemia morphology, 4
mcf3 oncogene, 334
Megakaryoblast, 102
  cytochemical reactions, 28
  identification, 2
Megakaryoblastic leukemia
  characterization, 5
  cytochemistry, 28
  monosomy 7, 13
Megakaryocyte
  colonies, 264
  phenotypic profile, 103
  PPO in endoplasmic reticulum, 101
Megakaryocytic cell identification, 24
Megaloblastic anemia, monocytic specific reaction, 26
Membrane
  antigens, 6–7
  immunofluorescence IF staining, 171–2, 174–6
  marker detection with McAbs and enzyme activities, 96–7, 99–106
  molecules expressed on T-cells, 234
Methods for study, 1–2
Methylcellulose, 258
Micromegakaryocyte, 56
  acute leukemia in Down's syndrome, *111*
  APAAP technic, 204
Microperoxisome, 96
Microplate method for McAbs, 171–2, 174–6
  interpretation, 174–6
  principle, *175*
Mini-satellite probes, *396*
Mitochondria in plasma cell leukemia, 152
Mixed leukocyte reaction, 234
Mixed lineage leukemia, chromosome analysis, 312–3
Mixed lineage membrane markers, 255
Mixed-erythroid colonies, 264
Molecular changes in leukemia, analysis, 392
  chromosomal translocation, 392–4
  future applications, 402
Molecular chimerism, 379–80
Monoclonal Antibodies, 168
Monoclonal antibodies, 1, 2, 8
  2H4, 238
  acute leukemia diagnosis, 7
  against TdT, 225
  analysis of nuclear TdT by flow cytometry, 188–90
  anti-B-cell, 135
  anti-class II, 244
  anti-idiotype in immunotherapy, 245
  anti-MPO, 8
  anti-My7 labeling, *101*
  B and T lineages of differentiation, 127
  C17 labeling, *109*
  CD11b(OKM1) recognition of T-CLL, 157
  cellular phenotypes of leukemic cells, 215
  cellular proliferative activity markers, 171
  clusters of differentiation (CD) classification, 168, *169–70* 171
  cytocentrifuge preparations and smears of cells, 177–85
  detection of aberrant leukemic features method, 185–6
  diagnosis of acute leukemia, 168, 171
  diagnostic reagents, *173*
  FMC7, 135
  FMC7 positivity with hairy cells, 148
  FMC7 reactivity of prolymphocytes, 147
  immunocytochemistry technics, 171
  immunological staining with colloidal gold, 186–8
  J5 (CD10) labeling, *116*
  Leu8, 237
  leukocyte differentiation antigen recognition, 234
  membrane immunofluorescence IF staining, 171–2, 174–6
  membrane labeling of leukemic blasts, 91
  membrane marker detection, 96–7, 99–106
  membrane molecules defined by, 234
  microplate method, 171–2, 174–6
  OKT10 (CD38), 135
  recognition of leukocyte-associated molecules (LFA), 6
  specific for myeloid lineage, 7
  stem-cell-related, 175
  to ADA, 226
  triple immunofluorescence using flow cytometry, 190–2
  two-colour immunofluorescence method, 176–7
  in ultrastructural cytochemistry technics, 5

INDEX   423

Monocyte-macrophage culture, 254
Monocytic cells
  colony-stimulating factor receptors, 256
  double esterase staining, pl 13
  identification, 24
Monocytic specific reaction, 26
Mononuclear cell analysis, 346
Monosomy 7, 13
MOPP (mustine, Oncovin, procarbazine, prednisolone) chemotherapy, 84
Morphology, *1*, 2–4
  acute leukemias, 2
  B-cell non-Hodgkin's lymphomas, 3–4
  chronic B-cell leukemias, 3–4
  chronic myeloid leukemias, 3
  mature T-cell leukemias, 4
Multi-CSF, 256
Multidrug resistant (mdr) phenotype, 17
Multiple abnormal lines
  in acute lymphoblastic leukemia (ALL), 315
  in AML, 320–1
Multiple myeloma, 135
  antigenic phenotype of neoplastic cells, pl 32
  bone marrow biopsy, 77, 79–81, *82*
  cytochemistry, 31
  diagnosis with APAAP technic, 207–8
  disease evolution, 79–81
  histological subdivisions, 79
Multipotential culture colonies, 254
Mycosis fungoides, 4
  cytogenetics, 331
  mature post-thymic phenotype, 327
Myeloblastic leukemia without maturation, undifferentiated blast cells, pl 1–4
Myeloblasts
  class II antigen expression, *183*
  with two nucleoli, *115*
Myelodysplastic syndrome, 2, 54–60
  bone marrow histology, 55–8
  chromosome 16 abnormalities, 317
  chromosome abnormalities, 13
  cytochemistry, 25–7
  diagnosis, 60
  disease evolution, 59–60
  fibrotic, 58, *59*
  histological subdivisions, 57–8
  monocytic specific reaction, 26
  sideroblastic, *58*
  topographic distortion, *56*, *57*
Myelofibrosis, *71*
  on chronic myeloid leukemia (CML), *69*
  on thrombocythemia, *70*
Myelofibrosis/osteomyelosclerosis, bone marrow biopsy, 67–70
Myeloid antigen co-expression, 8
Myeloid associated markers for acute leukemia, 174
Myeloid colony-forming cells (CFU-C), 101
  McAbs labeling, 101
Myeloid development, *183*
Myeloid differentiation, 5
Myeloid leukemia
  CSFs in induction, 279–80
  monoclonal, 255

suppression by CSFs, 280–1
Myeloid leukemia cells
  colony-stimulating factor provision in culture, 262
  liquid culture, 253
  primary culture, 253
  semisolid culture, 253
Myeloperoxidase (MPO), 94
  activity, 5, 6
  bactericidal function, 102
  genes coding for, 102
  localization in granules, 97, *98*, 99, 101, 102
  location in Golgi cisternae, 102
  reaction in acute granulocytic leukemia, 25–6
  substrate conditions, 199
Myeloperoxidase (MPO) method, 23, 33–4
  acute lymphoblastic leukemia (ALL), 30
  acute monocytic leukemia, 27
Myeloproliferative disorders, 54–70
  acute and subacute leukemias, 60–2
  chronic myeloid leukemia (CML), 66–7
  myelodysplastic syndromes, 54–60
  myelofibrosis/osteomyelosclerosis, 67–70
  polycythemia vera, 62–3
  primary thrombocythemia, 63–6
Myleran therapy, 270

N-ras gene, 398, *401*
  mutations, 16
N-region insertion, 344
Naphthol AS-D acetate esterase (NASDA), 24
  acute monocytic leukemia, 27
  acute myeloid leukemia (AML), 26
  method, 37
Naphthol AS-D chloracetate esterase (NASDCA)
  acute myeloid leukemia (AML), 26
  method, 24–5
  method in acute monocytic leukemia, 27
Naphthol phosphates, 24
α-Naphthyl acetate esterase (ANAE), 5, 26
  atypical reaction, 26
  chronic lymphoid leukemias, 31–2
α-Naphthyl butyrate esterase (ANBE) method, 36
  acute monocytic leukemia, 27
α-Naphthyl phosphate, 24
Natural killer
  activity, 239–40
  cells, 4
Neoplasias, hematological, 52, 56
Nick-translation, 357, 358–9
Non-hemopoietic neoplasms, APAAP diagnosis, 208
Non-Hodgkin's lymphoma
  bone marrow biopsy, 77
  centroblastic and immunoblastic malignant lymphoma, 77
  centroblastic/centrocytic malignant lymphoma, 77
  centrocytic malignant lymphoma, 77
  chromosome abnormalities, 321
  cytogenetics, 321

Non-Hodgkin's lymphoma (contd)
  markers, 9-10
  morphology, 4
  peripheral T-cell lymphoma (PTL), 330
  TdT in, 220
  transformation, 16
Non-lymphoid leukemias, ALL phenotypes, 215
Non-specific esterase (NSE), 24
Non-T-ALL, 215
  DNA synthetic activity, 187
  immunological staining with colloidal gold, 187
Nuclear TdT
  analysis by flow cytometry, 188-90
  detection, 188
  staining for flow cytometry, 189
Nucleic acid labeling for Ig and TCR gene analysis, 357-9
Nucleolus
  in chronic lymphocytic leukemia (B-CLL), 143
  in prolymphocytic leukemia (B-PLL), 147
  in T-prolymphocytic leukemia (T-PLL), 155
'Null'-ALL, 30, 179, 182

Oil red O method, 41
Oligolabeling, 359
Oligonucleotide
  priming, 357, 359, 402
  probe, 401
  probe hybridization, 406
  sequence, 400
Oncogene, 15
  chromosomal mapping, 392
  deregulation, 288
Osteomyosclerosis, 68, 71

^{32}P-labeled dCTP, 357
Paint-a-Gate program, 191
Pan-T antigen expression, 143
Parachute bands, 367
Pararosaniline method, 35-6
Period acid-Schiff (PAS) method, 25, 40-1
  acute lymphoblastic leukemia (ALL), 30
  acute monocytic leukemia, 27
  in acute myeloid leukemia (AML), 27
Peripheral blood, lymphocyte preparation, 127-8
Peripheral T-cell lymphoma (PTL), 330-1
  chromosome 3 abnormality, 330
  chromosome 6 abnormality, 331
  chromosome abnormalities, 330-1
  mature post-thymic phenotype, 327
  translocation, 336
Peroxisomal catalase, 95
Peroxisomes, 95
Phenotypic switch, 2, 9
  gene rearrangement, 16
  therapy implications, 13
Philadelphia chromosome, 3, 118, 269
  in acute lymphoblastic leukemia (ALL), 309, 315

in AML, 318
analysis, 394-5
prognosis, 313
translocation in CML, 395
translocation t(9;22), 392
Phorbol myristate acetate (PMA), 235
Phytohemagglutinin (PHA), 234
  culture system for AML, 273-4
  in cytogenetic studies on mature T-cell malignancies, 327
Phytohemagglutinin-stimulated leukocyte-conditioned media (PHA-LCM), 263
Plasma cell, 137
Plasma cell leukemia, 151-2, 153
  chromosome abnormalities, 14
  fibrils around nucleus, 151-2
  lymphoplasmacytoid cell, 153
  mitochondria, 152
  plasma cell differentiation, 151, 153
Platelet
  factor-4, 103, 104
  glycoproteins, 102
  markers in acute megakaryoblastic leukemia, 106
Platelet peroxidase (PPO), 94, 101-3
  activity, 28
  in acute megakaryoblastic leukemia diagnosis, 106
  in blasts for acute early erythroblastic leukemia, 113
  fixation to preserve activity, 95
  function, 102
  genes coding for, 102
  location in RER and SER, 101, 102
  megakaryocyte nature, 102
  platelet prostaglandin biosynthesis, 102
Ploidy
  in acute lymphoblastic leukemia (ALL), 305-6
  in ALL and AML, 316
Pokeweed mitogen (PWM), 234, 235
  cytogenetic studies on mature T-cell malignancies, 327
Polycythemia rubra vera, 10
Polycythemia vera
  bone marrow biopsy, 62-3
  diagnosis, 66
  disease evolution, 65
  histological subdivisions, 64-5
  histology of bone marrow, 62-3
  spent, 63
Polymerase chain reaction, 2, 15, 400, 402, 403-4
  ras mutation investigation, 16
Polyoma middle-T antigen, 280
Pre-B-ALL, 179, 182, 183, 185
  APAAP technic in diagnosis, 205
  CD34 marker, 184
Pre-T-ALL, 185
Primary thrombocythemia, bone marrow biopsy, 63-6
Proerythroblast, 104-5
Progenitor cells, 253, 254, 255
  absence in AML, 274

Progenitor cells (contd)
  detection problems, 261
  eosinophil in CML, 269
  My10(CD34) labeling, 268
Proliferative stimulation, 276
Prolymphocytes
  of CLL/PL, 148
  prolymphocytic leukemia (B-PLL), 147
Prolymphocytic leukemia (PLL), 3, 147
Prolymphocytoid cells, 148
  chronic lymphocytic leukemia (B-CLL), 143
Promegakaryoblasts, 102, *103*
  catalase-containing particles, 105
  glycoprotein expression, 103-4
  labeling, 103
  with phenotype 3, 110
  platelet peroxidase testing, *104*
  PMKB II characterization, 108
  PPO as marker of maturation, 108
Promegakaryocytes
  Golgi apparatus, *107*
  PPO activity, 106, *107, 108*
Promonocyte, 97, *98*
Promyelocyte, 97, *99*
  basophil, 99, 118, *119*
  eosinophil, *100*
  neutrophil, *100*
Promyelocytic leukemia
  α-napthyl acetate esterase reactivity, 5
  peripheral blood, pl 9
Protein kinase C activation, 235
Pseudodiploidy in childhood acute lymphoblastic leukemia (ALL), 314
Purine nucleoside phosphorylase (PNP)
  biochemical parameters, 217-18
  chemotherapeutic targets, 224
  functional immune system relationship, 216
  human gene coding, 217
  immune function development, 215
  inhibitors, 224, 227
  in leukemia, 222
  lymphoid cell immune function and differentiation, 222
  lymphopenia in deficiency, 216
  methods for detection, 226

5q–
  and –5 deletion, 318
  syndrome, 279

R bands, 378, 379
ras genes, 398, *399*, 400-2
  human mutations, *399*
  mutation detection, 398, 400-2, 402-7
  mutations, 16
  point mutations, 398, *401*
  polymerase chain reaction (PCR), 400-2
Reactive lymphocytosis, immunocytochemical staining, *207*
Rearranged fragments, 367
Restriction fragment length
  measurement, 354
  polymorphism (RFLP), 367, 370
Reverse transcriptase, 275
Reynold's lead citrate, 130
Rhabdomyosarcoma, 208
Rheumatoid arthritis, 4
Rhopheocytosis, 104-5
Ribosome-lamella complexes, hairy cells, *149*, 150
Richter's syndrome, 16, 73
RNA immunological markers and probes, 188
Rosetting tests, 5

S-phase of cell cycle, 267
  CML cells, 269, 270
Secondary leukemias
  after radiation and chemotherapy, 320-1
  chromosome abnormalities, 13
  gene rearrangement, 16
Semisolid cloning, 253-5
  heterogeneity of granulocyte-monocyte progenitors, 254-5
Semisolid cultures
  adherent cell removal, 261
  AML cells, 273
  cell collection, 260
  crude conditioned media, 263
  culture medium, 258-9
  culture preparation, 261-2
  culture technics, 260-64
  incubating conditions, 259-60
  pH maintenance, 259
  preculture fractionation, 260-1, 267
  purified colony-stimulating factors, 263-4
  scoring, 265-6
  spontaneous colony formation, 262
  staining, 265
  stimulation of colony formation by other cell types, 264
  technical procedures, 257-60
Serum for semi-solid cultures, 258-9
Sézary cell, 31, 32
  nucleus, 159, 160
  phenotype, 157, 159
  T-cell helper activity, 242
  T-cell nature, 157
Sézary syndrome, 4, 127, 242-3
  chromosome abnormalities, 331-2
  cytogenetics, 331-2
  lymphocytes, 142
  lymphoid cell, *159*
  mature post-thymic phenotype, 327
  small cell variant, 159-60
  ultrastructure, 157, 159-60
Skin, lymphocyte preparation, 128, 129
SmIg, 171
  monomorphic molecule association, 180
Smoldering leukemia, 61
Smoldering myeloma, 80
Somatic hypermutation, 344
Southern blot analysis, 344
  bacteriophage lambda DNA molecular weight markers, 353
  clone location, 378

Southern blot analysis (contd)
  DNA digestion, 349-50
  failure, 362-7
  fragment size, 363
  genetic variation in DNA, 367
  germline fragment size, 357
  incomplete DNA digestion, 362-3, 565
  J_γ TCR probe, 376
  non-genomic DNA contamination, 367
  procedure, 354-7
  restriction enzymes for gene rearrangement analysis, 351
  TCR β-chain gene locus, 374
  technic, 380
  variable resolving power, 366
Spermidine, 362
Splenic lymphoma with circulating villous lymphocytes (SLVL), 3, 150
  villous lymphocytes, 152
Stem cell, 254, 255
  colonies, 264
Subacute leukemia
  bone marrow biopsy, 60-2
  diagnosis, 62
  disease evolution, 61-2
Sudan black B method, 23, 25, 40
  in acute granulocytic leukemia, 25-6
  acute lymphoblastic leukemia (ALL), 30
  acute monocytic leukemia, 27
Suppressor T-cell activity, 237-8
  measurement, 237
Surface antigen staining, 197-8
Surface immunoglobulin staining, 196-7
Surface membrane antigen staining, 200-2
  slide storage, 204
Switching sequences, 341, 344

t(15;17)(q22;q21.1) chromosome translocation in acute promyelocytic leukemia, 317
t(4;11) chromosome translocation, prognosis, 313
t(6;9)(p22.2;q34.1) chromosome translocation in AML with increased basophils, 318
t(8;14) chromosome translocation, prognosis, 313
t(8;21)(q22;q22) chromosome translocation in AML, 317
t(9;22) chromosome translocation, prognosis, 313
t(9;22) translocation, 402
  in ALL, 397
  Philadelphia chromosome, 392
t(9;22)(q34;q11) chromosome translocation in AML, 318
T-cell
  activation, 240
  activation with major histocompatibility complex (MHC), 234
  antigens, 171
  antisera, 168
  associated markers for acute leukemia, 174
  cCD3 expression, 181
  CD3 complex as receptor, 180
  CD4+ malignancies functional analysis, 242-3
  CD7 expression on neoplasias, 242
  clonal neoplastic, 242
  cloned, 242
  cutaneous lymphomas, 4
  cytotoxic CD8, 238
  differentiation, 181
  differentiation antigens, 153
  differentiation stage identification, 234
  disorders and clonal markers, 15
  functional properties of subpopulations, 234
  helper activity, 235
  lymphoid malignancies, 11
  membrane molecules expressed on, 234
  mitogens, 327
  neoplastic, 242
  precursors in thymus, 180
  proliferation, 234-5, 375
  prolymphocytic leukemia (T-PLL), 4, 127
  regulatory activity, 237
  regulatory function evaluation, 235
  sequence of antigen expression during maturation, 203
  stimulation in mixed leukocyte reaction, 234
  triggering via TCR/CD3+ complex, 235
T-cell acute lymphoblastic leukemia (T-ALL)
  ADA in, 222
  anti-CD3 antibody reactions, 204
  APAAP technic in diagnosis, 205
  bone marrow aspirate procedure, 293
  cCD3 as marker, 179-80
  CD7 antigen expression, 180
  CD8 antigen expression, 185
  classification, 215
  leukemia markers, 171
  peripheral blood buffy-coat preparation, pl 19
  pre-T-ALL, 185
  T-cell antigen expression, pl 30
  TCR-associated antigen expression, 184, 185
T-cell chronic lymphocytic leukemia (T-CLL), 31, 141-2, 156-7, 158
  benign T-cell leukemia, 243
  cytogenetics, 333
  functional analysis, 243
  granular lymphocytes, 158
  mature post-thymic phenotype, 327
  natural killer activity of membrane antigens, 157
  phenotype, 157
  symptoms, 156
T-cell leukemias
  adult T-cell leukemia lymphoma, 160-2
  large granular lymphocyte leukemia, 156-7
  post-thymic (mature), 5, 154-62
  Sézary syndrome, 157, 159-60
  thymic (immature), 154
  ultrastructure, 153-62
T-cell malignancies, cytogenetic abnormalities, 327
  ATLL, 328-30
  cell separation, 327
  chromosome 14 abnormalities, 335-6
  conditioned medium preparation, 327-8
  CTLL, 331-2
  cultures, 328
  methods, 327-8
  PTL, 330-1

T-cell malignancies, cytogenetic abnormalities (contd)
  T-CLL, 333
  T-PLL, 332–3
  trisomy, 333–4
  trypsin-Giemsa banding, 328
T-cell receptor (TCR), 171
  α-chain genes, 335, 373
  αβ molecule, 340, 342
  antigen recognition, 339
  arrangement analysis, 344
  β molecule, 363
  β-chain genes, 373, *374*, 375
  C region of β-chain genes, 373, *374*, 375
  CD3 complex, 180
  γ-chain genes, 375, 378
  γβ molecule, 341, 342
  mapping, 327
  rearrangement in non-T-ALL, 215
  T-cell activation, 234
  thymic development, *182*
T-cell receptor (TCR) gene, 13, 15, 340, 342
  germline map of loci, *343*
  probes, *340*
  rearrangement as clonal markers, 15–16
T-cell receptor (TCR) gene analysis
  investigation of lymphoproliferative disorders, 339
  probes, *340*, 357
  solutions for, 381–3
T-cell-derived lymphokine interleukin-2, 234
T-helper activity
  antigen specific, 235
  enzyme-linked immunoassay (ELISA), 237
  kinetics, *238*
  measurement, 237
T-helper cell activation, 240
T-large cell malignant lymphoma, lymph node imprint, pl 20
T-lineage cells, CD3 antigens, 171
T-lymphocytes
  CD4 +, 140
  CD8 +, 140
  cerebriform, 142–3
  convoluted, 142–3
  E-rosettes for, 127
  functional gene rearrangement, 15
  functional studies, 242–5
  normal blood, *144*
  peripheral blood, *141*
  subsets, 140
  ultrastructural features, 140–3
T-lymphoid
  cell characterization, 2
  differentiation, *134*
T-lymphoma, 330
  of CD8 +, *331*
T-precursor-ALL, 185
T-prolymphocytes
  cytoplasmic features, 156
  Sézary syndrome, 160
  in T-prolymphocytic leukemia (T-PLL), 154, *155*, 156

T-prolymphocytic leukemia (T-PLL), 154–6, 332–3
  cells, 31, 32
  chromosome abnormalities, 332–3, 334
  cytogenetic abnormality, 156
  functional analysis, 243
  mature post-thymic phenotype, 327
  p40 (CD7) antigen expression, 154
  peripheral blood buffy-coat preparation, pl 21
  peripheral blood film, pl 24
  small cell variant, 156
T-suppressor effector cell induction, 238
Taq polymerase, 404
Tartrate-resistant acid phosphatase (TRAP) activity, 149
tcl-l oncogene, 335
[^{3}H]TdR, 267
Terminal deoxynucleotidyl transferase (TdT), 7
  acute lymphoblastic leukemia, 218
  acute myelogenous leukemia, 207, 220
  antisera, 168
  APAAP technic, 205, 207
  applications of assays, 221
  assay methods, 224–6
  biochemical parameters, 216–17
  chemotherapeutic targets, 222–3
  chronic myelogenous leukemia, 220
  double fluorochrome analysis, 225
  expression, 215
  expression in acute myeloid leukemia (AML), 207
  expression in leukemia, 181
  expression of nuclear, 178
  in hematologic disease, *219*
  human gene coding, 216, *217*
  immune function development, 215
  immunocytochemical detection, 224–6
  lymphoid marker, 7
  lymphoid progenitor cell marker, 215
  lymphomas, 220–1
  meningeal relapse in ALL, 7
  monoclonal antibodies against, 25
  mRNA abundance, 216
  in myeloid malignancies, 184
  N-region insertion, 344
  protein sequencing, 216
  quantitative biochemical assay, 224
  quantitative enzyme-linked immunoassays, 225–6
  single-cell immunocytochemical tests, 225
  solid-phase immunoassay, 226
  synthesis during B or T differentiation, 183
  T-cell malignancies, 153
  technic, 127
12-O-Tetradecanoylphorbol-13-acetate (TPA), 327
Tγ lymphocytosis
  clonality, 243
  discrimination, 243–4
  functional studies, 244
  spontaneous regression, 244
Tμ-lymphocytes, 140
Thiocarbohydrazide, 96

Thiosemicarbazide, 96
β-Thromboglobulin, 104
Thrombospondin, 103, 104
Thymic development, *182*
Thymocytes, 204
Thymus TdT + cells, 190
T_μ-lymphocytes, 140
Translocation
 in acute lymphoblastic leukemia (ALL), 305–7
 prognosis in ALL, 315
Transmission electron microscopy, 5, 127
Trephine, 49
Trilineage myelodysplasia, 2
Triple immunofluorescence using flow cytometry, 190–2
 interpretation, 190–2
 method, 190
Trisomy 8 in AML, 320
Two-colour immunofluorescence method for McAbs, 176–7

Ultrastructure of leukemic cell, 91
[^{14}C]Uric acid, 226

v-myc, 334
v-rafl oncogene, 334
Von Willebrand's factor, 103, 104

Waldenström's macroglobulinemia, 135
 bone marrow biopsy, 74, *76*, 77
WEH1-3B leukemia, 280

X hapten, 108, 114, 116

Yunis high resolution chromosome technic for bone marrow aspirate, 295–305

ZEISS integration eyepiece I, 54, *56*